Infectious Diseases in Children: Clinical Pediatrics

Infectious Diseases in Children: Clinical Pediatrics

Edited by Caroline Francis

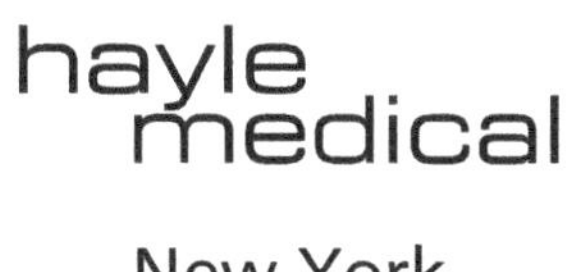

New York

Hayle Medical,
750 Third Avenue, 9th Floor,
New York, NY 10017, USA

Visit us on the World Wide Web at:
www.haylemedical.com

ISBN: 978-1-63241-734-3

Cataloging-in-Publication Data

Infectious diseases in children : clinical pediatrics / edited by Caroline Francis.
p. cm.
Includes bibliographical references and index.
ISBN 978-1-63241-734-3
1. Infection in children. 2. Children--Diseases--Diagnosis. 3. Children--Diseases--Treatment.
4. Bacterial diseases in children. 5. Pediatrics. 6. Infection. I. Francis, Caroline.

RJ401 .I54 2019
618.929--dc23

Table of Contents

Preface

This book aims to highlight the current researches and provides a platform to further the scope of innovations in this area. This book is a product of the combined efforts of many researchers and scientists, after going through thorough studies and analysis from different parts of the world. The objective of this book is to provide the readers with the latest information of the field.

The diseases caused by bacteria, fungi, viruses or parasites are known as infectious diseases. Children are more susceptible to such diseases as they come in contact with a variety of germs. Some of the common infectious diseases affecting children include influenza, tuberculosis, measles, meningitis, whooping cough and chicken pox, among others. Influenza in an infectious disease caused by influenza virus. Its common symptoms in children include diarrhea and vomiting. The infectious disease caused by Mycobacterium tuberculosis bacteria is called tuberculosis. Bacillus Calmette-Guérin is the most commonly used vaccine to prevent and reduce the risk of tuberculosis in children. The topics included in this book on infectious diseases in children are of utmost significance and bound to provide incredible insights to readers. It will also provide interesting topics for research, which interested readers can take up. The book is appropriate for students seeking detailed information in this area as well as for experts.

I would like to express my sincere thanks to the authors for their dedicated efforts in the completion of this book. I acknowledge the efforts of the publisher for providing constant support. Lastly, I would like to thank my family for their support in all academic endeavors.

Editor

Lactobacillus rhamnosus GG and *Bifidobacterium longum* Attenuate Lung Injury and Inflammatory Response in Experimental Sepsis

Ludmila Khailova, Benjamin Petrie, Christine H. Baird, Jessica A. Dominguez Rieg, Paul E. Wischmeyer*

Department of Anesthesiology, University of Colorado School of Medicine, Aurora, Colorado, United States of America

Abstract

Introduction: Probiotic use to prevent nosocomial gastrointestinal and potentially respiratory tract infections in critical care has shown great promise in recent clinical trials of adult and pediatric patients. Despite well-documented benefits of probiotic use in intestinal disorders, the potential for probiotic treatment to reduce lung injury following infection and shock has not been well explored.

Objective: Evaluate if *Lactobacillus rhamnosus* GG (LGG) or *Bifidobacterium longum* (BL) treatment in a weanling mouse model of cecal ligation and puncture (CLP) peritonitis will protect against lung injury.

Methods: 3 week-old FVB/N mice were orally gavaged with 200 μl of either LGG, BL or sterile water (vehicle) immediately prior to CLP. Mice were euthanized at 24 h. Lung injury was evaluated via histology and lung neutrophil infiltration was evaluated by myeloperoxidase (MPO) staining. mRNA levels of IL-6, TNF-α, MyD88, TLR-4, TLR-2, NFKB (p50/p105) and Cox-2 in the lung analyzed via real-time PCR. TNF-α and IL-6 in lung was analyzed via ELISA.

Results: LGG and BL treatment significantly improved lung injury following experimental infection and sepsis and lung neutrophil infiltration was significantly lower than in untreated septic mice. Lung mRNA and protein levels of IL-6 and TNF-α and gene expression of Cox-2 were also significantly reduced in mice receiving LGG or BL treatment. Gene expression of TLR-2, MyD88 and NFKB (p50/p105) was significantly increased in septic mice compared to shams and decreased in the lung of mice receiving LGG or BL while TLR-4 levels remained unchanged.

Conclusions: Treatment with LGG and BL can reduce lung injury following experimental infection and sepsis and is associated with reduced lung inflammatory cell infiltrate and decreased markers of lung inflammatory response. Probiotic therapy may be a promising intervention to improve clinical lung injury following systemic infection and sepsis.

Editor: Brenda Smith, Oklahoma State University, United States of America

Funding: This work was funded in part by National Institutes of Health (NIH) R01 GM078312 to P. Wischmeyer. The funders had no role in study design, data collection and analysis, decision to publish, or preparation of the manuscript. No additional external funding was received for this study.

Competing Interests: The authors declare that the only competing interest that exists for this work is that it was funded in part by a grant from the National Institutes of Health (R01 GM078312) to P. Wischmeyer.

* E-mail: Paul.Wischmeyer@ucdenver.edu

Introduction

Sepsis is a leading cause of death in infants and children despite the advances in medical and ICU care. Over 42,000 cases of severe sepsis are reported each year in the United States alone and millions are thought to occur worldwide [1]. Over 1 million deaths worldwide are associated with sepsis within the neonatal population [2,3]. Low birth weight infants are particularly at risk, where the mortality is reported to be ~50% [4]. Further the neonates who survive sepsis and septic shock continue to face substantial long term adverse effects [5]. Pediatric patients diagnosed with pneumonia or sepsis are also susceptible to acute lung injury or acute respiratory distress syndrome leading to a mortality rate of ~25% [6,7].

Critical illness and ICU care (broad spectrum antibiotics, poor nutrition deliver etc) creates a hostile environment in the gut and alter the microflora tilting the balance to favor pathogens [8]. Probiotics are living nonpathogenic bacteria colonizing intestine and providing benefit to the host with the potential to normalize the altered intestinal flora [9]. The use of probiotics in prevention of nosocomial gastrointestinal and respiratory tract infections in critical care has increased over the last few years and results from a growing number of randomized controlled trials within the adult and pediatric populations suggest their use as a promising treatment [10,11,12,13]. The need for alternative, non-antimicrobial interventions for prevention of infection in an age of increasing antimicrobial resistance also make probiotics a promising strategy. Specifically, lactobacilli and bifidobacteria alone or in combination are the most frequently used strains in the treatment of various gastrointestinal disorders [14,15,16] or as therapy for different clinical conditions including antibiotic associated diarrhea [17], acute pancreatitis [18], ventilator associated pneumonia [11,12,19], sepsis and postoperative infections [20,21].

Although probiotics are showing promise as an effective therapy in a growing number of illnesses, the mechanisms of their action are complex and still elusive [22]. Based on the results from several *in vivo* and *in vitro* studies, probiotics are able to decrease apoptosis in intestinal epithelial cells [23,24,25,26], improve intestinal integrity [27,28,29,30], prevent bacterial translocation [30,31], reduce the overgrowth of pathogenic bacteria and suppress cytokine production [32,33,34,35].

Despite the benefits of probiotic use in intestinal disorders, the effects of probiotic treatment to protect against lung injury following infection and sepsis are not well understood. We have recently shown the benefits of *Lactobacillus rhamnosus* GG (LGG) and *Bifidobacterium longum* (BL) on improved survival and intestinal homeostasis in weanling mouse model of cecal ligation and puncture (CLP) [36]. CLP is an experimental model of shock that mimics the pathology of sepsis occurring in the ICU patients [37]. Toll like receptors (TLRs) are pattern recognition receptors involved in the initial steps of signaling pathway leading to multiple organ failure in sepsis. TLRs bind to cell-wall components which activates nuclear factor (NF)-KB/IKB system resulting in release of pro-inflammatory cytokines [38]. In addition to cytokines, pathogens activating TLRs were also reported to induce Cox-2 expression [39,40].

In this study we hypothesized that LGG and BL will also have a protective effect against lung injury and will decrease the inflammatory response in the lungs potentially via the TLR/Myd88 pathway.

Methods

Probiotic treatment and septic peritonitis model

The animal protocol used in these studies was approved by the Institutional Animal Care and Use Committee of the University of Colorado Anschutz Medical Campus. Briefly, 3 weeks old FVB/N mice were orally gavaged with 200 µl of either LGG (1×10^9 CFU/ml), BL (1×10^7 CFU/ml), or sterile water (vehicle) immediately prior to initiation of the cecal ligation and puncture (CLP) procedure [41]. Briefly, a small midline abdominal incision was made, the cecum was ligated just distal to the ileocecal valve, and was then punctured twice with a 23-gauge needle. The cecum was squeezed to extrude a small amount of stool, replaced in the abdomen, and the peritoneum and skin were closed in layers. Sham mice were treated identically except the cecum was neither ligated nor punctured. All mice received 1.0 ml normal saline subcutaneously after the surgery to compensate for fluid loss. Mice received a single dose of probiotics prior to tissue collection. Animals were euthanized at 24 h.

Lactobacillus rhamnosus GG and *Bifidobacterium longum* culture

LGG (ATCC, Manassas, VA) was incubated in MRS broth (BD, Sparks, MD) for 24 hours at 37°C and 5% CO_2. BL (ATCC, Manassas, VA) was cultured in Trypticase soy broth (BD, Sparks, MD) for 72 hours in an anaerobic chamber at 37°C. A_{600} was measured to determine the number of colony forming units (CFU) per 1 ml. BL and LGG were pelleted from the broth (10,000 rpm; 10 min) and resuspended in distilled water.

Immunohistology

Lung tissue was collected from each animal at 24 h and fixed overnight in 10% formalin, paraffin-embedded, and sectioned at 4–6 µm. Serial sections were stained with hematoxylin-eosin (H&E) and evaluated for severity of lung injury by blinded evaluator using a grading scale from 0 (no abnormality) to 4 (severe lung injury) as described previously [42].

Neutrophil infiltration into the lungs was evaluated by staining for myeloperoxidase (MPO). After deparaffinization and rehydration, sections were blocked with 1.5% rabbit serum (Vector Laboratories, Burlingame, CA) in phosphate-buffered saline for 30 min, then incubated with goat polyclonal MPO (1:50; R&D Systems, Minneapolis, MN) antibody for 1 hour, washed with phosphate-buffered saline, and incubated with rabbit anti-goat biotinylated secondary antibody (Vector Laboratories) for 30 min. Vectastain Elite ABC reagent (Vector Laboratories) was then applied, followed by diaminobenzidine as substrate. Sections were counterstained with hematoxylin, dehydrated and cover-slipped. MPO positive cells were quantified in 10 random high-power fields per section. All counting was performed by a blinded evaluator.

RNA Preparation, RT, and Real-Time PCR

Total RNA was isolated from lung tissue (snap frozen in liquid N_2, collected at 24 h) using the RNeasy Plus Mini Kit (Qiagen, Santa Clarita, CA) as described in the manufacturer's protocol. RNA concentrations were quantified at 260 nm, and the purity and integrity were determined using a NanoDrop. RT and real-time PCR assays were performed to quantify steady-state mRNA levels of IL-6, TNF-α, MyD88, TLR-4, TLR-2, NFKB (p50/p105) and Cox-2. cDNA was synthesized from 0.2 µg of total RNA. Predeveloped TaqMan primers and probes (Applied Biosystems) were used for detection. Reporter dye emission was detected by an automated sequence detector combined with ABI Prism 7300 Real Time PCR System (Applied Biosystems). Real-time PCR quantification was performed with TaqMan GAPDH controls and relative mRNA expression calculated using the $2^{-\Delta\Delta CT}$ method [43].

IL-6 and TNF-α protein analysis in the lung tissue

Lung tissue was harvested and frozen immediately in liquid nitrogen. Samples were homogenized with a hand-held homogenizer in a 5× volume of ice-cold homogenization buffer (Tris HCl, 50 mm; pH, 7.4; NaCl, 100 mm; EDTA, 10 mm; Triton X-100, 0.5%) with added protease inhibitors (Roche Diagnostics, Mannheim, Germany). The homogenates were centrifuged at 10,000 rpm for 5 min at 4°C and the supernatant was collected. Total protein concentration was quantified using the Bradford protein assay. Enzyme-linked immunosorbent assay (ELISA) (R&D Systems, Mineapolis, MN) was used to determine the concentrations of TNF-α and IL-6 in lung tissue homogenates according to the manufacturer's instructions.

Statistics

Comparisons were performed with t test analysis (unpaired, two-tailed). To analyze the bacterial culture results, 2-tailed NPar, Mann-Whitney Test was used. No measurements or animals were lost to observation or missing in the analysis. Data were analyzed using Prism 4.0 (GraphPad Software, San Diego, CA) and reported as means ± SE. A p value≤0.05 was considered to be statistically significant.

Results

Probiotics improve lung injury and decrease the neutrophil infiltration during sepsis

We have previously shown in this model that probiotic treatment with LGG or BL can improve survival following CLP

[36]. In this study we hypothesized this may be associated with or be related to reduction in lung injury. Thus, the effect of probiotic treatment on lung pathology was assessed. Sepsis led to marked histological injury 24 hours after CLP surgery in septic animals. This injury was significantly improved in septic animals treated with LGG or BL (Figure 1A, B). Sepsis-mediated lung injury was associated with a significantly higher number of infiltrating neutrophils, represented by the number of MPO positive cells in the septic animals when compared to shams ($P<0.0001$). Treatment with LGG and BL normalized ($P<0.0001$) the number of MPO positive cells in the lungs to that observed in sham mice (Figure 2A, B).

Probiotics attenuate proinflammatory cytokine release in the lung after sepsis

To determine the effect of LGG and BL treatment on pro-inflammatory cytokine release in lungs after CLP-induced polymicrobial sepsis, mRNA levels of IL-6 and TNF-α were analyzed by Real-Time PCR and protein levels measured by ELISA. Gene expressions of IL-6 and TNF-α (Figure 3A, B) were significantly increased in lungs of septic animals ($P<0.05$) and normalized to sham levels in LGG or BL treated mice. Protein levels of IL-6 ($P<0.01$) (Figure 3C) and TNF-α ($P<0.05$) (Figure 3D) were also markedly elevated in septic mice and attenuated to sham levels in mice treated with either probiotic strain.

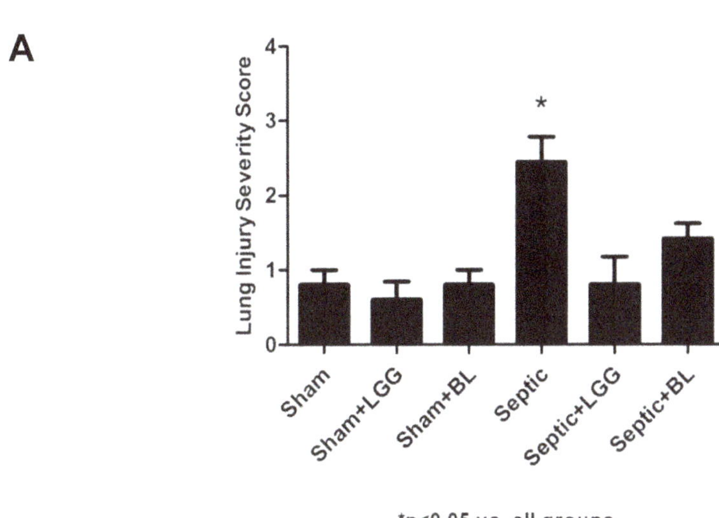

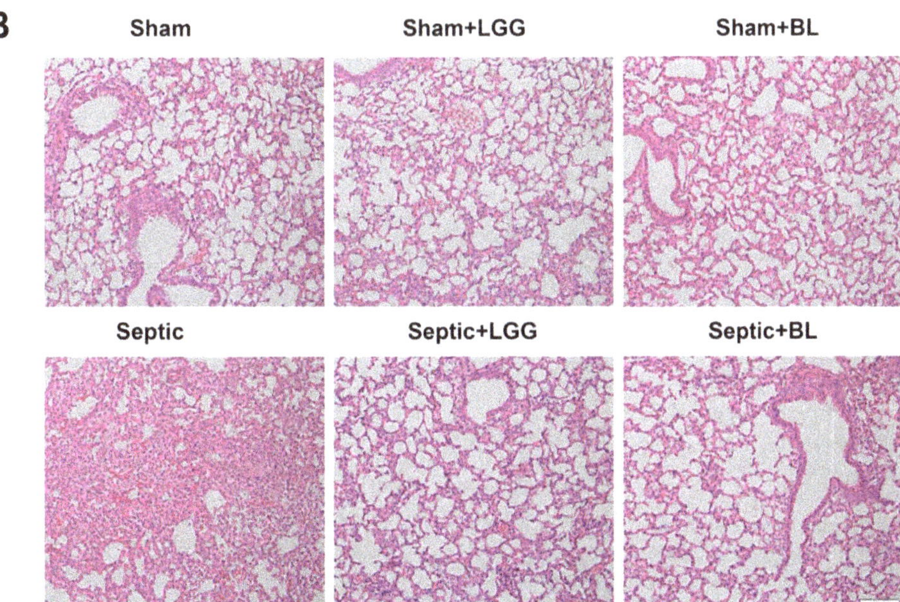

Figure 1. Probiotics improve lung pathology 24 hours post CLP. (A) The severity of pneumonia (from 0: no abnormality to 4: severe lung injury) was significantly reduced in the lungs of mice treated with LGG and BL ($P<0.05$). (B) Representative H&E stained sections of lung are shown. Original magnification ×100. Shams n = 4 per group, Septic, Septic+LGG, Septic+BL n = 5–8 per group.

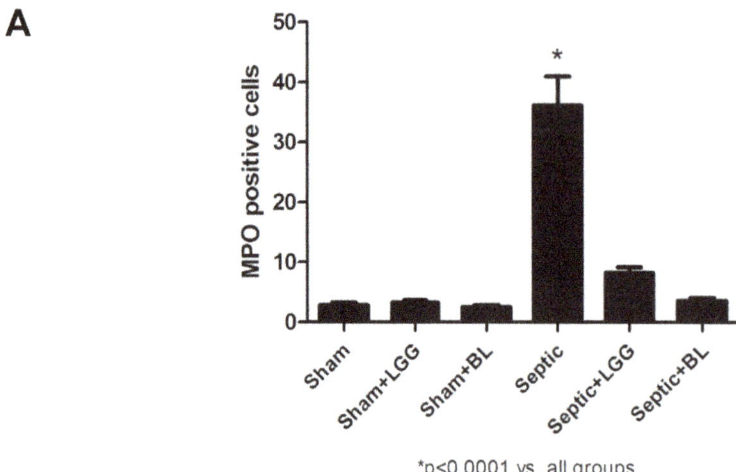

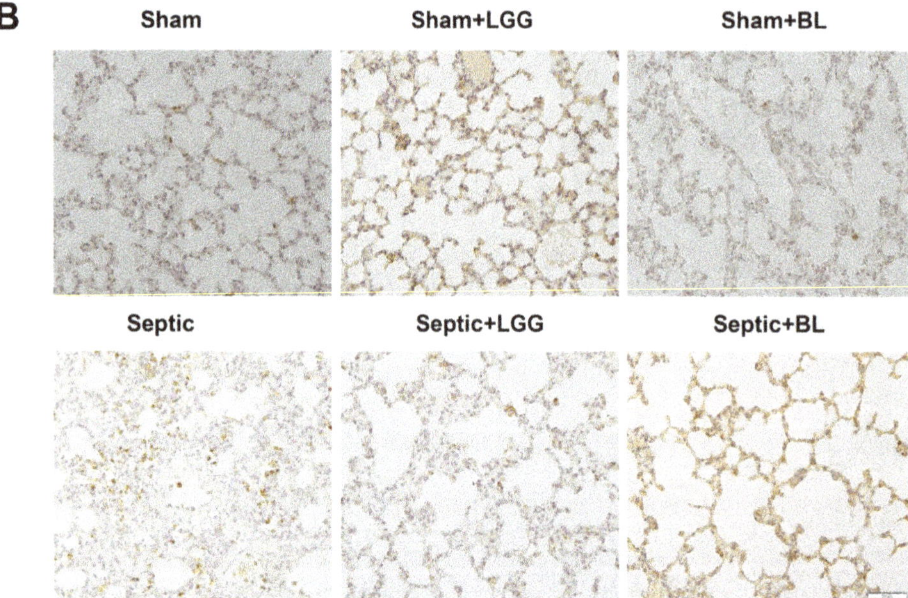

Figure 2. Probiotics decrease neutrophil infiltration in the lung 24 hours post CLP (A) Number of MPO positive cells in the lungs of septic mice were significantly increased compared to shams. LGG or BL treatment normalized these levels ($P<0.0001$). (B) Representative MPO stained sections of lung are shown. Original magnification ×200. Shams n = 4 per group, Septic, Septic+LGG, Septic+BL n = 6 per group.

Probiotics decrease Cox-2 expression and regulate toll-like receptor (TLR) pathway in the lung during sepsis

Cox-2 is rapidly induced in response to cytokines and is elevated at sites of inflammation. Gene expression of Cox-2 was significantly increased in lungs of septic mice ($P<0.05$) and treatment with LGG or BL significantly decreased ($P<0.05$) Cox-2 levels to those observed in the lung of sham animals (Figure 4).

TLRs signal via the MyD88 pathway that includes the NFKB transcriptional factor, which is a key activator of the cytokines involved in the innate immunity response. MyD88 has an important role in early recruitment of inflammatory cells and in the control of bacterial infection [44]. Gene expression of TLR-2, TLR-4, MyD88 and NFKB (p50/p105) was analyzed by Real-Time PCR. There was significant increase of TLR-2 MyD88 and NFKB (p50/p105) in the lungs of septic mice ($P<0.05$) (Figure 5A, C, D). LGG or BL treatment normalized the levels of TLR-2 and MyD88 to those in shams (Figure 5A, C). NFKB (p50/p105) was significantly decreased in the lung of LGG treated mice ($P<0.05$). The levels in BL treated mice were also decreased but did not reach statistical significance (Figure 5D). TLR-4 remained unchanged regardless of treatment (Figure 5B).

Discussion

This work demonstrates two probiotic strains, *Lactobacillus rhamnosus* GG and *Bifidobacterium longum*, can reduce lung injury and attenuate the inflammatory response in the lungs of weanling mice subjected to CLP.

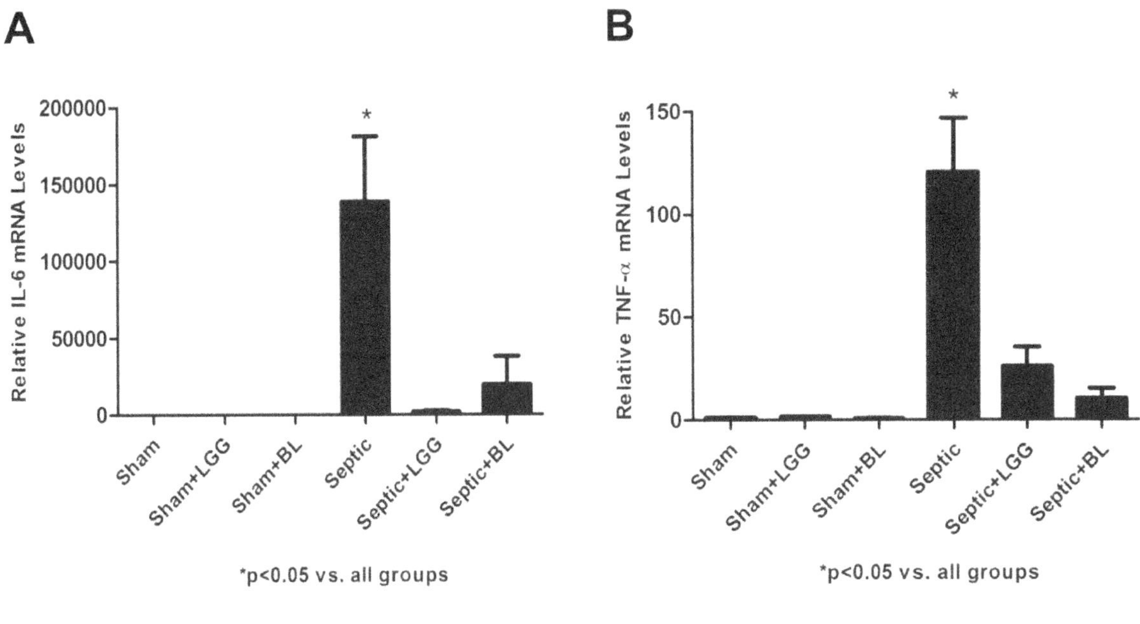

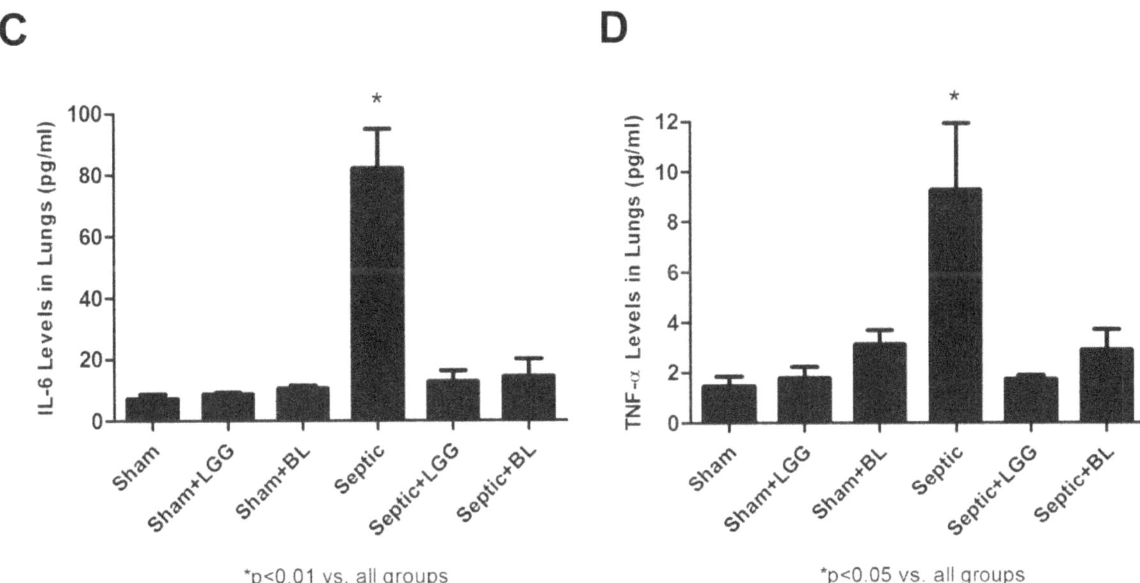

Figure 3. Probiotics attenuate proinflammatory cytokine release in lung 24 hours post CLP. Reverse transcription and real-time PCR assays were performed to quantify steady-state mRNA levels of pro-inflammatory cytokines. (A) IL-6 and (B) TNF-α were significantly increased in the lung of septic animals compare to shams ($P<0.05$). LGG or BL treatment normalized these levels to shams ($P<0.05$). Shams n = 4 per group; Septic, Septic+LGG, Septic+BL n = 5 per group. Data are expressed as the mean ± SE. Enzyme-linked immunosorbent assay (ELISA) was used to determine the protein concentrations of IL-6 and TNF-α in the lung. (C) IL-6 and (D) TNF-α were significantly elevated in the lung of septic mice compared to shams ($P<0.05$). Treatment with LGG or BL prior to CLP led to significantly reduced ($P<0.05$) levels of both cytokines compared to untreated septic mice. Shams n = 3 per group; Septic, Septic+LGG, Septic+BL n = 4 per group. Data are expressed as the mean ± SE.

Not surprisingly, the gut has been identified as an origin and promoter of nosocomial sepsis and multiorgan failure in the critically ill, the major determinant of ICU outcome [45].Critical illness and ICU-based therapies, such as vasopressors and broad spectrum antibiotics, create a hostile environment in the gut and alter the microflora favoring the growth of pathogens. This is in part due to the loss of key beneficial lactic acid bacteria [46] otherwise called probiotics that can inhibit the overgrowth of pathogens by production of bacteriocins, hydrogen peroxide, organic acids, ammonia and by increased competition for adhesion sites on intestinal epithelia [47,48]. Also, a number of bioactive factors secreted by probiotics, mainly by LGG, have been identified and their effects studied in intestinal injury as well as airway inflammation models [49,50]. Soluble protein p40 derived from LGG as published by Polk et al preserves barrier function and reduces apoptosis in the colon epithelium in an EGF

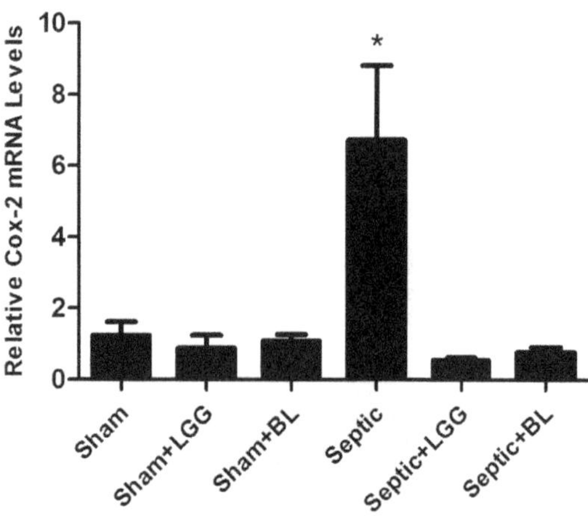

Figure 4. Probiotics downregulate Cox-2 expression in the lung 24 hours post CLP. Reverse transcription and real-time PCR assays were performed to quantify steady-state mRNA levels of Cox-2. Cox-2 was significantly elevated in the septic group compared to sham groups ($P<0.05$). Treatment with LGG or BL significantly reduced mRNA levels of Cox-2 compared to untreated septic mice ($P<0.05$). Shams n = 4 per group; Septic, Septic+LGG, Septic+BL n = 4–5 per group. Data are expressed as the mean ± SE.

receptor-dependent manner [51]. A study performed in healthy adults suggests how three different lactobacilli induce differential gene-regulatory networks and pathways in the human mucosa, showing that mucosal responses to LGG involve would healing, IFN response and ion homeostasis [52]. A recent review article provides detailed information on several probiotic strains and their ability to stimulate the immune system including activation of macrophages, natural killer cells, T-lymphocytes and release of cytokines in strain specific, dose dependent manner [53]. Several randomized controlled trials within adult and pediatric populations suggest the use of probiotics as a promising therapy for nosocomial gastrointestinal and respiratory tract infections [10,11,12,13] but there are still many questions to be answered about their mechanisms of action.

From current clinical studies of probiotic therapy, it appears that timing of probiotic administration may be important in their effectiveness with administration early in critical illness potentially being important. [27,54,55,56]. In our mouse model of sepsis, the animals were given LGG or BL immediately before the surgery to better reflect the common clinical setting where a patient presenting with peritonitis could be treated at the time of surgery to attempt to prevent future hospital acquired infections and acute lung injury. Our recently published data describe significant improvement of several outcomes including survival, bacteremia, systemic inflammatory response and intestinal homeostasis with administration of these probiotic strains in this immediate "surgical" timeframe. [36].

The pathophysiology of septic shock syndrome is characterized by hyperactive and dysregulated endogenous inflammatory mediators including cytokines such as IL-6, TNF-α, IL-1β, IL-12 and interferon γ [57,58]. It has been shown that early attenuation of transcription factor NFKB activation and cytokine message expression correlates with improved outcome in polymicrobial sepsis [59]. Controlling inflammatory mediated injury to distant organs is a key goal in sepsis to prevent the multiple organ dysfunction syndrome (MODS) which carries quite a high mortality. This is often observed in generalized peritonitis (as studied in our model), which accompanies surgical conditions such as gastrointestinal perforation [58]. Clinical and experimental data support an important role of the lung during the initial stages of the multiple organ dysfunction syndrome (MODS) [60]. The release of pro-inflammatory mediators can cause acute lung injury [61] and it has been reported that levels of pro-inflammatory cytokines such as IL-6 and TNF-α are significantly elevated in the lungs after CLP-induced peritonitis [59,62]. There are several publications reporting the protective effect of different probiotic strains against bacterial infection. A study done in the rat CLP peritonitis model demostrated a decrease of TNF-α and IL-1β in lungs of animals receiving a prolonged three week pre-treatment with probiotics and overall reduction of acute lung injury was also observed [35]. Racedo at al. used a mouse model of *Streptococcus pneumoniae* infection to evaluate the effect of *L. casei* and found that two days of pre-treatment could beneficially regulate the TNF-α and IL-10 balance, allowing a more effective immune response against infection and modulation the inflammatory response. This was associated with less damage to the lung in this model [63]. In our unique immediate pre-treatment model, we found significantly increased mRNA and protein levels of pro-inflammatory cytokines TNF-α, IL-6 in the lungs of septic mice. Treatment at the time of onset of peritonitis (rather than a prolonged pre-treatment period) with either *Lactobacillus rhamnosus GG* or *Bifidobacterium longum* normalized these cytokine levels to those seen in shams indicating the anti-inflammatory effect of both probiotic strains possibly contributing to better overall outcome.

In general, Cox-2 is not expressed in healthy tissues but is rapidly induced in response to cytokines and is elevated at sites of inflammation and injury [64] and is involved in pathogenesis of sepsis [65]. In mouse CLP model, Cox-2 expression was previously shown to increase in the lungs of septic mice [66,67,68], in addition dual inhibition of Cox-2 and 5-LOX successfully attenuated lung injury, reduced MPO activity and improved survival of these mice [69]. As shown in several *in vitro* and *in vivo* models, pathogens induce Cox-2 expression via activated Toll like receptors (TLRs) [39,40]. TLRs play a central role in the initiation of innate immune responses and in the development of a subsequent pro-inflammatory response, which can lead to inflammation induced organ injury. TLRs are activated by specific microbial ligands leading to an association with TIR domain containing MyD88 factor which mediates a signaling cascade that activates NFKB factor and results in upregulation of pro-inflammatory cytokines [70]. Markedly increased expression of TLR-2 and TLR-4 in monocytes [71,72] and leukocytes [73] has been reported in septic patients. In mouse CLP peritonitis models, TLR-2 and TLR-4 expressions were significantly upregulated in hepatic and splenic macrophages [74], in the lungs and liver [75,76] as well as in the intestine [77] when compared to sham mice. Here we demonstrate that Cox-2, TLR-2, MyD88 and NFKB (p50/p105) were significantly higher in the lungs of septic mice compared to healthy shams and lower in the lungs of LGG and BL mice. NFKB (p50/p105) in the lungs of BL treated septic mice showed only a decreasing trend. The expression of TLR-4 in the lungs remained unchanged among all experimental groups, similar to the observations of Williams et al. [75] in a CLP peritonitis model where TLR-4 expression increased at earlier time points but not at 24 hours. We speculate that downregulation of Cox-2 through TLR-2/TLR-4 (via MyD88) in the lungs of *Lactobacillus rhamnosus GG* or *Bifidobacterium longum* treated mice may play a protective role in attenuating inflammation induced lung injury following systemic sepsis and peritonitis.

In conclusion, probiotic therapy with LGG and BL can reduce lung injury following experimental peritonitis and sepsis and is

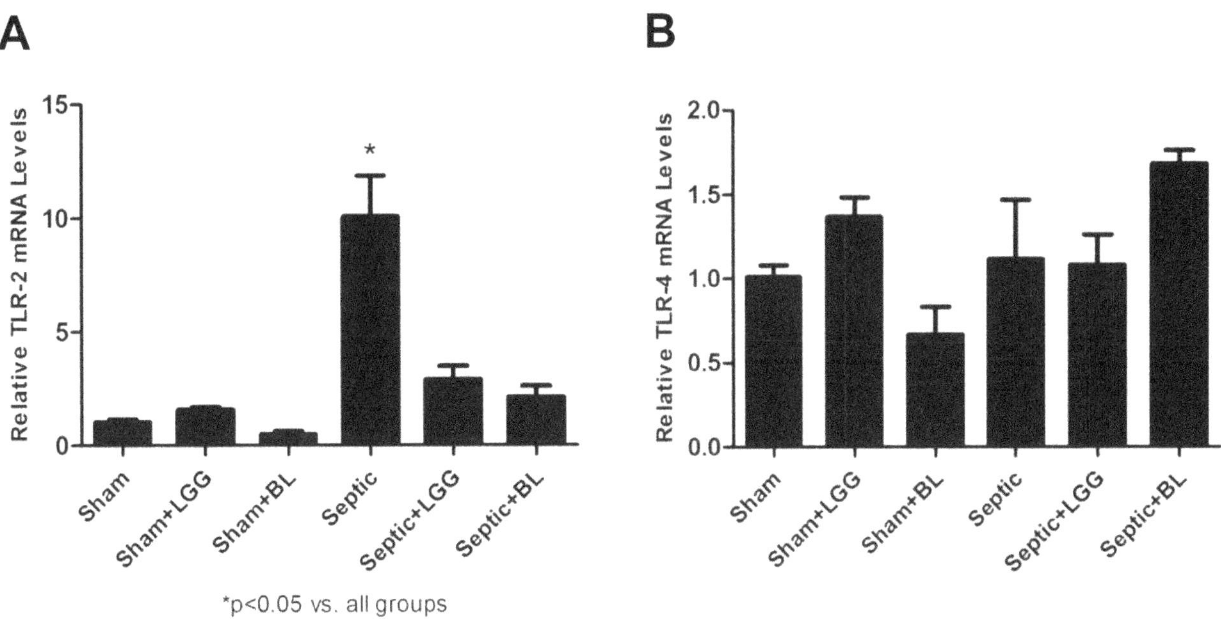

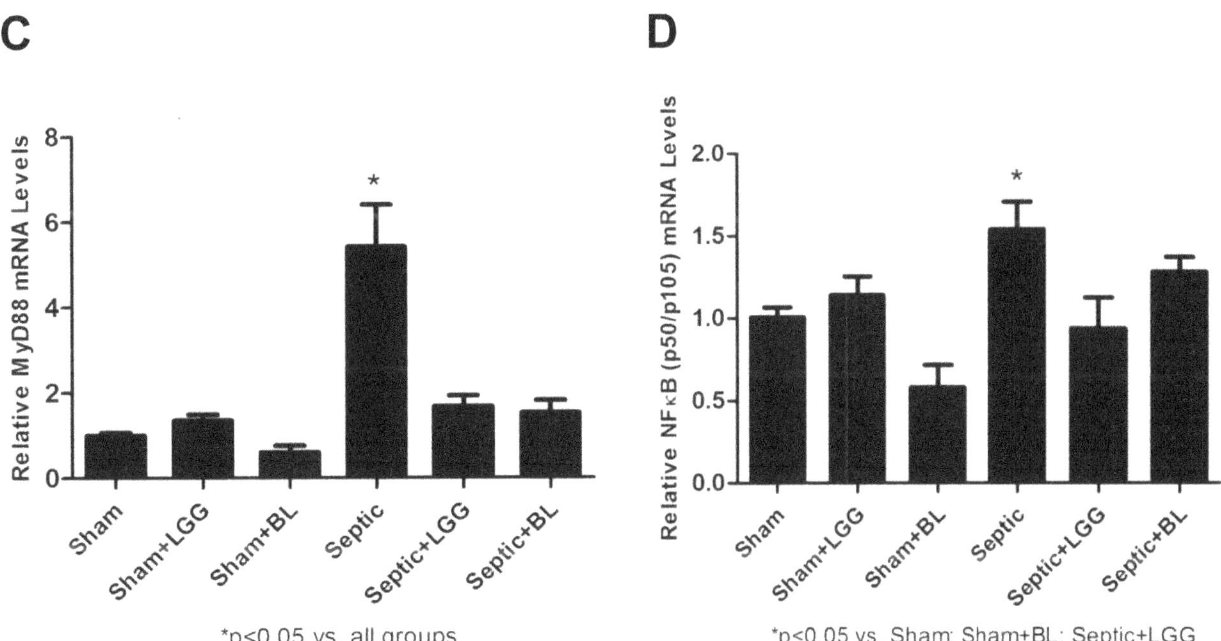

Figure 5. Probiotics regulate Toll-like receptor (TLR) pathway in the lung 24 hours post CLP. Reverse transcription and real-time PCR assays were performed to quantify steady-state mRNA levels of TLR-2, TLR-4, MyD88 and NFKB (p50/p105). (A) TLR-2 and (C) MyD88 were significantly upregulated in the septic group compared to shams ($P<0.05$) and significantly downregulated in the lungs of LGG and BL treated septic mice compared to untreated septic mice. (B) mRNA levels of TLR-4 remained unchanged in all groups. (D) NFKB (p50/p105) was significantly upregulated in the septic group compared to shams ($P<0.05$) and significantly downregulated in the lungs of LGG treated septic mice compared to untreated septic mice. The levels in BL treated mice were decreased but did not reach statistical significance. Shams n = 5 per group; Septic, Septic+ LGG, Septic+BL n = 5–7 per group. Data are expressed as the mean ± SE.

associated with reduced lung inflammatory cell infiltrate and decreased markers of lung inflammatory response activation. Probiotic therapy may be a promising intervention to improve clinical lung injury following systemic infection and sepsis.

Author Contributions

Conceived and designed the experiments: LK PW. Performed the experiments: LK BP. Analyzed the data: LK. Contributed reagents/materials/analysis tools: PW. Wrote the paper: LK PW CB JDR.

References

1. Watson RS, Carcillo JA, Linde-Zwirble WT, Clermont G, Lidicker J, et al. (2003) The epidemiology of severe sepsis in children in the United States. Am J Respir Crit Care Med 167: 695–701.
2. Lukacs SL, Schoendorf KC, Schuchat A (2004) Trends in sepsis-related neonatal mortality in the United States, 1985–1998. Pediatr Infect Dis J 23: 599–603.
3. Wynn JL, Scumpia PO, Delano MJ, O'Malley KA, Ungaro R, et al. (2007) Increased mortality and altered immunity in neonatal sepsis produced by generalized peritonitis. Shock 28: 675–683.
4. Kermorvant-Duchemin E, Laborie S, Rabilloud M, Lapillonne A, Claris O (2008) Outcome and prognostic factors in neonates with septic shock. Pediatr Crit Care Med 9: 186–191.
5. Adams-Chapman I, Stoll BJ (2006) Neonatal infection and long-term neurodevelopmental outcome in the preterm infant. Curr Opin Infect Dis 19: 290–297.
6. Dahlem P, van Aalderen WM, Bos AP (2007) Pediatric acute lung injury. Paediatr Respir Rev 8: 348–362.
7. Flori HR, Glidden DV, Rutherford GW, Matthay MA (2005) Pediatric acute lung injury: prospective evaluation of risk factors associated with mortality. Am J Respir Crit Care Med 171: 995–1001.
8. Singhi SC, Baranwal A (2008) Probiotic use in the critically ill. Indian J Pediatr 75: 621–627.
9. Hammerman C, Bin-Nun A, Kaplan M (2004) Germ warfare: probiotics in defense of the premature gut. Clin Perinatol 31: 489–500.
10. Hojsak I, Abdovic S, Szajewska H, Milosevic M, Krznaric Z, et al. (2010) Lactobacillus GG in the prevention of nosocomial gastrointestinal and respiratory tract infections. Pediatrics 125: e1171–1177.
11. Morrow LE, Kollef MH, Casale TB (2010) Probiotic prophylaxis of ventilator-associated pneumonia: a blinded, randomized, controlled trial. Am J Respir Crit Care Med 182: 1058–1064.
12. Siempos, II, Ntaidou TK, Falagas ME (2010) Impact of the administration of probiotics on the incidence of ventilator-associated pneumonia: a meta-analysis of randomized controlled trials. Crit Care Med 38: 954–962.
13. Pitsouni E, Alexiou V, Saridakis V, Peppas G, Falagas ME (2009) Does the use of probiotics/synbiotics prevent postoperative infections in patients undergoing abdominal surgery? A meta-analysis of randomized controlled trials. Eur J Clin Pharmacol 65: 561–570.
14. Bausserman M, Michail S (2005) The use of Lactobacillus GG in irritable bowel syndrome in children: a double-blind randomized control trial. J Pediatr 147: 197–201.
15. Bin-Nun A, Bromiker R, Wilschanski M, Kaplan M, Rudensky B, et al. (2005) Oral probiotics prevent necrotizing enterocolitis in very low birth weight neonates. J Pediatr 147: 192–196.
16. Drouault-Holowacz S, Bieuvelet S, Burckel A, Cazaubiel M, Dray X, et al. (2008) A double blind randomized controlled trial of a probiotic combination in 100 patients with irritable bowel syndrome. Gastroenterol Clin Biol 32: 147–152.
17. Arvola T, Laiho K, Torkkeli S, Mykkanen H, Salminen S, et al. (1999) Prophylactic Lactobacillus GG reduces antibiotic-associated diarrhea in children with respiratory infections: a randomized study. Pediatrics 104: e64.
18. Olah A, Belagyi T, Poto L, Romics L Jr, Bengmark S (2007) Synbiotic control of inflammation and infection in severe acute pancreatitis: a prospective, randomized, double blind study. Hepatogastroenterology 54: 590–594.
19. Schultz MJ (2010) Symbiotics as a preventive measure against ventilator-associated pneumonia. Crit Care Med 38: 1506–1507; author reply 1507.
20. Giamarellos-Bourboulis EJ, Bengmark S, Kanellakopoulou K, Kotzampassi K (2009) Pro- and synbiotics to control inflammation and infection in patients with multiple injuries. J Trauma 67: 815–821.
21. Kotzampassi K, Giamarellos-Bourboulis EJ, Voudouris A, Kazamias P, Eleftheriadis E (2006) Benefits of a synbiotic formula (Synbiotic 2000Forte) in critically Ill trauma patients: early results of a randomized controlled trial. World J Surg 30: 1848–1855.
22. Shanahan F (2002) Probiotics and inflammatory bowel disease: from fads and fantasy to facts and future. Br J Nutr 88 Suppl 1: S5–9.
23. Khailova L, Mount Patrick SK, Arganbright KM, Halpern MD, Kinouchi T, et al. (2010) Bifidobacterium bifidum reduces apoptosis in the intestinal epithelium in necrotizing enterocolitis. Am J Physiol Gastrointest Liver Physiol 299: G1118–1127.
24. Tao Y, Drabik KA, Waypa TS, Musch MW, Alverdy JC, et al. (2006) Soluble factors from Lactobacillus GG activate MAPKs and induce cytoprotective heat shock proteins in intestinal epithelial cells. Am J Physiol Cell Physiol 290: C1018–1030.
25. Yan F, Cao H, Cover TL, Whitehead R, Washington MK, et al. (2007) Soluble proteins produced by probiotic bacteria regulate intestinal epithelial cell survival and growth. Gastroenterology 132: 562–575.
26. Yan F, Polk DB (2002) Probiotic bacterium prevents cytokine-induced apoptosis in intestinal epithelial cells. J Biol Chem 277: 50959–50965.
27. Alberda C, Gramlich L, Meddings J, Field C, McCargar L, et al. (2007) Effects of probiotic therapy in critically ill patients: a randomized, double-blind, placebo-controlled trial. Am J Clin Nutr 85: 816–823.
28. Anderson RC, Cookson AL, McNabb WC, Kelly WJ, Roy NC (2010) Lactobacillus plantarum DSM 2648 is a potential probiotic that enhances intestinal barrier function. FEMS Microbiol Lett 309: 184–192.
29. Khailova L, Dvorak K, Arganbright KM, Halpern MD, Kinouchi T, et al. (2009) Bifidobacterium bifidum improves intestinal integrity in a rat model of necrotizing enterocolitis. Am J Physiol Gastrointest Liver Physiol 297: G940–949.
30. Zareie M, Johnson-Henry K, Jury J, Yang PC, Ngan BY, et al. (2006) Probiotics prevent bacterial translocation and improve intestinal barrier function in rats following chronic psychological stress. Gut 55: 1553–1560.
31. Luyer MD, Buurman WA, Hadfoune M, Speelmans G, Knol J, et al. (2005) Strain-specific effects of probiotics on gut barrier integrity following hemorrhagic shock. Infect Immun 73: 3686–3692.
32. Aguero G, Villena J, Racedo S, Haro C, Alvarez S (2006) Beneficial immunomodulatory activity of Lactobacillus casei in malnourished mice pneumonia: effect on inflammation and coagulation. Nutrition 22: 810–819.
33. Arribas B, Rodriguez-Cabezas ME, Comalada M, Bailon E, Camuesco D, et al. (2009) Evaluation of the preventative effects exerted by Lactobacillus fermentum in an experimental model of septic shock induced in mice. Br J Nutr 101: 51–58.
34. Matsumoto T, Ishikawa H, Tateda K, Yaeshima T, Ishibashi N, et al. (2008) Oral administration of Bifidobacterium longum prevents gut-derived Pseudomonas aeruginosa sepsis in mice. J Appl Microbiol 104: 672–680.
35. Tok D, Ilkgul O, Bengmark S, Aydede H, Erhan Y, et al. (2007) Pretreatment with pro- and synbiotics reduces peritonitis-induced acute lung injury in rats. J Trauma 62: 880–885.
36. Khailova L, Frank DN, Dominguez JA, Wischmeyer PE (2013) Probiotic Administration Reduces Mortality and Improves Intestinal Epithelial Homeostasis in Experimental Sepsis. Anesthesiology.
37. Annane D, Bellissant E, Cavaillon JM (2005) Septic shock. Lancet 365: 63–78.
38. Akira S, Uematsu S, Takeuchi O (2006) Pathogen recognition and innate immunity. Cell 124: 783–801.
39. Xu F, Xu Z, Zhang R, Wu Z, Lim JH, et al. (2008) Nontypeable Haemophilus influenzae induces COX-2 and PGE2 expression in lung epithelial cells via activation of p38 MAPK and NF-kappa B. Respir Res 9: 16.
40. Kirkby NS, Zaiss AK, Wright WR, Jiao J, Chan MV, et al. (2013) Differential COX-2 induction by viral and bacterial PAMPs: Consequences for cytokine and interferon responses and implications for anti-viral COX-2 directed therapies. Biochem Biophys Res Commun 438: 249–256.
41. Baker CC, Chaudry IH, Gaines HO, Baue AE (1983) Evaluation of factors affecting mortality rate after sepsis in a murine cecal ligation and puncture model. Surgery 94: 331–335.
42. Robertson CM, Perrone EE, McConnell KW, Dunne WM, Boody B, et al. (2008) Neutrophil depletion causes a fatal defect in murine pulmonary Staphylococcus aureus clearance. J Surg Res 150: 278–285.
43. Livak KJ, Schmittgen TD (2001) Analysis of relative gene expression data using real-time quantitative PCR and the 2(-Delta Delta C(T)) Method. Methods 25: 402–408.
44. Hajjar AM, Harowicz H, Liggitt HD, Fink PJ, Wilson CB, et al. (2005) An essential role for non-bone marrow-derived cells in control of Pseudomonas aeruginosa pneumonia. Am J Respir Cell Mol Biol 33: 470–475.
45. MacFie J, O'Boyle C, Mitchell CJ, Buckley PM, Johnstone D, et al. (1999) Gut origin of sepsis: a prospective study investigating associations between bacterial translocation, gastric microflora, and septic morbidity. Gut 45: 223–228.
46. Wang X, Andersson R, Soltesz V, Leveau P, Ihse I (1996) Gut origin sepsis, macrophage function, and oxygen extraction associated with acute pancreatitis in the rat. World J Surg 20: 299–307; discussion 307–298.
47. Cleveland J, Montville TJ, Nes IF, Chikindas ML (2001) Bacteriocins: safe, natural antimicrobials for food preservation. Int J Food Microbiol 71: 1–20.
48. Lee YK, Lim CY, Teng WL, Ouwehand AC, Tuomola EM, et al. (2000) Quantitative approach in the study of adhesion of lactic acid bacteria to intestinal cells and their competition with enterobacteria. Appl Environ Microbiol 66: 3692–3697.
49. Yan F, Cao H, Cover TL, Washington MK, Shi Y, et al. (2011) Colon-specific delivery of a probiotic-derived soluble protein ameliorates intestinal inflammation in mice through an EGFR-dependent mechanism. J Clin Invest 121: 2242–2253.
50. Harb H, van Tol EA, Heine H, Braaksma M, Gross G, et al. (2013) Neonatal supplementation of processed supernatant from Lactobacillus rhamnosus GG improves allergic airway inflammation in mice later in life. Clin Exp Allergy 43: 353–364.
51. Yan F, Polk DB (2012) Characterization of a probiotic-derived soluble protein which reveals a mechanism of preventive and treatment effects of probiotics on intestinal inflammatory diseases. Gut Microbes 3: 25–28.
52. van Baarlen P, Troost F, van der Meer C, Hooiveld G, Boekschoten M, et al. (2011) Human mucosal in vivo transcriptome responses to three lactobacilli indicate how probiotics may modulate human cellular pathways. Proc Natl Acad Sci U S A 108 Suppl 1: 4562–4569.
53. Ashraf R, Shah NP (2014) Immune system stimulation by probiotic microorganisms. Crit Rev Food Sci Nutr 54: 938–956.
54. Dani C, Biadaioli R, Bertini G, Martelli E, Rubaltelli FF (2002) Probiotics feeding in prevention of urinary tract infection, bacterial sepsis and necrotizing

enterocolitis in preterm infants. A prospective double-blind study. Biol Neonate 82: 103–108.

55. McNaught CE, Woodcock NP, Anderson AD, MacFie J (2005) A prospective randomised trial of probiotics in critically ill patients. Clin Nutr 24: 211–219.
56. Honeycutt TC, El Khashab M, Wardrop RM 3rd, McNeal-Trice K, Honeycutt AL, et al. (2007) Probiotic administration and the incidence of nosocomial infection in pediatric intensive care: a randomized placebo-controlled trial. Pediatr Crit Care Med 8: 452–458; quiz 464.
57. Netea MG, van der Meer JW, van Deuren M, Kullberg BJ (2003) Proinflammatory cytokines and sepsis syndrome: not enough, or too much of a good thing? Trends Immunol 24: 254–258.
58. Kono Y, Inomata M, Hagiwara S, Shiraishi N, Noguchi T, et al. (2011) A newly synthetic vitamin E derivative, E-Ant-S-GS, attenuates lung injury caused by cecal ligation and puncture-induced sepsis in rats. Surgery.
59. Williams DL, Ha T, Li C, Kalbfleisch JH, Laffan JJ, et al. (1999) Inhibiting early activation of tissue nuclear factor-kappa B and nuclear factor interleukin 6 with (1→3)-beta-D-glucan increases long-term survival in polymicrobial sepsis. Surgery 126: 54–65.
60. Regel G, Grotz M, Weltner T, Sturm JA, Tscherne H (1996) Pattern of organ failure following severe trauma. World J Surg 20: 422–429.
61. Farley KS, Wang LF, Razavi HM, Law C, Rohan M, et al. (2006) Effects of macrophage inducible nitric oxide synthase in murine septic lung injury. Am J Physiol Lung Cell Mol Physiol 290: L1164–1172.
62. Singleton KD, Wischmeyer PE (2007) Glutamine's protection against sepsis and lung injury is dependent on heat shock protein 70 expression. Am J Physiol Regul Integr Comp Physiol 292: R1839–1845.
63. Racedo S, Villena J, Medina M, Aguero G, Rodriguez V, et al. (2006) Lactobacillus casei administration reduces lung injuries in a Streptococcus pneumoniae infection in mice. Microbes Infect 8: 2359–2366.
64. Appleby SB, Ristimaki A, Neilson K, Narko K, Hla T (1994) Structure of the human cyclo-oxygenase-2 gene. Biochem J 302 (Pt 3): 723–727.
65. Rajapakse N, Kim MM, Mendis E, Kim SK (2008) Inhibition of inducible nitric oxide synthase and cyclooxygenase-2 in lipopolysaccharide-stimulated RAW264.7 cells by carboxybutyrylated glucosamine takes place via down-regulation of mitogen-activated protein kinase-mediated nuclear factor-kappaB signaling. Immunology 123: 348–357.
66. Zhang LN, Zheng JJ, Zhang L, Gong X, Huang H, et al. (2011) Protective effects of asiaticoside on septic lung injury in mice. Exp Toxicol Pathol 63: 519–525.
67. Li XH, Gong X, Zhang L, Jiang R, Li HZ, et al. (2013) Protective effects of polydatin on septic lung injury in mice via upregulation of HO-1. Mediators Inflamm 2013: 354087.
68. Ang SF, Sio SW, Moochhala SM, MacAry PA, Bhatia M (2011) Hydrogen sulfide upregulates cyclooxygenase-2 and prostaglandin E metabolite in sepsis-evoked acute lung injury via transient receptor potential vanilloid type 1 channel activation. J Immunol 187: 4778–4787.
69. Bitto A, Minutoli L, David A, Irrera N, Rinaldi M, et al. (2012) Flavocoxid, a dual inhibitor of COX-2 and 5-LOX of natural origin, attenuates the inflammatory response and protects mice from sepsis. Crit Care 16: R32.
70. Akira S, Takeda K (2004) Toll-like receptor signalling. Nat Rev Immunol 4: 499–511.
71. Tsujimoto H, Ono S, Hiraki S, Majima T, Kawarabayashi N, et al. (2004) Hemoperfusion with polymyxin B-immobilized fibers reduced the number of CD16+ CD14+ monocytes in patients with septic shock. J Endotoxin Res 10: 229–237.
72. Armstrong L, Medford AR, Hunter KJ, Uppington KM, Millar AB (2004) Differential expression of Toll-like receptor (TLR)-2 and TLR-4 on monocytes in human sepsis. Clin Exp Immunol 136: 312–319.
73. Harter L, Mica L, Stocker R, Trentz O, Keel M (2004) Increased expression of toll-like receptor-2 and -4 on leukocytes from patients with sepsis. Shock 22: 403–409.
74. Tsujimoto H, Ono S, Majima T, Kawarabayashi N, Takayama E, et al. (2005) Neutrophil elastase, MIP-2, and TLR-4 expression during human and experimental sepsis. Shock 23: 39–44.
75. Williams DL, Ha T, Li C, Kalbfleisch JH, Schweitzer J, et al. (2003) Modulation of tissue Toll-like receptor 2 and 4 during the early phases of polymicrobial sepsis correlates with mortality. Crit Care Med 31: 1808–1818.
76. Edelman DA, Jiang Y, Tyburski J, Wilson RF, Steffes C (2006) Toll-like receptor-4 message is up-regulated in lipopolysaccharide-exposed rat lung pericytes. J Surg Res 134: 22–27.
77. Yu M, Shao D, Liu J, Zhu J, Zhang Z, et al. (2007) Effects of ketamine on levels of cytokines, NF-kappaB and TLRs in rat intestine during CLP-induced sepsis. Int Immunopharmacol 7: 1076–1082.

2

Performance of Thirteen Clinical Rules to Distinguish Bacterial and Presumed Viral Meningitis in Vietnamese Children

Nguyen Tien Huy[1], Nguyen Thanh Hong Thao[2], Nguyen Anh Tuan[2,3], Nguyen Tuan Khiem[4], Christopher C. Moore[5], Doan Thi Ngoc Diep[2,3]*, Kenji Hirayama[1,6]*

1 Department of Immunogenetics, Institute of Tropical Medicine (NEKKEN), Nagasaki University, Nagasaki City, Japan, **2** Department of Pediatrics, University of Medicine and Pharmacy at Ho Chi Minh City, Ho Chi Minh City, Vietnam, **3** Children's Hospital No.1, Ho Chi Minh City, Vietnam, **4** Department of Pediatrics, Pham Ngoc Thach University of Medicine, Ho Chi Minh City, Vietnam, **5** Division of Infectious Diseases and International Health, Department of Medicine, University of Virginia, Charlottesville, Virginia, United States of America, **6** Global COE Program, Nagasaki University, Nagasaki City, Japan

Abstract

Background and Purpose: Successful outcomes from bacterial meningitis require rapid antibiotic treatment; however, unnecessary treatment of viral meningitis may lead to increased toxicities and expense. Thus, improved diagnostics are required to maximize treatment and minimize side effects and cost. Thirteen clinical decision rules have been reported to identify bacterial from viral meningitis. However, few rules have been tested and compared in a single study, while several rules are yet to be tested by independent researchers or in pediatric populations. Thus, simultaneous test and comparison of these rules are required to enable clinicians to select an optimal diagnostic rule for bacterial meningitis in settings and populations similar to ours.

Methods: A retrospective cross-sectional study was conducted at the Infectious Department of Pediatric Hospital Number 1, Ho Chi Minh City, Vietnam. The performance of the clinical rules was evaluated by area under a receiver operating characteristic curve (ROC-AUC) using the method of DeLong and McNemar test for specificity comparison.

Results: Our study included 129 patients, of whom 80 had bacterial meningitis and 49 had presumed viral meningitis. Spanos's rule had the highest AUC at 0.938 but was not significantly greater than other rules. No rule provided 100% sensitivity with a specificity higher than 50%. Based on our calculation of theoretical sensitivity and specificity, we suggest that a perfect rule requires at least four independent variables that posses both sensitivity and specificity higher than 85–90%.

Conclusions: No clinical decision rules provided an acceptable specificity (>50%) with 100% sensitivity when applying our data set in children. More studies in Vietnam and developing countries are required to develop and/or validate clinical rules and more very good biomarkers are required to develop such a perfect rule.

Editor: Chaoyang Xue, University of Medicine & Dentistry of New Jersey – New Jersey Medical School, United States of America

Funding: This work was supported in part by a Grant-in-Aid for Young Scientists (17301870, 2008–2010 for NTH) from Ministry of Education, Culture, Sports, Science and Technology (MEXT, Japan), and was supported in part by a Grant-in-Aid for Scientific Research from Nagasaki University to NTH (2007–2009). This study was also supported in part by Global COE Program (2008–2012) and Japan Initiative for Global Research Network on Infectious Diseases (J-GRID) for KH. The funders had no role in study design, data collection and analysis, decision to publish, or preparation of the manuscript.

Competing Interests: The authors declare no competing interests of the manuscript due to commercial or other affiliations.

* E-mail: hiraken@nagasaki-u.ac.jp (KH); diepkhanh93@vnn.vn (DTND)

Introduction

Accurate and rapid diagnosis of acute bacterial meningitis (ABM) is essential as successful disease outcome is dependent on immediate initiation of appropriate antibiotic therapy [1,2]. Differentiating ABM from presumed acute viral meningitis (pAVM) often proves challenging for clinicians as their symptoms and laboratory tests are often similar and overlapping. Classical clinical manifestations of ABM in infants and children are usually difficult to recognize given the absence of meningeal irritation signs and delayed elevation of intracranial pressure. In addition, the various parameters examined in the cerebral spinal fluid (CSF) are less discriminative in children than in adults, especially in enterovirus meningitis where the CSF parameters may be similar to bacterial meningitis values. The vast majority of patients with acute meningitis are administered broad-spectral antibiotics targeting ABM while awaiting results of definitive CSF bacterial cultures. In the absence of ABM, this practice may enhance the local frequency of antibiotic resistance [3], cause adverse antibiotic effects [4], and high medical costs [5]. Thus, it is not only important to recognize ABM patients who promptly require antimicrobial therapy, but also pAVM patients who do not need antibiotics or hospital admission at all. An ideal diagnostic rule should demonstrate 100% sensitivity in detecting bacterial meningitis [6], while retaining a high specificity.

Unfortunately, no single clinical symptom or laboratory test has differentiated ABM from pAVM with 100% sensitivity and high specificity [7,8]. More recently, numerous researchers have investigated potential clinical decision rules that recognize ABM from pAVM including: Thome [9], Spanos [10], Hoen [11] (also called Jaeger et al [12]), Freedman [13], Nigrovic [14], Oostenbrink [15], Bonsu 2004 [16], Brivet [17], Schmidt [18], De Cauwer [19], Chavanet [20], Dubos [21], Bonsu 2008[22], Tokuda [23], and Lussiana [24]. A few rules have included complicated multivariate models that require the use of a computer [10,11], while others have used scoring systems [9,15], tree model decisions [23], or a simple list of items [13,14,17,18,19,20,21,22]. These clinical decision rules require extensive test prior to their use in hospitals [25] and have rarely been compared in a single study. In addition, several rules are yet to be tested by independent researchers [17,21,22,23,24] or tested in children [17,23]. The Nigrovic's rule, also called Bacterial Meningitis Score (BMS) [14], performed perfectly in several studies [8,26,27,28,29,30], but failed to provide 100% sensitivity in other independent data sets [7,19,20,31]. Simultaneous test and comparison of these rules is required to enable clinicians to select an optimal rule to limit the number of patients being unnecessarily treated with antibiotics, and to guarantee that patients with bacterial meningitis receive appropriate antibiotics.

Materials and Methods

Identification of clinical rules

Two electronic databases including PubMed and Scopus were searched for suitable clinical rules. The search terms used were as follows: "dengue AND (rule OR score)". We supplemented these searches with a manual search of articles that developed and/or compared clinical rules. Since we aimed to find the clinical rule that could be applied in our hospital and test the generalizability of clinical rules [32], no restrictions were applied with respect to country, year, and language of studies that developed clinical rules. A total of 15 clinical rules were identified. Among them the Bonsu 2008 [22] and Dubos rules [21] were not tested as band leukocytes and procalcitonin were not available in our hospital.

Study design

The current study was performed at the Infectious Department of Pediatric Hospital Number 1, Ho Chi Minh City, Vietnam. The hospital is a tertiary pediatric hospital in southern Vietnam with 1200 beds. It was a retrospective cross-sectional analysis of the clinical signs and laboratory tests obtained from previously healthy children (≤15 years) that were diagnosed with acute meningitis. Discharge diagnosis was reviewed to identify meningitis patients based on the International Classification of Diseases, 10th Revision (ICD-10) with the following codes: G00, G00.x, G01*, G02.0*, G03, and G03.x. The study was approved in advance by the Ethical Review Committee of the Pediatric Hospital Number 1, Ho Chi Minh City, Vietnam. Written informed consent from the patients or their parents was waived by the Committee, because all data were retrospectively collected after the discharge of patients and numerically coded to ensure patient anonymity.

The entry criteria were as follows: children with proven acute bacterial meningitis (ABM) or presumed acute viral meningitis (PAVM), who had received a lumbar puncture between December 2003 and December 2008. Patients exhibiting blood-contaminated CSF (CSF erythrocyte count >10,000 cells/μL) [33], tuberculous meningitis, HIV infection, immune depression, and those found to have histories of pulmonary tuberculosis, liver diseases such as autoimmune disease, alcoholic liver disease and metabolic disease, kidney disease, neurosurgical disease or had undergone recent neurosurgery were excluded from the study. Neonates (less than 28 days old) and patients with missing laboratory variables listed in Table 1 were also excluded.

Proven ABM was diagnosed if the patient demonstrated CSF pleocytosis (CSF leukocyte count >7 cells/μL) [34,35] in addition to one of the following test results: (1) positive CSF culture for bacterial pathogens, (2) positive CSF latex agglutination test, or (3) positive blood culture. PAVM was defined as patients with a pleocytosis in the CSF (CSF leukocyte count >7 cells/μL) in addition to positive culture for viral pathogens or rapid remission without extensive antibiotic therapy combined with an absence of any four criteria of proven ABM [10,14,20,26,36,37].

Blood cultures were performed using 5% sheep blood agar before 2005 and a BACTEC 9240 system instrument (BD Biosciences, China) from 2005. CSF culture was done on 7% horse blood agar and 5% chocolate blood agar plates and incubated at 36°C for 24 h. Observed colonies were further identified by standard microbiological methods. Viral culture was not routinely performed, only five CSF samples were sent to Pasteur Institute (Ho Chi Minh City, Vietnam) for virus isolation.

At the time of admission, the relevant patient history regarding clinical symptoms and signs, and laboratory parameters listed in the Table 1 was collected. Clinical signs and symptoms that were not noted in the patient medical record were coded as normal.

Data analysis

All information was entered into a Microsoft Office Excel 2007 computerized database. Missing clinical signs and symptoms were not included and the number of patients per group was also adjusted before analysis. Our analysis showed that there were no significant differences in selected variables between patients with and without missing data." into the data analysis (page 6).

A score, judge, or probability of ABM (pABM) was calculated from each patient for each of the clinical decision rules according to the authors of the rules (Method S1). The overall accuracy of these rules represented by area under a receiver operating characteristic curve (ROC-AUC) was compared by the method of DeLong [38] using MedCalc statistical software (11.0, MedCalc Software bvba, Belgium). AUC values ≥0.5, 0.75, 0.93, or 0.97 were considered as fair, good, very good, or excellent accuracy [39]. The sensitivity and specificity of each rule was then calculated using our patient data set. To do so, we applied the thresholds indicated by the authors of the rules and by our own ROC analyses. The rules demonstrating 100% sensitivity were further analyzed to compare their specificity using the McNemar test [8].

The minimal required sample size and power of comparison were calculated using the MedCalc statistical software based on 5% type I error rate and 20% type II error rate. Assuming that ROC-AUCs of all clinical rules are at least 90% compared to the null hypothesis value 70% [22] , the required sample size was 48 subjects per group in this case.

In order to explain the limitation of Nigrovic's rule, we calculated the theoretical sensitivity and specificity of simple list of items rule with cut-off value at one item. Since selected variable demonstrated an independent predictor of ABM [14], the theoretical sensitivities and specificities of the simple list of items rule with cut-off value ≥1 can be derived from individual sensitivity and specificity of each variable as presented by equation 1 and 2, respectively (Figure 1). The individual sensitivity and specificity of each variable were derived from the current study

Table 1. Characteristic of variables used in the clinical decision rules to distinguish ABM from pAVM.

Variables	Scores using equation			List of items					Classified scores				Tree model
	Spanos (1989)	Hoen (1995)	Bonsu (2004)	Freedman (2001)	Nigrovic (2002)	Brivet (2005)	Schmidt (2006)	De Cauwer (2007)	Thome (1980)	Oostenbrink (2004)	Chavanet (2007)	Lussiana (2011)	Tokuda (2009)
Clinical variables													
Age	⊕		⊕	⊕									
Admission month	⊕												
Symtoms duration										⊕			
Seizure					⊕	⊕			⊕				
Vomit										⊕			
Body temperature									⊕				
Disturbed consciousness						⊕			⊕	⊕			⊕
Focal neurological						⊕							
Shock						⊕							
Meningeal irritation										⊕			
Cyanosis										⊕			
Purpura or petechiae									⊕	⊕			
Blood variables													
WBC		⊕							⊕				
Neutrophils %													
Neutrophil count				⊕	⊕								
Neutrophil band count													
Glucose		⊕											
CRP								⊕		⊕			
CSF variables													
Gram stain	⊕			⊕	⊕								⊕
WBC				⊕			⊕		⊕		⊕	⊕	
Neutrophils %								⊕	⊕		⊕		⊕
Neutrophil count	⊕	⊕	⊕		⊕								⊕
Protein		⊕	⊕	⊕	⊕		⊕	⊕	⊕		⊕	⊕	
Glucose				⊕				⊕	⊕		⊕	⊕	
CSF/blood glucose ratio	⊕			⊕									
Lactate							⊕						
Threshold	pABM* ≥0.1			≥1 item					Complex judge				

*Probability of ABM (pABM).

- Equation 1: Theoretical sensitivity of rule = 1- $\prod_{i=1}^{n}(1 - Sens_i)$
- Equation 2: Theoretical specificity of rule = $\prod_{i=1}^{n}(Spec_i)$

Where *n*, Sens*i*, and Spec*i* are number of variables, sensitivity, and specificity of variable *i*, respectively.

Figure 1. Equation for calculation of theoretical sensitivity and specificity of simple list of items rule with cut-off value at one item.

unless otherwise stated. The method calculation was described in the (Figure 2).

Results

Characteristic of patient population

Between December 2003 and December 2008, 192 patients met our inclusion criteria. A total of 63 patients were excluded from the final analysis due to the following reasons: (1) age of 0–28 days (n = 34), (2) traumatic lumbar puncture (n = 14), (3) recent neurosurgery or head injury (n = 12), or (4) HIV infection (n = 3). The high number of excluded patients could be explained by the characteristics of the tertiary hospital. A total of 129 patients including 80 ABM (62%) and 49 PAVM (38%) patients were selected for the final analysis (Table 2). Among the 80 patients with proven ABM, death occurred in 6.3% (n = 5), and neurological sequelae was observed in 25% (n = 15, Table 2). Of the 80 ABM cases, bacterial pathogen was identified in the CSF Gram-stain of 34 cases (43%), in the CSF culture of 39 cases (49%), blood culture of 18 patients (23%), in the blood culture alone of one patient (1.2%), and by latex agglutination in 65 patients (81%). Bacterial infections were caused by *Haemophilus influenzae* (n = 49, 61.3%), *Streptococcus pneumoniae* (n = 26, 32.5%), *Streptococcus agalactiae* (n = 1, 1.3%), *Neisseria meningitides* (n = 1, 1.3%), *Escherichia coli* (n = 2, 2.5%) and *Morganella morganii* (n = 1, 1.3%). Of the 49 PAVM cases, Herpes simplex virus 1 was the only viral pathogen isolated (n = 2).

Comparison of clinical rules

The overall accuracy of the rules was explored by calculation of the ROC-AUCs. All 13 clinical rules possessed AUC values between 0.75 and 0.94, indicating good accuracy (Table 3 and Figure S1) [39]. The Spanos rule had the highest AUC at 0.938. However, when comparing with the other four best rules (De Cauwer, Freedman, Nigrovic, and Thome), the Spanos rule was not significantly better by Delong method [38] ($P>0.05$, Figure 3).

When applying the thresholds indicated by the authors of the rules, no rule demonstrated 100% sensitivity, as prediction rules failed to identify six ABM patients by Thome, one ABM patient by Spanos, 19 ABM patients by Hoen, one ABM patients by Freedman, three ABM patients by Nigrovic, 18 ABM patients by Oostenbrink, seven ABM patients by Bonsu, 15 by Brivet, 33 ABM patients by Schmidt, one ABM patient by De Cauwer, 18 ABM patients by Chavanet, ten by Tokuda, and eight by Lussiana's rule. When applying the thresholds computed by our ROC analysis to achieve 100% sensitivity, all rules showed low specificity (< 25%). The Spanos's rule demonstrated the highest specificity at 24%, followed by Oostenbrink (8%), Bonsu (8%),

1. *Theoretical sensitivity of a clinical rule that combines n varialbes:*

- Probability of a ABM patient is missed by test *i* = (FN*i*)/(TP*i* + FN*i*) = 1- (TP*i*)/ TP*i* + FN*i*) = 1- Sens*i*

Where *n*, TP*i*, FN*i*, and Sens*i* are number of tests (variables), true positive, false negative, and sensitivity of test *i*, respectively.

- Probability of a ABM patient is missed by all *n* test (test*1*, *2*, ..*i*,..*n*) = $\prod_{i=1}^{n}(1 - Sens_i)$
- Sensitivity of simple list of items rule with cut-off value ≥ 1 is equal to probability of a ABM patient met by any test =1- $\prod_{i=1}^{n}(1 - Sens_i)$

2. *Specificity of simple list of items rule:*

- Probability of a pAVM patient is missed (diagnosed as pAVM) by test *i* = (TN*i*)/(FP*i* + TN*i*) = Spec*i*

Where TN*i*, FP*i*, and Spec*i* are true negative, false positive and specificity of test *i*, respectively.

- Specificivity of simple list of items rule with cut-off value ≥ 1 is equal to probability of a pAVM patient that is missed by all n test (test*1*, *2*, ..*i*,..*n*) = $\prod_{i=1}^{n}(Spec_i)$

Figure 2. Explanation for calculation of theoretical sensitivity and specificity. The theoretical sensitivity is the likelihood of sensitivity of the clinical rule after combining *n* tests, thus its values is depend on the individual sensitivity of each test. For example, a clinical rule combining two tests with sensitivities at 90% and 80%, respectively, the likelihood of the combined sensitivity (of the clinical rule of two tests) is calculated as 1–(1–0.90)×(1–0.80) = 0.98 or 98%. Therefore, combination of several tests will enhance the rule's sensitivity. In contrast, a clinical rule combining two tests with specificities at 80% and 70%, the likelihood of the combined specificity (of the clinical rule of two tests) will be decreased as the follow calculation: 0.80×0.70 = 0.56 or 56%.

Table 2. Characteristics of the 129 patients in this study.

Characteristic	ABM n (%) or mean ± SD	pAVM n (%) or mean ± SD
Number of patients	80	49
Age ≤ 12 month	49 (62)	13 (28)
> 12 month	31 (38)	36 (72)
Sex: male	50 (63)	33 (67)
Duration of illness (days, median, 95% CI for the median)	3 (3–5)	2 (2–3)
Hospitalization days	16.3±8.8	5.3±2.6
Nausea	3 (4)	4 (8)
Vomiting	47 (60)	31 (62)
Fever	78 (98)	48 (96)
Purpura	0 (0)	0 (0)
Cyanosis	7 (9)	1 (2)
Seizure	54 (68)	11(22)
Fever	59 (74)	36 (72)
Cyanosis	13 (16)	1 (2)
Purpura or petechiae	4(5)	0 (0)
Meningeal signs	28 (35)	20 (40)
Bulging fontanelle	37 (46)	11 (22)
Altered mental status	35 (44)	4 (8)
Focal neurological deficits	23 (29)	5 (10)
Shock	3 (4)	0 (0)
Blood WBC	15,398±9,033	13.420±4,989
Blood neutrophil %	58.5±18.1	53.0±21.4
Blood neutrophil count	9,776±8,224	7.298±4,709
Blood glucose (mg%)	84.5±30.4	89.8±18.2
Blood CRP	136.7±97.5	25.0±47.9
CSF WBC	2,946±5,809	136±215
CSF neutrophils %	71±21	36±23
CSF neutrophil count	2,469±4,920	36±48
CSF protein (g/L)	1.13±0.70	0.39±0.31
CSF glucose (mg%)	26.1±19.6	56.9±12.9
CSF/blood glucose ratio	0.34±0.26	0.65±0.19
CSF lactate (mmol/L)	7.0±4.3	2.1±0.7
Blood culture (+)	18 (23)	
Gram-stain (+)	34 (43)	
CSF culture (+)	39 (49)	
Latex (+)	65 (82)	
Death	5 (6)	0 (0)
Neurological sequelae or death	20 (25)	0 (0)

Hoen's rules (4%), while the Freedman, Nigrovic, Thome, Brivet, Schmidt, De Cauwer, Chavanet, Tokuda, and Lussiana's rules could not achieve 100% sensitivity.

Our calculation showed that the theoretical sensitivity of Nigrovic's rule was 96.6% when computing the variables' sensitivity values observed in our study. The strength of the theoretical sensitivities was in the following order: Freedman = De Cauwer > Nigrovic > Schmidt > Brivet > Chavanet, which was almost identical to the order of real sensitivities performed in our data set (Table S1). The theoretical sensitivity of Nigrovic's rule was just slightly increased (98.1%) upon computing the variables' sensitivity values observed in Nigrovic's studies [14], further supporting that the rule is not perfect. Similarly, the strength of theoretical specificities was in the following order: Chavanet > Schmidt > Brivet > Nigrovic > De Cauwer > Freedman. These findings were similar to the order of real specificities in the data set. Furthermore, the correlation between the theoretical and real accuracy was analyzed by a Spearman rank test. Our results demonstrated that the theoretical sensitivity and specificity were highly correlated with real sensitivity and

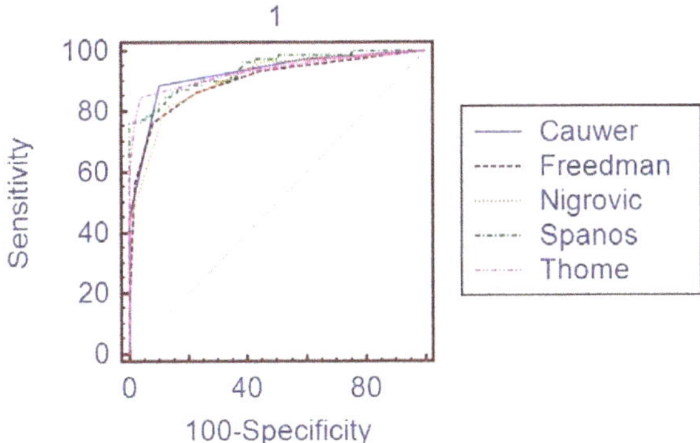

Figure 3. ROC curves of five best clinical rules for differential diagnosis of ABM from PAVM. The AUCs of ROC curves were 0.927 for De Cauwer rule, 0.900 for Freedman, 0.907 for Nigrovic, 0.938 for Spanos, and 0.935 for Thome. Pairwise comparison of all ROC-AUCs showed no significant difference of the five selected rules.

specificity, respectively (Figure S2). Overall, there was no statistical difference between theoretical calculations and real values in data sets in regards to sensitivity and specificity, suggesting that our calculation was correct.

Discussion

To our knowledge, this is the first study that simultaneously tested more than ten prediction rules for clinical practice in meningitis. No clinical rule had superior overall accuracy compared to other rules. In addition, no rule provided 100% sensitivity with acceptable specificity (>50%). The overall accuracy of the two earliest rules (Spanos and Thomas rules) was not outperformed by recent developed rules, probably due to the similar epidemiology to the pre-vaccination era [10]. The high frequency of *H. influenzae* in our study could be explained by the lack of conjugate Hib vaccine in the Vietnamese national vaccination policy, and only a small number of children (0.5%) reportedly received conjugate Hib vaccine [40].

Among reported clinical decision models, the Nigrovic's rule [14] is the only rule that has been tested by more than three independent groups, and performed perfectly in several studies [8,26,27,28,29,30]. However, it only provided 96.3% sensitivity in our study, which is also in the range of other independent data sets [7,19,20,31] and well agreed with the theoretical sensitivity (96.64%) and specificity values (53.35%), explaining that the Nigrovic's rule could not identify all ABM patients in several data sets.

Based on these evidences and our equations, an ideal simple list of items clinical rule with theoretical sensitivity >99.99% and theoretical specificity >50% should include at least four independent variables that posses both sensitivity and specificity >85–90%. In addition, to improve the rule sensitivity without significantly reducing its specificity, we recommend adding additional variables with extremely high specificity (approximately 100%). We are not aware of more than three such conventional parameters to derive such an ideal rule. However, recent studies have proposed that blood procalcitonin [21,41], CSF lactate [42,43,44], and blood C-reactive protein (CRP) [45] are very good biomarkers for bacterial meningitis. Upon addition of procalcitonin test (99% sensitivity and 83% specificity [37]), the theoretical sensitivity of Nigrovic's rule would be significantly increased from 96.64% to 99.77% (Calculation: $1-(1-0.9664)\times(1-0.99)=0.9997$), while the theoretical specificity value would be dropped

Table 3. Accuracy comparison of clinical rules.

Rule	AUC	Cut-off values	Sensitivity % (95% CI)	Number of ABM patients missed by the rule	Specificity % (95% CI)
Thome	0.935	≥2#	92.5 (84.4–97.2)	6	65.3 (51.2–78.8)
Spanos	0.938	**pABM>0.04***	**100 (96.3–100)**	**0**	**a24 (13.1–38.2)**
		pABM≥0.10#	98.7 (93.2–99.9)	1	34 (21.2–48.8)
Hoen	0.883	pABM>0.0026	**100 (96.3–100)**	0	a4 (0.5–13.7)
		pABM≥0.10#	77.2 (65.4–85.1)	19	80 (67.7–89.2)
Freedman	0.900	≥1#	98.7 (93.2–99.9)	1	12.2 (5.8–26.7)
Nigrovic	0.907	≥1#	96.3 (91.2–98.7)	3	55.1 (46.9–59.0)
Oostenbrink	0.758	≥2⊕	100 (96.3–100)	0	a8 (2.2–19.2)
		≥8.5#	78.5 (66.8–86.1)	18	50 (35.5–64.5)
Bonsu	0.812	**pABM≥0.014**	**100 (96.3–100)**	0	**a8 (2.2–19.2)**
		pABM≥0.10#	92.4 (82.8–96.4)	7	28 (16.2–42.5)
Brivet	0.790	≥1#	81.3(71.0–89.1)	15	70 (55.4–82.1)
Schmidt	0.880	≥2#	58.8 (47.2–69.7)	33	100 (92.9–100)
De Cauwer	0.927	≥1#	98.7 (93.2–99.9)	1	40.8 (33.3–43.7)
Chavanet	0.878	≥2#	78.5 (66.8–86.1)	18	96 (86.3–99.5)
Tokuda	0.876	High risk	87.5 (78.2–93.8)	10	88 (75.7–95.5)
Lussiana	0.868	High risk	90.0 (81.2–95.6)	8	75.5 (61.1–86.7)

#Thresholds indicated by the authors of the rules.
⊕Thresholds computed by ROC analysis to achieve 100% sensitivity.
*Probability of ABM (pABM).
Numbers in boldface indicate rule with 100% sensitivity.

from 53.35% to 44.28% (Calculation: 0.5335×0.83 = 0.4428). However, these three parameters have rarely been measured in the same study and their usefulness and independent contribution in the differential diagnosis of ABM from pAVM are rarely evaluated [46,47]. Thus, further studies are required to evaluate the contribution of these variables in the performance of clinical rules.

There were several limitations in our study. The first limitation was that the design was retrospective. Secondly, we only analyzed data from only one hospital. Therefore our results would be different from other hospitals, particularly in high-resources countries, where the epidemiology, clinical characteristics and outcome are different. Thirdly, our study focused on hospitalized patients in a big city. Therefore, further studies recruiting patients in clinics or local hospitals are required to further test these clinical rules. Fourthly, we could not confirm all pAVM patients as aseptic meningitis due to limited diagnosis in our hospital, which may affect the result. Another limitation is that the number of pAVM patients was much smaller than that of ABM, because several patients with extensive antibiotic therapy were excluded from criteria of pAVM. Finally, we were unable to include band leukocytes and blood procalcitonin, thus we could not test two promising Bonsu 2008 [22] and Dubos's [21] rules in the current study.

In conclusion, accurate bacterial meningitis is serious and the outcome is dependent on immediate initiation of appropriate antibiotic therapy. The best method for differentiating accurate bacterial meningitis from viral meningitis remains unclear. Several clinical decision rules have been derived to assist clinicians to distinguish between bacterial meningitis and viral meningitis, but barely tested and compared by independent studies. When applying our data set, no clinical rule provided an acceptable specificity (>50%) with 100% sensitivity. More studies in developing countries are required to confirm due to several limitations related to population and more accurate biomarkers are required to develop such a perfect rule.

Supporting Information

Figure S1 ROC curves of 13 clinical rules for differential diagnosis of ABM from PAVM when applying our data set. The AUCs of ROC curves were 0.812 for Bonsu 2004, 0.790 for Brivet, 0.927 for De Cauwer, 0.878 for Chavanet, 0.900 for Freedman (upper panel), 0.883 for Hoen, 0.868 for Lussiana, 0.907 for Nigrovic, 0.758 for Oostenbrink (middle panel), 0.880 for Schmidt, 0.938 for Spanos, 0.935 for Thome, and 0.876 for Tokuda rule (lower panel). Pairwise comparison of all ROC-AUCs was shown as the follow: -Spanos rule was significantly better than Schmidt, Chavanet, Tokuda, Lussiana, Bonsu, Brivet, and Oostenbrink rule. -Thome rule was significantly better than Hoen, Chavanet, Tokuda, Lussiana, Bonsu, Brivet, and Oostenbrink rule. -De Cauwer rule was significantly better than Bonsu 2004, Brivet, and Oostenbrink rule. -Nigrovic rule was significantly better than Brivet and Oostenbrink rule. -Freedman rule was significantly better than Bonsu 2004, Brivet, and Oostenbrink rule. -Hoen rule was significantly better than Bonsu 2004, Brivet, and Oostenbrink rule. -Schmidt rule was significantly better than Bonsu 2004, Brivet, and Oostenbrink rule. -Chavanet rule was significantly better than Brivet and Oostenbrink rule. -Tokuda rule was significantly better than Bonsu 2004, Brivet, and Oostenbrink rule. -Lussiana rule was significantly better than Oostenbrink rule. -Other pairwise comparison showed no significant difference.

Figure S2 Correlation between real and theoretical accuracy of six simple list of items rules. The Spearman correlation showed an r value of 0.971, P = 0.001, n = 6 for sensitivity correlation, and r value of 1.0, P<0.001, n = 6.

Method S1 Description and calculation of clinical rules. The rules were derived from original studies.

Table S1 Theoretical sensitivities and specificities of simple list of items rule calculated and compared using our data set.

Author Contributions

Conceived and designed the experiments: NTH NTHT DTND KH. Performed the experiments: NTHT NTH NTK DTND. Analyzed the data: NTH NTHT NAT CCM DTND KH. Wrote the paper: NTH NTHT DTND CCM KH.

References

1. Saez-Llorens X, McCracken GH Jr (2003) Bacterial meningitis in children. Lancet 361: 2139–2148.
2. Zimmerli W (2005) How to differentiate bacterial from viral meningitis. Intensive Care Med 31: 1608–1610.
3. Wise R, Hart T, Cars O, Streulens M, Helmuth R, et al. (1998) Antimicrobial resistance. Is a major threat to public health. Bmj 317: 609–610.
4. Raymond J (2000) [Epidemiology of nosocomial infections in pediatrics]. Pathol Biol (Paris) 48: 879–884.
5. Parasuraman TV, Frenia K, Romero J (2001) Enteroviral meningitis. Cost of illness and considerations for the economic evaluation of potential therapies. Pharmacoeconomics 19: 3–12.
6. Haruda FD (2003) Meningitis–viral versus bacterial. Pediatrics 112: 447–448; author reply 447–448.
7. Dubos F, De la Rocque F, Levy C, Bingen E, Aujard Y, et al. (2008) Sensitivity of the bacterial meningitis score in 889 children with bacterial meningitis. J Pediatr 152: 378–382.
8. Dubos F, Lamotte B, Bibi-Triki F, Moulin F, Raymond J, et al. (2006) Clinical decision rules to distinguish between bacterial and aseptic meningitis. Arch Dis Child 91: 647–650.
9. Thome J, Bovier-Lapierre M, Vercherat M, Boyer P (1980) [Bacterial or viral meningitis? Study of a numerical score permitting an early etiologic orientation in meningitis difficult to diagnose]. Pediatrie 35: 225–236.
10. Spanos A, Harrell FE Jr, Durack DT (1989) Differential diagnosis of acute meningitis. An analysis of the predictive value of initial observations. Jama 262: 2700–2707.
11. Hoen B, Viel JF, Paquot C, Gerard A, Canton P (1995) Multivariate approach to differential diagnosis of acute meningitis. Eur J Clin Microbiol Infect Dis 14: 267–274.
12. Jaeger F, Leroy J, Duchene F, Baty V, Baillet S, et al. (2000) Validation of a diagnosis model for differentiating bacterial from viral meningitis in infants and children under 3.5 years of age. Eur J Clin Microbiol Infect Dis 19: 418–421.
13. Freedman SB, Marrocco A, Pirie J, Dick PT (2001) Predictors of bacterial meningitis in the era after Haemophilus influenzae. Arch Pediatr Adolesc Med 155: 1301–1306.
14. Nigrovic LE, Kuppermann N, Malley R (2002) Development and validation of a multivariable predictive model to distinguish bacterial from aseptic meningitis in children in the post-Haemophilus influenzae era. Pediatrics 110: 712–719.
15. Oostenbrink R, Moons KG, Derksen-Lubsen AG, Grobbee DE, Moll HA (2004) A diagnostic decision rule for management of children with meningeal signs. Eur J Epidemiol 19: 109–116.
16. Bonsu BK, Harper MB (2004) Differentiating acute bacterial meningitis from acute viral meningitis among children with cerebrospinal fluid pleocytosis: a multivariable regression model. Pediatr Infect Dis J 23: 511–517.
17. Brivet FG, Ducuing S, Jacobs F, Chary I, Pompier R, et al. (2005) Accuracy of clinical presentation for differentiating bacterial from viral meningitis in adults: a multivariate approach. Intensive Care Med 31: 1654–1660.
18. Schmidt H, Heimann B, Djukic M, Mazurek C, Fels C, et al. (2006) Neuropsychological sequelae of bacterial and viral meningitis. Brain 129: 333–345.

19. De Cauwer HG, Eykens L, Hellinckx J, Mortelmans LJ (2007) Differential diagnosis between viral and bacterial meningitis in children. Eur J Emerg Med 14: 343–347.
20. Chavanet P, Schaller C, Levy C, Flores-Cordero J, Arens M, et al. (2007) Performance of a predictive rule to distinguish bacterial and viral meningitis. J Infect 54: 328–336.
21. Dubos F, Moulin F, Raymond J, Gendrel D, Breart G, et al. (2007) [Distinction between bacterial and aseptic meningitis in children: refinement of a clinical decision rule]. Arch Pediatr 14: 434–438.
22. Bonsu BK, Ortega HW, Marcon MJ, Harper MB (2008) A decision rule for predicting bacterial meningitis in children with cerebrospinal fluid pleocytosis when gram stain is negative or unavailable. Acad Emerg Med 15: 437–444.
23. Tokuda Y, Koizumi M, Stein GH, Birrer RB (2009) Identifying low-risk patients for bacterial meningitis in adult patients with acute meningitis. Intern Med 48: 537–543.
24. Lussiana C, Loa Clemente SV, Pulido Tarquino IA, Paulo I (2011) Predictors of bacterial meningitis in resource-limited contexts: an Angolan case. PLoS One 6: e25706.
25. McGinn TG, Guyatt GH, Wyer PC, Naylor CD, Stiell IG, et al. (2000) Users' guides to the medical literature: XXII: how to use articles about clinical decision rules. Evidence-Based Medicine Working Group. Jama 284: 79–84.
26. Nigrovic LE, Kuppermann N, Macias CG, Cannavino CR, Moro-Sutherland DM, et al. (2007) Clinical prediction rule for identifying children with cerebrospinal fluid pleocytosis at very low risk of bacterial meningitis. Jama 297: 52–60.
27. Doolittle BR, Alias A (2009) Application of a prediction rule to discriminate between aseptic and bacterial meningitis in adults. Hosp Pract (Minneap) 37: 93–97.
28. Aguero G, Davenport MC, Del Valle Mde L, Gallegos P, Kannemann AL, et al. (2010) [Validation of a clinical prediction rule to distinguish bacterial from aseptic meningitis]. Arch Argent Pediatr 108: 40–44.
29. Pierart J, Lepage P (2006) [Value of the "Bacterial Meningitis Score" (BMS) for the differential diagnosis of bacterial versus viral meningitis]. Rev Med Liege 61: 581–585.
30. Torres OL, González GM, López JM, Terciado OV, Milián JDB, et al. (2011) Retrospective application of the score for bacterial meningoencephalitis in patients admitted with infectious neurological syndrome during 5 years. Provincial Teaching Pediat ric Hospital. Matanzas. 2001, 2003-2006. Rev Med Electrón vol33 no3 Matanzas mayo-jun 33: 293–301.
31. Boulanger C, Weynants D, Zakrzewska-Jagiello K, Van der Linden D, Bodart E, et al. (2009) External validation of the bacterial meningitis score Proceedings of European Society for Paediatric Infectious Diseases, 27th Annual Meeting 9–13 June.
32. Toll DB, Janssen KJ, Vergouwe Y, Moons KG (2008) Validation, updating and impact of clinical prediction rules: a review. J Clin Epidemiol 61: 1085–1094.
33. Bonsu BK, Harper MB (2006) Corrections for leukocytes and percent of neutrophils do not match observations in blood-contaminated cerebrospinal fluid and have no value over uncorrected cells for diagnosis. Pediatr Infect Dis J 25: 8–11.
34. Greenlee JE (1990) Approach to diagnosis of meningitis. Cerebrospinal fluid evaluation. Infect Dis Clin North Am 4: 583–598.
35. Saez-Llorens X, McCracken GH Jr (1990) Bacterial meningitis in neonates and children. Infect Dis Clin North Am 4: 623–644.
36. Oostenbrink R, Moll HA, Moons KG, Grobbee DE (2004) Predictive model for childhood meningitis. Pediatr Infect Dis J 23: 1070–1071.
37. Dubos F, Korczowski B, Aygun DA, Martinot A, Prat C, et al. (2008) Serum procalcitonin level and other biological markers to distinguish between bacterial and aseptic meningitis in children: a European multicenter case cohort study. Arch Pediatr Adolesc Med 162: 1157–1163.
38. DeLong ER, DeLong DM, Clarke-Pearson DL (1988) Comparing the areas under two or more correlated receiver operating characteristic curves: a nonparametric approach. Biometrics 44: 837–845.
39. Jones CM, Athanasiou T (2005) Summary receiver operating characteristic curve analysis techniques in the evaluation of diagnostic tests. Ann Thorac Surg 79: 16–20.
40. Anh DD, Kilgore PE, Kennedy WA, Nyambat B, Long HT, et al. (2006) Haemophilus influenzae type B meningitis among children in Hanoi, Vietnam: epidemiologic patterns and estimates of H. Influenzae type B disease burden. Am J Trop Med Hyg 74: 509–515.
41. Dubos F, Moulin F, Gajdos V, De Suremain N, Biscardi S, et al. (2006) Serum procalcitonin and other biologic markers to distinguish between bacterial and aseptic meningitis. J Pediatr 149: 72–76.
42. Cunha BA (2006) Distinguishing bacterial from viral meningitis: the critical importance of the CSF lactic acid levels. Intensive Care Med 32: 1272–1273; author reply 1274.
43. Huy NT, Thao NT, Diep DT, Kikuchi M, Zamora J, et al. (2010) Cerebrospinal fluid lactate concentration to distinguish bacterial from aseptic meningitis: a systemic review and meta-analysis. Crit Care 14: R240.
44. Sakushima K, Hayashino Y, Kawaguchi T, J LJ, Fukuhara S (2011) Diagnostic Accuracy Of Cerebrospinal Fluid Lactate For Differentiating Bacterial Meningitis From Aseptic Meningitis: A Meta-Analysis. J Infect.
45. Rajs G, Finzi-Yeheskel Z, Rajs A, Mayer M (2002) C-reactive protein concentrations in cerebral spinal fluid in gram-positive and gram-negative bacterial meningitis. Clin Chem 48: 591–592.
46. Gerdes LU, Jorgensen PE, Nexo E, Wang P (1998) C-reactive protein and bacterial meningitis: a meta-analysis. Scand J Clin Lab Invest 58: 383–393.
47. Prasad K, Sahu JK (2011) Cerebrospinal fluid lactate: Is it a reliable and valid marker to distinguish between acute bacterial meningitis and aseptic meningitis? Crit Care 15: 104.

3

Human Bocaviruses Are Not Significantly Associated with Gastroenteritis: Results of Retesting Archive DNA from a Case Control Study in the UK

Sameena Nawaz, David J. Allen, Farah Aladin, Christopher Gallimore, Miren Iturriza-Gómara*¤

Virus Reference Department, Health Protection Agency, London, United Kingdom

Abstract

Gastroenteritis is a common illness causing considerable morbidity and mortality worldwide. Despite improvements in detection methods, a significant diagnostic gap still remains. Human bocavirus (HBoV)s, which are associated with respiratory infections, have also frequently been detected in stool samples in cases of gastroenteritis, and a tentative association between HBoVs, and in particular type-2 HBoVs, and gastroenteritis has previously been made. The aim of this study was to determine the role of HBoVs in gastroenteritis, using archived DNA samples from the case-control Infectious Intestinal Disease Study (IID). DNA extracted from stool samples from 2,256 cases and 2,124 controls were tested for the presence of HBoV DNA. All samples were screened in a real time PCR pan-HBoV assay, and positive samples were then tested in genotype 1 to 3-specific assays. HBoV was detected in 7.4% but no significantly different prevalence was observed between cases and controls. In the genotype-specific assays 106 of the 324 HBoV-positive samples were genotyped, with HBoV-1 predominantly found in controls whilst HBoV-2 was more frequently associated with cases of gastroenteritis ($p<0.01$). A significant proportion of HBoV positives could not be typed using the type specific assays, 67% of the total positives, and this was most likely due to low viral loads being present in the samples. However, the distribution of the untyped HBoV strains was no different between cases and controls. In conclusion, HBoVs, including HBoV-2 do not appear to be a significant cause of gastroenteritis in the UK population.

Editor: Yury E. Khudyakov, Centers for Disease Control and Prevention, United States of America

Funding: The authors have no support or funding to report.

Competing Interests: The authors have declared that no competing interests exist.

* E-mail: M.Iturriza-Gomara@liverpool.ac.uk

¤ Current address: Institute of Infection and Global Health, University of Liverpool, Liverpool, United Kingdom

Introduction

In 2005 a novel parvovirus was discovered in respiratory secretions of young children and was termed Human Bocavirus (HBoV-1) [1]. Other important members of the parvoviridae family include B19 which causes fith disease and human parvovirus 4 (Parv 4) which has not yet been associated with a disease [2]. Parvoviruses in animals are generally associated with systemic disease but also with respiratory and enteric symptoms [3,4]. Since the discovery of HBoV-1 three other HBoV genotypes have been described, HBoV-2, HBoV-3 and HBoV-4. The association between HBoV-1 and respiratory disease has previously been well established [5,6,7,8,9,10,11,12,13,14,15,16,17,18,19]. Although all HBoVs have also been detected in stool samples with prevalences ranging from <1% to 20%, only HBoV-2 has been reported to be associated with symptoms of gastroenteritis [20]. Nevertheless, the role of HBoV2 as an aetiological agent of gastroenteritis has not been clearly confirmed, furthermore, to date, no clear association between the presence of HBoV-3 and HBoV-4 and disease has been established [21,22].

Recent seroepidemiological studies indicate that exposure to HBoVs occurs early in life and 90% of the population are seropositive by the age of 5, although differences were reported in the seroprevalence of type-specific antibodies to the different HBoVs, which suggested that HBoV-1 infections are more prevalent [23].

The Infectious Intestinal Disease Study (IID Study) was a large case control study of gastroenteritis carried out in the UK between 1993–1996 [24] with the aim to determine the burden and aetiology of sporadic cases IID in the UK population. Initially, the use of classical microbiology diagnostic methods and electron microscopy (for virus detection) failed to detect a potential aetiological agent or toxin in 49% of the cases [25]. Retesting of the archived samples from this study using molecular methods for the detection of enteric viruses, bacteria and protozoa revealed viruses to be the most common aetiological agents of gastroenteritis,the diagnostic gap for IID was reduced to 25% from 49% [26]. The aim of the present study was to evaluate the role of HBoVs in IID in the UK population, using archived DNA samples from the matched case-control IID-1 study [26]. In addition, the presence specifically of HBoV-1, 2 or 3 was investigated in order to determine any possible associations between specific HBoV genotypes and IID.

Materials and Methods

Samples

A total of 4,380 archived DNA from the IID study [26,27] were tested for the presence of HBoV DNA. This archive comprised DNA extracted from stool samples from 2,256 cases and 2,124 controls.

Pan- HBoV Detection Assay

The qPCR assay targeted the NS1 gene (Ratcliff et al., unpublished method, personal communication) and was performed using an ABI Taqman7500. Oligonucleotide primer and probe sequences and positions are described in table 1.

The reaction consisted of 0.1 M DDT (Invitrogen), 1X Platinum Quantitative PCR Supermix-UDG (Invitrogen), Pan-HBoV-F and Pan-HBoV-R primers each at a concentration of 100 µm, Pan-HBoV-NS1 probe at 10 µm concentration, ROX 25 µm (Invitrogen) 2.5 µl of template DNA and RNase free water to a final reaction volume of 25 µl. The amplification consisted of an initial denaturation at 95°C for 10 min, followed by 40 cycles with denaturation at 95°C for 15 sec, annealing at 55°C for 30 sec and extension at 60°C for 45 sec.

HBoV1, 2 and 3 Genotyping qPCR Assays

HBoV-1, 2 and 3-specific primer pair and probes were designed in house through alignment of sequence data available in GenBank. The reaction conditions are as follows; 1X Platinum Quantitative PCR Supermix-UDG (Invitrogen), HBoV-NS1-1F, HBoV-1R, HBoV2-R and HBoV3R primers each at a concentration of 20 µm, the HBoV1,2 and 3 probe at 10 µm concentration, ROX 25 µm (Invitrogen), 2.5 µl of template and RNase free water was added to a final reaction volume of 25 µl. The amplification conditions for the typing assay are the same as those described in the HBoV NS1 detection assay above.

Plasmid Controls

Plasmids containing a 1773 bp and a 1737 bp region of the NS1 encoding gene of HBoV-1 and HBoV-3 respectively were used for assay optimisation and as controls. Control material was kindly provided by R. Ratcliff, Adelaide, Australia.

The controls were also used in order to generate a standard curve for use with the pan-HBoV assay in order to allow for normalisation of the data generated including the comparison of relative sensitivities of the different assays and for quantitation of DNA present in each of the positive samples. The standard curve was generated using the plasmid containing a genome segment of the HBoV-1 and consisted of a series of 10 fold dilution containing from 300,000 copies/µl down to 3 copies/µl. Inter- and intra-assay reproducibility was analysed by performing replicate testing of the standards in a single run (X11) and repeated runs (X2), and the standard curve was also included in each assay run for quality control and normalisation of results.

Untypable Strains

A subset of 17 samples positive in the Pan-HBoV assay but which failed to amplify in the type-specific assays were confirmed using an alternative method published elsewhere [28,29], and 6 were further confirmed though direct sequencing of the amplicons obtained after purification either from solution or agarose gels using Agencourt AMPure (Beckman Coulter, USA) and GeneClean Spin kit (QBiogene), respectively, following manufactures protocols.

Statistical Analysis

The chi-squared test was used in order to evaluate the significance of differences observed between groups. For comparison of median values (analysis of CT values) the Mann Witney U-test was used. Prevalence Odds Ratio (POR = Pcases/(1-Pcases)/ Pcontrols/(1-Pcontrols)) was calculated in the total cohorts and by age group.

Table 1. HBoV-specific oligonucleotide primers and probes (all located at the NS gene).

Primers	Sequence (5′-3′)	Nt positions	reference
Pan qpcr primers			
Pan-HBoV-F	ATA AAG TTC CAA ACT CAT TTC CTC TTG	1994–2020	Ratcliff et al*
Pan-HBoV-R	AGT GCA GWA TCC GTT TTC GTG	2079-2059	Ratcliff et al*
Pan HBoV1-F	TCT CC GGC GAG TGA ACA TC	201–219	This study
Type-specific qpcr primers (anti-sense)			
HBoV1-R	CAT CCG GAT GAG GAG CGC	424-407	This study
HBoV2-R	CTT CAG GAT GTG GTG CGC	427-410	This study
HBoV3-R	CAT CCG GAT GAG GA CAC	405-392	This study
Generic PCR primers for sequencing			
HBoV01.2F	TAT GGC CAA GGC AAT CGT CCA AG	2091	[29]
HBoV02.2R	GCC GCG TGA ACA TGA GAA ACA GA	1791	[29]
Probes			
pan HBoV-NS1	6FAM-CCT TTG TCC TAC WCA TTC-MGBBNFQ	2025–2042	Ratcliff et al*
HBoV-1	6Fam- TAT CAT AGA TTG TTC AGT TCC AGT AGC-MGBBNFQ	393-372	This study
HBoV-2	6Vic- TT GGA TCA TGA GAC GTT CAG TCC C-MGBBNFQ	399-376	This study
HBoV-3	6Ned- CTG GAT CAT GGC TTG CTC GGT A-MGBBNFQ	377-351	This study

*Unpublished method, personal communication.

Table 2. Age distribution of HBoV positive samples in cases and controls of IID.

	CASES			CONTROLS				ALLTOTAL		
Age Group (years)	HBoV pos	%	TOTAL	HBoV pos	%	TOTAL	POR	HBoV pos	%	TOTAL
<1	34	26.2	130	62	34.8	178	0.66514	96	31.2	308
1–4	58	12.2	476	91	18.0	506	0.633	149	15.2	982
5–9	9	6.9	131	8	6.0	134	1.16112	17	6.4	265
10–19	5	4.4	114	2	1.9	103	2.37635	7	3.2	217
20–29	7	2.4	286	2	1.1	177	2.21088	9	1.9	463
30–39	8	2.2	365	3	1.0	294	2.22699	11	1.7	659
40–49	11	4.4	249	2	0.8	240	5.70711	13	2.7	489
50–59	8	4.0	199	1	0.5	192	8.29167	9	2.3	391
60–69	5	2.9	175	3	1.7	177	1.72696	8	2.3	352
>70	4	3.1	131	1	0.8	123	3.96698	5	2.0	254
TOTAL	**149**	**6.6**	**2256**	**175**	**8.2**	**2124**	**0.79109**	**324**	**7.4**	**4380**

POR = prevalence odds ratio.

Results

Prevalence of Infection with HBoVs

A total of 7.4% of the samples tested were positive for HBoV. No statistically significant differences were seen in the prevalence of HBoV between cases and asymptomatic controls, POR = 0.79 (Table 2). Peak HBoV infection was observed in children under the age of 5, both in cases and controls, with significantly higher HBoV incidence in children between 1 and 4 in asymptomatic controls than in the cases of gastroenteritis (POR = 0.6; $p<0.02$). The number of HBoV positives in older age groups was too small for meaningful statistical analysis.

Viral Load

The average CT values were 34.5 and 34.8, and the median CT values were 36.3 and 37.4 in cases and controls respectively (see distribution in Figure 1). The majority of HBoV-positives in both cases and controls had copy numbers ranging between 30 and 299 copies/reaction (or between 4.5×10^3 and 4.5×10^4 copies/ml of feaces). The distribution of HBoV viral loads between cases and controls was comparable and the median CT values between cases and controls were not significantly different (U-test; z = 0.458139, $p>0.05$).

HBoV in the Presence of Other Enteric Pathogens

HBoV DNA was found in 149 (46%) samples in the absence of other co-pathogens (Table 3). No statistically significant differences were observed in the proportion of cases or controls in which HBoV was found as a single organism or in the presence of one or more pathogens in the cohort as a whole, however in the 1–4 years of age group, HBoV in the absence of any other enteric pathogens

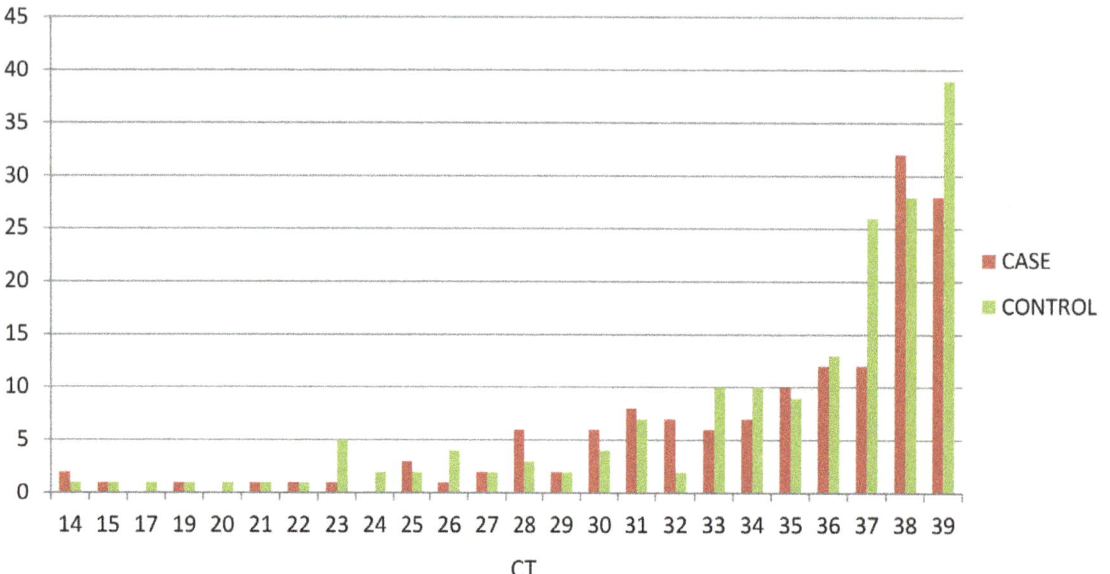

Figure 1. HBoV detection assays, CT distribution in cases and controls.

Table 3. Distribution of HBoV-positive samples in cases and controls with or without a co-infection.

	CASES		CONTROLS		TOTAL	
Age Group	**Single HBoV**	**Multiple infections**	**Single HBoV**	**Multiple infections**	**Single HBoV**	**All HBoV positives**
<1	18	16	24	38	42	96
1–4	17	41	51	40	68	149
5–9	2	7	4	4	6	17
10–19	0	5	1	1	1	7
20–29	4	3	2	0	6	9
30–39	4	4	2	1	6	11
40–49	6	5	2	0	8	13
50–59	5	3	1	0	6	9
60–69	3	2	1	2	4	8
>70	2	2	0	1	2	5
TOTAL	61	88	88	87	149	324
% of total positives	**40.9**	**59.1**	**50.3**	**49.7**	**46.0**	

was found in 29% of the cases, but in 56% of the controls ($p<0.05$).

Temporal Distribution of HBoV Infections

HBoV infections were detected year round although a peak was observed in the spring/early summer months, between April and June 1994 (Figure 2).

Distribution of HBoV by Gender

HBoV DNA was found in 48.8% and 45.7% of female cases and controls, respectively. The distribution of HBoV among females and males was not significantly different from the distribution of females and males in the entire cohort which was 53% and 47%, respectively.

Distribution of HBoV Genotypes

A total of 106 (32.7%) HBoV positives were genotyped, whilst 218 (67.3%) remained untyped after testing in the HBoV types 1, 2 or 3 specific assays (Table 4). HBoV-1 detection was found predominantly in controls, ($p<0.001$) and HBoV-2 was predominantly associated with cases ($p<0.01$). The prevalence of HBoV-3 was not significantly different between cases and controls.

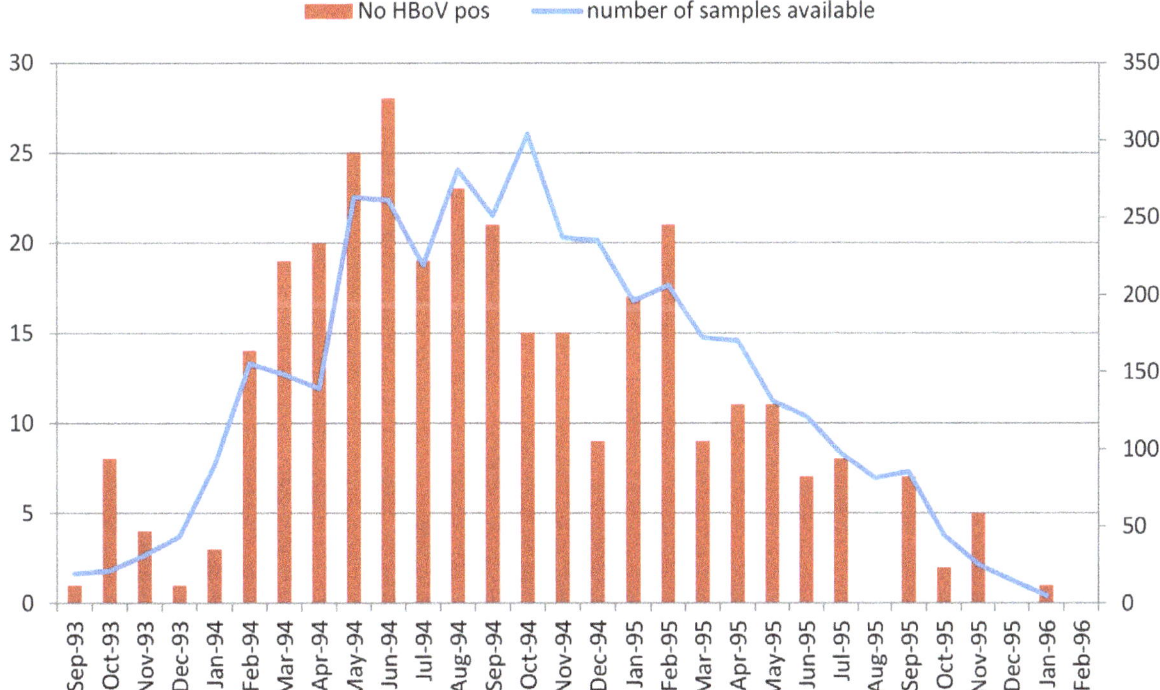

Figure 2. Temporal distribution of HBoV infections.

Table 4. Distribution of HBoV genotypes in cases and controls.

COHORT	Age Group (years)	HBoV-1	HBoV-1+HBoV-2	HBoV-2	HBoV-3	Untyped	TOTAL
CASES	<1	1	1	9	2	21	34
	1–4	3	1	8	6	40	58
	5–9			1	1	7	9
	10–19			2	1	2	5
	20–29			2		5	7
	30–39			3		5	8
	40–49			2		9	11
	50–59			3		5	8
	>70			2		2	4
	60–69					5	5
CASES Total		4	2	32	10	101	149
Percent		**2.7**	**1.3**	**21.5**	**6.7**	**67.8**	**100.0**
CONTROLS	<1	10	1	10	4	37	62
	1–4	14		8	6	63	91
	5–9				1	7	8
	10–19					2	2
	20–29					2	2
	30–39				2	1	3
	40–49					2	2
	50–59				1		1
	60–69			1		2	3
	>70					1	1
CONTROLS Total		24	1	19	14	117	175
Percent		**13.7**	**0.6**	**10.9**	**8.0**	**66.9**	**100.0**
GRAND TOTAL		**28**	**3**	**51**	**24**	**218**	**324**
Percent		**8.6**	**0.9**	**15.7**	**7.4**	**67.3**	**100.0**

HBoV-1 and -3 were predominantly found in children (Table 4). HBoV-2 in the absence of any other pathogen was detected in 17 (81.3%) of the cases, compared to 9 (47.4%) of the controls. In cases, HBoV-2 was found across the age groups, although more frequently in children <5, whereas in controls they were found predominantly in children <5 with only 1 example in an adult (Table 4). The prevalence of HBoV-2 in children <5 years old was however not significantly different between cases and controls, 2.8% and 2.6%, respectively.

A subset of HBoV that were negative in the type 1,2 or 3-specific assays were confirmed in an alternative pan-HBoV PCR, and sequencing of a small number confirmed them as types 1, 2 or 3. The majority of the untyped samples (70%) had a CT value of >37 in the screening pan-HBoV PCR, indicative of low viral loads being present in the samples.

Discussion

This represents the largest study to date investigating the role and distribution of HBoVs infections in community acquired sporadic gastroenteritis and in asymptomatic controls. The prevalence of HBoV infection in the UK population was found to be 7.4% across all ages, with a higher percentage of the infections occurring in children <5 years of age (19%). However, the prevalence of HBoV infections was comparable in cases of gastroenteritis and in age-matched asymptomatic controls. Although the presence of enteric pathogens, eg norovirus or rotavirus, in asymptomatic individuals is well documented, a significantly higher prevalence of the pathogen is seen in cases than in the controls [26]. Therefore, our data suggests that HBoV are not causally associated with gastrointestinal disease in the UK population as a whole, nor in children. The prevalence of detection of HBoV in stool samples in previous studies varies widely (see summary in Table 5), but most coincide in reporting the highest prevalence in children.

HBoV infections were detected all year round in the UK although a tentative peak was observed in the spring/early summer months in 1994 (between April and June). Different seasonal patterns in the peak prevalence of HBoV have been reported in different countries (see Table 5),

Of the 324 HBoV positive samples, 106 (32.7%) were genotyped in the type-specific assays. HBoV-1 was found predominantly in controls ($p<0.001$) and the prevalence of HBoV-3 was similar in cases and controls. Both HBoV-1 and -3 were predominantly found in children. HBoV-2 was predominantly associated with gastroenteritis cases ($p<0.01$). The overall prevalence in cases was 1.4% and 0.8% in controls, however, in children <5 year of age, the prevalence in cases and controls was similar, 2.8% and 2.6%, respectively. The prevalence of HBoV-2 in children in the UK was significantly lower than that reported in

Table 5. Summary of published studies on the prevalence of HBoV in stool samples.

Country	Sampling date	Cases No	Controls No	Population studied	% Cases HBoV-pos	% Controls HBoV-pos	Main Conclusion	Ref
Australia	Jan-Dec 2001.	186	186	Paediatric	17.20%	8.10%	HBoV-2 associated with gastroenteritis (only if cases with a concomitant bacterial infection included).	[22]
					(HBoV-2)	(HBoV-2)	Temporal pattern observed : summer months.	
Brazil	Jan 2003–Dec 2005.	705	ND	Paediatric	2.0% (HBoV)	ND	No obvious temporal clustering of the HBoV-positive patients.	[39]
China	July 2006–Sept 2007.	397	115	Paediatric	3.50% (HBoV)	3.50% (HBoV)	HBoV not associated with gastroenteritis. Temporal patterns observed : winter months.	[28].
China	July 2006–June 2008.	632	162	Paediatric	20.40% (HBoV-2)	12.30% (HBoV-2)	No statistically significant association between HBoV detection and gastroenteritis.	[32]
Germany	Jan-Feb and Sept–Dec 2007.	307	ND	Paediatric (daycare outbreaks)	4.60% (HBoV)		HBoV was not associated with outbreaks of gastroenteritis in children in day care.	[40]
Hong Kong	Nov 2004–Oct 2005.	1,435	ND	ND	2.10%		Same virus found in respiratory and stool samples.	[13]
Korea	Jan 2005–Dec 2006.	962	ND	Paediatric	0.80% (HBoV)		Temporal patterns observed : summer months.	[41]
South Korea	May 2008–April 2009.	358	ND	Paediatric	0.5% (HBoV-1) 3.6% (HBoV-2)		Temporal pattern observed : winter months.	[31]
Spain	Dec 2005–Mar 2006.	527	ND	Paediatric	9.10% (HBoV)		Prevalence of HBoVs in respiratory and stool samples was similar.	[42]
Thailand	Nov 2005–Sep 2006.	225	202	Paediatric	0.90% (HBoV)	0	Low prevalence. No statistically significant difference between cases and controls ($p = 0.17$).	[43]
USA	Dec 1–Marc 31 2008.	479	ND	Paedriatic and adult	1.30% (HBoV2)		0.7% children and 1.5% adults.	[45]

a study in Australia, in which HBoV-2 was detected in 17.2% and 8.1% of the cases and controls, respectively [22]. The findings of the study in Australia lead to the proposal of HBoV-2 as an important aetiological agent of infantile gastroenteritis. It is noteworthy however, that in the Australian study, the association of HBoV-2 with gastroenteritis was only significant when cases with a bacterial co-pathogen were included in the analysis. Although in the present study HBoV-2 in the absence of other enteric pathogens was found more frequently in cases than in controls, the small numbers found in such large study suggest that the role of these viruses in IID, if any, is likely to be small. A lack of correlation between HBoVs or HBoV-2 and paediatric gastroenteritis was also reported in several smaller studies published elsewhere [30,31,32].

A total of 67% of the HBoV-positive samples could not be genotyped using the genotype-specific PCR assays. The majority of these untyped samples (70%) had CT values >37. This suggests that failure to type may be associated with low viral loads and differences in the relative sensitivities of the genotyping assays compared to the detection assay. Although under experimental conditions and using plasmid controls the sensitivities of all assays were comparable, it is likely that when applied to true clinical samples the sensitivity of the type-specific assays was inferior, possibly due to as yet not identified strain variability within genotypes. Also, a HBoV type 4-specific assay was not included in this study, therefore, any possible HBoV4 infections would not have been typed. Of the panel of samples that were tested in an alternative pan-HBoV PCR, the strains typed through sequencing were HBoV-1 (2 samples), HBoV-2 (1 sample) and HBoV-3 (3 samples). Furthermore, the distribution of untyped HBoVs was not significantly different in cases and controls.

HBoVs in the absence of other enteric pathogens were seen in 46% of the HBoV-positive samples, and more frequently in the controls, 50.3% vs 40.9% in cases. No significant difference in HBoV load was observed between cases and controls, or between the samples positive for HBoV alone or in the presence of other pathogens. Previous studies have investigated the relationships between viral load and disease severity [33,34,35,36,37]. In respiratory infections significantly higher HBoV loads were seen in samples collected from children positive for HBoV alone than in those from children with co-infections. In respiratory infections also, viral loads $>10^4$ were associated with disease, whereas loads $<10^4$ were associated with asymptomatic children [33,38]. This lead to the suggestion that higher viral loads are indicative of a causative role of HBoV in respiratory infections [33,38]. However, Brieu et al [38] found no significant correlation between viral load and clinical symptoms or disease severity.

In conclusion, the results obtained from investigating for the presence of HBoV DNA in archived DNA samples from a large and previously well described case-control study of IID suggest that HBoV, including HBoV-2,do not appear to be a significant cause of gastroenteritis in the UK population, and particularly in the paediatric population. Although HBoVs are relatively frequent across all ages, and in particular in preschool age children, they are found just as frequently among children and adults without symptoms of gastroenteritis.

Acknowledgments

This study was conducted using existing material and data form the IID-1 study, which was funded by the Food Standards Agency. We would like to thank the IID study executive committee for their support in approving the use of the archive DNA material for this study.

Author Contributions

Conceived and designed the experiments: MIG. Performed the experiments: SN DJA FA CG. Analyzed the data: SN DJA MIG. Contributed reagents/materials/analysis tools: SN DJA CG MIG. Wrote the paper: SN DJA MIG.

References

1. Allander T, Tammi MT, Eriksson M, Bjerkner A, Tiveljung-Lindell A, et al. (2005) Cloning of a human parvovirus by molecular screening of respiratory tract samples. Proc Natl Acad Sci U S A 102: 12891–12896.
2. Jones MS, Kapoor A, Lukashov VV, Simmonds P, Hecht F, et al. (2005) New DNA viruses identified in patients with acute viral infection syndrome. J Virol 79: 8230–8236.
3. Durham PJ, Johnson RH, Isles H, Parker RJ, Holroyd RG, et al. (1985) Epidemiological studies of parvovirus infections in calves on endemically infected properties. Res Vet Sci 38: 234–240.
4. Carmichael LE, Schlafer DH, Hashimoto A (1994) Minute virus of canines (MVC, canine parvovirus type-1): pathogenicity for pups and seroprevalence estimate. J Vet Diagn Invest 6: 165–174.
5. Arden KE, McErlean P, Nissen MD, Sloots TP, Mackay IM (2006) Frequent detection of human rhinoviruses, paramyxoviruses, coronaviruses, and bocavirus during acute respiratory tract infections. J Med Virol 78: 1232–1240.
6. Arnold JC, Singh KK, Spector SA, Sawyer MH (2006) Human bocavirus: prevalence and clinical spectrum at a children's hospital. Clin Infect Dis 43: 283–288.
7. Bastien N, Chui N, Robinson JL, Lee BE, Dust K, et al. (2007) Detection of human bocavirus in Canadian children in a 1-year study. J Clin Microbiol 45: 610–613.
8. Chieochansin T, Chutinimitkul S, Payungporn S, Hiranras T, Samransamruajkit R, et al. (2007) Complete coding sequences and phylogenetic analysis of Human Bocavirus (HBoV). Virus Res 129: 54–57.
9. Choi EH, Lee HJ, Kim SJ, Eun BW, Kim NH, et al. (2006) The association of newly identified respiratory viruses with lower respiratory tract infections in Korean children, 2000–2005. Clin Infect Dis 43: 585–592.
10. Fry AM, Lu X, Chittaganpitch M, Peret T, Fischer J, et al. (2007) Human bocavirus: a novel parvovirus epidemiologically associated with pneumonia requiring hospitalization in Thailand. J Infect Dis 195: 1038–1045.
11. Jacques J, Moret H, Renois F, Leveque N, Motte J, et al. (2008) Human Bocavirus quantitative DNA detection in French children hospitalized for acute bronchiolitis. J Clin Virol 43: 142–147.
12. Kesebir D, Vazquez M, Weibel C, Shapiro ED, Ferguson D, et al. (2006) Human bocavirus infection in young children in the United States: molecular epidemiological profile and clinical characteristics of a newly emerging respiratory virus. J Infect Dis 194: 1276–1282.
13. Lau SK, Yip CC, Tsoi HW, Lee RA, So LY, et al. (2007) Clinical features and complete genome characterization of a distinct human rhinovirus (HRV) genetic cluster, probably representing a previously undetected HRV species, HRV-C, associated with acute respiratory illness in children. J Clin Microbiol 45: 3655–3664.
14. Ma X, Endo R, Ishiguro N, Ebihara T, Ishiko H, et al. (2006) Detection of human bocavirus in Japanese children with lower respiratory tract infections. J Clin Microbiol 44: 1132–1134.
15. Manning A, Russell V, Eastick K, Leadbetter GH, Hallam N, et al. (2006) Epidemiological profile and clinical associations of human bocavirus and other human parvoviruses. J Infect Dis 194: 1283–1290.
16. Naghipour M, Cuevas LE, Bakhshinejad T, Dove W, Hart CA (2007) Human bocavirus in Iranian children with acute respiratory infections. J Med Virol 79: 539–543.
17. Qu XW, Duan ZJ, Qi ZY, Xie ZP, Gao HC, et al. (2007) Human bocavirus infection, People's Republic of China. Emerg Infect Dis 13: 165–168.
18. Smuts H, Hardie D (2006) Human bocavirus in hospitalized children, South Africa. Emerg Infect Dis 12: 1457–1458.
19. Weissbrich B, Neske F, Schubert J, Tollmann F, Blath K, et al. (2006) Frequent detection of bocavirus DNA in German children with respiratory tract infections. BMC Infect Dis 6: 109.
20. Kapoor A, Slikas E, Simmonds P, Chieochansin T, Naeem A, et al. (2009) A newly identified bocavirus species in human stool. J Infect Dis 199: 196–200.
21. Kapoor A, Simmonds P, Slikas E, Li L, Bodhidatta L, et al. (2010) Human bocaviruses are highly diverse, dispersed, recombination prone, and prevalent in enteric infections. J Infect Dis 201: 1633–1643.
22. Arthur JL, Higgins GD, Davidson GP, Givney RC, Ratcliff RM (2009) A novel bocavirus associated with acute gastroenteritis in Australian children. PLoS Pathog 5: e1000391.
23. Kantola K, Hedman L, Arthur J, Alibeto A, Delwart E, et al. (2011) Seroepidemiology of human bocaviruses 1–4. J Infect Dis 204: 1403–1412.
24. Agency FS (2000) A report of the study of infectious intestinal disease in England.: Food Standard Agency. The Stationery Office, London.

25. Tompkins DS, Hudson MJ, Smith HR, Eglin RP, Wheeler JG, et al. (1999) A study of infectious intestinal disease in England: microbiological findings in cases and controls. Commun Dis Public Health 2: 108–113.
26. Amar CF, East CL, Gray J, Iturriza-Gomara M, Maclure EA, et al. (2007) Detection by PCR of eight groups of enteric pathogens in 4,627 faecal samples: re-examination of the English case-control Infectious Intestinal Disease Study (1993–1996). Eur J Clin Microbiol Infect Dis 26: 311–323.
27. Amar CF, East CL, Grant KA, Gray J, Iturriza-Gomara M, et al. (2005) Detection of viral, bacterial, and parasitological RNA or DNA of nine intestinal pathogens in fecal samples archived as part of the english infectious intestinal disease study: assessment of the stability of target nucleic acid. Diagn Mol Pathol 14: 90–96.
28. Cheng WX, Jin Y, Duan ZJ, Xu ZQ, Qi HM, et al. (2008) Human bocavirus in children hospitalized for acute gastroenteritis: a case-control study. Clin Infect Dis 47: 161–167.
29. Sloots TP, McErlean P, Speicher DJ, Arden KE, Nissen MD, et al. (2006) Evidence of human coronavirus HKU1 and human bocavirus in Australian children. J Clin Virol 35: 99–102.
30. Han TH, Chung JY, Hwang ES (2009) Human bocavirus 2 in children, South Korea. Emerg Infect Dis 15: 1698–1700.
31. Han TH, Kim CH, Park SH, Kim EJ, Chung JY, et al. (2009) Detection of human bocavirus-2 in children with acute gastroenteritis in South Korea. Arch Virol 154: 1923–1927.
32. Jin Y, Cheng WX, Xu ZQ, Liu N, Yu JM, et al. (2011) High prevalence of human bocavirus 2 and its role in childhood acute gastroenteritis in China. J Clin Virol 52: 251–253.
33. Allander T, Jartti T, Gupta S, Niesters HG, Lehtinen P, et al. (2007) Human bocavirus and acute wheezing in children. Clin Infect Dis 44: 904–910.
34. Campanini G, Percivalle E, Baldanti F, Rovida F, Bertaina A, et al. (2007) Human respiratory syncytial virus (hRSV) RNA quantification in nasopharyngeal secretions identifies the hRSV etiologic role in acute respiratory tract infections of hospitalized infants. J Clin Virol 39: 119–124.
35. Kang G, Iturriza-Gomara M, Wheeler JG, Crystal P, Monica B, et al. (2004) Quantitation of group A rotavirus by real-time reverse-transcription-polymerase chain reaction: correlation with clinical severity in children in South India. J Med Virol 73: 118–122.
36. Phillips G, Lopman B, Tam CC, Iturriza-Gomara M, Brown D, et al. (2009) Diagnosing rotavirus A associated IID: Using ELISA to identify a cut-off for real time RT-PCR. J Clin Virol 44: 242–245.
37. Phillips G, Lopman B, Tam CC, Iturriza-Gomara M, Brown D, et al. (2009) Diagnosing norovirus-associated infectious intestinal disease using viral load. BMC Infect Dis 9: 63.
38. Brieu N, Guyon G, Rodiere M, Segondy M, Foulongne V (2008) Human bocavirus infection in children with respiratory tract disease. Pediatr Infect Dis J 27: 969–973.

4

Soil-Transmitted Helminth Infections and Correlated Risk Factors in Preschool and School-Aged Children in Rural Southwest China

Xiaobing Wang[1], Linxiu Zhang[1]*, Renfu Luo[1], Guofei Wang[2], Yingdan Chen[2], Alexis Medina[3], Karen Eggleston[3], Scott Rozelle[3], D. Scott Smith[4,5]

1 Center for Chinese Agricultural Policy, Institute for Geographical Sciences and Natural Resources Research, Chinese Academy of Sciences, Beijing, China, **2** National Institute of Parasitic Diseases, Chinese Center for Disease Control and Prevention, Shanghai, China, **3** Freeman Spogli Institute, Stanford University, Stanford, California, United States of America, **4** Stanford University School of Medicine, Stanford, California, United States of America, **5** Department of Internal Medicine, Kaiser Permanente Medical Group, Redwood City, California, United States of America

Abstract

We conducted a survey of 1707 children in 141 impoverished rural areas of Guizhou and Sichuan Provinces in Southwest China. Kato-Katz smear testing of stool samples elucidated the prevalence of ascariasis, trichuriasis and hookworm infections in pre-school and school aged children. Demographic, hygiene, household and anthropometric data were collected to better understand risks for infection in this population. 21.2 percent of pre-school children and 22.9 percent of school aged children were infected with at least one of the three types of STH. In Guizhou, 33.9 percent of pre-school children were infected, as were 40.1 percent of school aged children. In Sichuan, these numbers were 9.7 percent and 6.6 percent, respectively. Number of siblings, maternal education, consumption of uncooked meat, consumption of unboiled water, and livestock ownership all correlated significantly with STH infection. Through decomposition analysis, we determined that these correlates made up 26.7 percent of the difference in STH infection between the two provinces. Multivariate analysis showed that STH infection is associated with significantly lower weight-for-age and height-for-age z-scores; moreover, older children infected with STHs lag further behind on the international growth scales than younger children.

Editor: Jennifer Keiser, Swiss Tropical and Public Health Institute, Switzerland

Funding: This study was funded by two private individual donors (husband and wife), Eric Hemel and Barbara Morgen. The funders had no role in study design, data collection and analysis, decision to publish, or preparation of the manuscript.

Competing Interests: The authors have declared that no competing interests exist.

* E-mail: lxzhang.ccap@igsnrr.ac.cn.

Introduction

Historically, controlling soil-transmitted helminth (STH) infections has been a challenge in China. Tremendous progress over the last 60 years has been made to control these parasites [1]. As recently as the 1960s many development experts applauded China's health care system for its effective delivery of basic health services, including STH control, in rural populations [2]. Minimally-trained "barefoot doctors" lived in and visited remote villages, offering free treatment of common diseases and educating the population about disease prevention and healthy behaviors [3,4]. These local health personnel often treated large numbers of children in schools, since schools have a concentration of the targeted population, making care programs accessible and inexpensive [5]. Treating STH infections was on their list of priorities [6].

In the 1980s, however, public funding for rural health declined precipitously [7]. The barefoot doctor system collapsed and rural residents were largely left to fend for themselves. It is only in the past several years that China has once again turned its attention to rural health. In the interim, many diseases that had been managed and better controlled appear to have re-emerged [1]. STH infections–perhaps due to their less clinically obvious and largely asymptomatic nature have re-emerged with marked increase in prevalence, especially in remote, impoverished and rural areas [8–11].

Over the last decade, high STH prevalence rates in various regions of China from Yunnan [8] to Fujian [9] to Hunan [10] have been observed. Nearly all of these studies have been small in size, typically limited to a single township or even a single village. The notable exception to this otherwise fragmented look at helminths across China is a large-scale national survey conducted by the Chinese Ministry of Health from 2001 to 2004 [11]. This survey included both urban and rural areas, and found national prevalence of STH infections to be 19.6%.

The aim of our study was to determine the prevalence and correlates of STH infections in over 1700 preschool and elementary school children in six rural and impoverished counties in Sichuan and Guizhou Provinces–defining the scope of the problem across a fairly large swath of rural China. Using multivariate regression and decomposition analyses, we identified: 1) correlates of infection that explain variance in the data, and 2) the independent association of the presence of STH infections with anthropometric measures, which are important markers of child development.

Methods

Study Design and Setting

A cross-sectional survey of impoverished children in rural Guizhou and Sichuan Provinces in Southwestern China was carried out in April and June of 2010. These two provinces were chosen because of their high rates of poverty and a humid climate that is conducive to STH infection. Three rural counties were randomly selected using computer-generated selection in each of these two provinces based on income level. The six counties were selected from the bottom quartile of the counties based on average net per capita incomes. The setting was defined as impoverished based on average net per capita incomes (2750 RMB/year in Guizhou and 4750 RMB/year in Sichuan), putting the individuals surveyed at the bottom quartile of China's rural income distribution [12,13].

Study Population, Sample Size and Sampling Strategy

Children were studied with respect to socialization (before school and in school) and exposure to school environments. We identified two groups of children: a 3–5 year old group and an 8–10 year old group.

A total of 141 areas, including 95 villages and 46 schools were studied in the survey. Details of the selection schema are shown in Figure 1.

In each of the six selected counties, we ranked all towns according to net income per capita, and then randomly chose four towns: two with income per capita above the mean for all towns in that county, and two with income per capita below the mean for all towns in that county. For each of the four chosen towns, two sample schools were chosen: the central primary school (which also serves as the local Bureau of Education's administrative representative for all educational affairs in the town) and a randomly selected primary school. (Two of our sample towns had only one primary school, therefore the total number of sample schools is 46, rather than 48).

For each school, we obtained a list of all local villages that feed into the school. We ranked this list of villages by the number of 8–10 year old students (henceforth called ***school-aged*** children) enrolled at the school. We randomly selected two villages from the list (henceforth called ***sample villages***) that had 16 or more students enrolled at the school. We then randomly chose 11 enrolled students from each sample village. In each sample school, a total of 22 students were surveyed.

Next, we went to the sample villages to conduct the sampling of the 3–5 year old children. We obtained a list of all the 3–5 year old children in each sample village from the Registry of Child Immunization (which is recorded and stored in the town's health center) and randomly chose 11 children from each of the sample villages (henceforth called ***preschool-aged children***).

In three of our sample schools, we were unable to find the requisite number of 3–5 year old children from the two corresponding sample villages. In those cases, we randomly selected a third village from the list of villages that feed into the school, and continued to select sample children from that village. This is why the total number of sample villages is 95, rather than 92 (46×2).

Our power calculations indicated that for our primary outcome variable, STH infection status, to estimate a 95% confidence interval with precision of 0.05 around a population prevalence of 40% and assuming an intra-cluster correlation (ICC) of 0.15, we required 8 children in each age group per village. We increased this to 11 children to account for attrition.

Overall then, in each sample village we randomly sampled 11 preschool-aged children, and 11 school-aged children. This led to sampling from a total of 817 pre-school aged children, and 890 school-aged children. Because some students refused to produce fecal samples, some sample villages had fewer than 22 observations with fecal samples. In no case were there fewer than 8 pre-school aged children and 8 school-aged children. On average, there were 9.75 school-aged children per sample village and 9.09 preschool-aged children per sample village.

Data Collection and Survey

The primary outcome variable was STH infection status, which was determined by a single stool sample from each child participant. In addition, the intensity of every infection by egg density per gram was measured using WHO standard protocol [5]. Other variables and characteristics like household eating and sanitation information were collected on a socio-economic survey form. This survey contained data on each child's age, gender, parental levels of education, health and sanitation behavior and other household characteristics. The survey also asked whether the child had taken anti-helminthic medication in the past 18 months. The school-aged children completed the survey themselves, in writing, under the direct supervision of trained enumerators from the Chinese Academy of Sciences. The preschool-aged children's data was obtained by interviews with the parents, also by these trained enumerators.

Body height and weight were measured and recorded by trained nurses from Xi'an Jiaotong University according to WHO recommendations [14]. The children were measured in light clothing without shoes. Weight was measured with a calibrated electronic scale recommended by the medical department at Xi'an Jiaotong University. Body height was measured using a standard tape measure. The nursing team was trained to make sure the weighing station was set up on level ground to ensure accuracy of the equipment. Two nurses manned each measurement station, with one responsible for preparing subjects for measurement (removing shoes, offering instruction, reassuring parents, positioning children, etc.) and the other responsible for conducting and recording the actual measurements.

Stool Sample Collection and Laboratory Testing

Stool samples of each of the children included in the study were collected once and sent to the local county Center for Disease Control & Prevention (CDC). There was one lab per county, or three labs per province, for a total of six labs. The majority of the samples were tested the same day that they were collected. Due to time and labor constraints, a small fraction of samples were tested the day after collection. These samples were stored overnight in the CDC laboratory refrigerator, which is kept at a constant 4°C. The Kato-Katz smear method was used for species specific identification of parasite eggs, including *Ascaris lumbricoides* (ascariasis), *Trichuris trichiuria* (whipworm) and hookworm. A single smear test was performed on each sample. Samples found to be positive for any of these three parasites underwent egg burden counts to determine eggs per gram (epg) of feces using standard WHO protocol [15].

CDC employees at the county level examined the samples and performed the tests. As a quality control, ten percent of samples were also checked by a parasite expert from the National Institute for Parasitic Disease to verify the initial diagnosis.

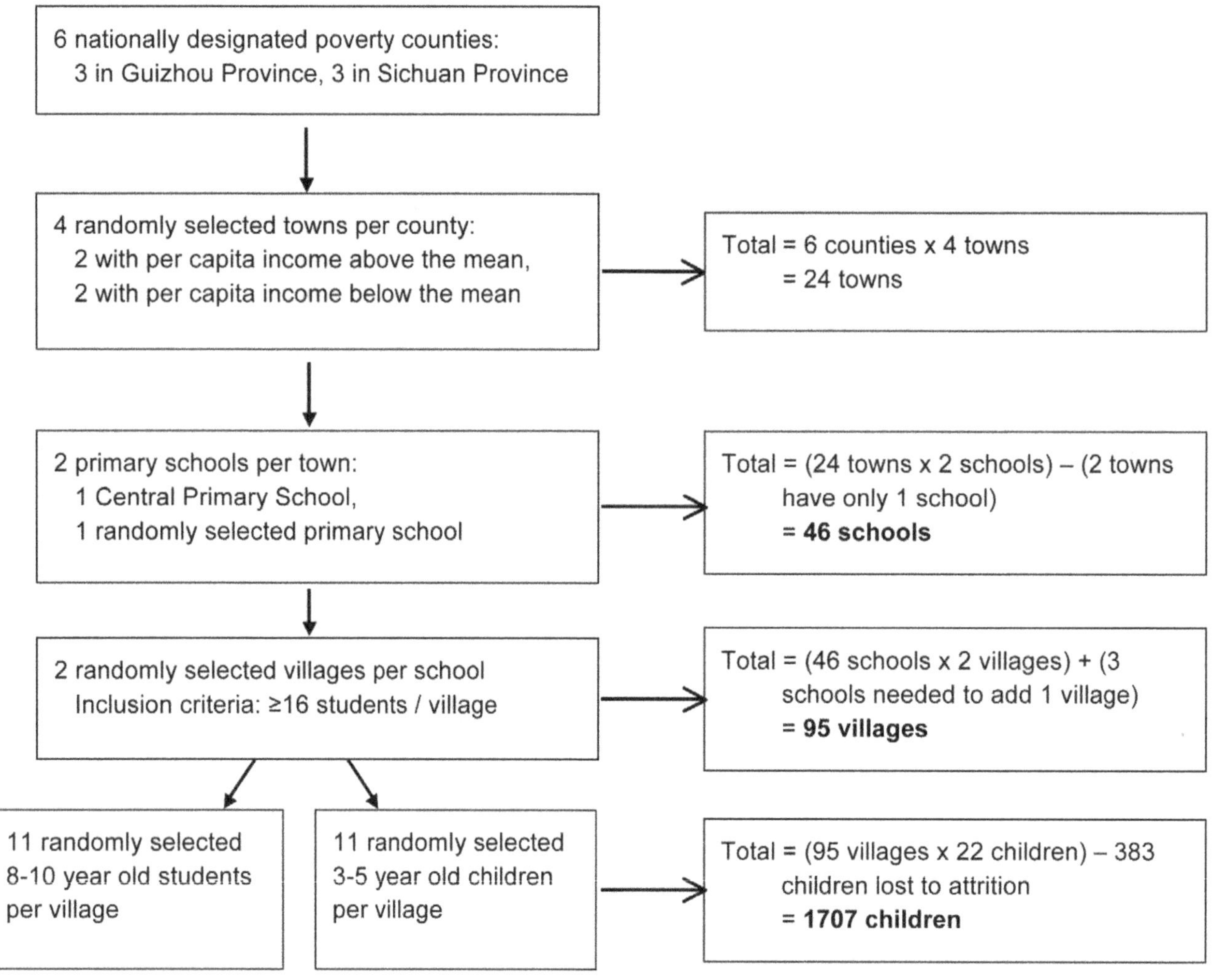

Figure 1. Sample selection schema.

Ethical Considerations

This study was approved by the Stanford University Institutional Review Board (IRB) on May 18th, 2010 and was assigned study protocol number 18780. The legal guardians (either parents or school principals) of all subjects provided informed oral consent, and the children themselves provided oral assent. The IRB approves the use of oral consents in rural China, to clarify understanding because many rural villagers are illiterate and it is culturally unusual to sign in writing. Our study enumerators recorded the consents on a list of names which is stored in a locked filing cabinet at the study center in Beijing, China.

Stool sampling falls within the regular purview of the Chinese Center for Disease Control & Prevention. They are professionally trained and perform routine stool sampling in the study areas as part of their national responsibilities. The stool sampling conducted as part of this study was approved and sanctioned by the national Chinese CDC as well as the local CDCs in the sample areas.

At the conclusion of the study, all participating children were treated with 200 mg of albendazole, per Chinese CDC national guidelines [16].

Data Management and Statistical Analysis

To make sense of our data, we conduct both descriptive (univariate) and multivariate analyses.

As part of our univariate analysis, we grouped risks into four sets of factors: (1) deworming history; (2) individual characteristics; (3) eating and sanitation behaviors; and (4) household characteristics. Individual characteristics include age, gender, number of siblings and parental education. Eating and sanitation behaviors include handwashing after using the bathroom or before eating, the consumption of undercooked meat or vegetables, and the consumption of unboiled drinking water. Household characteristics include the type of toilet used by the household (either soil-based pits, including open defecation, or "other", where "other" includes cement-lined pits or troughs, portable containers, and flush toilets); the material used to construct the floor of the home; the use of human fecal matter in household crop production; and whether the household raises livestock.

In order to better understand the strength of the correlations between each potential explanatory factor and infection prevalence, we conducted a multivariate regression analysis. Using a probit estimator (since our dependent variable is binary in nature–infected with STHs or not), we regressed STH treatment history; individual characteristics; health and sanitation behaviors; and household characteristics on STH infection, which we define as: "infection with any of the three types of STH." The results of this analysis will help shed light on which factors are most strongly associated with STH infection.

Through our multivariate analysis, we will identify factors that influence STH infection. This information combined with any observed differences across survey regions can be used to identify factors that contribute to the variation in STH infection rates across different areas. This analysis, known as a decomposition analysis, uses a combination of the marginal impact of a variable on STH infection and the variation in that variable across regions to understand what share of the total variation in STH infection rate can be attributed to each variable.

Results

Prevalence of Intestinal Parasitic Infections

Overall, 21.2 percent of preschool-aged children and 22.9 percent of school-aged children were infected with one or more of the three types of STH tested for in the survey (Table 1). In Guizhou province, 33.9 percent of preschool-aged children and 40.1 percent of school-aged children tested positive for infection with one or more types of STH. In Sichuan province, only 9.7 percent of preschool-aged children and 6.6 percent of school-aged children were tested positive for infection.

Variation in prevalence across both villages and schools was observed in Sichuan (Figure 2). Seven of the 48 sample villages and two of the 23 sample schools have prevalence of 20 percent or higher. Twenty-five of the 48 sample villages and 11 of the 23 sample schools show STH infection rates greater than 0 percent. In Guizhou, ten of the 47 sample villages and seven of the 23 sample schools have infection rates of over 50 percent.

The results of the worm burden testing (eggs per gram of stool sample) are shown in Table 2. We find that for *A. lumbricoides*, 50.0% (n = 57) of preschool-aged children are characterized with having low intensity infections according to WHO guidelines, compared with 45.0% (n = 9) in Sichuan. Slightly higher percentages of school-aged children have low intensity *A. lumbricoides* infections in both provinces, at 52.9% (n = 74) in Guizhou and 81.8% (n = 9) in Sichuan. In both provinces, children with high intensity *A. lumbricoides* infections make up the smallest proportion of the total sample, at 13.2% (n = 15) and 10.7% (n = 15) among preschool-aged and school-aged children, respectively, in Guizhou, and 25.0% (n = 5) and 0.0% (n = 0) among children in Sichuan. Similar trends can be seen in the burden data for hookworm and *T. trichiura*: across both age groups and both provinces, the majority of sampled children have low intensity infections. The single exception to this rule is preschool-aged children infected with hookworm in Guizhou. Among this group, children with high intensity infections account for 66.6% (n = 4) of infected children, versus only 33.3% (n = 2) for children with low intensity infections; however, the sample size here is too small to allow the drawing of any meaningful conclusions.

Univariate Analysis

We grouped risks into four sets of factors: (1) deworming history; (2) individual characteristics; (3) eating and sanitation behaviors; and (4) household characteristics (Table 3). 49 percent of the sample population in Guizhou and 46 percent in Sichuan took anti-helminth medication in the past 18 months.

Individual characteristics included age, gender, number of siblings and parental education. In Guizhou, 45 percent of the sample is female and 55 percent is male; in Sichuan these numbers are 54 percent and 46 percent, respectively. Children in Guizhou have 1.18 siblings, on average, while children in Sichuan have 0.93. Only 33 percent of mothers in Guizhou finished secondary school, compared with 56 percent in Sichuan. For fathers, these numbers were 51 percent and 65 percent, respectively.

Eating and sanitation behaviors include handwashing after using the bathroom or before eating, the consumption of undercooked meat or vegetables, and the consumption of unboiled drinking water. In Sichuan, 86 percent of children reported washing their hands before dinner and 70 percent reported washing their hands after using the toilet. In Guizhou, these numbers were 67 percent and 59 percent, respectively. In Sichuan, 87 percent of children had never eaten uncooked meat, and 47 percent had never drunk unboiled water. In Guizhou, these numbers were 80 percent and 19 percent, respectively.

Household characteristics include the type of toilet used by the household (either soil-based pits, including open defecation, or "other", where "other" includes cement-lined pits or troughs, portable containers, and flush toilets); the material used to construct the floor of the home; the use of human fecal matter in household crop production; and whether the household raises livestock. Households in Guizhou and Sichuan look fairly similar except for two factors. First, 68 percent of households in Guizhou use a soil-based latrine, versus 79 percent in Sichuan. Second, 76 percent of households in Guizhou raise livestock, versus 69 percent in Sichuan.

Table 1. Prevalence of soil-transmitted helminth infections for two age cohorts in Guizhou and Sichuan, 2010.

	Preschool-aged children (Aged 3–5 years)			School-aged children (Aged 8–10 years)		
	Total (n = 815)	**Guizhou (n = 386)**	**Sichuan (n = 429)**	**Total (n = 886)**	**Guizhou (n = 435)**	**Sichuan (n = 451)**
Ascaris lumbricoides (%)	16.4[a]	29.5	4.7	18.6	32.2	2.4
Hookworm (%)	2.9	1.6	4.2	6.2	6.4	2.9
Trichuris trichiura (%)	4.9	6.7	3.3	9.7	14.3	2.2
Any soil-transmitted helminth infection	**21.2**	**33.9**	**9.8**	**26.1**	**39.8**	**6.7**
Prevalence of single infection	18.9	31.1	7.9	17.6	29.8	5.8
Prevalence of double infection	1.8	1.8	1.3	8.5	6.7	0.8
Prevalence of triple infection	0.7	1.0	0.5	0.0	3.2	0.0

[a]Totals may not sum exactly due to rounding.

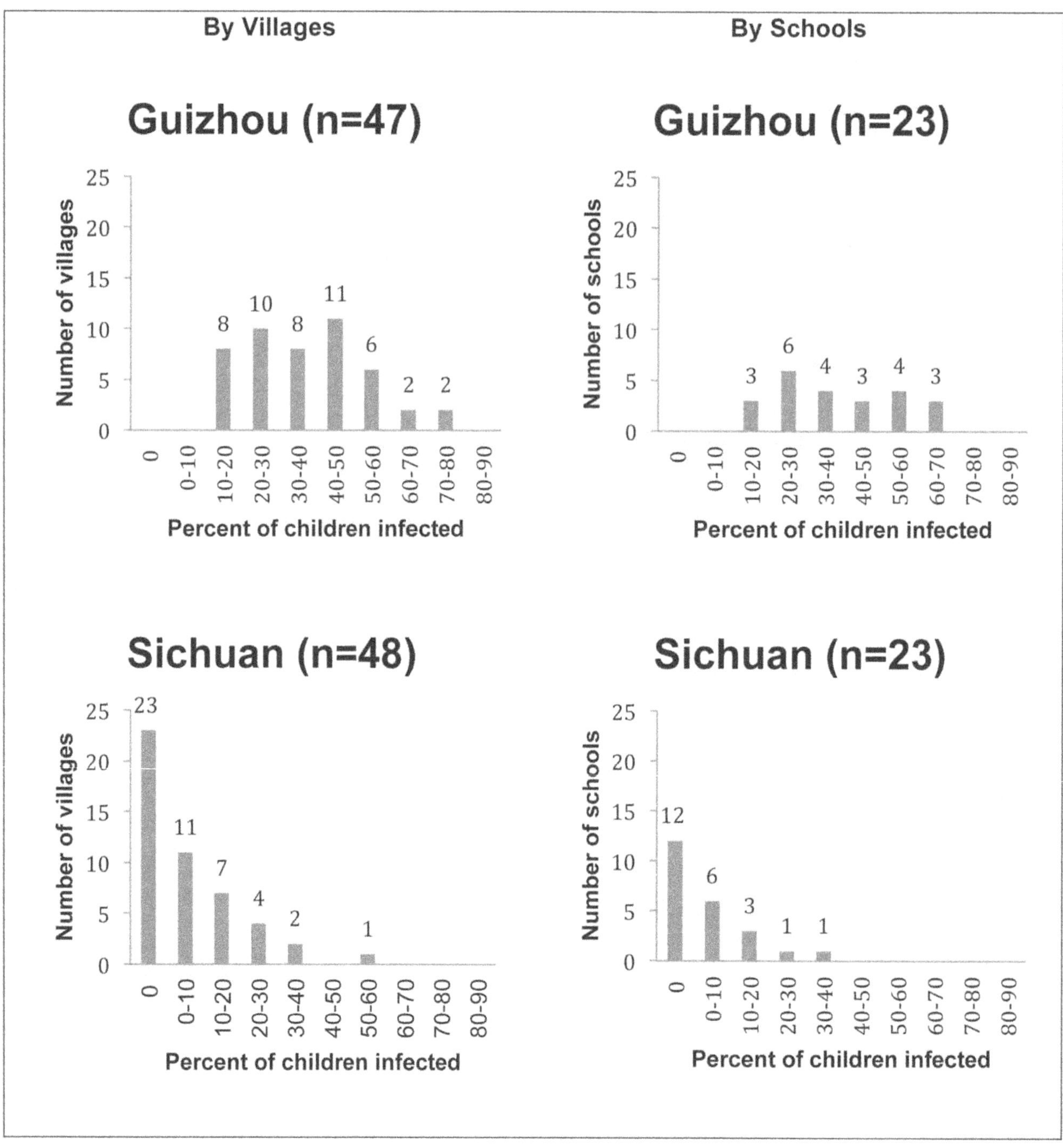

Figure 2. Numbers of villages and schools by prevalence of infection with A. lumbricoides, hookworm, T. trichiura, or any combination thereof in Guizhou and Sichuan, 2010.

Multivariate Analysis

Recall of whether a child has taken anti-helminth medication in the past 18 months has no significant effect on observed infection status (Table 4).

Mothers' education is negatively correlates with children's infection status. Specifically, the more educated the mother is, the less likely it is that her children are infected. With each additional year of maternal education, the probability of infection decreases by 7 percent (marginal effect is −0.07). In contrast, father's education level has no impact on the probability of STH infection.

Health and sanitation behaviors were observed to correlate with STH infections. The consumption of undercooked meat is significantly and positively correlated with the probability of STH infection. Drinking unclean (unboiled) water is associated with a significant increase in the likelihood of infection.

Finally, soil-based latrine use is significantly and negatively correlated with infection, indicating that children living in households with soil-based latrines are *less* likely to have a child with STH infection. In addition, raising livestock is associated with

Table 2. Eggs per gram in stool samples of infected children, by A. lumbricoides, hookworm and T. trichiura and by WHO category for two age cohorts in Sichuan and Guizhou, 2010.

	Preschool-aged children (Aged 3–5 years)		School-aged children (Aged 8–10 years)	
	Guizhou	**Sichuan**	**Guizhou**	**Sichuan**
A. lumbricoides				
Low (1–4,999)	57 (50.0%)	9 (45.0%)	74 (52.9%)	9 (81.8%)
Medium (5,000–49,999)	42 (36.8%)	6 (30.0%)	51 (36.4%)	2 (18.2%)
High (50,000+)	15 (13.2%)	5 (25.0%)	15(10.7%)	0 (0.0%)
Total	**114 (100%)**	**20 (100%)**	**140 (100%)**	**11 (100%)**
Hookworm				
Low (1–4,999)	2 (33.3%)	16 (88.9%)	20 (71.4%)	12 (92.3%)
Medium (5,000–49,999)	0 (0.0%)	0 (0.0%)	0 (0.0%)	0 (0.0%)
High (50,000+)	4 (66.6%)	2 (11.1%)	8 (28.6%)	1 (7.7%)
Total	**6 (100%)**	**18 (100%)**	**28 (100%)**	**13 (100%)**
T. trichiura				
Low (1–4,999)	22 (84.6%)	10 (71.4%)	52 (83.9%)	10 (100.0%)
Medium (5,000–49,999)	0 (0.0%)	2 (14.3%)	2 (3.2%)	0 (0.0%)
High (50,000+)	4 (15.4%)	2 (14.3%)	8 (12.9%)	0 (0.0%)
Total	**26 (100%)**	**14 (100%)**	**62 (100%)**	**10 (100%)**

a significant increase in the probability of STH infection of 8.0 percent.

Decomposition Analysis

The difference in STH prevalence between Guizhou and Sichuan is 30.0 percent (Table 5). Table 5 shows that the

Table 3. Descriptive statistics of independent variables used in the study, by province.

	Guizhou (n = 821)		Sichuan (n = 880)	
	Mean	**95% Confidence Interval**	**Mean**	**95% Confidence Interval**
Child has taken anti-helminth medicine in past 18 months (1 = yes, 0 = no)	50%	(46%–53%)	46%	(43%–49%)
Individual characteristics				
Gender (1 = male, 0 = female)	55%	(52%–59%)	46%	(43%–49%)
No. of family members (person)	5.1	(5.0–5.3)	5.2	(5.1–5.3)
No. of siblings (person)	1.2	(1.1–1.2)	0.9	(0.9–1.0)
Mother finished secondary school or above (1 = yes, 0 = no)	33%	(30%–36%)	56%	(53%–60%)
Father finished secondary school or above (1 = yes, 0 = no)	51%	(48%–55%)	64%	(61%–68%)
Eating and sanitation habits				
Wash hands before dinner (1 = yes, 0 = no)	67%	(64%–70%)	86%	(84%–89%)
Wash hands after using toilet (1 = yes, 0 = no)	59%	(56%–62%)	70%	(67%–73%)
Eat uncooked vegetables (1 = never, 0 otherwise)	25%	(22%–28%)	42%	(39%–45%)
Eat uncooked meat (1 = never, 0 otherwise)	80%	(78%–83%)	87%	(84%–89%)
Drink un-boiled water (1 = never, 0 otherwise)	19%	(16%–22%)	47%	(44%–50%)
Household characteristics				
Dirt floor (1 = yes, 0 = no)	17%	(15%–20%)	18%	(15%–20%)
Household has own toilet (1 = yes, 0 = no)	95%	(93%–96%)	96%	(95%–98%)
Soil-based latrine (1 = yes, 0 = no)	68%	(65%–71%)	79%	(76%–82%)
Use of human fecal material in household crop production (1 = yes, 0 = no)	77%	(74%–80%)	80%	(78%–83%)
Household owns livestock (1 = yes, 0 = no)	76%	(73%–79%)	69%	(66%–72%)
Use of human fecal material in household garden (1 = no, 0 = yes)	33%	(30%–36%)	30%	(27%–33%)

Table 4. Univariate and multivariate analyses of risk factors for STH infection (dependent variable) for sampled children in Guizhou and Sichuan, 2010.

Dependent Variable: STH infection (1 = yes, 0 = no)

	Case	Controls	Univariate		Multivariate	
Variables	(n = 376)[a]	(n = 1325)[a]	Adjusted OR (95% CI)	P-value	Adjusted OR (95% CI)	P-value
Child has taken anti-helminth medicine in past 18 months (1 = yes, 0 = no)	164 (43.6)	647 (48.8)	0.81 (0.64–1.02)	0.07	0.85 (0.67–1.09)	0.20
Individual characteristics						
Gender (1 = male, 0 = female)	208 (55.3)	651 (49.1)	1.29 (1.02–1.62)	0.03	1.20 (0.94–1.52)	0.15
Age	6.9 (2.8)	6.7 (2.7)	1.03 (0.99–1.07)	0.15	0.99 (0.94–1.04)	0.63
Number of family members	5.2 (1.6)	5.1 (1.5)	1.04 (0.96–1.12)	0.34	0.99 (0.91–1.07)	0.72
Number of siblings	1.2 (0.9)	1.0 (0.9)	1.28 (1.13–1.45)	<0.001	1.18 (1.02–1.36)	0.03
Mother finished secondary school or above (1 = yes, 0 = no)	118 (31.4)	648 (48.9)	0.48 (0.37–0.61)	<0.001	0.63 (0.48–0.83)	<0.001
Father finished secondary school or above (1 = yes, 0 = no)	186 (49.5)	803 (60.6)	0.64 (0.51–0.80)	<0.001	0.90 (0.67–1.17)	0.44
Eating and sanitation habits						
Wash hands before dinner (1 = yes, 0 = no)	258 (68.6)	1053 (79.5)	0.56 (0.44–0.73)	<0.001	0.78 (0.58–1.05)	0.11
Wash hands after using toilet (1 = yes, 0 = no)	226 (60.1)	872 (65.8)	0.78 (0.62–0.99)	0.04	0.99 (0.74–1.33)	0.95
Eat uncooked vegetables (1 = never, 0 otherwise)	114 (30.3)	465 (35.1)	0.80 (0.63–1.03)	0.09	1.05 (0.81–1.37)	0.72
Eat uncooked meat (1 = never, 0 otherwise)	296 (78.7)	1128 (85.1)	0.65 (0.49–0.87)	0.004	0.73 (0.53–1.00)	0.05
Drink un-boiled water (1 = never, 0 otherwise)	70 (18.6)	500 (37.7)	0.38 (0.29–0.50)	<0.001	0.48 (0.35–0.64)	<0.001
Household characteristics						
Dirt floor (1 = yes, 0 = no)	70 (18.6)	227 (17.1)	1.11 (0.83–1.50)	0.48	0.85 (0.62–1.18)	0.34
Household has own toilet (1 = yes, 0 = no)	358 (95.2)	1269 (95.8)	0.86 (0.50–1.49)	0.59	0.73 (0.41–1.30)	0.28
Soil-based latrine (1 = yes, 0 = no)	247 (65.7)	1004 (75.8)	0.61 (0.48–0.78)	<0.001	0.71 (0.54–0.93)	0.01
Use of human fecal material in household crop production (1 = yes, 0 = no)	304 (80.9)	1034 (78.0)	1.18 (0.89–1.58)	0.24	0.83 (0.59–1.18)	0.30
Household owns livestock (1 = yes, 0 = no)	306 (81.4)	926 (69.9)	1.88 (1.42–2.50)	<0.001	1.68 (1.19–2.36)	0.00
Use of human fecal material in household garden (1 = no, 0 = yes)	103 (27.4)	427 (32.2)	0.79 (0.62–1.02)	0.08	0.96 (0.73–1.27)	0.79

NOTE. [a]Categorical data are no. (%) of subjects, continuous data are expressed as mean (SD)
OR = odds ratio; CI = confidence interval.

statistically significant variables in Table 4 made up 24.14 percent of the difference in STH infection between the two provinces. Consistent with other studies [17,18], 5.83 percent of the provincial difference in prevalence is due to differences in maternal education. The percentage of mothers with at least a secondary school education is 20 percent lower in Guizhou than in Sichuan. More siblings would have caused the infection rate in Sichuan to be 2.26 percent higher. The difference in infection rates between provinces derived from eating uncooked meat was 1.31 percent. Drinking unboiled water explains 10.69 percent of the difference. While the percentage of children who drink unboiled water was 81 percent in Guizhou, it was only 53 percent in Sichuan. Household characteristics explained 4.05 percent of the provincial difference in prevalence: soil-based latrines explained 2.18 percent, while owning livestock explained 1.87 percent.

Overall, our data only explain 24.14 percent of the provincial difference in infection rates. This means that 75.86 percent of the difference is due to unexplained factors that we have not measured.

Effect on Student Growth

Infection with one or more of the three STHs (*A. lumbricoides*, hookworm, or *T. trichiura*) is associated with significantly lower weight-for-age and height-for-age (Table 6). Moreover, there is a statistically significant negative coefficient on the age variable, indicating that older children infected with STHs lag further behind on the international growth scales than younger children.

Discussion

This study examines the prevalence and correlates of intestinal parasitic infection in children in impoverished rural regions of China where there is little published data or rigorous definition of the scope of the problem. We find that 33.9 percent of preschool-aged children and 40.1 percent of school-aged children in Guizhou tested positive for infection with one or more types of STH, while these numbers were 9.7 percent and 6.6 percent, respectively, in Sichuan. The national Ministry of Health survey of helminth prevalence from 2001–2004 included 356,629 individuals across China, and encompassed several studies by local Centers for Disease Control and Prevention (CDC), including in

Table 5. Decomposition analysis of the difference in STH infection rates between Guizhou and Sichuan, 2010.

	Explanatory variables	Rate in Guizhou	Rate in Sichuan	Marginal Effect (on infection)	Explained infection rate	
		A	B	C	(A–B)*C	%
	% INFECTED	38%	8%		0.3	100
1	Number of siblings	1.18	0.93	0.026	−0.65	2.26
2	Percent with mother who finished secondary school or above	33	56	−0.073	−1.68	5.83
3	Percent who ever eat uncooked meat	20	13	−0.054	−0.38	1.31
4	Percent who ever drink un-boiled water	81	53	−0.110	−3.08	10.69
5	Percent with soil-based latrine	68	79	−0.057	−0.63	2.18
6	Percent whose household owns livestock	76	0.69	0.077	−0.54	1.87
	Explained infection rate (sum of rows 1–6)					**24.14**
	Residual (all else)					*75.86*

Table 6. Ordinary Least Square (OLS) estimates of growth measures for sampled children in Guizhou and Sichuan, 2010.

Dependent variables	Weight-for-age z-score		Height-for-age z-score	
	OLS Coefficient (95% CI)	*P*-value	OLS Coefficient (95% CI)	*P*-value
Infected with any of three STHs (1 = yes, 0 = no)	−0.148 (−0.260–0.036)	0.009	−0.148 (−0.293–0.003)	0.046
Individual characteristics				
Gender (1 = male, 0 = female)	0.191 (0.101–0.282)	0.000	0.001 (−0.117–0.119)	0.987
Age	−0.024 (−0.043–0.005)	0.013	−0.041 (−0.066–0.016)	0.001
Number of family members	−0.019 (−0.050–0.013)	0.245	−0.013 (−0.054–0.028)	0.539
Number of siblings	−0.012 (−0.069–0.044)	0.665	0.028 (−0.045–0.102)	0.449
Mother finished secondary school or above (1 = yes, 0 = no)	0.146 (0.044–0.248)	0.005	0.097 (−0.036–0.231)	0.152
Father finished secondary school or above (1 = yes, 0 = no)	0.012 (−0.090–0.114)	0.816	0.097 (−0.035–0.230)	0.150
Eating and sanitation habits				
Wash hands before dinner (1 = yes, 0 = no)	0.193 (0.071–0.315)	0.002	0.195 (0.036–0.354)	0.017
Wash hands after using toilet (1 = yes, 0 = no)	−0.037 (−0.149–0.075)	0.519	0.079 (−0.067–0.225)	0.287
Eat uncooked vegetables (1 = never, 0 otherwise)	0.019 (−0.079–0.117)	0.704	0.115 (−0.012–0.242)	0.076
Eat uncooked meat (1 = never, 0 otherwise)	0.051 (−0.077–0.179)	0.432	0.018 (−0.149–0.185)	0.832
Drink un-boiled water (1 = never, 0 otherwise)	0.140 (0.037–0.242)	0.008	−0.079 (−0.213–0.054)	0.242
Household characteristics				
Dirt floor (1 = yes, 0 = no)	0.042 (−0.082–0.167)	0.507	−0.107 (−0.269–0.056)	0.198
Household has own toilet (1 = yes, 0 = no)	−0.002 (−0.226–0.222)	0.987	−0.159 (−0.451–0.132)	0.284
Soil-based latrine (1 = yes, 0 = no)	0.128 (0.019–0.237)	0.021	0.049 (−0.093–0.190)	0.501
Use of human fecal material in household crop production (1 = yes, 0 = no)	−0.032 (−0.160–0.097)	0.629	−0.039 (−0.206–0.128)	0.644
Household owns livestock (1 = yes, 0 = no)	−0.085 (−0.204–0.034)	0.160	−0.161 (−0.317–0.006)	0.042
Use of human fecal material in household garden (1 = no, 0 = yes)	−0.079 (−0.179–0.022)	0.124	−0.023 (−0.154–0.108)	0.732
Constant	−0.615	0.001	−0.632	0.008
Adj-R^2	0.051		0.024	
No. of obs.	1,699		1,697	

our study areas. The prevalence of *A. lumbricoides*, hookworm, and *T. trichiura* that we identify here support the results of these local CDC surveys, and indicate little change between 2002 and present-day. For example, Tang et al. (2005) found infection rates of 10.4%, 21.1%, and 2.6% for hookworm, *A. lumbricoides*, and *T. trichiura*, respectively, among 625 children under 5 years old in hilly regions of Sichuan province [19]. For children aged 5–9 years, these numbers were 11.0%, 23.0%, and 5.6%, respectively. In 2005, the Sichuan Provincial CDC reported an overall STH infection rate of 39.2%, among 6684 children under age 14 from 18 randomly selected counties [20]. The Guizhou Provincial CDC found STH prevalence of 53.8% among 4091 primary and middle school students, and prevalence of 48.3% among 1748 children of preschool age [21]. A more localized study in Guizhou found similar rates in 2007; specifically, the authors reported STH prevalence of 50.0% among children aged 2–12 years in a rural, mountainous county in western Guizhou [22].

We also identify factors that correlate with STH infection. Many of the correlates are not surprising, like the number of siblings, maternal education, consumption of uncooked meat, and consumption of unboiled water. These factors have been identified in other studies of STH infection elsewhere [23–25].

We found two unexpected results. Our first surprising result was the statistically insignificant effect of deworming treatment on STH infection. Why might this be? One possibility is that individuals who take deworming medicine may be taking an insufficient dose of the medication. National guidelines released by the Chinese CDC [25] recommend the annual administration of only 200 mg of albendazole for children aged 2–12 years, only half of the 400 mg dose recommended by the World Health Organization (WHO) [15]. Giving this lower dosage may have under-treated, thus leading to the ineffectiveness of the deworming treatment and probably sooner re-infection.

A second reason may be related to the frequency of treatment. The WHO treatment guidelines recommend that in communities with infection rates of 20% to 50% (the rate observed in our study areas), school-aged children should be treated once a year, since for the STHs considered in this study, reinfection occurs rapidly after treatment [26]. However, our survey asked individuals about their deworming history over the past 18 months, more than sufficient time for reinfection to have occurred.

In the context of the observed high rates of infection more frequent or structured and formalized population-level deworming efforts may be needed to better manage the observed infections. Currently, intestinal parasite control is left to the individual and there is no population-level regular intervention. Such programs have been successful in the past in China [6], and in other settings [17]. Health education and environmental sanitation programs have also been successful at reducing reinfection rates in other settings, and may be a prudent addition to China's anti-helminth efforts [26].

Our second surprising result was that the use of soil-based latrines is negatively correlated with roundworm infection. Soil-based latrines are usually thought of as dirty environments conducive to STH survival and spread. However, it may be that soil-based latrines are actually *cleaner* than the alternative. In our sample villages, the two predominant types of latrine are soil-based and water-based. Soil-based latrines are, at their most basic, simply a large hole in the ground. Water-based latrines are large, lined troughs in the ground that are partially filled with water. The waste in water-based latrines is periodically drained to a nearby cesspool. Although soil leeching at the point of defecation is less likely in water latrines, the waste eventually covers a larger area, potentially offering more opportunities for contamination to occur. Few, if any, rural households have porcelain flush toilets that are commonplace in wealthier areas with plumbing.

Through our decomposition analysis we identify the correlating factors primarily responsible for the difference in prevalence between the two study areas. Unclean drinking water is the most important correlate, accounting for over 10 percent of the difference in prevalence between Guizhou and Sichuan.

Another important factor contributing to the difference in provincial infection rates is maternal education. Because mothers are often responsible for both food preparation and the health education of children in the family, they significantly influence the health of their children. If a child's mother is educated, she is more likely to know about the dangers of STH infection and how to prevent it, and thus more likely to incorporate safe health behaviors into the home, including boiling water.

Our study also offers a quantitative look at the physical effects of STH infection. Children infected with STHs have significantly lower weight-for-age and height-for-age z-scores than do healthy children, putting them at risk for a number of conditions associated with undernutrition.

Unfortunately, the STH problem is receiving little attention from health officials, teachers or parents. Contrary to WHO guidelines, the decision to deworm in rural China is typically made at the individual level, rather than at the community level. The few deworming campaigns that exist appear to be ineffective, since deworming at the observed frequency appears to be uncorrelated with infection rates. The primary factors correlated with infection are low levels of maternal education and poor food preparation techniques such as drinking unclean water or eating undercooked meat. Accordingly, for intestinal roundworms to be effectively controlled, it appears that a two-pronged approach is needed: first, educating parents and students about how to prevent infection, and then ensuring that deworming programs offer anthelminthic medicines regularly so that children remain STH-free. This is consistent with the official recommendations of the World Health Organization [5].

Limitations

Because only a single stool sample was collected on each child in this study, using the Kato-Katz preparation to determine infection status, there is likely a significant underestimation of infection. This underestimation is based on the fact that a single sample misses infection in an individual because of the temporal variation in egg excretion over hours and days. It has been shown that obtaining only a single sample for *A. lumbricoides* and *T. trichiura* can underestimate infection rates by up to 50% [18]. Similarly, in areas of lower endemicity for STHs, it is observed that a single smear sample may not be reliable in determining infection status, due to fewer shed eggs, again giving falsely low prevalence estimates in the population. Because only a single slide from the stool sample was prepared, this is a limitation in that it results in under-reporting of infection rates. It has been reported that sensitivity for low infection rates increases from 20 to 54% when going from a single sample to three fecal samples on separate days [27]. (The usual practice would be to obtain 3 specimens on separate days for immediate microscopic analysis.) Lastly, because the samples had to be obtained then transported to the central lab for each province, some time elapsed before their review and thus specifically in the case of hookworm, fewer cases were likely identified. This occurs because of the observed rapid desiccation of hookworm eggs in the stool samples, and has been shown to lead to severe underestimates of the density of this pathogen if samples cannot be examined immediately [28]. Thus because of single sampling and the time lapse between stool collection and expert review, there are likely significant underestimates of the actual rates and densities of intestinal parasitic infections in our population.

Another potential source of bias may have come from the administration of the socioeconomic survey forms. School-aged children answered questions about their individual, household, and health behavior characteristics on their own, while the same information was collected about preschool children by asking their parents. It is possible that this may have led to fundamental differences between the two age groups in the types of answers we received, although there is no reason to think that either group would systematically overestimate or underestimate in their responses. Regardless, any differences between the age groups should not affect our results since we control for the age of the child in our multivariate analyses.

Conclusions

Our study shows an unexpectedly high prevalence of STH infections among children in impoverished areas of rural Guizhou and Sichuan provinces. There is considerable variation in prevalence rates between the two provinces that we sampled. We identified several factors that contribute to the difference in infection prevalence between Guizhou and Sichuan. Health and sanitation behaviors explain most of the explained difference; unclean drinking water and failing to wash hands before eating are among the most important correlates. Maternal education also plays an important role.

Student and parent recall about deworming treatments appear to indicate no significant correlation between deworming treatment and STH infection. This result hints at the ineffectiveness of sporadic deworming measures at an individual level, which allows for high rates of reinfection. It underscores the importance of a long-term, consistent deworming regimen.

Our study shows that STH infections still pose a significant health challenge to children in some poor, rural areas of China. Children infected with STHs have significantly lower weight-for-age and height-for-age z-scores than do non-infected children, putting them at risk for a number of conditions known to be associated with undernutrition.

We hope that this study will be the first of a series of studies that will start to define the scope of the problem, not only reporting the numbers observed, but also adverse outcomes such as the effects of infection on measures of nutritional status and school performance.

Acknowledgments

We are grateful for expert assistance from the National Institute of Parasitic Diseases at the Chinese Center for Disease Control & Prevention in Shanghai, and the dedication and cooperation of the health professionals at the local Centers for Disease Control in Guizhou and Sichuan provinces. Thank you also to the Walter H. Shorenstein Asia-Pacific Research Center and the Asia Health Care Initiative at the Freeman Spogli Institute for International Studies at Stanford University. Finally, we would like to extend special thanks to Eric Hemel and Barbara Morgen for their generous support of our work on health in rural China.

Author Contributions

Conceived and designed the experiments: XW LZ RL KE SR. Performed the experiments: XW LZ RL GW YC SR. Analyzed the data: XW RL AM KE DSS SR. Contributed reagents/materials/analysis tools: XW RL YC GW SR LZ. Wrote the paper: XW AM SR DSS YC GW LZ.

References

1. Wu G (2005) Medical Parasitology in China: A Historical Perspective. Chinese Medical Journal 118(9): 759–761.
2. Wagstaff A, Lindelow M, Wang S, Zhang S (2009a) Reforming China's Rural Health System. Washington, DC: The World Bank.
3. Zhang D, Unschuld PU (2008) China's Barefoot Doctor: Past, Present, and Future. Lancet 372(9653): 1865–1867.
4. Valentine V (2005) Health for the Masses: China's 'Barefoot Doctors'. National Public Radio, broadcast November 4.
5. Montresor A, Crompton DWT, Gyorkos TW, Savioli L (2002) Helminth control in school-age children. Geneva: World Health Organization.
6. Li T, He S, Zhao H, Zhao G, Zhu XQ (2010) Major trends in human parasitic diseases in China. Trends in Parasitology 26: 264–270.
7. Wagstaff A, Yip W, Lindelow M, Hsiao W (2009) China's health system and its reform: A review of recent studies. Health Economics 18: S7–S23.
8. Steinmann P, Du ZW, Wang LB, Wang XZ, Jiang JY, et al. (2008) Extensive multiparasitism in a village of Yunnan province, People's Republic of China, revealed by a suite of diagnostic methods. Am. J. Trop. Med. Hyg. 78: 760–769.
9. Xu L, Pan B, Lin J, Chen L, Yu S, et al. (2000) Creating health-promoting schools in rural China: a project started from deworming. Health Promotion International 15: 197–206.
10. Zhou H, Watanabe C, Ohtsuka R (2007) Impacts of dietary intake and helminth infection on diversity in growth among schoolchildren in rural south China: A four-year longitudinal study. American Journal of Human Biology 19: 96–106.
11. Coordinating Office of the National Survey on the Important Human Parasitic Diseases (2005) A National Survey on Current Status of the Important Parasitic Diseases in Human Population, China Journal of Parasitology and Parasitic Diseases 23: 332–340.
12. National Statistical Bureau of China (2009a) Guizhou Statistical Yearbook. China Statistical Press.
13. National Statistical Bureau of China (2009b) Sichuan Statistical Yearbook. China Statistical Press.
14. de Onis M, Onyango AW, Van den Broeck J, Chumlea WC, Martorell R (2004) Measurement and standardization protocols for anthropometry used in the construction of a new international growth reference. Food and Nutrition Bulletin 25: S27–S36.
15. World Health Organization (2006) Preventive chemotherapy in human helminthiasis: Coordinated use of anthelminthic drugs. Geneva: World Health Organization.
16. Center for Disease Control & Prevention (2010) Treatment guidelines for soil-transmitted helminth infections. Official Disease Control Publication of the Administrative Office of the Ministry of Health 98. [in Chinese].
17. Kasai T, Nakatani H, Takeuchi T, Crump A (2007) Research and control of parasitic diseases in Japan: current position and future perspectives. Trends in Parasitology 23: 230–235.
18. Knopp S, Mgeni AF, Khamis IS, Steinmann P, Stothard JR, et al. (2008) Diagnosis of soil-transmitted helminths in the era of preventive chemotherapy: Effect of multiple stool sampling and use of different diagnostic techniques. PLoS Neglected Tropical Diseases 2: e331.
19. Tang Z, Tian H, Yang W, Liu C, Zheng D, et al. (2005) Investigation on Human Intestinal Helminthiasis in Hilly Areas of Sichuan Province from 2002 to 2003. Parasitoses and Infectious Diseases 3: 161–164. [in Chinese].
20. Xie H, Zheng D, Yang W, Liu C, Tang Z, et al. (2005) Parasitic Infections among Children in Sichuan Province. Parasitoses and Infectious Diseases 3: 181–183. [in Chinese].
21. Wang S, Chen Z, Li A, Tang L, Xu L, et al. (2008) Current status and analysis of important human parasitic diseases in Guizhou Province. Journal of Pathogen Biology 2: 450–453. [in Chinese].
22. Chen X, Xia X (2010) Survey of intestinal nematode infection among children visiting a hospital in Puding County. Journal of Medical Pest Control 26. [in Chinese].
23. Olsen A, Samuelsen H, Onyango-Ouma W (2001) A study of risk factors for intestinal helminth infections using epidemiological and anthropological approaches. J. Biosoc. Sci. 33: 569–584.
24. Norhayati M, Oothuman P, Fatmah MS (1998) Some risk factors of Ascaris and Trichuris infection in Malaysian aborigine (Orang Asli) children. Med J Malaysia 53: 401–7.
25. Nyarango RM, Aloo PA, Kabiru EW, Nyanchongi BO (2008) The risk of pathogenic intestinal parasite infections in Kisii Municipality, Kenya. BMC Public Health 8: 237–242.
26. Jia T-W, Melville S, Utzinger J, King CH, Zhou X-N (2012) Soil-transmitted helminth reinfection after drug treatment: A systematic review and meta-analysis. PLoS Negl Trop Dis 6(5): e1621.
27. Cartwright CP (1999) Utility of multiple-stool-specimen ova and parasite examinations in a high-prevalence setting. Journal of Clinical Microbiology 37(8): 2408–2411.
28. Tarafder MR, Carabin H, Joseph L, Balolong E Jr, Olveda R, et al. (2010) Estimating the sensitivity and specificity of Kato-Katz stool examination technique for detection of hookworms, Ascaris lumbricoides and Trichuris trichiura infections in humans in the absence of a 'gold standard'. International Journal for Parasitology 40: 399–404.

5

Determining *Mycobacterium tuberculosis* Infection among BCG-Immunised Ugandan Children by T-SPOT.TB and Tuberculin Skin Testing

Gyaviira Nkurunungi[1]*, Jimreeves E. Lutangira[1], Swaib A. Lule[1], Hellen Akurut[1], Robert Kizindo[1], Joseph R. Fitchett[2], Dennison Kizito[1], Ismail Sebina[1], Lawrence Muhangi[1], Emily L. Webb[3], Stephen Cose[1,2], Alison M. Elliott[1,2]

1 Co-infection Studies Programme, Medical Research Council/Uganda Virus Research Institute Uganda Research Unit on AIDS, Entebbe, Uganda, **2** Department of Clinical Research, London School of Hygiene and Tropical Medicine, London, United Kingdom, **3** Department of Infectious Disease Epidemiology, London School of Hygiene and Tropical Medicine, London, United Kingdom

Abstract

Background: Children with latent tuberculosis infection (LTBI) represent a huge reservoir for future disease. We wished to determine *Mycobacterium tuberculosis (M.tb)* infection prevalence among BCG-immunised five-year-old children in Entebbe, Uganda, but there are limited data on the performance of immunoassays for diagnosis of tuberculosis infection in children in endemic settings. We therefore evaluated agreement between a commercial interferon gamma release assay (T-SPOT.TB) and the tuberculin skin test (TST; 2 units RT-23 tuberculin; positive defined as diameter ≥10 mm), along with the reproducibility of T-SPOT.TB on short-term follow-up, in this population.

Methodology/Principal Findings: We recruited 907 children of which 56 were household contacts of TB patients. They were tested with T-SPOT.TB at age five years and then re-examined with T-SPOT.TB (n = 405) and TST (n = 319) approximately three weeks later. The principal outcome measures were T-SPOT.TB and TST positivity. At five years, 88 (9.7%) children tested positive by T-SPOT.TB. More than half of those that were T-SPOT.TB positive at five years were negative at follow-up, whereas 96% of baseline negatives were consistently negative. We observed somewhat better agreement between initial and follow-up T-SPOT.TB results among household TB contacts ($\kappa = 0.77$) than among non-contacts ($\kappa = 0.39$). Agreement between T-SPOT.TB and TST was weak ($\kappa = 0.28$ and $\kappa = 0.40$ for T-SPOT.TB at 5 years and follow-up, respectively). Of 28 children who were positive on both T-SPOT.TB tests, 14 (50%) had a negative TST. Analysis of spot counts showed high levels of instability in responses between baseline and follow-up, indicating variability in circulating numbers of T cells specific for certain *M.tb* antigens.

Conclusions/Significance: We found that T-SPOT.TB positives are unstable over a three-week follow-up interval, and that TST compares poorly with T-SPOT.TB, making the categorisation of children as TB-infected or TB-uninfected difficult. Existing tools for the diagnosis of TB infection are unsatisfactory in determining infection among children in this setting.

Editor: Madhukar Pai, McGill University, Canada

Funding: The study was funded by Wellcome Trust (www.wellcome.ac.uk) grant numbers 064693, 079110 and 086801. E. Webb was supported in part by the UK Medical Research Council (www.mrc.ac.uk). The funders had no role in study design, data collection and analysis, decision to publish, or preparation of the manuscript.

Competing Interests: The authors have declared that no competing interests exist.

* E-mail: gyaviira.nkurunungi@mrcuganda.org

Introduction

Worldwide, tuberculosis (TB) remains one of the most important infectious causes of mortality. In 2010, there were an estimated 8.8 million incident cases and approximately 1.4 million people died from this disease [1]. Uganda is designated by the World Health Organisation (WHO) to be one of the 22 high burden countries for TB. A vast pool of individuals with latent tuberculosis infection (LTBI) persists in developing countries, posing a major barrier to global TB control [2]. The overall lifetime risk of LTBI reactivation is approximately 5–10% among older children and adults, but in infants and young children, the risk of progression to active disease is increased; most disease cases occur within 12 months of infection [3,4]. Moreover, infection in childhood establishes the reservoir for future epidemics, making proper diagnosis and treatment of LTBI in this vulnerable group important for TB control [5].

For many years, the standard technique used to diagnose LTBI has been the tuberculin skin test (TST). Although the TST has proven to be useful in clinical practice, it has several known limitations [3,6]. Perhaps the most significant of these is the cross reactivity of the purified protein derivative of tuberculin used in the TST with antigens from several nontuberculous mycobacteria, and also with those from the *Mycobacterium bovis* bacille Calmette-

Guérin (BCG) vaccine [7,8]. This means that the skin test may not reliably discern LTBI from prior immunisation or infection with other mycobacteria. Work done in the last decade has suggested that *in vitro* T-cell based interferon gamma release assays (IGRAs) may offer a suitable alternative approach to LTBI diagnosis [6,9]. One such assay is an Enzyme-linked immunosorbent spot (ELISpot) assay, commercially known as T-SPOT.TB, whose antigens (early secretory antigenic target 6, ESAT-6 and culture filtrate protein 10, CFP-10) are coded by the Region of Difference 1 (RD1) genes of the *Mycobacterium tuberculosis* (*M.tb*) complex which is absent from the majority of nontuberculous isolates, as well as from BCG [7,10].

These immunoassays have been widely studied and reviewed in adults and in contacts of infectious cases [3,9–17], yet very little data exist about their performance in children from the general population, and whether their diagnostic accuracy is superior to that of TST, especially in endemic settings. In a recent systematic review and meta-analysis, it was observed that IGRAs are less sensitive and less specific in areas of high TB burden [18]. It is not known whether IGRAs can replace TST surveys as a tool for estimating the annual incidence of infection with *M.tb*. Lack of a "gold standard" reference test for LTBI has made it difficult to assess performance of IGRAs, prompting adoption of surrogate indicators such as evaluation of efficacy of preventive therapy based on test results, predictive value of a test for active TB, correlation with exposure gradient, sensitivity and/or specificity among patients with active TB, and concordance between the IGRA and other LTBI tests [19]. Some studies, mostly in adults, have shown that after *M.tb* exposure, IGRA results fluctuate when serial testing is done [14,20,21], and this has been attributed to variations in laboratory procedures, within subject variability and biological and environmental causes [22].

Within the structure of an existing study [23], we set out to measure the prevalence of LTBI among BCG-immunised five-year olds in Entebbe, Uganda, using the T-SPOT.TB assay. We performed repeat T-SPOT.TB assays approximately three weeks later to determine stability of responses, as well as the more conventional TST to allow comparison with T-SPOT.TB results. We present findings detailing T-SPOT.TB and TST test agreement, stability of T-SPOT.TB responses on short-term follow-up, and analysis of spot forming units in *M.tb* exposed and unexposed children in a high prevalence African setting.

Methods

Study Design and Participants

This was an observational, cross sectional study. From March 2009 to April 2011, participants were prospectively recruited at the fifth annual visit within the framework of the Entebbe Mother and Baby Study (EMaBS), a population-based birth cohort in Entebbe, Wakiso district, Central Uganda [23]. EMaBS was originally established to evaluate the impact of maternal and childhood helminth infections and of anthelminthic treatment on immune responses to vaccines and childhood infections. The study setting was an area with a moderately high background rate of TB: unpublished data from the Uganda National TB and Leprosy Programme (NTLP) indicates that 929 new pulmonary and extra-pulmonary TB cases were detected in Wakiso district (estimated population 1,205,000) in 2009, an incidence of 77 per 100,000.

Participants in EMaBS were enrolled at the Entebbe Hospital antenatal clinic. Follow-up and enrolment into this sub-study of TB infection was done at the EMaBS outpatient clinic within the hospital grounds. Assessment of the household TB contacts, and verification of the TB cases they were exposed to, was done at the study clinic through verbal interviews of the children's parents or guardians. T-SPOT.TB assays were performed in the main immunology research laboratory at the Uganda Virus Research Institute, a five minute drive from the hospital. Demographic, socioeconomic, and health-related information was collected prospectively from enrolment through to follow-up at five years. Participants were medically examined and anthropometric measurements recorded. All the children were enrolled into the parent study and into the T-SPOT.TB sub-study reported here following informed and documented written consent by their parents or formal guardian. Children were included in this sub-study if they were five years of age, in good health and BCG-immunised. They were excluded if they had moved outside the study area and could not comply with the required procedures, or if the parent or guardian did not give permission for the additional procedures required for this study. Children enrolled in the larger EMaBS study received BCG as neonates [24,25]: 94% of these immunisations were given under observation at Entebbe Hospital, the remainder were given elsewhere. Records were present at the EMaBS study clinic. In the event of active disease or suspected TB infection due to positive immunodiagnostic testing, they were referred to a physician for medical examination, chest X-ray, and treatment if required.

Our initial objective for the study was to estimate the prevalence of LTBI in five year olds. At first we anticipated that T-SPOT.TB could be used to accurately achieve this. For confirmation of the results, and of the repeatability of the T-SPOT.TB test, the initial protocol (Protocol 1) identified three groups of children to undergo, in addition to T-SPOT.TB at age five years, a TST and repeat T-SPOT.TB at follow-up three weeks later: 1) children who were T-SPOT.TB-positive at 5 years, 2) children who were reported to have had household contact with a TB patient, no matter the initial test result, and 3) a comparison sample of approximately 50 T-SPOT.TB-negative children, selected as the first T-SPOT.TB-negative child, willing to undergo the additional procedures, who was seen each week by the study doctor (SAL). Once variations between the initial and repeat T-SPOT.TB results from the same individuals became evident, it was clear that we could not rely on the initial positive result to determine the infection status of a child. The protocol was then amended and all children who underwent the T-SPOT.TB test at five years were asked to undergo the follow-up T-SPOT.TB and TST tests (Protocol 2). By doing this, we hoped to determine whether children with current LTBI could be identified by using T-SPOT.TB as a screening assay, followed by confirmation with repeat T-SPOT.TB combined with TST.

The study was approved by ethics committees of the Uganda Virus Research Institute and London School of Hygiene and Tropical Medicine, and by the Uganda National Council for Science and Technology.

Procedures

T-SPOT.TB assays. Blood samples were processed within eight hours of collection. The assays were carried out according to the manufacturer's instructions (Oxford Immunotec, Abingdon, UK). Briefly, peripheral blood mononuclear cells were isolated by centrifugation, washed twice and the cell concentration was adjusted such that each of four wells of the assay plate contained 250,000 cells. The cells were stimulated for 16–20 hours (under 5% carbon dioxide at 37°C) with media (negative control), phytohaemagglutinin (positive control) or peptides from the TB-specific antigens ESAT-6 or CFP-10. The interferon gamma released by single cells was observed as spots. Automated spot counting was performed using an ELISpot plate reader (AID,

Strassberg, Germany). At the time of performing and reading the assays, persons responsible for reading the test were blind to TST results and other health related information.

Tuberculin skin tests. TST is unlikely to induce false positive T-SPOT.TB responses [26], but might enhance sub-threshold responses, so it was performed after drawing blood for the repeat T-SPOT.TB assay at the follow-up study visit, three weeks after the five-year visit. As recommended by the manufacturer, 2 tuberculin units of RT-23 purified protein derivative (PPD) (Statens Serum Institut, Copenhagen, Denmark) were injected intradermally into the forearm and the diameter of induration was read 48–72 hours later. Tuberculin injections were performed along the longitudinal axis of the forearm, and the diameter of reaction was measured transversely. Reaction sizes greater or equal to 10 mm were considered positive, based on evidence from studies in Malawi that reactions of this size are associated with increased risk of tuberculosis disease in both BCG-immunised and non-immunised individuals, implying that these individuals are latently infected with *M.tb* [27]. The team performing the TSTs was trained by a highly experienced nurse. Dual readings of a proportion of the TSTs (27.9%) were made by two trained study nurses. The readings were made independently by the two nurses and were not shown subsequently to either reader. They showed a very close agreement between the readers: there was a difference in induration in only two of the readings and in both cases the difference was 1 mm. Because of this close agreement, only the readings which were made by the first reader will be included in our analysis. Tuberculin was kept under refrigeration when not in use.

Data Analysis

Personal data and TST results were captured into Microsoft Access databases. Data were double-entered and then checked by the study data manager for integrity and consistency. Spot counts were retrieved from the automated plate reader and entered into Microsoft Excel. In accordance with the manufacturer's instructions, T-SPOT.TB responses were considered positive if either or both of panel A (containing ESAT-6 peptides) or panel B (containing CFP-10 peptides) had six or more spot forming units (SFUs) above the negative control when the negative control had five or less SFUs. In cases where the negative control had six to 10 SFUs, the result was defined as positive when either the ESAT-6- or CFP-10- stimulated well contained at least twice as many SFUs as the negative control well. The result was considered indeterminate if the positive control had less than 20 SFUs (unless either panel A or panel B was positive, as described above, in which case the result was valid), or if the negative control well had 10 or more SFUs. Data analysis was performed with STATA 10.0 (StataCorp, College Station, Texas, USA). Concordance between baseline and repeat T-SPOT.TB, and between T-SPOT.TB and TST was calculated using the kappa (κ) statistic, and assessed according to the criteria suggested by Landis and Koch [28]. Strength of association between SFUs recorded for the two RD1 antigens was estimated by calculating Spearman's rank correlation coefficient (r_s). Proportions with positive TST results were compared between groups defined by T-SPOT.TB results using a chi-squared test. The chi-squared test was also used to compare the number of participants for whom the two T-SPOT.TB results agreed, and for whom T-SPOT.TB and TST results agreed, between household contacts and non-household contacts. A 5% significance level (two-sided $p = 0.05$) was used for all tests.

Results

Characteristics of the Study Population

The Entebbe Mother and Baby Study (EMaBS) recruited 2507 pregnant women. Information was obtained on 2345 live births and 1622 were under follow-up at five years, of whom 1438 were seen by the study physicians at age five. Of these, 907 took part in the T-SPOT.TB study. Of the 531 who did not take part in the study, 186 had passed age five before the study began, the parents or guardians of 237 did not give consent, and 108 had moved outside the study area and could not comply with the required procedures. Mothers of participants who took part in the T-SPOT.TB study were on average older, more educated, and of higher socio-economic status than mothers of those who were not included in this study. The participants themselves were less likely to be HIV infected than those who were not included in this study. Of the 907 participants, 432 (47.6%) were female and 475 (52.4%) were male. In total, 56 (6.2%) were household contacts of TB patients, defined as being reported to have been in household contact with a known TB case at any time during the past five years. Analysis of anthropometric data showed a low level of undernutrition, with prevalence of wasting (weight-for-height z-score <-2) at 5.4%. Only 13 (1.4%) of the participants were HIV infected, and prevalence of other infections was relatively low, with 4.0% of children having asymptomatic malaria infection and 9.6% of children having a helminth infection. Where relevant, we assessed the results from Protocol 1 (before amendment; 546 participants), and Protocol 2 (after amendment; 361 participants) separately. The flow of participants in Protocol 1 and Protocol 2 is shown in Figure 1 and Figure 2. The prevalence of wasting was higher for children recruited under Protocol 1 compared to those recruited under Protocol 2 (prevalence 7.6% versus 1.9%, $p = 0.001$). The prevalence of HIV, asymptomatic malaria, and any helminth infection did not differ between the two Protocols ($p = 0.92$, 0.46 and 0.49, respectively). Only one child, among those that were household TB contacts, or those that were T-SPOT.TB and/or TST positive, was diagnosed with active TB.

T-SPOT.TB at Five Years and at Follow-up

Overall, at five years, 88 (9.7%) children were positive for T-SPOT.TB, 770 (84.9%) were negative, and the remaining 49 (5.4%) were indeterminate. We re-examined 405 children at follow-up approximately three weeks later (Figure 1 and Figure 2). Excluding indeterminate results from both tests, 356 children were eligible for direct comparison between the baseline and the repeat T-SPOT.TB assay. For both protocols, agreement between T-SPOT.TB at five years and T-SPOT.TB at follow-up was weak (protocol 1, $\kappa = 0.37$; protocol 2, $\kappa = 0.35$). More than half of those that were positive on the first test were negative on the second in both protocols, whereas, excluding indeterminate results, 96% of the baseline negatives were consistently negative at follow-up (Figure 1 and Figure 2).

In order to ascertain whether spot counts were concentrated around the diagnostic test cut-off level for participants whose T-SPOT.TB result varied between age five and follow-up, we analysed median changes in spot counts for each RD-1 antigen according to whether participants were T-SPOT.TB positive on the first test and negative on the second test (+/−) or T-SPOT.TB negative on the first test and positive on the second (−/+) (Table 1). Although some spot counts were close to the cut-off on the repeat assay, many of the children who were either +/− or −/+ had SFUs considerably above the cut-off for their positive test: the median change in spot counts between the two tests ranged from six to 17.5 SFUs.

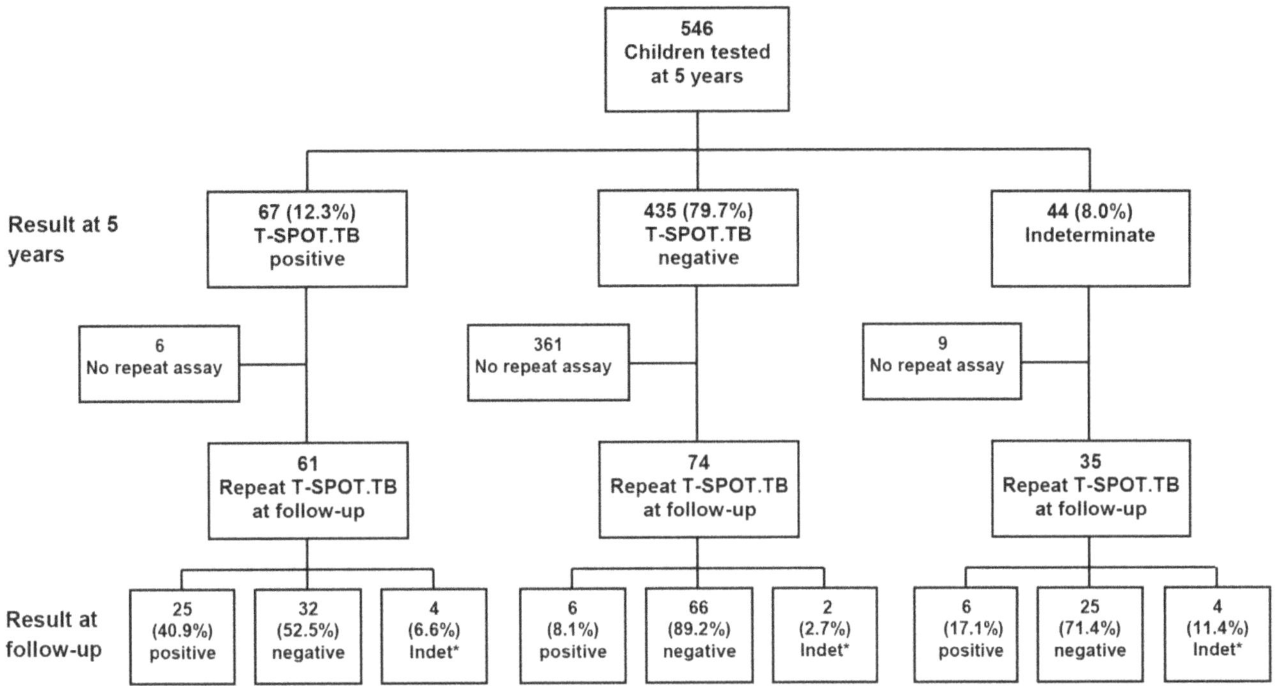

Figure 1. T-SPOT.TB assay results at five years and at follow-up: Protocol 1.

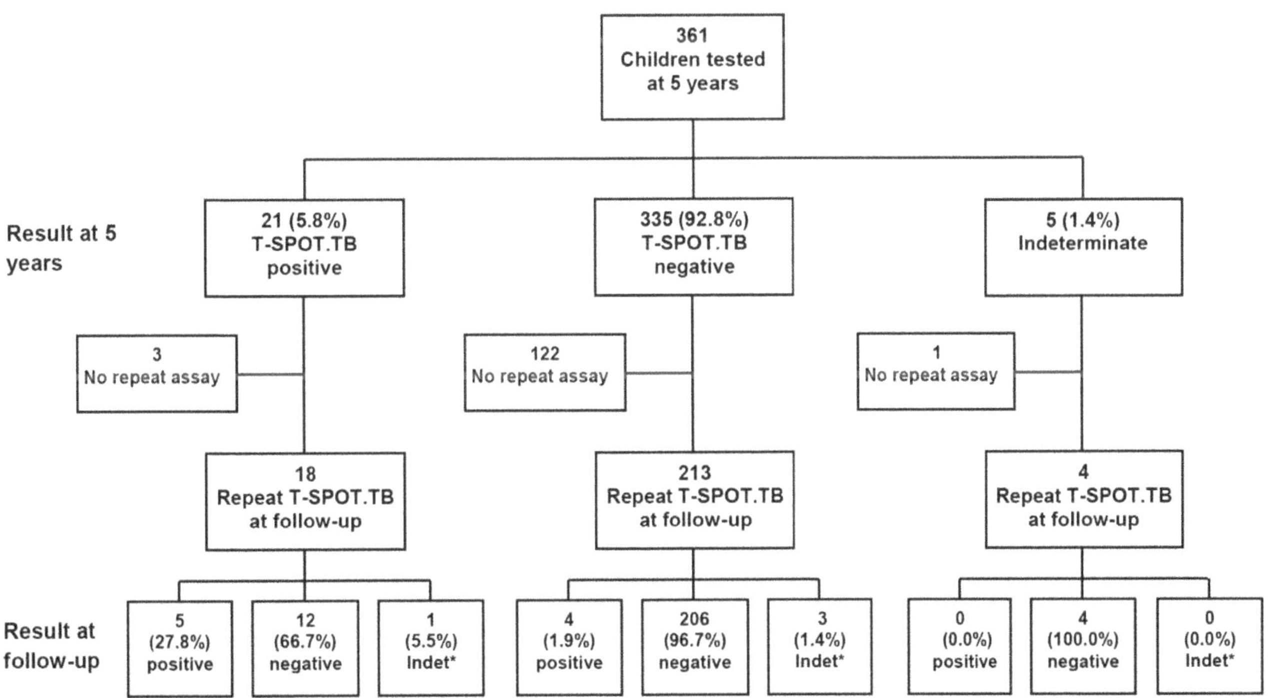

Figure 2. T-SPOT.TB assay results at five years and at follow-up: Protocol 2.

Table 1. Median difference in spot counts to ESAT-6 and CFP-10 for participants whose T-SPOT.TB result varied between age five and follow-up.

	T-SPOT.TB result Initial/follow-up	Observations	Median difference in SFUs	IQR
ESAT-6				
Protocol 1	+/−	32	−12.00	−32.25, −4.00
	−/+	6	10.50	3.75, 13.50
Protocol 2	+/−	12	−9.50	−12.00, −7.25
	−/+	4	6.50	1.25, 11.00
CFP-10				
Protocol 1	+/−	32	−17.50	−25.75, −8.50
	−/+	6	6.00	2.5, 17.75
Protocol 2	+/−	12	−6.50	−11.75, −3.00
	−/+	4	7.00	2.25, 11.00

SFUs: spot forming units; IQR: interquartile range; + indicates positive result; − indicates negative result.

T-SPOT.TB and TST at Follow-up

Having demonstrated that variations between the initial and repeat T-SPOT.TB results were not characteristic only of protocol 1, we combined results from both protocols to compare T-SPOT.TB and TST results. Data for this analysis were therefore biased towards children with a positive first T-SPOT.TB result, and with a history of contact with a TB patient. Results from all three tests (T-SPOT.TB at five years and at follow-up, and TST at follow-up) were available for 319 children (Table 2). Agreement between T-SPOT.TB and TST was weak ($\kappa = 0.28$ for T-SPOT.TB assay at 5 years and $\kappa = 0.40$ for T-SPOT.TB at follow-up). Combining T-SPOT.TB results, among children who were negative on both T-SPOT.TB tests, 5 (2.2%) had a positive TST; of those who were positive on only one T-SPOT.TB test, 4 (8.2%) had a positive TST; and of those who were positive on both tests, 14 (50%) had a positive TST ($p<0.001$: Table 2). The 14 children who were positive on all three tests constituted only 4.4% of the 319 children who had all three tests done.

We evaluated sizes of TST induration among children who had differing T-SPOT.TB and TST results (Table 3), to establish whether discordant results were associated with sizes close to the 10 mm cut-off. Children who were TST positive but T-SPOT.TB negative at both time points tended to have TST indurations close to the cut-off. By contrast, all but one of the 14 children who were TST negative but T-SPOT.TB positive at both time points had no detectable induration. Children who were T-SPOT.TB positive at only one time point had large sizes of TST induration if they were TST positive, but small or no detectable induration if they were TST negative. These results paint a general picture that the high level of disagreement between T-SPOT.TB and TST was not due to threshold TST values.

Table 2. Agreement between T-SPOT.TB and TST results.

T-SPOT.TB result at 5 years	T-SPOT.TB result at follow-up	TST result −	TST result +	Total
-	-	218 (97.8%)	5 (2.2%)	223
-	+	8 (88.9%)	1 (11.1%)	9
+	-	37 (92.5%)	3 (7.5%)	40
+	+	14 (50.0%)	14 (50.0%)	28
Indeterminate at either time point		18 (94.7%)	1 (5.3%)	19

+ indicates positive result; − indicates negative result.

Correlation between RD1 Antigens

To determine whether there was a correlation between ESAT-6 and CFP-10 RD1 antigens, we analysed spot counts in greater detail (Figure 3). Correlation between ESAT-6 and CFP-10 spot counts at five years was high ($r_s = 0.75$), as was correlation at follow-up ($r_s = 0.78$). By contrast, correlation between ESAT-6 spot counts at five years and at follow-up was low ($r_s = 0.35$), as was correlation between CFP-10 spot counts at five years and at follow-up ($r_s = 0.31$). Thus, ESAT-6 and CFP-10 strongly correlated with each other at a given time point, but each individual antigen correlated poorly with itself at the two distinct time points. This was also observed when analysis of spot counts was done separately for each protocol (data not shown). These results indicate that the same individuals were responding to both RD1 antigens at a given time point, but that different individuals were responding at different time points. This was consistent with the high levels of unstable responses observed between baseline and follow-up.

Household Contacts of TB Patients

We enrolled 56 household contacts (HHC) of TB patients at five years. Of these, 41 had a repeat T-SPOT.TB test at follow-up and a TST result was available for 35. Excluding indeterminate results, there was better agreement between initial and follow-up T-SPOT.TB results among household TB contacts than among non-contacts ($\kappa = 0.77$ and 0.39 respectively; $p = 0.15$): of those HHC who were positive at five years, 70% were also positive at follow-up, and all the HHC who were negative at five years were also negative at follow-up. However, agreement between positive T-SPOT.TB and TST was still weak: of the six HHC who were positive on both T-SPOT.TB tests, only two had a positive skin test. All the 27 HHC who were negative on both T-SPOT.TB tests

Table 3. Assessment of size of TST in relation to T-SPOT.TB and TST results.

T-SPOT.TB result at 5 years	T-SPOT.TB result at follow-up	TST result	Number of children	Median size of TST induration (mm)	IQR
–	–	–	218	0.0	0.0, 0.0
–	–	+	5	11.0	10.0, 13.0
+	+	+	14	15.0	13.7, 17.5
+	+	–	14	0.0	0.0, 0.0
positive at either time point		+	4	16.5	11.0, 19.7
positive at either time point		–	45	0.0	0.0, 0.0

IQR: interquartile range; + indicates positive result; – indicates negative result.

were also negative with the TST. Household TB contacts also experienced somewhat higher proportions of T-SPOT.TB positivity (17.8% vs. 9.2%; p = 0.045 at baseline and 17.1% vs. 10.7%; p = 0.265 at follow-up) and TST positivity (11.4% vs. 7.0%; p = 0.353), than non-contacts. Age of first exposure was available for 36 (64%) HHC. Five children were exposed as infants, two as one-year olds, seven as three-year olds, five as four-year olds and 17 were exposed in the year preceding enrolment in this study.

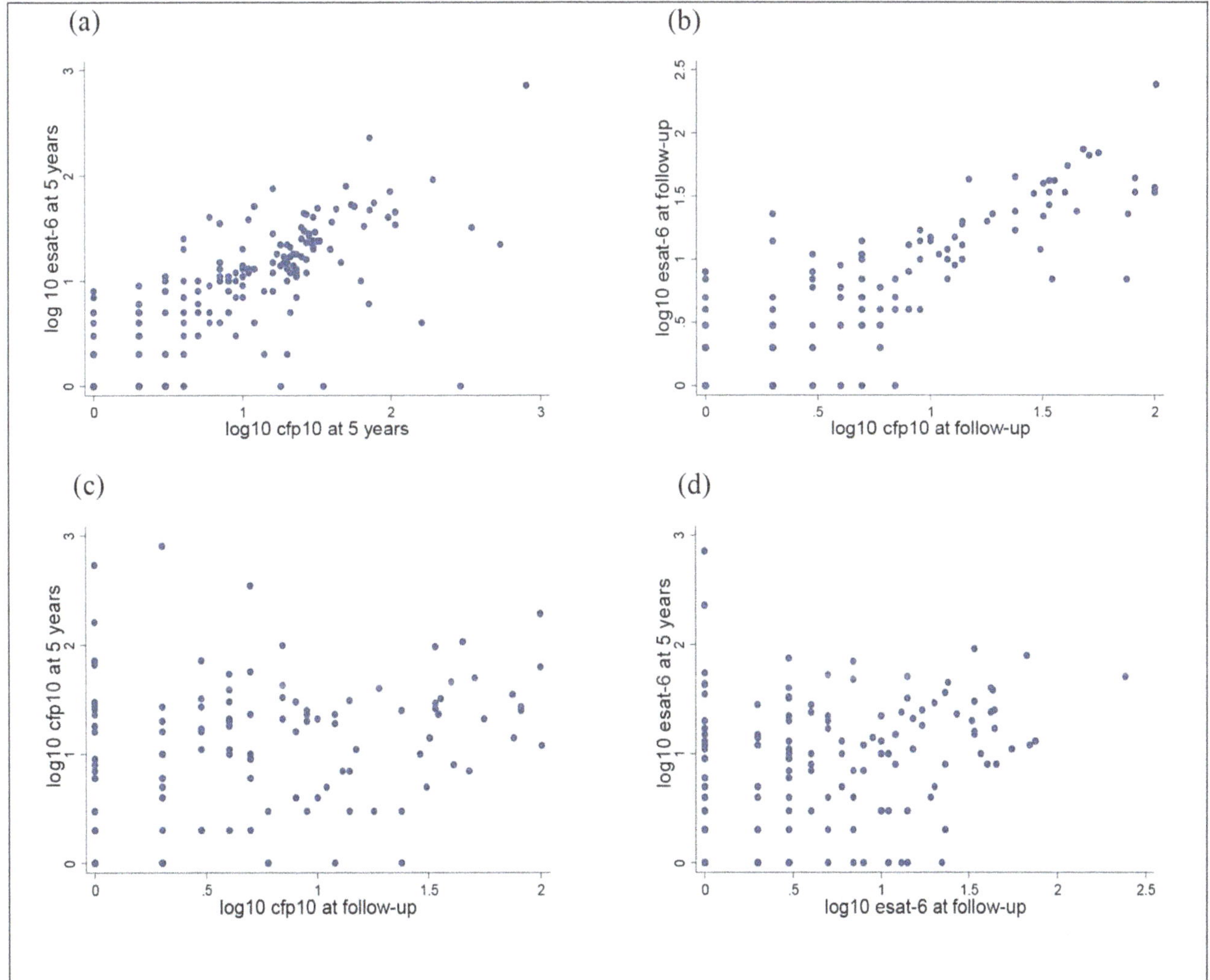

Figure 3. Association between RD1 antigens at five years and at follow-up. Results are presented as logs (to base 10) of spot forming units for the two RD1 antigens. (a) ESAT-6 at five years vs.CFP-10 at five years (n = 179); $r_s = 0.7548$ (b) ESAT-6 follow-up vs. CFP-10 follow-up (n = 158); $r_s = 0.7838$ (c) CFP-10 at five years vs. CFP-10 at follow-up (n = 127); $r_s = 0.3125$ (d) ESAT -6 at five years vs. ESAT-6 at follow-up (n = 163); $r_s = 0.3576$.

There was no evidence of a trend in probability of a positive test result with age of exposure for T-SPOT.TB ($p = 0.44$ at enrolment, $p = 0.36$ at follow-up) or for TST ($p = 0.80$).

Tuberculosis Infection Prevalence Estimates

The infection prevalence estimates by different measures are shown in Table 4. A single T-SPOT.TB result at five years would estimate infection prevalence at 9.7% among children in our study, whereas a more stringent criterion of a positive TST and positive T-SPOT.TB at both time points would put the prevalence at 1.5%. From our data, the true infection prevalence in this population of children lies somewhere between 1.5% and 11.2%, highlighting the complexity of estimating LTBI in this age group and setting, using T-SPOT.TB and/or TST.

Discussion

Our aim was to use the T-SPOT.TB assay to determine *M.tb* infection prevalence among *M.tb* exposed and unexposed five year old children in Entebbe, Uganda. We anticipated that positive responses would be confirmed with a second T-SPOT.TB assay and a TST. However, we have demonstrated a high level of instability in positive T-SPOT.TB responses between baseline and a three week follow-up and poor agreement between T-SPOT.TB and TST responses, making the categorisation of children as LTB-infected or LTB-uninfected difficult.

Analysis of SFUs showed that positive responses were not concentrated around the diagnostic test cut-off level for children whose T-SPOT.TB result varied between the first and second tests. Instead, some children showed large changes in response – both increases and decreases in SFUs – between the two assessments. In contrast, ESAT-6 and CFP-10 spot counts correlated well at each time point. Together these findings suggest that our results may reflect a true change in the immune response to the *M.tb* antigens in peripheral blood. Several other studies, albeit with longer term follow-up, have observed variations in responses between baseline and follow-up [14,21,29]. In a bid to explain changes on follow-up when using IGRAs, Hill *et al.* suggested that IGRA responses are not long-lived and generally require sustained, continuous exposure to *M.tb* antigens to maintain high frequencies [14]. They hypothesized that the decline in response following exposure to *M.tb* may be a reflection of the lifecycle of *M.tb* and the dynamic interaction with the host immune system. As the mycobacteria enter a state of dormancy, secretion of ESAT-6 and CFP-10 may decline leading to a decrease in circulating memory T cells specific for the antigens used in the assay [14,30]. The weak association between T-SPOT.TB and TST in our study raises a further question as to whether the responses observed indicate LTBI at all. It may be that the unstable positive T-SPOT.TB responses in this young age group reflect a weak (perhaps transient) response to *M.tb* antigens in BCG-immunised children who resist the establishment of latent infection. However, the short time between the two assessments in our study make it unlikely that a change in TB exposure could account for the effects observed.

Some studies have described a rather high rate of changes from negative to positive IGRA response during follow-up in high-risk populations in endemic settings [29,30]. Incident infections might explain this, especially in studies involving contacts of TB patients, or, again, the intermittent secretion of ESAT-6 and CFP-10 by *M.tb*. However, in our study, changes from negative to positive were very few compared to changes from positive to negative.

Fluctuation in IGRA results upon serial testing has sometimes been attributed to technical factors. These factors may include blood volume (for QuantiFERON assays), different staff performing the assay, preanalytical delays and reagents. The T-SPOT.TB assay uses blood volumes as low as 2 ml; we collected 4 ml on average. Most of the assays were performed by the study laboratory technologists (GN and JEL), and any other staff performing the assay were given specialist training and worked under the supervision of the study laboratory technologists. Doberne *et al.* [31] recently demonstrated that preanalytical delay resulted in increased positive-to-negative reversions in as little as six hours. Such delays were not characteristic of our study (median time after sample collection = 1.4 hours, IQR 50 min-2.2 hours), so time to processing is unlikely to explain our observed fluctuations. A recent systematic review [20] showed that tuberculin skin testing has a boosting effect on IGRA responses, but this cannot explain the observed fluctuations in our study because we drew blood before performing the TST.

Longitudinal assessments for IGRAs in published literature have mainly been in contacts of TB patients [11,29,32,33]. Our study investigated children, most of whom had no known TB contacts. We hypothesize that the intense exposure that TB contacts experience, compared to non-contacts, may explain the more stable responses observed in those studies. In keeping with this hypothesis, we found that household TB contacts in our study showed better agreement between the baseline and repeat test although the number of contacts was too small to provide good power for sub-group analyses.

T-SPOT.TB has been dubbed the "100-year upgrade" to the well-established TST for the diagnosis of TB infection [34].

Table 4. *Mycobacterium tuberculosis* infection prevalence estimates by different measures.

Measure of infection	Number	Prevalence estimate (95% CI)
Positive on all three tests (T-SPOT.TB at baseline and follow-up, TST at follow-up)*	14	1.5% (0.8%–2.6%)
Positive T-SPOT.TB result at either or both time points, and a positive TST**	18	2.0% (1.2%–3.1%)
Positive T-SPOT.TB result at both time points*	30	3.3% (2.2%–3.7%)
Positive T-SPOT.TB result at baseline	88	9.7% (7.9%–11.8%)
Any one positive T-SPOT.TB result**	98	10.8% (8.9%–13.0%)
Any one positive result (T-SPOT.TB or TST)**	102	11.2% (9.3%–13.5%)

The denominator is 907 for all the estimates.
*All but 9 of the baseline T-SPOT.TB positives were followed up. Prevalence doesn't change when the 9 are subtracted from the denominator.
**Does not take into account the baseline T-SPOT.TB negatives that were not followed up, yet might have turned positive on follow-up. This is not likely to change the prevalence estimates, since most (96%) of the baseline negatives that were followed up remained negative.

However, we report a high level of disagreement between the TST and T-SPOT.TB in our cohort of children. Previous studies have shown that levels of agreement are varied depending on the study and outcome measurement. For example, in four investigations that analysed agreement between the two tests, the κ scores ranged from -0.15 to 0.76 [16,35–37]. In our group, recent unpublished data from adult women in Entebbe showed that T-SPOT.TB performed better as an indicator of LTBI among adults. Among 23 women who tested T-SPOT.TB positive, 21 (91%) were TST positive as well. All these findings support the perception that agreement between the TST and the IGRA in the diagnosis of TB infection might vary depending on several factors such as age, history of previous BCG vaccination [38], and infection with other mycobacteria.

The immunological inferences that can be drawn from the observed discordance between T-SPOT.TB and TST in our study are unclear. TST results may be falsely negative in children due to the influence of factors such as malnutrition, concurrent viral and/or parasitic infections, and concurrent medical conditions and diseases [39]. However, these factors were not characteristic of our participants. For example, we had TST data for six of the 13 HIV positive participants, and none of these had discordant T-SPOT.TB and TST results. The children in this study were BCG-immunised, making it possible that the discordances observed were due to false TST positives, but this is unlikely because we observed fewer positives by TST than by T-SPOT.TB. Furthermore, there was a general lack of intermediate sized TST responses, which have been attributed to BCG vaccination and infection with mycobacteria other than tuberculosis [40–42]. The discordances may therefore be due to the unstable T-SPOT.TB responses between baseline and follow-up, rather than a result of the known shortcomings of the TST.

Tuberculin surveys carried out in the 1970s suggested that the annual risk infection (ARI) with TB in Uganda was approximately 3%, although rates were lower than this in young children [43]. Recent national reports and other studies continue to quote this estimate [44–47] although some surveys have indicated a steady decline in ARI – for example, a survey in northern Uganda in 1994 estimated ARI at 1.4% [48]. Our results suggest that this may now be a more realistic figure for young children in Central Uganda also. However, our study cohort was derived from a small area, and those who participated in this study showed some biases. New *M.tb* infection surveys of broader scope may be warranted for Uganda.

The principal limitation of our study was the change in protocol, resulting in variation in sample sizes for T-SPOT.TB at five years (n = 907), repeat T-SPOT.TB at follow-up (n = 405) and TST (n = 319) making it difficult to compare the three tests directly. Secondly, the proportions of children followed up were different depending on the child's T-SPOT.TB result at five years: this was expected with Protocol 1 but not with Protocol 2, where 85.7% of the children who were initially positive were followed up compared to 63.6% of those who were initially negative. Data analysis was therefore biased towards children with a positive first T-SPOT.TB result. We attempted to overcome this limitation by presenting results from Protocol 1 and Protocol 2 separately where it was relevant, and by comparing the participants' characteristics between the two protocols.

Our data provide a valuable insight into the usefulness of IGRAs in the diagnosis of TB infection among children living in endemic settings. It has been suggested that recommendations on use of IGRAs in children younger than five years and in immunocompromised children should be taken with caution because of a lack of adequate published data on their efficacy in these groups [49,50]. Our study has contributed to the increasing evidence that IGRAs may not be superior to TST in children in high incidence settings and cannot be used alone to diagnose TB infection in these settings. Diagnosis of TB infection and estimating TB infection prevalence among children in high incidence settings remains a challenge; better diagnostic tests are still needed.

Acknowledgments

We thank all staff and participants of the Entebbe Mother and Baby Study. We are also grateful to Patrice Mawa for contributing unpublished data for the discussion.

Author Contributions

Conceived and designed the experiments: AME. Performed the experiments: GN JEL IS DK. Analyzed the data: GN JRF LM ELW. Wrote the paper: GN ELW JRF SC AME. Recruited, did follow-up, investigated and provided clinical care for participants: SAL HA RK.

References

1. WHO (2011) Global tuberculosis control: WHO report 2011. Geneva: WHO.
2. Pai M, Joshi R, Dogra S, Mendiratta DK, Narang P, et al. (2006) Persistently elevated T cell interferon-gamma responses after treatment for latent tuberculosis infection among health care workers in India: a preliminary report. J Occup Med Toxicol 1: 7.
3. Cruz AT, Geltemeyer AM, Starke JR, Flores JA, Graviss EA, et al. (2011) Comparing the tuberculin skin test and T-SPOT.TB blood test in children. Pediatrics 127: e31–38.
4. Lucas M, Nicol P, McKinnon E, Whidborne R, Lucas A, et al. (2010) A prospective large-scale study of methods for the detection of latent Mycobacterium tuberculosis infection in refugee children. Thorax 65: 442–448.
5. Newton SM, Brent AJ, Anderson S, Whittaker E, Kampmann B (2008) Paediatric tuberculosis. Lancet Infect Dis 8: 498–510.
6. Ewer K, Deeks J, Alvarez L, Bryant G, Waller S, et al. (2003) Comparison of T-cell-based assay with tuberculin skin test for diagnosis of Mycobacterium tuberculosis infection in a school tuberculosis outbreak. Lancet 361: 1168–1173.
7. Lalvani A (2007) Diagnosing tuberculosis infection in the 21st century: new tools to tackle an old enemy. Chest 131: 1898–1906.
8. Lalvani A, Nagvenkar P, Udwadia Z, Pathan AA, Wilkinson KA, et al. (2001) Enumeration of T cells specific for RD1-encoded antigens suggests a high prevalence of latent Mycobacterium tuberculosis infection in healthy urban Indians. J Infect Dis 183: 469–477.
9. Lalvani A, Pathan AA, Durkan H, Wilkinson KA, Whelan A, et al. (2001) Enhanced contact tracing and spatial tracking of Mycobacterium tuberculosis infection by enumeration of antigen-specific T cells. Lancet 357: 2017–2021.
10. Chee CB, KhinMar KW, Gan SH, Barkham TM, Pushparani M, et al. (2007) Latent tuberculosis infection treatment and T-cell responses to Mycobacterium tuberculosis-specific antigens. Am J Respir Crit Care Med 175: 282–287.
11. Menzies D, Pai M, Comstock G (2007) Meta-analysis: new tests for the diagnosis of latent tuberculosis infection: areas of uncertainty and recommendations for research. Ann Intern Med 146: 340–354.
12. Joshi R, Narang U, Zwerling A, Jain D, Jain V, et al. (2011) Predictive value of latent tuberculosis tests in Indian healthcare workers: a cohort study. Eur Respir J 38: 1475–1477.
13. Shams H, Weis SE, Klucar P, Lalvani A, Moonan PK, et al. (2005) Enzyme-linked immunospot and tuberculin skin testing to detect latent tuberculosis infection. Am J Respir Crit Care Med 172: 1161–1168.
14. Hill PC, Brookes RH, Fox A, Jackson-Sillah D, Jeffries DJ, et al. (2007) Longitudinal assessment of an ELISPOT test for Mycobacterium tuberculosis infection. PLoS Med 4: e192.
15. Mutsvangwa J, Millington KA, Chaka K, Mavhudzi T, Cheung YB, et al. (2010) Identifying recent Mycobacterium tuberculosis transmission in the setting of high HIV and TB burden. Thorax 65: 315–320.
16. Soysal A, Millington KA, Bakir M, Dosanjh D, Aslan Y, et al. (2005) Effect of BCG vaccination on risk of Mycobacterium tuberculosis infection in children with household tuberculosis contact: a prospective community-based study. Lancet 366: 1443–1451.
17. Okada K, Mao TE, Mori T, Miura T, Sugiyama T, et al. (2008) Performance of an interferon-gamma release assay for diagnosing latent tuberculosis infection in children. Epidemiol Infect 136: 1179–1187.

18. Machingaidze S, Wiysonge CS, Gonzalez-Angulo Y, Hatherill M, Moyo S, et al. (2011) The utility of an interferon gamma release assay for diagnosis of latent tuberculosis infection and disease in children: a systematic review and meta-analysis. Pediatr Infect Dis J 30: 694–700.
19. WHO (2011) Use of tuberculosis interferon gamma release assays (IGRAs) in low- and medium- income countries: Policy statement. Geneva: WHO.
20. van Zyl-Smit RN, Zwerling A, Dheda K, Pai M (2009) Within-subject variability of interferon-g assay results for tuberculosis and boosting effect of tuberculin skin testing: a systematic review. PLoS One 4: e8517.
21. Pai M, Joshi R, Dogra S, Zwerling AA, Gajalakshmi D, et al. (2009) T-cell assay conversions and reversions among household contacts of tuberculosis patients in rural India. Int J Tuberc Lung Dis 13: 84–92.
22. Herrera V, Perry S, Parsonnet J, Banaei N (2011) Clinical application and limitations of interferon-gamma release assays for the diagnosis of latent tuberculosis infection. Clin Infect Dis 52: 1031–1037.
23. Elliott AM, Kizza M, Quigley MA, Ndibazza J, Nampijja M, et al. (2007) The impact of helminths on the response to immunization and on the incidence of infection and disease in childhood in Uganda: design of a randomized, double-blind, placebo-controlled, factorial trial of deworming interventions delivered in pregnancy and early childhood [ISRCTN32849447]. Clin Trials 4: 42–57.
24. Anderson EJ, Webb EL, Mawa PA, Kizza M, Lyadda N, et al. (2012) The influence of BCG vaccine strain on mycobacteria-specific and non-specific immune responses in a prospective cohort of infants in Uganda. Vaccine 30: 2083–2089.
25. Elliott AM, Mawa PA, Webb EL, Nampijja M, Lyadda N, et al. (2010) Effects of maternal and infant co-infections, and of maternal immunisation, on the infant response to BCG and tetanus immunisation. Vaccine 29: 247–255.
26. Sauzullo I, Massetti AP, Mengoni F, Rossi R, Lichtner M, et al. (2011) Influence of previous tuberculin skin test on serial IFN-gamma release assays. Tuberculosis (Edinb) 91: 322–326.
27. Fine PE, Sterne JA, Ponnighaus JM, Rees RJ (1994) Delayed-type hypersensitivity, mycobacterial vaccines and protective immunity. Lancet 344: 1245–1249.
28. Landis JR, Koch GG (1977) The measurement of observer agreement for categorical data. Biometrics 33: 159–174.
29. Pai M, Joshi R, Dogra S, Mendiratta DK, Narang P, et al. (2006) Serial testing of health care workers for tuberculosis using interferon-gamma assay. Am J Respir Crit Care Med 174: 349–355.
30. Pai M, O'Brien R (2007) Serial testing for tuberculosis: can we make sense of T cell assay conversions and reversions? PLoS Med 4: e208.
31. Doberne D, Gaur RL, Banaei N (2011) Preanalytical delay reduces sensitivity of QuantiFERON-TB gold in-tube assay for detection of latent tuberculosis infection. J Clin Microbiol 49: 3061–3064.
32. Detjen AK, Loebenberg L, Grewal HM, Stanley K, Gutschmidt A, et al. (2009) Short-term reproducibility of a commercial interferon gamma release assay. Clin Vaccine Immunol 16: 1170–1175.
33. Perry S, Sanchez L, Yang S, Agarwal Z, Hurst P, et al. (2008) Reproducibility of QuantiFERON-TB gold in-tube assay. Clin Vaccine Immunol 15: 425–432.
34. Barnes PF (2001) Diagnosing latent tuberculosis infection: the 100-year upgrade. Am J Respir Crit Care Med 163: 807–808.
35. Codecasa L, Mantegani P, Galli L, Lazzarin A, Scarpellini P, et al. (2006) An in-house RD1-based enzyme-linked immunospot-gamma interferon assay instead of the tuberculin skin test for diagnosis of latent Mycobacterium tuberculosis infection. J Clin Microbiol 44: 1944–1950.
36. Ferrara G, Losi M, D'Amico R, Roversi P, Piro R, et al. (2006) Use in routine clinical practice of two commercial blood tests for diagnosis of infection with Mycobacterium tuberculosis: a prospective study. Lancet 367: 1328–1334.
37. Hesseling AC, Mandalakas AM, Kirchner HL, Chegou NN, Marais BJ, et al. (2009) Highly discordant T cell responses in individuals with recent exposure to household tuberculosis. Thorax 64: 840–846.
38. Bakir M, Millington KA, Soysal A, Deeks JJ, Efee S, et al. (2008) Prognostic value of a T-cell-based, interferon-gamma biomarker in children with tuberculosis contact. Ann Intern Med 149: 777–787.
39. Kakkar F, Allen U, Ling D, Pai M, Kitai I (2010) Tuberculosis in children: New diagnostic blood tests. Can J Infect Dis Med Microbiol 21: e111–115.
40. Wang L, Turner MO, Elwood RK, Schulzer M, FitzGerald JM (2002) A meta-analysis of the effect of Bacille Calmette Guerin vaccination on tuberculin skin test measurements. Thorax 57: 804–809.
41. Chee CB, Soh CH, Boudville IC, Chor SS, Wang YT (2001) Interpretation of the tuberculin skin test in Mycobacterium bovis BCG-vaccinated Singaporean schoolchildren. Am J Respir Crit Care Med 164: 958–961.
42. Tissot F, Zanetti G, Francioli P, Zellweger JP, Zysset F (2005) Influence of bacille Calmette-Guerin vaccination on size of tuberculin skin test reaction: to what size? Clin Infect Dis 40: 211–217.
43. Stott H, Patel A, Sutherland I, Thorup I, Smith PG, et al. (1973) The risk of tuberculous infection in Uganda, deprived from the findings of national tuberculin surveys 1958 and 1970. Tubercle 54: 1–22.
44. National Tuberculosis and Leprosy Program (2005) Uganda National Program surveillance Report for 2004. Kampala, Uganda.
45. Uganda MoH (2006) National Policy Guidelines for TB/HIV Collaborative Activities in Uganda. Ministry of Health.
46. Uganda MoH (2010) Manual of the National Tuberculosis and Leprosy Programme. Uganda: Ministry of Health.
47. Stein CM, Zalwango S, Malone LL, Won S, Mayanja-Kizza H, et al. (2008) Genome scan of M. tuberculosis infection and disease in Ugandans. PLoS One 3: e4094.
48. Migliori GB, Borghesi A, Spanevello A, Eriki P, Raviglione M, et al. (1994) Risk of infection and estimated incidence of tuberculosis in Northern Uganda. Eur Respir J 7: 946–953.
49. Mazurek GH, Jereb J, Vernon A, LoBue P, Goldberg S, et al. (2010) Updated guidelines for using Interferon Gamma Release Assays to detect Mycobacterium tuberculosis infection - United States, 2010. MMWR Recomm Rep 59: 1–25.
50. Report CCD (2008) Updated recommendations on interferon gamma release assays for latent tuberculosis infection. An Advisory Committee Statement (ACS). Can Commun Dis Rep 34: 1–13.

6

Predominance of Norovirus and Sapovirus in Nicaragua after Implementation of Universal Rotavirus Vaccination

Filemón Bucardo[1], Yaoska Reyes[1], Lennart Svensson[2], Johan Nordgren[2*]

1 Department of Microbiology, University of León (UNAN-León), León, Nicaragua, 2 Division of Molecular Virology, Department of Clinical and Experimental Medicine, Linköping University, Linköping, Sweden

Abstract

Background: Despite significant reduction of rotavirus (RV) infections following implementation of RotaTeq vaccination in Nicaragua, a large burden of patients with diarrhea persists.

Methods: We conducted a community- and hospital-based study of the burden of RV, norovirus (NV) and sapovirus (SV) infections as cause of sporadic acute gastroenteritis (GE) among 330 children ≤ 5 years of age between September 2009 and October 2010 in two major cities of Nicaragua with a RotaTeq coverage rate of 95%.

Results: We found that NV, SV and RV infections altogether accounted for 45% of cases of GE. Notably, NV was found in 24% (79/330) of the children, followed by SV (17%, 57/330) and RV (8%, 25/330). The detection rate in the hospital setting was 27%, 15% and 14% for NV, SV and RV respectively, whereas in the community setting the detection rate of RV was < 1%. Among each of the investigated viruses one particular genogroup or genotype was dominant; GII.4 (82%) for NV, GI (46%) for SV and G1P[8] (64%) in RV. These variants were also found in higher proportions in the hospital setting compared to the community setting. The GII.4.2006 Minerva strain circulating globally since 2006 was the most common among genotyped NV in this study, with the GII.4-2010 New Orleans emerging in 2010.

Conclusions: This study shows that NV has become the leading viral cause of gastroenteritis at hospital and community settings in Nicaragua after implementation of RV vaccination.

Editor: Li-Min Huang, National Taiwan University Hospital, Taiwan

Funding: This study was supported by grants from the Network for Research and Training in Tropical Diseases in Central America (NeTropica, Grant:05-N-2010) and Swedish Research Council (grants 10392 and 348-2011-7420). The funders had no role in study design, data collection and analysis, decision to publish, or preparation of the manuscript.

Competing Interests: The authors have declared that no competing interests exist.

* E-mail: johan.nordgren@liu.se

Introduction

Acute gastroenteritis (GE) is one of the leading causes of morbidity and mortality in children in the developing countries, with rotavirus (RV) and norovirus (NV) being the major causes of pediatric viral GE, altogether associated with approximately 800,000 deaths in young children every year [1–3]. In contrast, sapovirus (SV) infections are more rarely reported and generally considered to cause milder symptoms, with detection rates rarely reaching 10% [4–8].

A major reduction of severe RVGE has been observed in countries with high vaccine coverage but comprehensive analysis in several clinical trials indicates the vaccine efficacy to be lower in countries with high RV mortality [9,10]. In October 2006, the Nicaraguan Expanded Program of Immunization (EPI) initiated universal RV vaccination with the pentavalent RV vaccine from Merck (RotaTeq), which is orally administrated in a 3-dose regimen to children at 2, 4, and 6 months of age. Vaccine coverage rapidly reached over > 90% in eligible Nicaraguan children [11]. A case control study evaluating RotaTeq in 2007–2008 in Nicaragua showed that vaccination was associated with a lower risk of RVGE in children younger than 2 years [12], but to a lesser extent than observed in clinical trials in Europe and USA [13]. The efficacy in Nicaragua against severe RV diarrhea was only 58%, which is similar to other studies from Asian and African countries [12,14,15]. In the post-vaccine period, a study found that 3.5% of outpatient children seeking care for diarrhea were positive for RV [16]. However, while RV incidence has decreased in Nicaragua, the overall number of GE cases of any etiology has remained at high levels after RV vaccine introduction [17]. A recent paper reports that a pre-vaccine community cohort experienced 36 episodes of watery diarrhea per 100 child-years, whereas a vaccine cohort experienced 25 episodes per 100 child-years, indicating a 60% persistence of watery diarrhea at community level during the vaccine era [18].

A non-specific effect of RV vaccine on GE of other etiologies has been suggested in a few studies [19–21]. However, this effect is still speculative and whether RV vaccination has any effect on NVGE or SVGE remains to be established.

In this study we investigated the virological causes behind the burden of diarrhea that persists after implementation of universal RV vaccination in Nicaragua. We thus explored the relative frequency of NV, SV and RV, both at hospital and community level in Nicaragua during 2009/2010 in the context of high RV vaccination rates. In addition we explored the association of these relative frequencies with RV vaccination status, dehydration status, and virus genotypes/genogroups.

Materials and Methods

Ethics statement

The study protocol and consent procedure was approved by the local ethical committee for biometrics research (Comite de Etica para Investigaciones Biomedicas [CEIB]; registration number: 61-2005, 73-2010). Informed written consent was given by parents or child guardians before samples were collected as described below. After the consent was given, personal details, as well as, epidemiological data were recorded in a paper file.

Study Design

Through a community- and hospital-based passive surveillance of sporadic acute diarrhea, a total of 330 children of ≤ 5 years of age with acute diarrhea were enrolled in a longitudinal, prospective manner from September 2009 to October 2010. In the hospital setting children (n = 175) were enrolled at the pediatric wards and emergency rooms from main hospitals of León and Jinotega, Nicaragua (Hospital Escuela "Oscar Danilo Rosales and Victoria Motta, respectively). Community children (n = 155) were outpatients consulting for diarrhea at two clinics of León.

Clinical assessment

All children involved in the study were clinically evaluated by pediatricians (hospital) or general practitioners (community) and classified by dehydration status, following the WHO protocol for integrated management of childhood illness (IMCI), into one of the following categories: "severe-dehydration", "some-dehydration", and "without-dehydration".

RotaTeq immunization assessment

The dates each child received vaccine doses in Nicaragua were registered by an EPI nurse on the child's vaccination-card. The RotaTeq immunization data used in this study were collected from the children's vaccination-cards. A child was considered "unvaccinated" if their vaccination card showed no recorded doses. If the child's vaccination card was not available, immunization status was considered unknown.

Collection of stool specimens

Fecal specimens were collected in sterile containers ≤ 24 h after admission, and transported either weekly (Jinotega) or daily (León) at 4°C to the microbiology laboratory of UNAN-León. At the two outpatient clinics, fecal samples were collected by a nurse during the visit. Before transportation, samples were stored at 4°C at the collection site to ensure quality of virological testing. A 10% (wt/vol) suspension of stool material was prepared with phosphate-buffered saline (pH = 7.2), and two aliquots were frozen at −20°C for later examination of RV, NV and SV.

RV antigen detection

A direct enzyme immunoassay for detection of RV in fecal specimens, OXOID ProSpecT R240396 (Cambridge, UK), was used according to the manufacturer's instructions. The results were visually read and confirmed by absorbance measurements.

RNA extraction from stool specimens

Viral RNA was extracted from stool suspensions (200 µl) following the manufacturer's instructions using High Pure Viral RNA Kit (Roche Applied Science, Indianapolis, USA). A total of 50 µl of RNA was collected and stored at −20°C until reverse transcription (RT).

Reverse transcription

Reverse transcription (RT) was carried out as described previously [22]. Briefly, 28 µl of purified RNA was mixed with 50 pmol of random hexadeoxynucleotides [pd(N)6] (GE Healthcare Life Sciences), and the mixture was denatured at 97°C for 5 min and quickly chilled on ice for 2 min, followed by the addition of one RT bead (Amersham Biosciences, UK) and RNase-free water to a final volume of 50 µl. RT reaction mixtures were incubated for 30 min at 42°C to produce complementary DNA (cDNA).

RV G and P multiplex genotyping

The G and P genotypes of RVs recovered from stool samples were determined by PCR. The generic and genotype-specific primers used for detecting VP7 genotypes G1, G2, G3, G4, G8, G9, G10, and G12 were described previously [23,24]. Primers used for detecting VP4 genotypes P[4], P[6], P[8], and P[9] were also described previously [23,25]. Genotypes and full genomic analysis of RV found in RotaTeq vaccinated children from Jinotega has been described previously [26].

NV detection by real-time PCR

In brief, 2.5 µl of purified RNA was added to a reaction mixture consisting of 12.5 µl of FastStart Universal SYBR Green Master (ROX) (Roche Applied Science, IN, USA), 1 µl (10 pmol) of each non-labeled GI and GII primers (NVG1f1b and NVG1rlux, NVG2flux1 and COG2R), [27] and 8 µl of RNAse free water, to final volume of 25 µl. The real-time PCR reactions were performed in a 96-well reaction plate using the ABI 7500 Real Time PCR System (Applied Biosystems, Foster, CA). PCR was performed under the following conditions: 95°C for 5 min, followed by 40 cycles of 95°C for 15 s, 55°C for 30 s and 72°C for 1 min. Melting curve analysis, to confirm amplicon specificity, was performed immediately after PCR completion.

NV GI and GII genogrouping

All NV-positive samples were re-analyzed by genogroup specific SYBR Green real-time PCR, in separate tubes, following the procedure described for NV screening but using specific primers for either GI or GII [27]. A sample was considered of NV GI and/or GII if the Ct value was ≤ 40 and Tm of 76.1 ± 0.6°C for GI and 77.1 ± 0.6°C for GII.

NV genotyping

A subset of NV-positive samples with sufficient viral load were sequenced in the N-terminal region of the capsid gene as described [22]. The 380-bp and 378-bp amplicons obtained from GI and GII NVs, respectively were sequenced by Macrogen Inc. (Seoul, South Korea)., using NVG1f1b, G1SKR, NVG2flux1 and G2SKR primers as sequencing primers [27,28]. Sequence alignment was performed by using the ClustalW algorithm, version 1.83, with default parameters on the European Bioinformatics Institute server (EMBL-EBI). Phylogenetic analysis was performed using the MEGA 5.03 software package and the tree was constructed using the neighbor-joining method with the Kimura two-parameter model [29]. The significance of phylogenetic relationships was assessed by bootstrap resampling analysis (1,000 replications). The assignment of genotypes was done using pairwise nucleotide distance measurements [30].

SV detection by real-time PCR

SV screening was carried out following a modification of the method described by Chan et al 2006 [31]. In brief, 2.5 µl of purified RNA was added to a reaction mixture consisting of 12.5 µl of 2X RT-PCR Buffer and 1 µl 25X RT-PCR Enzyme Mix (AgPath-ID One-Step RT-PCR kit, Life Technologies, NY, USA), 1 µl (10 pmol) of each forward (CUSVF1 and CUSVF2) and reverse primer (CUSVR), 1 µl (10 pmol) of SV TaqMan Probe (TaqMan MGB was replaced with [6FAM] TGG TTY ATA GGY GGT AC [BHQ1]), 1.67 µl of detection enhancer and 4.33 µl of RNAse free water, to final volume of 25 µl. The real-time PCR reactions were performed on a 7500 Real-Time PCR System (Applied Biosystems, Foster City, CA). A sample with Ct value ≤ 40 was considered positive.

SV genogrouping

The cDNA of SV-positive specimens were amplified by an outer PCR using a primer pool that consisted of two forward (SV-F13 and SV-F14), and two reverse (SV-R13 and SV-R14) primers with PCR conditions as described elsewhere [32]. Genogroups, GI, GII, GIV and GV, were examined by nested PCR under identical conditions to the outer PCR using a primer pool that consisted of universal forward primers (SV-F13/-F14) and genogroup specific reverse primers (SV-G1-R, SV-G2-R, SV-G4-R and SV-G5-R). The 500-bp, 430-bp, 360-bp and 290-bp amplicons obtained from GI, GII, GIV and GV viruses, respectively, were visualized by 2% agarose gel electrophoresis followed by ethidium bromide staining. Co-infections with SV of different genogroups was confirmed by allele specific PCR.

SV genotyping

The N-terminal region of the capsid gene (~ 420 bp) was sequenced in a subset of 23 SV-positive samples. A total of 1 µl of PCR product from the outer PCR reaction, described in SV genogrouping section, 10 pmol of each of forward (F22) and reverse (R2) primers [32] and RNase-free water were added to one Illustra PuReTaq Ready-To-Go PCR Bead (GE Healthcare, Uppsala, Sweden) to a final volume of 25 µl. The PCR reaction was performed following the conditions described previously [32]. The 420-bp amplicons obtained from SV-positive samples were sequenced by Macrogen Inc. (Seoul, South Korea) using F22 and R2 primers as sequencing primers. The assignment of genotypes was done using pairwise nucleotide distance measurements.

Statistical analysis

Relative frequencies between viral etiologies and genetic variants were analyzed for setting, clinical and epidemiological variables to investigate trends or statistical differences. Unadjusted Odds ratios (OR) were used to determine the degree of association and Fisher's exact test was used to compare frequencies of qualitative variables. Differences were considered to be statistically significant when the level of two-tailed significance was < 0.05.

The softwares SPSS (Statistical Program for Social Science version 14.0 for Windows; Chicago, IL) and GraphPad Prism (version 5.00 for Windows, GraphPad Software, San Diego California USA) were used for statistical analysis.

Nucleotide sequence accession numbers

The nucleotide sequences for NV, SV and RV determined in this work were submitted to GenBank and the following accession numbers were assigned for Norovirus: KF361389 to KF361442; Sapovirus: KF361366 to KF361388 and Rotavirus: JN129124, JN129096, JN129110, JN129054, JN129068, JN129082, JN128984, JN128998, JN129012, JN129026, JN129040.

Results

High detection rates of viruses among children with diarrhea vaccinated with RotaTeq

In total, viral GE was associated with 147 (45%) of the 330 diarrheal children investigated. The RV vaccine coverage observed in the current study was 95% (270/284; Table 1). Of these, 213 (79%), 43 (16%) and 14 (5%) had received 3, 2 and 1 vaccine dose(s) respectively. For 46 children, the vaccination status was not known.

Norovirus was the major cause of pediatric gastroenteritis

NV was observed in 79 (24%) of the 330 children with diarrhea investigated in this study. In the hospital setting, NV was observed in 27% (n = 47) of the children and in the community setting NV was observed in 21% (n = 32) (OR = 1.4, p = 0.2). NV was furthermore observed in 15 (26%) of 57 children with severe dehydration (Table 1). NVGE was not gender-dependent and most children with NVGE were less than 24 months of age with a mean age of 12.2 months (median = 10.1) (Table 1). The major peak for NVGE was observed in June 2010, corresponding to the early rainy season in Nicaragua (Fig. 1). Similar rates of NVGE (24% vs 21%) were observed in RV vaccinated compared to non-vaccinated children.

The majority of norovirus were of genotype GII.4

Genogroups analysis showed that a total of 71 (90%) NV-positive belonged to GII followed by GI with 7 (9%) and co-infection with both GI:GII in one case (Table 2). To investigate the relative predominance of NV genotypes in hospital and community settings a subset of 55 NV-positive were genotyped by nt sequencing analysis (Table 2). The globally dominant GII.4 genotype was observed in 82% (45/55) of all genotyped cases. The GII.4 genotype was observed in 30 (94%) of the 32 genotyped cases from the hospital and in 15 (65%) of the 23 genotyped cases from the community (Table 2) (OR = 8.0, p = 0.012). Other detected genotypes were; GII.6, GII.14, GII.9, GI.3 and GI.2 all found in lesser proportions and mainly in the community (Table 1). The pandemic variant GII.4-2006b also known as Minerva was dominant among GII.4 (35/45) and circulated in 2009 and 2010 with high detection rates during the rainy season of 2010. The other detected GII.4 variant, GII.4-2010 (10/45), also known as New Orleans emerged in 2010. The epidemiological peak of GII.4 Minerva and New Orleans variants corresponded with the peak of NVGE and peak of total GE cases (Fig. 1).

Sapovirus was the second major cause of pediatric gastroenteritis

SV was observed in 57 (17%) of the 330 children with diarrhea investigated in this study (Table 1). In the hospital setting, SV was observed in 15% (n = 27) of the children, and in the community setting SV was observed in 19% (n = 30) (OR = 0.76, p = 0.38). Most of the SV were observed in children with no or mild dehydration (48/57; 84%). Similar to NV, SVGE was not gender-

Table 1. Epidemiological profile and dehydration status of norovirus, sapovirus and rotavirus infections in a population with high RotaTeq coverage in Nicaragua, 2009–2010.

Parameter	Total	Norovirus n (%)	Sapovirus n (%)	Rotavirus n (%)
All children	330[a]	79 (24)	57 (17)	25 (8)
Site				
León	227	57 (25)	44 (19)	8 (4)
Jinotega	103	22 (21)	13 (13)	17 (16)
Setting				
Hospital	175	47 (27)	27 (15)	24 (14)
Community	155	32 (21)	30 (19)	1 (1)
Gender				
Male	190	45 (24)	34 (18)	13 (7)
Female	140	34 (24)	23 (17)	12 (9)
Age range (mo)				
≤ 6	64	16 (25)	8 (12)	4 (6)
7–12	108	31 (29)	21 (19)	9 (8)
13–24	107	25 (23)	24 (22)	7 (7)
25–60	51	7 (14)	4 (8)	5 (10)
RV vaccination status				
Vaccinated	270	64 (24)	51 (19)	16 (6)
Unvaccinated	14	3 (21)	0 (0)	2 (14)
Unknown	46	12 (26)	6 (13)	7 (15)
Dehydration status				
Severe dehydration[b]	57	15 (26)	9 (16)	16 (28)
Some dehydration	98	28 (29)	14 (14)	7 (7)
No dehydration	175	36 (21)	34 (19)	2 (1)

[a]Detection rates of norovirus, sapovirus and rotavirus is calculated per line in the table; thus for the total number of children per parameter
[b]All children with severe dehydration required intravenous rehydration.

dependent, with the majority of children with SVGE (45/57, 79%) being 7–24 months of age (Table 1) (OR = 2.3, p = 0.02), with the mean age of 12.7 months (median = 11.8). As for NVGE; the epidemiological peak of SVGE was in June 2010 corresponding to the early rainy season (Fig. 1). SV infections occurred in (51/270) children having received at least one RotaTeq dose and nil (0/14) in non-immunized children (OR = 6.8, p = 0.08) (Table 1).

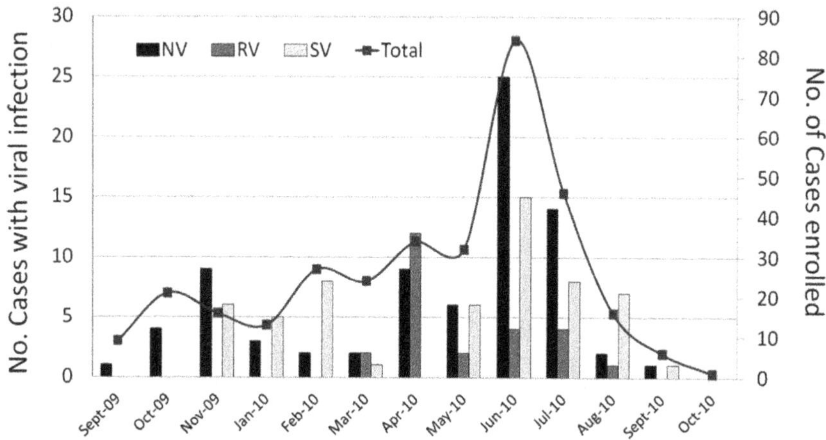

Figure 1. Temporal distribution of norovirus (NV), sapovirus (SV) and rotavirus (RV) infections in children with diarrhea ≤ 5 years of age, after national RotaTeq vaccination in Nicaragua, 2009–2010. Left Y axis; the black, grey and white bars represent monthly frequencies of NV, RV and SV, respectively. Right Y axis; the line represent monthly frequencies of gastroenteritis cases enrolled. The X axis represents seasonality, with the early rainy season typically starting in May and lasting until July.

Table. 2. Relative predominance between genetic variants of norovirus, sapovirus and rotavirus among children with gastroenteritis at hospital and community settings in Nicaragua, 2009–2010.

Genetic Variants	Both settings n (%)	Setting		OR[a] [95%, CI]; *p-value*[a]
		Hospital n (%)	Community n (%)	
Norovirus Genogroups				
GII	71 (90)	44 (94)	27 (84)	4.1 [0.74–22.5]; *0.12*
GI	7 (9)	2 (4)	5 (16)	0.25 [0.04–1.4]; *0.12*
GI:GII	1 (1)	1 (2)	0 (0)	NA[e]
Total	79 (100)	47 (100)	32 (100)	
Norovirus Genotypes				
GII.4[b]	45 (82)	30 (94)	15 (65)	8.0 [1.5–42]; *0.012*
GII Non-GII.4[c]	7 (13)	1 (3)	6 (26)	0.09 [0.01–0.82]; *0.017*
GI.3	2 (4)	1 (3)	1(4)	0.71 [0.04–12]; *1.0*
GI.2	1 (2)	0	1 (4)	NA
Total	55 (100)	32 (100)	23 (100)	
Sapovirus Genogroups				
GI	26 (46)	14 (52)	12 (40)	2.3[0.67–8.1]; *0.23*
GII	16 (28)	5 (19)	11 (37)	0.39 [0.11–1.4]; *0.21*
GIV	2 (3)	1 (4)	1 (3)	1.2 [0.07–21]; *1.0*
Mixed[d]	5 (9)	3 (11)	2 (7)	NA
Not genogrouped	8 (14)	4 (15)	4 (13)	NA
Total	57 (100)	27 (100)	30 (100)	
Sapovirus Genotypes				
GI/1	6 (27)	5 (36)	1 (12)	4.4 [0.42–47]; *0.34*
GI/2	8 (36)	7 (50)	1 (12)	8.0 [0.78–82]; *0.086*
GII/2	4 (14)	1 (7)	3 (25)	0.15 [0.01–1.8]; *0.26*
GII/3	5 (23)	1 (7)	4 (50)	0.1 [0.01–1.08]; *0.056*
Total	23 (100)	14 (100)	9 (100)	
Rotavirus Genotypes				
G1P[8]	16 (64)	16 (67)	0 (0)	NA
G3 P[8]	5 (20)	5 (21)	0 (0)	
G4 P[4]	1 (4)	1 (4)	0 (0)	
Not genotyped	3 (12)	2 (8)	1 (100)	
Total	25 (100)	24 (100)	1 (100)	

[a]Fisher's exact test with unadjusted odds ratio. Relative frequencies of genetic variants in hospital vs community setting. Mixed and non-typed infections were excluded from analysis.
[b]Only GII.4-2006 Minerva (n = 35) and GII.4-2009 New Orleans (n = 10) genetics variants were detected among GII.4.
[c]GII.6 (n = 3), GII.14 (n = 3) and GII.9 (n = 1).
[d]GI:GII (n = 3), GI:GIV (n = 1) and GI:GV(n = 1).
[e]Not applicable.

The most common SV genogroup was GI (46%), followed by GII (28%), GIV (3%) and mixed infections (9%). In 8 (14%) SV-positive samples, the genogroup could not be determined with the reagents used. To investigate if a particular genetic variant of SV contributed to the unusual high detection rate of SV in the current study, a subset of 23 SV-positives were genotyped by nt sequencing analysis (Table 2). In the hospital setting, GI/1 and GI/2 were the dominant genotypes (12/14), while SV of genotypes GII/2 and GII/3 were mainly found in community cases (7/9) (Table 2).

Rotavirus gastroenteritis was uncommon but severe in RotaTeq vaccinated children

RV was observed in 25 (8%) of the 330 children with diarrhea investigated. Interestingly, in the community setting, RV was observed in <1% (n = 1) of the cases whereas in the hospital setting RV was observed in 14% of the cases (n = 24) (OR = 24.5, $p < 0.001$), including 16 children with documented RV vaccination. Furthermore, the majority of RV infections were observed in children with severe dehydration (Table 1) (OR = 11.5, $p < 0.001$). In contrast to NV and SV infections however, there was an equal distribution of RV infections in all age groups (Table 1). Of note is also that the mean age for children with RVGE was high (14.6 months: median = 10.6). RVGE was observed in 16 (6%) of 270 children vaccinated with RotaTeq and in 2 (14%) of the 14 non-vaccinated children (OR = 0.38; p = 0.22). RV was also observed in 7 (15%) of 46 children with unknown vaccination status. In RV-positive children having received 3 and 2 RotaTeq doses, the RVGE episode occurred 193 and 65 days (median) post vaccination, respectively.

Rotavirus of genotypes G1P[8] and G3P[8] infected RotaTeq vaccinated children

Most RV genotypes (16/17), from hospitalized children of Jinotega were G1P[8], whereas the RV genotypes from León were G3P[8] (n = 4), G9P[4] (n = 1) and non-typeable (n = 3) with the reagents used. Full genome sequencing analysis of a G3P[8] RV strain (125L) from León, showed a Wa-like genome (G3-P[8]-I1-R1-C1-M1-A1-N1-T1-E1-H1). Similar genome constellations were previously observed after full genome sequencing of 12 RV-positive from Jinotega, of which 11 were G1P[8] and 1 was G3P[8]; as published elsewhere [26].

Co-infections with NV and SV

In total 14 (4%) children with GE shed more than one of the virus investigated. Of these, 11 shed SV-NV, 2 SV-RV, and 1 NV-RV, no triple virus infection was observed, but SVGI-SVGII-NVGI was observed. More than 50% (8/14) of the children with co-infections were observed in hospitalized children. Co-infections were confirmed by either secondary PCR or sequencing analysis.

Discussion

The burden of diarrhea after universal RV vaccination in Nicaragua remains high, despite reduction of RV infections and transmission in the community [12,16,18,33]. In the current study we investigated the role of NV, SV and RV in pediatric gastroenteritis in hospital and community settings in two cities with high RV vaccine coverage (>90%) in Nicaragua.

Our findings show that after RV vaccine implementation, NV has become the leading viral cause (24%) of medically attended acute GE among Nicaraguan children younger than 5 years of age. This is in agreement with recent studies carried out in Finland and USA [34–36]. SV was the second most common cause of acute GE (17%), followed by RV (8%). Altogether, these observations indicate that the etiology of viral gastroenteritis at hospital and community settings in Nicaragua has been altered by RV vaccine implementation and that NV and SV strongly contribute to the burden of diarrhea that still persists in the country [17,18]. Since a viral cause of GE was found in only approximately one half of the children investigated in this study, further surveillance studies of other etiologies are recommended to close this diagnostic gap in these settings [37,38].

NVGE has been generally described as a mild disease of short duration but new evidence suggests that the illness can be severe, especially among vulnerable populations [39,40]. The current study is in agreement with such new evidence as 27% of children in the hospital setting had NVGE and many of these required medical attention for mild and severe dehydration. The GII.4 genotypes comprised 94% of all genotyped NV in children in the hospital setting; compared to 65% in the community setting (p=0.012). In a study carried out in Nicaragua in 2005, we observed that most NV cases requiring intravenous treatment were associated with GII.4 (Hunter), and that the same variant was less common in asymptomatic children [22,41]. Altogether, these observations suggest that besides vulnerable populations, not yet described virulence factors of GII.4 variants contribute to illness severity, a suggestion supported by a recent review of outbreaks associated with GII.4 viruses [39]. A potential bias of our comparison is that community samples were only collected from one city, León, and not Jinotega. However, due to the close geographical location of the cities which have good logistic connections and the long-term nature of the study, it is likely that GII.4 variants circulated in similar proportion in the communities of the two cities.

We further investigated the non-specific effect of RV vaccine against GE from other etiologies, previously suggested in one of the largest clinical trial of RotaTeq [13]. We found no significant differences between rates of NV infection and RV vaccination (24% vs 21%), and NV and SV together, were found in almost a half (24% and 19%, respectively) of the children with diarrhea having received one vaccination dose, with SV only observed in children vaccinated with RotaTeq. These observations strongly suggest that RV-vaccination do not reduce the incidence of NVGE and SVGE.

In previous surveillance studies of pediatric diarrhea in developed and developing countries, prevalence rates of SVGE barely reached 10% [4–8]. Despite significant progress on methods for SV detection, it remains poorly recognized as a cause of GE, probably because infection is generally believed mild and few cases need medical care [42]. In the current study, we report that SV infections were the second most common cause (17%) of pediatric GE in the vaccinated population investigated and that SV infections were detected less frequent in children with dehydration as compared to NV and RV. To demonstrate the clinical significance of SaV infections in RV5 vaccinated children; more studies (case – control) should be performed including more non-vaccinated children as well as asymptomatic children. A previous report from Nicaragua found asymptomatic shedding of SaV in ~9% of children < 5 years of age [8]. A possible explanation for the increased SV prevalence in this study (17%), as compared with a prevalence rate of 12% in 2005–2006 before RV-vaccination in Nicaragua [8] is that there is a higher relative likelihood of finding non-RV enteropathogens in this study where most children had been vaccinated for RV, compared to the time period before RV vaccination. Another reason could be the use of more sensitive methods enhancing detection of most genetic variants. The real-time PCR used in this study was proven to be 10-fold more sensitive than the conventional RT-PCR that uses first generation SV primers (JV33 and SR80) [31,43].

In line with previous studies we observed a decline of RVGE after introduction of universal RV vaccination [34–36], with RV observed in 14% of hospitalized children and less than 1% in community children with diarrhea. This data is also in line with the reduction of incidence of watery diarrhea in the community after RV vaccine introduction in Nicaragua [18]. These observations suggest that RotaTeq implementation has dramatically decreased the number of RVGE in primary care setting in Nicaragua, which is consistent with the low prevalence of RV at environmental level [33].

We investigated whether RV vaccinated children with severe RVGE in the current study were infected with RV strains different from those included in the vaccine. However, genomic analysis of a subset of the strains showed that all RV strains analyzed had genotype specificities typical for human G1P[8] and G3P[8] RVs, similar to genotypes present in the RotaTeq vaccine. This suggests that viral factors alone were not responsible for the vaccine failures in this study population. Another possible explanation could be a short duration of RotaTeq vaccine protection in some children. In this study we observed that RVGE occurred about 6 or 2 months post 3rd and 2nd vaccine dose respectively. A third possible explanation might be that host genetic factors in some children influence vaccine take. A particular attention has now been put on histo-blood group antigens, and remains to be elucidated [44].

To conclude, this study shows that NV has become the leading viral cause of pediatric viral gastroenteritis at hospital and community settings in Nicaragua after universal implementation of RotaTeq vaccine; and that NV together with SV infections strongly contribute to the high burden of diarrhea remaining after RV vaccination.

Acknowledgments

We would like to express our appreciation to Licdas. Angelica Castro and Cristel Escoto for help in collecting samples and epidemiological information in children from Jinotega, Dr. Gioconda Ramirez and Dra. Rafaela Briceno, for providing diarrhea surveillance data from Hospital Victoria Motta in Jinotega and HEODRA in León, respectively, Silvia Altamirano for valuable assistance on fieldwork activities, Eliana Espinoza, for collaboration on norovirus methods optimization and Patricia Blandon for her valuable assistance on laboratory activities.

Author Contributions

Conceived and designed the experiments: FB YR LS JN. Performed the experiments: FB YR. Analyzed the data: FB YR JN. Contributed reagents/materials/analysis tools: FB LS. Wrote the paper: FB YR LS JN.

References

1. Patel MM, Widdowson MA, Glass RI, Akazawa K, Vinje J, et al. (2008) Systematic literature review of role of noroviruses in sporadic gastroenteritis. Emerg Infect Dis 14: 1224–1231.
2. Parashar UD, Gibson CJ, Bresse JS, Glass RI (2006) Rotavirus and severe childhood diarrhea. Emerg Infect Dis 12: 304–306.
3. Tate JE, Burton AH, Boschi-Pinto C, Steele AD, Duque J, et al. (2012) 2008 estimate of worldwide rotavirus-associated mortality in children younger than 5 years before the introduction of universal rotavirus vaccination programmes: a systematic review and meta-analysis. Lancet Infect Dis 12: 136–141.
4. Johnsen CK, Midgley S, Bottiger B (2009) Genetic diversity of sapovirus infections in Danish children 2005-2007. J Clin Virol 46: 265–269.
5. Khamrin P, Maneekarn N, Peerakome S, Tonusin S, Malasao R, et al. (2007) Genetic diversity of noroviruses and sapoviruses in children hospitalized with acute gastroenteritis in Chiang Mai, Thailand. J Med Virol 79: 1921–1926.
6. Podkolzin AT, Fenske EB, Abramycheva NY, Shipulin GA, Sagalova OI, et al. (2009) Hospital-based surveillance of rotavirus and other viral agents of diarrhea in children and adults in Russia, 2005-2007. J Infect Dis 200 Suppl 1: S228–233.
7. Sakai Y, Nakata S, Honma S, Tatsumi M, Numata-Kinoshita K, et al. (2001) Clinical severity of Norwalk virus and Sapporo virus gastroenteritis in children in Hokkaido, Japan. Pediatr Infect Dis J 20: 849–853.
8. Bucardo F, Carlsson B, Nordgren J, Larson G, Blandon P, et al. (2012) Susceptibility of children to sapovirus infections, Nicaragua, 2005-2006. Emerg Infect Dis 18: 1875–1878.
9. Soares-Weiser K, Maclehose H, Bergman H, Ben-Aharon I, Nagpal S, et al. (2012) Vaccines for preventing rotavirus diarrhoea: vaccines in use. Cochrane Database Syst Rev 11: CD008521.
10. Vesikari T, Karvonen A, Ferrante SA, Ciarlet M (2010) Efficacy of the pentavalent rotavirus vaccine, RotaTeq(R), in Finnish infants up to 3 years of age: the Finnish Extension Study. Eur J Pediatr 169: 1379–1386.
11. Khawaja S, Cardellino A, Klotz D, Kuter BJ, Feinberg MB, et al. (2012) Evaluating the health impact of a public-private partnership: to reduce rotavirus disease in Nicaragua. Hum Vaccin Immunother 8: 777–782.
12. Patel M, Pedreira C, De Oliveira LH, Tate J, Orozco M, et al. (2009) Association between pentavalent rotavirus vaccine and severe rotavirus diarrhea among children in Nicaragua. JAMA 301: 2243–2251.
13. Vesikari T, Matson DO, Dennehy P, Van Damme P, Santosham M, et al. (2006) Safety and efficacy of a pentavalent human-bovine (WC3) reassortant rotavirus vaccine. N Engl J Med 354: 23–33.
14. Zaman K, Dang DA, Victor JC, Shin S, Yunus M, et al. (2010) Efficacy of pentavalent rotavirus vaccine against severe rotavirus gastroenteritis in infants in developing countries in Asia: a randomised, double-blind, placebo-controlled trial. Lancet 376: 615–623.
15. Madhi SA, Cunliffe NA, Steele D, Witte D, Kirsten M, et al. (2010) Effect of human rotavirus vaccine on severe diarrhea in African infants. N Engl J Med 362: 289–298.
16. Becker-Dreps S, Paniagua M, Zambrana LE, Bucardo F, Hudgens MG, et al. (2011) Rotavirus prevalence in the primary care setting in Nicaragua after universal infant rotavirus immunization. Am J Trop Med Hyg 85: 957–960.
17. Becker-Dreps S, Paniagua M, Dominik R, Cao H, Shah NK, et al. (2011) Changes in childhood diarrhea incidence in nicaragua following 3 years of universal infant rotavirus immunization. Pediatr Infect Dis J 30: 243–247.
18. Becker-Dreps S, Melendez M, Liu L, Zambrana LE, Paniagua M, et al. (2013) Community diarrhea incidence before and after rotavirus vaccine introduction in Nicaragua. Am J Trop Med Hyg 89: 246–250.
19. Pang XL, Koskenniemi E, Joensuu J, Vesikari T (1999) Effect of rhesus rotavirus vaccine on enteric adenovirus—associated diarrhea in children. J Pediatr Gastroenterol Nutr 29: 366–369.
20. Pang XL, Zeng SQ, Honma S, Nakata S, Vesikari T (2001) Effect of rotavirus vaccine on Sapporo virus gastroenteritis in Finnish infants. Pediatr Infect Dis J 20: 295–300.
21. Zeng SQ, Halkosalo A, Salminen M, Szakal ED, Karvonen A, et al. (2010) Norovirus gastroenteritis in young children receiving human rotavirus vaccine. Scand J Infect Dis 42: 540–544.
22. Bucardo F, Nordgren J, Carlsson B, Paniagua M, Lindgren PE, et al. (2008) Pediatric norovirus diarrhea in Nicaragua. J Clin Microbiol 46: 2573–2580.
23. Iturriza-Gomara M, Kang G, Gray J (2004) Rotavirus genotyping: keeping up with an evolving population of human rotaviruses. J Clin Virol 31: 259–265.
24. Samajdar S, Varghese V, Barman P, Ghosh S, Mitra U, et al. (2006) Changing pattern of human group A rotaviruses: emergence of G12 as an important pathogen among children in eastern India. J Clin Virol 36: 183–188.
25. Gentsch JR, Glass RI, Woods P, Gouvea V, Gorziglia M, et al. (1992) Identification of group A rotavirus gene 4 types by polymerase chain reaction. J Clin Microbiol 30: 1365–1373.
26. Bucardo F, Rippinger CM, Svensson L, Patton JT (2012) Vaccine-derived NSP2 segment in rotaviruses from vaccinated children with gastroenteritis in Nicaragua. Infect Genet Evol 12: 1282–1294.
27. Nordgren J, Bucardo F, Dienus O, Svensson L, Lindgren PE (2008) Novel light-upon-extension real-time PCR assays for detection and quantification of genogroup I and II noroviruses in clinical specimens. J Clin Microbiol 46: 164–170.
28. Kojima S, Kageyama T, Fukushi S, Hoshino FB, Shinohara M, et al. (2002) Genogroup-specific PCR primers for detection of Norwalk-like viruses. J Virol Methods 100: 107–114.
29. Kimura M (1980) A simple method for estimating evolutionary rates of base substitutions through comparative studies of nucleotide sequences. J Mol Evol 16: 111–120.
30. Zheng DP, Ando T, Fankhauser RL, Beard RS, Glass RI, et al. (2006) Norovirus classification and proposed strain nomenclature. Virology 346: 312–323.
31. Chan MC, Sung JJ, Lam RK, Chan PK, Lai RW, et al. (2006) Sapovirus detection by quantitative real-time RT-PCR in clinical stool specimens. J Virol Methods 134: 146–153.
32. Okada M, Yamashita Y, Oseto M, Shinozaki K (2006) The detection of human sapoviruses with universal and genogroup-specific primers. Arch Virol 151: 2503–2509.
33. Bucardo F, Lindgren PE, Svensson L, Nordgren J (2011) Low prevalence of rotavirus and high prevalence of norovirus in hospital and community wastewater after introduction of rotavirus vaccine in Nicaragua. PLoS One 6: e25962.
34. Payne DC, Vinje J, Szilagyi PG, Edwards KM, Staat MA, et al. (2013) Norovirus and medically attended gastroenteritis in U.S. children. N Engl J Med 368: 1121–1130.
35. Hemming M, Rasanen S, Huhti L, Paloniemi M, Salminen M, et al. (2013) Major reduction of rotavirus, but not norovirus, gastroenteritis in children seen in hospital after the introduction of RotaTeq vaccine into the National Immunization Programme in Finland. Eur J Pediatr 172: 739–746.
36. Koo HL, Neill FH, Estes MK, Munoz FM, Cameron A, et al. (2013) Noroviruses: The Most Common Pediatric Viral Enteric Pathogen at a Large University Hospital After Introduction of Rotavirus Vaccination. J Pediatric Infect Dis Soc 2: 57–60.
37. Tam CC, O'Brien SJ, Tompkins DS, Bolton FJ, Berry L, et al. (2012) Changes in causes of acute gastroenteritis in the United Kingdom over 15 years: microbiologic findings from 2 prospective, population-based studies of infectious intestinal disease. Clin Infect Dis 54: 1275–1286.
38. Simpson R, Aliyu S, Iturriza-Gomara M, Desselberger U, Gray J (2003) Infantile viral gastroenteritis: on the way to closing the diagnostic gap. J Med Virol 70: 258–262.
39. Desai R, Hembree CD, Handel A, Matthews JE, Dickey BW, et al. (2012) Severe outcomes are associated with genogroup 2 genotype 4 norovirus outbreaks: a systematic literature review. Clin Infect Dis 55: 189–193.
40. Glass RI, Parashar UD, Estes MK (2009) Norovirus gastroenteritis. N Engl J Med 361: 1776–1785.
41. Bucardo F, Nordgren J, Carlsson B, Kindberg E, Paniagua M, et al. (2010) Asymptomatic norovirus infections in Nicaraguan children and its association with viral properties and histo-blood group antigens. Pediatr Infect Dis J 29: 934–939.
42. Moreno-Espinosa S, Farkas T, Jiang X (2004) Human caliciviruses and pediatric gastroenteritis. Semin Pediatr Infect Dis 15: 237–245.

43. Vinje J, Deijl H, van der Heide R, Lewis D, Hedlund KO, et al. (2000) Molecular detection and epidemiology of Sapporo-like viruses. J Clin Microbiol 38: 530–536.

44. Hu L, Crawford SE, Czako R, Cortes-Penfield NW, Smith DF, et al. (2012) Cell attachment protein VP8* of a human rotavirus specifically interacts with A-type histo-blood group antigen. Nature 485: 256–259.

A Randomized, Non-Inferiority Study Comparing Efficacy and Safety of a Single Dose of Pegfilgrastim versus Daily Filgrastim in Pediatric Patients after Autologous Peripheral Blood Stem Cell Transplant

Simone Cesaro[1]*, Francesca Nesi[2], Gloria Tridello[1], Massimo Abate[3], Irene Sara Panizzolo[1], Rita Balter[1], Elisabetta Calore[4]

1 Pediatric Hematology Oncology, Azienda Ospedaliera Universitaria Integrata, Verona, Italy, **2** Pediatric Hematology Oncology, Ospedale Infantile Regina Margherita, Torino, Italy, **3** Chemotherapy Unit, Istituto Ortopedico Rizzoli, Bologna, Italy, **4** Department of Pediatrics, Pediatric Hematology Oncology, Padova, Italy

Abstract

Purpose: To assess the non-inferiority of pegfilgrastim versus filgrastim in speeding the recovery of polymorphonuclear cells (PMN) in pediatric patients who underwent autologous peripheral blood stem cell transplant (PBSCT).

Methods: The sample size of this randomized, multicenter, phase III study, was calculated assuming that a single dose of pegfilgrastim of 100 ug/kg was not inferior to 9 doses of filgrastim of 5 ug/kg/day. Randomization was performed by a computer-generated list and stored by sequentially numbered sealed envelopes.

Results: Sixty-one patients, with a median age of 11.5 years, were recruited: 29 in the filgrastim arm and 32 in the pegfilgrastim arm. Twenty percent were affected by lymphoma/leukaemia and eighty percent by solid tumors. The mean time to PMN engraftment was 10.48 days (standard deviation [SD] 1.57) and 10.44 days (SD 2.44) in the filgrastim and pegfilgrastim arms, respectively. Having fixed a non-inferiority margin Delta of 3, the primary endpoint of non-inferiority was reached. No differences were observed for other secondary endpoints: platelet engraftment, mean time to platelet recovery (28 days vs. 33 days), fever of unknown origin (79% vs. 78%), proven infection (34% vs. 28%), mucositis (76% vs. 59%). After a median follow-up of 2.3 years (95% C.I.: 1.5, 3.3), 20 deaths were observed due to disease progression.

Conclusions: We conclude that pegfilgrastim was not inferior to daily filgrastim in pediatric patients who underwent PBSCT.

Editor: John W. Glod, Robert Wood Johnson Medical School, United States of America

Funding: The authors have no support or funding to report.

Competing Interests: The authors have declared that no competing interests exist.

* E-mail: simone.cesaro@ospedaleuniverona.it

Introduction

In autologous transplantation in the last 2 decades, peripheral blood stem cells (PBSC) have progressively become the preferred source of stem cells in place of bone marrow cells [1]. The most important reason is their capability to shorten the period of aplasia, accelerating neutrophil recovery and reducing infectious morbidity. Notwithstanding that myeloid engraftment may be influenced by the quality and quantity of progenitor cells, the use of granulocyte-colony stimulating factor (G-CSF) is recommended for autologous PBSC, regardless of the number of CD34+/kg of patient body weight infused [2]. Most retrospective and prospective studies have confirmed that the use of G-CSF reduced the period of severe neutropenia compared to untreated controls or placebo, without affecting platelet engraftment; moreover, most of randomized prospective studies found additional advantages in reduction of days of intravenous administration of antibiotics and length of hospitalization [3],[4]. The choice of G-CSF, filgrastim, lenograstim, and more recently biosimilars is left to the physician's discretion because they are considered equally efficacious; but the availability of pegfilgrastim, the pegylated form of filgrastim that has a longer half-life, make it possible to cover the entire period of aplasia with just a single injection. As shown in a recent meta-analysis, the use of pegfilgrastim is attractive because it has been associated with clinical advantages in terms of a shorter duration of severe neutropenia and of febrile neutropenic episodes [5].

All these studies were performed in adult patients whereas there are limited data regarding the use of pegfilgrastim in pediatric patients. We report the results of a prospective, randomized study assessing the non-inferiority of pegfilgrastim versus filgrastim as support agent for pediatric PBSC transplant.

Materials and Methods

The protocol for this trial and supporting CONSORT checklist are available as supporting information; see Checklist S1 and Protocol S1.

Patients

This was a prospective, randomized, open label, phase III, non-inferiority study, designed by the working group for supportive care of the Italian Association of Pediatric Hematology Oncology (AIEOP) that was conducted in four transplant centres from May 2007 to June 2011. The main endpoint was the hypothesis that a single dose of pegfilgrastim of 100 ug/kg (maximun 6 mg) was not inferior to 9 or more doses of filgrastim of 5 ug/kg/day (maximum 300 ug/day) in speeding recovery of PMN. Both drugs were administered beginning from day +3 after PBSC infusion. The doses of pegfilgrastim and filgrastim, and timing of their administration, were chosen on the basis of previous pediatric studies regarding the off-label use of pegfilgrastim for stem cell mobilization or prophylaxis of severe neutropenia after chemotherapy and the use of filgrastim after autologous stem cell transplantation [6–9],[10–15]. The secondary endpoints were the time to platelet engraftment, the incidence and severity of mucositis according to World Health Organization (WHO) score, the incidence of febrile neutropenia and proven infection, the duration of parenteral nutrition and intravenous antibiotic therapy, the duration of hospitalization, and overall survival. Eligible patients were aged between 0–17 years, affected by leukemia, lymphoma or solid tumor who underwent a first autologous PBSC transplant.

The study was registered at European Clinical Trial Register (Eudract number 2007-001430-14), approved by each Ethics Committee of participating centres, and all parents or patients (where applicable) gave their written informed consent before entering the study. Follow-up data are as at December 2011.

Transplant procedures and definitions

Recruited patients were randomly assigned to the treatment arm, pegfilgrastim versus filgrastim, in the period between admission for transplant and the day of PBSC infusion (day 0). Myeloablation followed by autologous PBSC infusion was performed in high-efficiency particulate- air rooms or isolation rooms according the policy of each centre. Standard supportive care and prophylactic measures were adopted to prevent infectious complications during the neutropenic phase, i.e., fluconazole for anti-fungal prophylaxis, acyclovir and cotrimoxazole for prophylaxis of HSV and *Pneumocystis* infections, respectively. Fever, defined as the presence of an oral or axillary temperature >38.5°C in a single measurement, or >38.0°C on two or more occasions taken at least 1 hour apart, was treated empirically with broad spectrum antibiotics.

Erythrocyte and platelet products were filtered to remove leukocytes and irradiated (25 Gray). PMN and PLT recovery were defined as the first of 3 and 7 consecutive days in which the counts were $>0.5\times10^3$/l and 50×10^9/l (and unsupported by transfusion), respectively.

Statistical analysis

To calculate the sample size we assumed that the mean time of PMN engraftment was 11 days for patients treated with filgrastim (control arm), as reported in a previous AIEOP randomized study [7]. Considering a standard deviation of 3.5, we hypothesised that the time to PMN engraftment in patients treated with pegfilgrastim (experimental group) was not longer than the non-inferior margin (Delta) of 3 days compared to the control group. Considering a beta = 0.1 and an alpha = 0.05, a total of 60 patients were needed to verify this hypothesis.

To verify the primary endpoint, the 95% confidence interval (CI) of the difference between the two arms (experimental and standard) was considered. Being the delta (experimental – standard) set at 3 days, the non-inferiority is established if the upper limit of the difference in means of the 95% CI is smaller than delta, as a shorter time to PMN is considered as a better outcome. The confidence interval will be computed according to the student's t distribution.

A computer-generated randomisation list was drawn up at Data Office Centre of AIEOP in Bologna, Italy, by a statistician not involved in patient management. Simple randomization was used. The list was stored by sequentially numbered sealed envelopes that was concealed to investigators until the completion of recruitment. The local investigator, after written informed consent of parents, assigned each eligible patient to randomization list by phoning to AIEOP Data Office Centre.

Information was collected by a specific case report form containing information on demographics (sex, age), disease (type, date of diagnosis, remission status), type of mobilizing chemotherapy and complications (occurrence and duration of severe neutropenia, mucositis and infections) and PBSC transplant (type of conditioning regimen, CD34+ cells infused, PMN and PLT engraftment, early post-transplant complications, mucositis, infection, follow-up); for patients who died, date and cause of death were also recorded. To calculate early (≤100 days) post-transplant overall survival and transplant-related mortality, death by any cause and death by toxic complications were used. Descriptive statistics were reported as percentages for categorical variables and median and ranges for continuous variables. Characteristics of patients whose mobilization was successful were compared with patients whose mobilization failed using chi-square or Fisher's exact test (as appropriate) in the case of discrete variables or the Mann-Whitney test, in the case of continuous variables. The level of significance was set at 0.05. The 1-year overall survival was computed using the Kaplan Meier estimator. Median follow-up was calculated according to the inverted Kaplan-Meier technique [16].

Results

During the study period 61 eligible patients were enrolled, 38 (62%) males and 23 (38%) females with a median age at diagnosis of 10.5, range 1.1–16.8. Figure 1 shows the progress of the patients through the phases of the study. Twenty-nine patients were assigned by randomization to filgrastim (control arm) whilst 32 patients were assigned to pegfilgrastim (experimental arm). Twenty percent of the patients were affected by leukemia and lymphoma: acute lymphoblastic leukaemia (ALL), 3, non-Hodgkin lymphoma (NHL), 4, and Hodgkin lymphoma (HD), 5, whilst the remaining patients were affected by a solid tumor: neuroblastoma 10, Ewing sarcoma/Peripheral neutroectodermal tumor, 27, medulloblastoma, 5, Wilms tumor, 3; central nervous system tumor, 4. The main demographic and patient clinical characteristics before PBSC transplant are shown in Table 1. No differences were found due to gender, diagnosis, status of the disease at transplant, age at transplant, and body weight.

Table 2 shows in detail the type and doses of drugs used for myeloablative conditioning regimens. Total body irradiation was used in only 4 patients at a dose of 12 Gy followed by etoposide 1800 mg/m^2 in 1 case and 14.4 Gy in 3 patients followed by cytarabine 24 g/m^2.

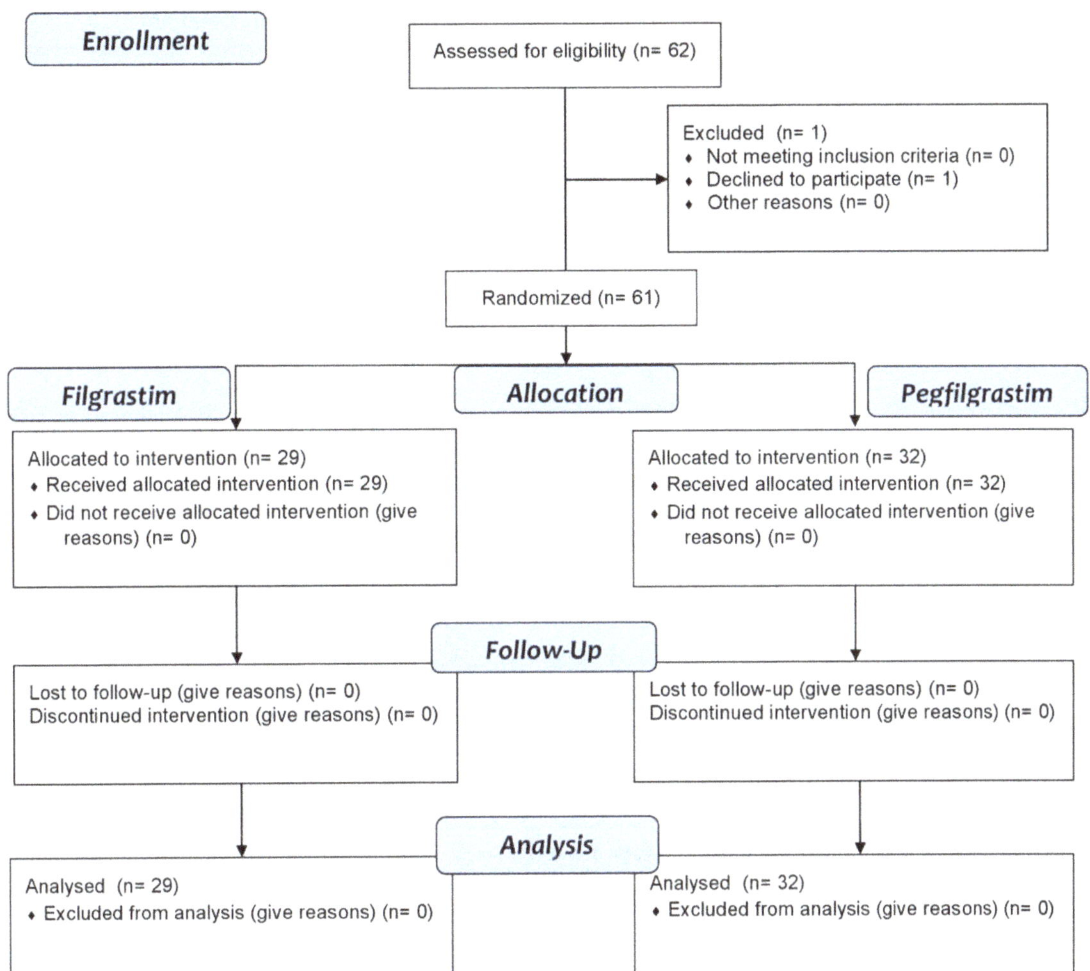

Figure 1. CONSORT 2010 Flow Diagram.

Patients of the control group were treated with filgrastim for a median of 9 days, range 6–17. In table 3, the comparison of main transplant variables between the 2 treatment groups is shown, ie. type of conditioning regimen, number of CD34+ cells infused, mucosal and infectious morbidity, PMN and PLT engraftment, use and duration of parenteral nutrition, need and duration of antibiotic therapy, time to discharge and mortality rate. Mean time to engraftment was 10.48 days (standard deviation (SD) 1.57) and 10.44 days (SD 2.44) in filgrastim and pegfilgrastim groups, respectively. The mean of the difference is equal to −0.045 (95% CI: −1.1–1.0). Considering that the upper limit is below 3, the primary endpoint was reached and the non inferiority of pegfilgrastim was established.

Regarding the secondary endpoints, no differences were found in PLT engraftment, episodes of fever of unknown origin (FUO), proven infections, mucositis, days of intravenous antibiotics and parenteral nutrition and days of hospitalization. Both pegfilgrastim and filgrastim were well tolerated and no significant adverse effects were associated with their use. Moreover, no toxic death was reported within the first 100 days post-PBSCT.

After a median follow-up of 2.3 years (95% C.I.: 1.5, 3.3), 41 patients were alive and 20 deaths were observed, 9 in the filgrastim and 11 in the pegfilgrastim group, all due to disease progression. The 1-year overall survival was 84.1% (95% C.I.: 62.9–93.8) in the filgrastim group vs. 74.5% (C.I.: 53.7–87.0) in the pegfilgrastim group, respectively ($p = 0.8$) (Figure 2).

Cost analysis. Considering that no centre had a centralised preparation of supportive drugs and that the discarding of the unused part of the vial was common practice, the cost of treatment was calculated comparing the price of pegfilgrastim and filgrastim vials. On the basis of current acquisition prices in Italy by hospital pharmacies that buy these drugs with a discount >50% off official prices, the costs were 622 euros for a vial of pegfilgrastim (official price 1489,50 euros) and 77.53 euros (official price 127,95 euros) for a vial of the original filgrastim. Given that 1 vial of pegfilgrastim equates to a median of 9 vials of filgrastim found in this study, the median cost of treatment with filgrastim was 698 euros (range 542–1318). This translated into a median saving of 76 euros for every patient treated with pegfilgrastim in addition to the reduced use of health personnel resources for its administration.

Discussion

The introduction of G-CSF in the late 1980's has radically changed the modality of performing HSCT and of pre-engraftment supportive care. This is true especially for autologous HSCT where the use of G-CSF-mobilized peripheral stem cells and pre-engraftment G-CSF reduced the time of myeloid recovery and, consequently, the incidence of infectious complications and

Table 1. The main demographic and clinical characteristics of two groups are shown according to treatment arm.

	Filgrastim N = 29 (%)	Peg-filgrastim N = 32 (%)	p
Gender			
Male	17 (58.6)	21 (65.6)	0.6
Female	12 (41.4)	11 (34.4)	
Body weight			
Median	38.0	31.8	0.8
Range	9.6–103.0	11.0–106.0	
Underlying disease			
Leukemia/Lymphoma	5 (17.2)	7 (21.9)	0.6
Solid tumors	24 (82.8)	25 (78.1)	
Status of underlying disease at transplant			
Complete remission	18 (62.1)	14 (43.8)	0.2
* Other status	11 (37.9)	18 (56.3)	
Age at diagnosis (years)			
Median	11.1	9.2	0.8
Range	1.1–16.8	1.4–16.8	
Age at SCT (years)			
Median	11.9	11.1	0.9
Range	1.6–17.2	1.7–17.4	
Time from diagnosis to transplant (days)			
Median	216.0	249.5	0.4
Range	67.0–1520.0	102.0–1136.0	

*other status comprised very good partial remission (16), partial remission (11), stable disease (2) before transplant.

duration of hospital stay [3]. Pegfilgrastim, the pegylated form of filgrastim, is considered equally effective as filgrastim with the advantage of allowing a smooth recovery of neutrophils, and in neutropenic adult patients, reducing the incidence of febrile episodes after chemotherapy [17]. Further advantages are the easier method of administration, one shot of pegfilgrastim

Table 2. Type and dose of drugs used for conditioning regimen.

N of drugs	Drug	Peg-filgrastim	Filgrastim	Total
1	*Cytarabine 24 mg/m^2	2	1	3
	*Etoposide 1800 mg/m^2		1	1
	Thiotepa 900 mg/m^2	3	3	6
2	Busulfan 16 mg/kg, Melphalan 140 mg/m^2	17	11	28
	Carboplatin 1500 mg/m^2, Etoposide1500–1800 mg/m^2	2	5	7
	Carboplatin 800 mg/m^2, Melphalan 140 mg/m^2	1		1
	Thiotepa 900 mg/m^2, Melphalan 140 mg/m^2	1		1
	Thiotepa 900 mg/m^2, Etoposide 1500 mg/m2	1		1
3	Thiotepa 10 mg/kg, Etoposide 1600 mg/m^2, Cyclophosphamide 7200 mg/m^2	3	2	5
	Carboplatin 800–1200 mg/m^2, Etoposide 800 mg/m^2, Melphalan 140–180 mg/m^2		3	3
	Carboplatin 1500 mg/m2, Etoposide 1000 mg/m2, Ifosfamide 12 g/m^2		1	1
	Busulfan 16 mg/kg, Etoposide 900 mg/m^2, Cyclophosphamide 120 mg/kg		2	2
4	BCNU 300 mg/m^2, Etoposide 800 mg/m^2, Cytarabine 1600 mg/m^2, Melphalan 140 mg/m^2	2		2

*with total body irradiation, 12–14.4Gray.

Table 3. No differences were found in the main parameters of transplant outcome according to treatment groups.

	Filgrastim N = 29, (%)	Peg-filgrastim N = 32, (%)	p
Type of conditioning regimen With TBI	2	2	-
Type of conditioning regimen Without TBI, high-dose chemotherapy			
>3 drugs	19 (70.4)	25 (83.3)	0.2
<2 drugs	8 (29.6)	5 (16.7)	
CD34+ infused			
Median	6.7	6.0	0.4
Range	3.0–299.6	3.4–78.9	
PMN engraftment			
Yes	29 (100.0)	32 (100.0)	-
Time to PMN engraftment (days)			
Mean (SD)	10.48 (1.57)	10.44 (2.44)	0.3
Median	10.0	10.0	
Range	8.0–17.0	8.0–23.0	
PLT engraftment			
Yes	29 (100.0)	32 (100.0)	-
Time to PLT engraftment (days)			
Mean (SD)	28.10 (17.83)	33.09 (25.51)	0.5
Median	22.0	28.5	
Range	10.0–84.0	10.0–132.0	
FUO			
No	6 (20.7)	7 (21.9)	0.9
Yes	23 (79.3)	25 (78.1)	
No. of episodes			
Median	1.0	1.0	0.6
Range	1.0–2.0	1.0–2.0	
Proven infectious			
No	19 (65.5)	23 (71.9)	0.6
Yes	10 (34.5)	9 (28.1)	
TPN			
Yes	29 (100.0)	32 (100.0)	-
Duration of TPN (days)			
Median	13.0	14.0	0.8
Range	5.0–26.0	7.0–30.0	
Mucositis			
No	5 (17.2)	5 (15.6)	1
Yes	24 (82.8)	27 (84.4)	
Mucositis WHO grade			
0–I	7 (24.1)	13 (40.6)	0.2
II–IV	22 (75.9)	19 (59.4)	
Mucositis duration (days)			
Median	9.5	9.0	0.7
Range	3.0–19.0	3.0–23.0	
Antibiotic therapy			
No	2 (6.9)	3 (9.4)	1
Yes	27 (93.1)	29 (90.6)	
Duration of antibiotic therapy			
Median	14.0	11.0	0.2
Range	5.0–41.0	5.0–27.0	

Table 3. Cont.

	Filgrastim N = 29, (%)	Peg-filgrastim N = 32, (%)	p
Time from SCT to discharge			
Median	15.0	15.5	0.7
Range	11.0–48.0	12.0–32.0	
Follow up			
Alive	20 (69.0)	21 (65.6)	0.8
Died	9 (31.0)	11 (34.4)	
Follow-up from SCT (days)			
Median	894	816	1
95% CI	261–1323	534–1294	
Time from SCT to death (days)			
Median	614.0	317.0	0.6
Range	71.0–1300.0	157.0–973.0	

TBI, total body irradiation; WHO, World Health organization; TPN, total parenteral nutrition.

compared with daily delivering of filgrastim, and the potential cost-savings because the efficacy of one dose of pegfilgrastim is equivalent to up to 11 doses of filgrastim [18],[19]. The safety and efficacy of pegfilgrastim versus filgrastim after high-dose chemotherapy and autologous HSCT has been assessed in 14 studies of adult patients, 5 of them prospective randomized studies [20–24] and the remaining 9 studies being retrospective or prospective with historical-controls [25–33]. Pegfilgrastim was demonstrated to be as efficacious as 7 to 12 doses of filgrastim and it achieved faster neutrophil engraftment, with a median gain of one day, and in shortening the duration of febrile episodes. No differences were found for other post-transplant outcomes such as need for transfusion, infection rate, transplant-related mortality, and length of hospital stay [5],[22]. Interestingly, the analysis of costs in 2 randomized trials, one single-centre, double-blind, placebo-controlled, and one multicenter, open-label, showed that the use of pegfilgrastim was less expensive than filgrastim [22],[23]. Pegfilgrastim is still off-label for pediatric patients despite several authors having documented its efficacy and safety for prophylaxis of febrile neutropenia post-chemotherapy and as the mobilizing agent for peripheral blood stem cell collection [6–10],[12–15],[34]. No data have been published so far on the role of pegfilgrastim as a supportive agent after pediatric autologous HSCT. The main motivation for conducting such a clinical study is the possibility of reducing the costs of supportive post-HSCT drugs [5],[22], considering the increasing demands on health to rationalize and better allocate drug expenditure. For this reason we designed a non-inferiority study between the 2 molecules. Patient groups were comparable for all demographic and clinical characteristics. The homogeneity of the study population is an important issue to avoid the potential bias effect due to type of underlying disease, doses and types of chemotherapy used as conditioning regimen, the main post-HSCT outcomes such as recovery of neutrophils, incidence of febrile episodes, incidence of mucositis, and duration of febrile episodes. A single dose of pegfilgrastim was shown to be not inferior to a median of 9 doses of filgrastim in terms of

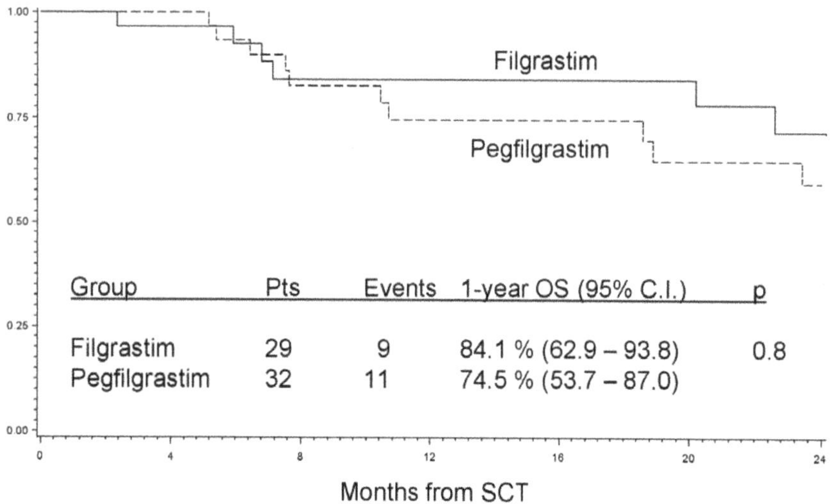

Figure 2. One-year overall survival curve for filgrastim and pegfilgrastim group, respectively. The 1-year overall survival in the in the filgrastim group and in the pegfilgrastim group is shown. No difference was found in the two groups.

neutrophil recovery and without any differences for all other variables analysed. Interestingly, as well as this non-inferiority, the use of pegfilgrastim provided a small cost reduction for G-CSF added to reduced health personnel resources in eliminating daily administration of filgrastim. The recent introduction of biosimilars of G-CSF has changed the scenario [35] Biosimilars of G-CSF, that were not available at the time of designing this study, are less expensive than filgrastim and therefore nullify the advantage of pegfilgrastin over filgrastim. No formal study has investigated the cost/benefit ratio of biosimilars over pegfilgrastim as regards unit cost and use of health personnel time.

Another point that is still a matter of debate is the time of initiation of filgrastim, early at day +1 vs. delayed at day +5 or day +7. It is generally accepted that both strategies are equally effective although some studies found an advantage of early G-CSF administration in terms of neutrophil engraftment, number of days of intravenous antibiotics, and length of hospital stay [3]. Despite the fact that this advantage is not completely clear, current guidelines recommend the use of G-CSF from day +1 post-HSCT [36].The delayed initiation of filgrastim is based on the concept that late-committed neutrophilic progenitors responsive to filgrastim are not yet present in the first days after HSCT. As far as pegfilgrastimis concerned, in the literature, the timing of administration ranges from day +1 (most of authors) to day +4 or day +5 [9], [25], [28], [37]. The advantage of a delayed administration of pegfilgrastim is to reduce the clearance by neutrophils obtaining a higher serum level during the period of aplasia. In fact, it is possible that at day +1 the myeloablative effects of conditioning regimen is not complete and the nadir of neutrophils is not achieved yet. To avoid any bias related to a different time of stimulation of myeloid progenitors we decided to start pegfilgrastim and filgrastim at the same time after transplant SCT. Day +3 was chosen because it was considered neither too late to compromise the biologic potential of pegfilgrastim nor too early to compromise the cost/effectiveness of filgrastim. Although this choice could have reduced the potential for a quicker neutrophil recovery with pegfilgrastim, the mean time to neutrophil engraftment was 10 days for both pegfilgrastin and filgrastim which is comparable to that observed in previous studies [3],[5].

In conclusion, this study showed that in pediatric autologous HSCT pegfilgrastim is not inferior to filgrastim for all post-transplant outcomes assessed, with the advantage of lower drug expenditure. The advent of biosimilars nullifies this advantage although prospective randomized studies are needed to compare the costs of 2 different therapeutic choices both in terms of drug expenditure and use of health personnel resources.

Acknowledgments

We thank Roberto Rondelli, M.D, for the help in the design of the study and Rodney Seddom for reviewing the English style.

Author Contributions

Conceived and designed the experiments: SC. Performed the experiments: SC FN GT MA ISP RB EC. Analyzed the data: SC GT ISP. Wrote the paper: SC GT ISP.

References

1. Passweg JR, Baldomero H, Gratwohl A, Bregni M, Cesaro S et al. (2012) The EBMT activity survey: 1990–2010. Bone Marrow Transplant 47: 906–923.
2. Aapro MS, Bohlius J, Cameron DA, Dal Lago L, Donnelly JP et al. (2011) 2010 update of EORTC guidelines for the use of granulocyte-colony stimulating factor to reduce the incidence of chemotherapy-induced febrile neutropenia in adult patients with lymphoproliferative disorders and solid tumours. Eur J Cancer 47: 8–32.
3. Trivedi M, Martinez S, Corringham S, Medley K, Ball ED. (2009) Optimal use of G-CSF administration after hematopoietic SCT. Bone Marrow Transplant 43: 895–908.
4. Samaras P, Blickenstorfer M, Siciliano RD, Haile SR, Buset EM et al. (2011) Pegfilgrastim reduces the length of hospitalization and the time to engraftment in multiple myeloma patients treated with melphalan 200 and auto-SCT compared with filgrastim. Ann Hematol 90: 89–94.
5. Ziakas PD, Kourbeti IS. (2012) Pegfilgrastim vs. filgrastim for supportive care after autologous stem cell transplantation: can we decide? Clin Transplant 26: 16–22.
6. Cesaro S, Zanazzo AG, Frenos S, Luksch R, Pegoraro A et al. (2011) A Phase II study on the safety and efficacy of a single dose of pegfilgrastim for mobilization and transplantation of autologous hematopoietic stem cells in pediatric oncohematology patients. Transfusion 51: 2480–7.
7. Dallorso S, Rondelli R, Messina C, Pession A, Giorgiani G et al. (2002) Clinical benefits of granulocyte colony-stimulating factor therapy after hematopoietic stem cell transplant in children: results of a prospective randomized trial. Haematologica 87: 1274–80.
8. te Poele EM, Kamps WA, Tamminga RY, Leeuw JA, Postma A et al. (2005) Pegfilgrastim in pediatric cancer patients. J Pediatr Hematol Oncol 2005; 27: 627–9.
9. Wendelin G, Lackner H, Schwinger W, Sovinz P, Urban C. (2005) Once-per-cycle pegfilgrastim versus daily filgrastim in pediatric patients with Ewing sarcoma. J Pediatr Hematol Oncol 27: 449–51.
10. André N, Kababri ME, Bertrand P, Rome A, Coze C et al. (2007) Safety and efficacy of pegfilgrastim in children with cancer receiving myelosuppressive chemotherapy. Anticancer Drugs 18: 277–81.
11. Borinstein SC, Pollard J, Winter L, Hawkins DS. (2009) Pegfilgrastim for prevention of chemotherapy-associated neutropenia in pediatric patients with solid tumors. Pediatr Blood Cancer 53: 375–8.
12. Milano-Bausset E, Gaudart J, Rome A, Coze C, Gentet JC et al. (2009) Retrospective comparison of neutropenia in children with Ewing sarcoma treated with chemotherapy and granulocyte colony-stimulating factor (G-CSF) or pegylated G-CSF. Clin Ther 31: 2388–95.
13. Spunt SL, Irving H, Frost J, Sender L, Guo M et al. (2010) Phase II, randomized, open-label study of pegfilgrastim-supported VDC/IE chemotherapy in pediatric sarcoma patients. J Clin Oncol 28:1329–36
14. Dallorso S, Berger M, Caviglia I, Emanueli T, Faraci M et al. (2008) Prospective single-arm study of pegfilgrastim activity and safety in children with poor-risk malignant tumours receiving chemotherapy. Bone Marrow Transplant 42: 507–13.
15. Fritsch P, Schwinger W, Schwantzer G, Lackner H, Sovinz P et al. (2010) Peripheral blood stem cell mobilization with pegfilgrastim compared to filgrastim in children and young adults with malignancies. Pediatr Blood Cancer 54: 134–7.
16. Schemper M, Smith TL, (1996) A note on quantifying follow-up studies of failure time. Control Clin Trials17:343–6
17. Siena S, Piccart MJ, Holmes FA, Glaspy J, Hackett J et al. (2003) A combined analysis of two pivotal randomized trials of a single dose of pegfilgrastim per chemotherapy cycle and daily Filgrastim in patients with stage II–IV breast cancer. Oncol Rep 10: 715–24.
18. Holmes FA, O'Shaughnessy JA, Vukelja S, Jones SE, Shogan J et al. (2002) Blinded, randomized, multicenter study to evaluate single administration pegfilgrastim once per cycle versus daily filgrastim as an adjunct to chemotherapy in patients with high-risk stage II or stage III/IV breast cancer. J Clin Oncol 20: 727–31.
19. Green MD, Koelbl H, Baselga J, Galid A, Guillem V et al. (2003) A randomized double-blind multicenter phase III study of fixed-dose single-administration pegfilgrastim versus daily filgrastim in patients receiving myelosuppressive chemotherapy. Ann Oncol 14: 29–35.
20. Martino M, Praticò G, Messina G, Irrera G, Massara E et al. (2006) Pegfilgrastim compared with filgrastim after high-dose melphalan and autologous hematopoietic peripheral blood stem cell transplantation in multiple myeloma patients. Eur J Haematol 77: 410–5.
21. Castagna L, Bramanti S, Levis A, Michieli MG, Anastasia A et al. (2010) Pegfilgrastim versus filgrastim after high-dose chemotherapy and autologous peripheral blood stem cell support. Ann Oncol 21: 1482–5.
22. Gerds A, Fox-Geiman M, Dawravoo K, Rodriguez T, Toor A et al. (2010) Randomized phase III trial of pegfilgrastim versus filgrastim after autologus peripheral blood stem cell transplantation. Biol Blood Marrow Transplant 16: 678–85.

23. Sebban C, Lefranc A, Perrier L, Moreau P, Espinouse D et al. (2012) A randomised phase II study of the efficacy, safety and cost-effectiveness of pegfilgrastim and filgrastim after autologous stem cell transplant for lymphoma and myeloma (PALM study). Eur J Cancer 48: 713–20.
24. Rifkin R, Spitzer G, Orloff G, Mandanas R, McGaughey D et al. (2010) Pegfilgrastim appears equivalent to daily dosing of filgrastim to treat neutropenia after autologous peripheral blood stem cell transplantation in patients with non-Hodgkin lymphoma. Clin Lymphoma Myeloma Leuk 10: 186–91.
25. Ferrara F, Izzo T, Criscuolo C, Riccardi C, Viola A et al. (2011) Comparison of fixed dose pegfilgrastim and daily filgrastim after autologous stem cell transplantation in patients with multiple myeloma autografted on a outpatient basis. Hematol Oncol 29: 139–43.
26. Mathew S, Adel N, Rice RD, Panageas K, Duck ET et al. (2010) Retrospective comparison of the effects of filgrastim and pegfilgrastim on the pace of engraftment in auto-SCT patients. Bone Marrow Transplant 45: 1522–7.
27. Musto P, Scalzulli PR, Terruzzi E, Rossini F, Iacopino P et al. (2007) Pegfilgrastim versus filgrastim after autologous stem cell tranplantation: case-control study in patients with multiple myeloma and review of the literature. Leuk Res 31: 1487–93.
28. Ballestrero A, Boy D, Gonella R, Miglino M, Clavio M et al. (2008) Pegfilgrastim compared with filgrastim after autologous peripheral blood stem cell transplantation in patients with solid tumours and lymphomas. Ann Hematol 87: 49–55.
29. Jagasia MH, Greer JP, Morgan DS, Mineishi S, Kassim AA et al. (2005) Pegfilgrastim after high-dose chemotherapy and autologous peripheral blood stem cell transplant: phase II study. Bone Marrow Transplant 35: 1165–9.
30. Staber PB, Holub R, Linkesch W, Schmidt H, Neumeister P. (2005) Fixed-dose single administration of Pegfilgrastim vs daily Filgrastim in patients with haematological malignancies undergoing autologous peripheral blood stem cell transplantation. Bone Marrow Transplant 35: 889–93.
31. Vanstraelen G, Frère P, Ngirabacu MC, Willems E, Fillet G et al. (2006) Pegfilgrastim compared with Filgrastim after autologous hematopoietic peripheral blood stem cell transplantation. Exp Hematol 34: 382–8.
32. Samaras P, Blickenstorfer M, Siciliano RD, Haile SR, Buset EM et al. (2011) Pegfilgrastim reduces the length of hospitalization and the time to engraftment in multiple myeloma patients treated with melphalan 200 and auto-SCT compared with filgrastim. Ann Hematol 90: 89–94.
33. Samaras P, Buset EM, Siciliano RD, Haile SR, Petrausch U et al. (2010) Equivalence of pegfilgrastim and filgrastim in lymphoma patients treated with BEAM followed by autologous stem cell transplantation. Oncology 79: 93–7.
34. Borinstein SC, Pollard J, Winter L, Hawkins DS. (2009) Pegfilgrastim for prevention of chemotherapy-associated neutropenia in pediatric patients with solid tumors. Pediatr Blood Cancer 53: 375–8.
35. Niederwieser D, Schmitz S. (2011) Biosimilar agents in oncology/haematology: from approval to practice. Eur J Haematol 86:277–88
36. Smith TJ, Khatcheressian J, Lyman GH, Ozer H, Armitage JO et al. (2006) 2006 update of recommendations for the use of white blood cell growth factors: an evidence-based clinical practice guideline. J Clin Oncol 24: 3187–205.
37. Zwick C, Hartmann F, Zeynalova S, Poschel V, Nickenig C, et al. (2011) Randomized comparison of pegfilgrastim day 4 versus day 2 for the prevention of chemotherapy-induced leucytopenia. Ann Oncol 22; 1872–877

8

Dynamics of *Streptococcus pneumoniae* Serotypes Causing Acute Otitis Media Isolated from Children with Spontaneous Middle-Ear Drainage over a 12-Year Period (1999–2010) in a Region of Northern Spain

Marta Alonso[1], José M. Marimon[1,2], María Ercibengoa[1], Eduardo G. Pérez-Yarza[3,4], Emilio Pérez-Trallero[1,2,4]*

1 Microbiology Department, Hospital Universitario Donostia-Instituto Biodonostia, San Sebastián, Spain, **2** Biomedical Research Center Network for Respiratory Diseases, San Sebastián, Spain, **3** Pediatric Department, Hospital Universitario Donostia-Instituto Biodonostia, San Sebastián, Spain, **4** Faculty of Medicine, University of the Basque Country, San Sebastián, Spain

Abstract

The aim of this study was to determine the serotype and clonal distribution of pneumococci causing acute otitis media (AOM) and their relationship with recurrences and mixed infections with other microorganisms under the influence of the 7-valent pneumococcal conjugate vaccine (PCV7). To do this, all pneumococcal isolates collected from the spontaneous middle-ear drainage of children <5 years old diagnosed of AOM by their pediatrician or their general practitioner from 1999 to 2010 were phenotypically characterized and the most frequent serotypes were genotyped. In the 12-year study, 818 episodes of pneumococcal AOM were detected, mostly (70.5%) in children younger than 2 years old. In 262 episodes (32%), the pneumococci were isolated with another bacterium, mainly (n = 214) *Haemophilus influenzae*. Mixed infections were similar in children under or over 2 years old. The most frequent serotypes were 19A (n = 227, 27.8%), 3 (n = 92, 11.2%) and 19F (n = 74, 9%). Serotypes included in the PCV7 sharply decreased from 62.4% in the pre-vaccination (1999–2001) to 2.2% in the late post-vaccination period (2008–2010). Serotype diversity steadily increased after the introduction of the PCV7 but decreased from 2008–2010 due to the predominant role of serotype 19A isolates, mostly ST276 and ST320. The prevalence of serotype 3 doubled from 6.1% (20/326) in 1999–2004 to 14.6% (72/492) in 2005–2010. Relapses mainly occurred in male infants infected with isolates with diminished antimicrobial susceptibility. Reinfections caused by isolates with the same serotype but different genotype were frequent, highlighting the need for genetic studies to differentiate among similar strains. In conclusion, the main change in pneumococcal AOM observed after the introduction of the PCV7 was the sharp decrease in vaccine serotypes. Also notable was the high burden of serotype 19A in total pneumococcal AOM before and especially after the introduction of the PCV7, as well as in relapses and reinfections.

Editor: Herminia de Lencastre, Rockefeller University, United States of America

Funding: This work was supported in part by grants from the University of the Basque Country (UPV/EHU; grant no. GIU 09/59) and from the Department of Health, Basque Country (grant 2009-111 012). The funders had no role in study design, data collection and analysis, decision to publish, or preparation of the manuscript.

Competing Interests: The authors have declared that no competing interests exist.

* E-mail: mikrobiol@terra.es

Introduction

Acute otitis media (AOM) is one of the most common infections during childhood and nearly every child has experienced an episode of AOM by the age of 5 years [1,2]. The etiology of AOM varies with age, the most frequently implicated agents being viruses such as rhinoviruses, influenza viruses, or respiratory syncytial viruses and bacteria, such as non-encapsulated *Haemophilus influenzae*, *Streptococcus pneumoniae* and *Moraxella catarrhalis*. Due to the high frequency of AOM, this infection accounts for one of the highest expenditures in health care, including direct (physician visits and antibiotics) or indirect (lost hours of work, etc.) costs [3]. *S. pneumoniae* is one of the main agents causing bacterial AOM, directly or as complication of a viral upper respiratory tract infection [4]. Since the introduction of the 7-valent pneumococcal conjugate vaccine (PCV7) for the prevention of invasive pneumococcal disease, many researchers have demonstrated a reduction in AOM cases in vaccinated as well as in non-vaccinated children as a consequence of herd protection [2,5]. However, an increase in the proportion of AOM caused by non-vaccine serotypes, especially of serotype 19A, has also been reported [5,6].

The main aim of this work was to analyze the epidemiology of pneumococcal AOM infection in relation to the serotype and clonal distribution of isolates in San Sebastián, northern Spain, over a 12-year period. As a secondary aim, the frequency of coinfection with other bacteria and the possible association of specific pneumococcal serotypes with recurrences were also studied.

Methods

Patients and Isolates

The study was conducted at Hospital Universitario Donostia, located in the city of San Sebastián, Basque Country, northern Spain which attends an estimated population of around 350,000 inhabitants from the region of Donostialdea and adjacent areas. The study included all *S. pneumoniae* isolates recovered from 1999 to 2010 from the spontaneous middle-ear drainage of children aged <5 years old diagnosed of AOM by their pediatrician or their general practitioner. Samples were sent to the Microbiology Department of Donostia Hospital where all microbiological procedures were performed. Publication of the results was approved by the Ethical Committee for Clinical Research of the Health Area of Gipuzkoa with a waiver of informed consent documentation since this was a retrospective study and patients' identities were safeguarded.

The middle ear fluid was processed by Gram-staining and culture. Pneumococci were identified by their colony morphology, optochin susceptibility and bile solubility. Bacteria others than *S. pneumoniae* were identified using standard microbiological procedures (requirement of X and V factors for growth of *H. influenzae* and coaglutination with specific b and a, c-f antisera; bacitracin-susceptibility and latex agglutination with specific group A streptococci antisera for *Streptococcus pyogenes;* oxidase-test and carbohydrate fermentation tests for *M. catarrhalis*; coagulase test for *Staphylococcus aureus*). Serotyping was performed with the Quellung reaction, an antibody-based microarray serotyping technique (Pneumoarray, Abyntek, Spain) and/or multiplex polymerase chain reaction (PCR) [7]. Isolates giving a negative serotype reaction and not amplifying the capsular-gene locus [8] were defined as non-encapsulated. The serotype of all 19F and 19A isolates serotyped with the Quellung reaction or the Pneumoarray was confirmed by a PCR specific for the 19F and 19A capsular loci [9].

This study was performed between 1999 and 2010 and was divided into four time periods: one pre-vaccination period, from 1999 to 2001 and three post-PCV7 periods: from 2002 to 2004 (early post-PCV7 period), from 2005 to 2007 (intermediate post-PCV7 period) and from 2008 to 2010 (late post-PCV7 period). The PCV7 has not been included in the official vaccination schedule of the public health system of the Basque Country, and was only dispensed in private practice. Its use had progressively increased from 2002, with a vaccine coverage rate in children under 2 years of age estimated to be close to 50% before 2006 [10]) and 60% in 2009, based on the number of doses sold in Gipuzkoa.

Minimal inhibitory concentrations were determined by the broth microdilution assay according to Clinical and Laboratory Standards Institute (CLSI) guidelines [11].

Molecular Characterization of Pneumococcal Isolates

To study the clonal relationship of the most frequent serotypes, pulsed-field gel electrophoresis (PFGE) and multi-locus sequence typing (MLST) were performed. PFGE was carried out according to previously described protocols [12] and MLST according to the protocol described on the pneumococcal MLST web site (http://www.mlst.net). PFGE characterization was performed in a random sample of approximately half of all isolates of the two most prevalent serotypes. Moreover, PFGE was also performed in all isolates causing relapses or reinfections by the same serotype in the same children and in selected multidrug-resistant isolates (penicillin MIC >0.06 µg/ml and non-susceptibility to a further two or more antimicrobial classes). PFGE similarity patterns of <85% were considered as different and were arbitrarily named in this study with a capital letter, from A to Z. After *Sma*I digestion, PFGE patterns were analyzed and a dendrogram was constructed using the Diversity Database software (Bio-Rad Laboratories, USA), with a band tolerance of 1%, the Dice coefficient and the unweighted pair group method with arithmetic averages (UPGMA). Isolates of the most prevalent PFGE patterns were further characterized by determining the MLST of two to three representative isolates.

Statistical Analyses

Differences in the distribution of serotypes were analyzed by the chi squared test or by Fisher's exact test when appropriate. Analysis of trends over time was calculated using the chi squared test for trend (GraphPad Instat ver 3.05. La Jolla, CA, USA). A p value of <0.05 was considered as statically significant. Diversity was calculated by Simpson's Index of Diversity 1− D, where $D = \sum n * (n-1)/N * (N-1)$, with n being the number of isolates of a specific serotype in each period and N the total number of isolates (sample size) in each period. The on-line tool: darwin.phyloviz.net/ComparingPartitions/was used. The value of this index ranges between 0 and 1 and the greater the value, the greater the sample diversity.

Recurrences, Relapses and Reinfections

In this study, recurrences encompassed both relapses and reinfections: a relapse was defined as a second episode of AOM caused by the same serotype and genotype with an interval between 7 and 89 days from the first episode. A reinfection was defined as a second episode produced by a different serotype or by the same serotype but with a different genotype, or as a second episode caused by the same serotype and genotype but taking place after 90 or more days. In this study, reinfections, but not relapses, were included as distinct episodes.

Results

Between 1999 and 2010, 1,006 non-duplicated *S. pneumoniae* isolates were cultured from the middle ear exudates collected from patients diagnosed with AOM. Of these, 818 (81.3%) belonged to 708 children aged <5 years old. A single episode of pneumococcal AOM was observed in 622/708 (87.9%) children and two or more episodes in 86 (12.1%) (Table 1). Age at the time of the first AOM episode, was less than 1 year in 229 infants (55.9% boys), 1 year in 270 (54.1% boys) children, 2 years in 105 (56.2% boys), 3 years in 63 (58.7% boys) children and 4 years in 41 (63.4% boys) children. By episodes, 69.1% (565/818) occurred before the child's second birthday.

Serotype Distribution

Overall, the three most frequent serotypes were 19A (n = 227, 27.8%), 3 (n = 92, 11.2%) and 19F (n = 74, 9.0%).

The prevalence of PCV7 serotypes causing AOM sharply decreased after the introduction of the PCV7 in 2001, from 62.4% in the 1999–2001 pre-vaccination period to 2.2% in the 2008–2010 late post-vaccination period (p value for trend p<0.001). Individually, each of the four most prevalent PCV7 serotypes (6B, 14, 19F and 23F) significantly decreased from 1999–2001 to 2008–2010 (p<0.001), with the fall in the percentage of serotypes 19F, 14, 6B and 23F across the four study periods being particularly striking (Fig. 1). The prevalence of serotypes 1, 5 and 7F, included in the 10-valent PCV (PCV10) but not in the PCV7, was low (equal to or under 4% for each serotype); however, when considered all together, these serotypes showed an increasing

Table 1. General characteristics of patients and pneumococcal acute otitis media (AOM) episodes.

No. patients (% males)	708 (55.9)
No. episodes	818
Age of patients in months at the time of the first AOM episode [median (interquartile range)]	12 (10–24)
No. (%) episodes with *Streptococcus pneumoniae* alone	556 (68.0)
No. (%) episodes with mixed infections	262 (32.0)
No. (%) patients with only 1 AOM episode	622 (87.8)
No. patients with reinfections	86
No. patients with 1 episode of reinfection	68
No. patients with 2 episodes of reinfection	13
No. patients with 3 episodes of reinfection	4
No. patients with 5 episodes of reinfection	1
No. patients with relapses[1]	*21*
No. patients relapsing with an interval of 7–20 days	*14*
No. patients relapsing with an interval of 21–30 days	*6*
No. patients relapsing with an interval of 31–89 days	*1*

[1]Relapses were not included as distinct episodes.

trend over the study period (p for trend $p = 0.003$). The number of AOM caused by the two most prevalent serotypes (3 and 19A), included in the PCV13 but not in the PCV7 nor in the PCV10, also increased throughout the study period (p for trend $p<0.001$ for each serotype). Specifically, the prevalence of serotype 19A increased from 17.9% to 37.9% between 1999–2001and 2008–2010 ($p<0.001$) and that of serotype 3 increased from 5.1% to 15.0% ($p = 0.007$). AOM caused by serotype 6A did not vary but those caused by serotype 6C showed a striking increase (p for trend $p<0.001$). Only 9 of the 818 pneumococci were non-encapsulated.

Serotype Diversity

The overall number of different serotypes causing pneumococcal AOM in young children increased after the introduction of the PCV7 (Table 2). In the 1999–2001 period, only 21 serotypes were identified but in the next three periods, 31 or more serotypes were found (33 in 2002–2004, 38 in 2005–2007 and 31 in 2008–2010).

Diversity increased from the pre-vaccine period to the 3 post-vaccine periods: 0.642 (95%CI 0.507–0.776) in the pre-vaccine period (1999–2001) to 0.844 (95%CI 0.782–0.907) in the second, 0.899 (95%CI 0.864–0.933) in the third period, and 0.844 (95%CI 0.774–0.915) in 2008–2010. When the PCV7 serotypes were excluded the significant difference between the pre-vaccine and the post-vaccine periods remained: 0.524 (95%CI 0.360–0.687), 0.814 (95%CI 0.733–0.894), 0.885 (95%CI 0.835–0.935), and 0.876 (95%CI 0.813–0.938) for the 1999–2001, 2002–2004, 2005–2007 and 2008–2010 periods, respectively.

Mixed Infections

Among the 818 isolates, in 556 (68.0%), *S. pneumoniae* was isolated alone, in 214 (26.2%) with *H. influenzae* and in 48 (5.9%) with microorganisms other than *H. influenzae*: *S. aureus* ($n = 23$), *S. pyogenes* ($n = 9$), *M. catarrhalis* ($n = 6$), etc. Triple mixed infections were found in 12 episodes (1.5%), most of them ($n = 7$) with *S. aureus*.

When we divided the study in four 3-year periods, we observed 117 episodes in 108 children in 1999–2001, 209 episodes in 187 children in 2002–2004, 265 episodes in 215 children in 2005–2007 and 227 episodes in 198 children in 2008–2010. Thirty children had two or more AOM episodes in different periods.

By periods, the percentages of episodes with mixed infections were similar in the four study periods: 31.6% ($n = 37/117$) in the pre-PCV7 period and 31.6% (66/209), 32.8% (87/265) and 31.7% (72/227) for the early, intermediate and late post-PCV7 periods. The percentages of pneumococci and *H. influenzae* mixed infections showed no differences (23.1%, 28.2%, 29.1% and 22.5% for 1999–2001, 2002–2004, 2005–2007 and 2008–2010, respectively). No *H. influenzae* group b was found.

By age, the frequency of episodes of overall mixed infections or mixed infections with *H. influenzae* was similar in children under or over 2 years old: 175/565 (31.0%) overall and 140/565 (24.8%) with *H. influenzae* versus 87/253 (34.4%) overall and 74/253 (29.2%) with *H. influenzae* ($p = 0.3$ and $p = 0.2$ for overall and for *H. influenzae* mixed infections respectively). By gender, the frequency remained non-significant: 133 overall mixed infections and 111 with *H. influenzae* in 453 episodes in boys and 129 ($p = 0.07$) and 103 ($p = 0.2$) in 365 episodes in girls, respectively.

Together or individually, PCV7 serotypes were similarly found as single etiology or as mixed infections (total 125/556 and 68/262, respectively, $p = 0.3$). Serotypes 1 (20/556 versus 1/262, $p = 0.004$), 3 (75/556 versus 17/262, $p = 0.003$) and 19A (170/556 versus 57/262, $p = 0.01$) were found mainly as a single etiology. In contrast, serotype 15B was more frequently found in mixed cultures (13/262 versus 12/556, $p = 0.03$). No differences were found among others serotypes.

Genotyping

Overall, 31 different PFGE patterns were identified among the random selection of 115 serotype 19A isolates characterized by PFGE (11, 27, 34, and 43 isolates per each study period, respectively). The high heterogeneity found within serotype 19A isolates was found in the four study periods with changes in the prevalence of specific clones throughout the study period. ST276 was the major clone circulating from 1999–2001 (3/11 isolates), 2002–2004 (9/27 isolates) and 2005–2007 (5/34 isolates). During the last period, 2008–2010, ST320 (19/43 studied isolates) was slightly more frequent than ST276 (15/43 isolates) which was the

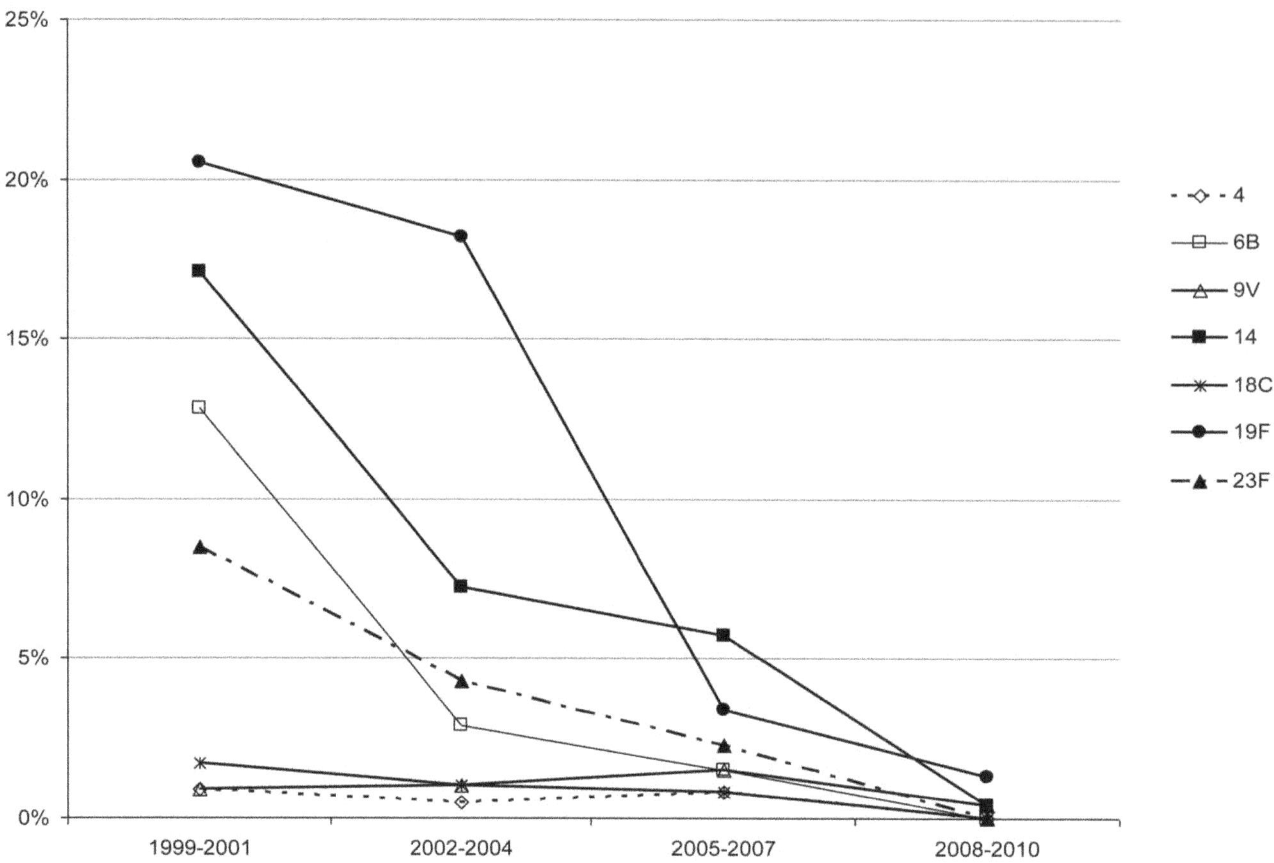

Figure 1. Percentage evolution of serotypes (number of a specific serotype/total isolates in each period) included in the 7-valent pneumococcal conjugate vaccine.

second most common genotype. ST320 was detected for the first time in this series in 2005. ST193 and ST199 clones were found in the four study periods, but minority clones such as ST62, ST63, ST202, ST220, ST994 and ST1201were only occasionally present. When all multidrug-resistant serotype 19A isolates (whether included or not in the random selection) were grouped, ST276 was the most prevalent clone (n = 69), followed by ST320 (n = 29). ST276 showed penicillin, erythromycin, tetracycline, and trimethoprim-sulfamethoxazole (SXT) MICs of 1–2, >4, >4 and 1–2 µg/mL, respectively. All ST320 isolates showed multiresistance with penicillin, erythromycin and SXT resistance and showed amoxicillin MICs ≥2 µg/ml (25/29, 88.2%, amoxicillin MICs were ≥4 µg/ml).

The 46 serotype 3 isolates characterized by PFGE showed three different patterns, corresponding to ST180, ST260 and ST1220. The most prevalent clone was ST180 (61.4%) and the least prevalent clone was ST1220 (4.5%), which belonged to the same clonal complex as ST260 (34.1%). ST180 and ST260 isolates were homogeneously distributed in the different periods. All serotype 3 isolates were penicillin- and erythromycin-susceptible (MICs <0.12 µg/ml and <0.5 µg/ml, respectively).

Recurrences

Relapses. Relapses occurred in 21 children (Table 3). Fourteen children relapsed with an interval of less than 3 weeks, six between 21 and 30 days and one relapsed after 43 days. Risk factors for relapses were detected in only three children: adenoids and obstructive sleep apnea, atopy, Down syndrome and obstructive sleep apnea.

In the first two study periods (1999–2001 and 2002–2004), relapses were produced mainly by PCV7 serotypes and the percentage of relapses progressively decreased: there were five relapses among 108 children (4.6%) in the pre-PCV7 period, decreasing to 7/187 (3.7%) and 2/215 (0.9%) in the early and intermediate post-PCV7 periods (p for trend p = 0.04). In the late post-PCV7 period, relapses increased, with seven relapses among 198 (3.5%) children, all of them caused by serotype 19A isolates. Only seven relapsing children had previously received the PCV7 and all of them were infected with serotype 19A isolates. One of these vaccinated children relapsed four times at intervals of between 23 and 30 days with the multiresistant ST320 clone. Five months after the last relapse, this child had a fifth episode with the same clone, which was classified as a reinfection, based on the definition described in Material and Methods. No modification in the susceptibility pattern of relapsing isolates was observed in any of the children. Diminished susceptibility to penicillin (MIC >0.06 µg/mL) was observed in 76.2% of isolates from relapsing children, and amoxicillin resistance (MIC >2 µg/mL) in 33.3% (n = 7). Isolates from another four children showed an amoxicillin MIC of 1–2 µg/mL (52.4% of relapsing children had isolates with an amoxicillin MIC >0.5 µg/mL). Moreover, erythromycin resistance was observed in isolates from 71.4% of relapsing children.

Reinfections. There were 86 children (48.8% boys) with at least two episodes of infection: 68 children had one episode of

Table 2. Serotype distribution of pneumococci isolated from 818 episodes of acute otitis media from children less than 5 years of age in Gipuzkoa, Northern Spain (1999–2010).

Serotype	1999–2001		2002–2004		2005–2007		2008–2010		Total	
	n	%	n	%	n	%	n	%	n	%
4	1	0.9	1	0.5	2	0.8	0		4	0.5
6B	15	12.8	6	2.9	4	1.5	0		25	3.1
9V	1	0.9	2	1.0	4	1.5	1	0.4	8	1.0
14	20	17.1	15	7.2	15	5.7	1	0.4	51	6.2
18C	2	1.7	2	1.0	2	0.8	0		6	0.7
19F	24	20.5	38	18.2	9	3.4	3	1.3	74	9.0
23F	10	8.5	9	4.3	6	2.3	0		25	3.1
PCV7[1]	**73**	**62.4**	**73**	**34.9**	**42**	**15.8**	**5**	**2.2**	**193**	**23.6**
1	1	0.9	3	1.4	10	3.8	7	3.1	21	2.6
5	0		0		2	0.8	5	2.2	7	0.9
7F	1	0.9	7	3.3	8	3.0	9	4.0	25	3.1
PCV10[2]	**2**	**1.7**	**10**	**4.8**	**20**	**7.5**	**21**	**9.3**	**53**	**6.5**
3	6	5.1	14	6.7	38	14.3	34	15.0	92	11.2
6A	2	1.7	8	3.8	9	3.4	4	1.8	23	2.8
19A	21	17.9	53	25.4	67	25.3	86	37.9	227	27.8
PCV13[3]	**29**	**24.8**	**75**	**35.9**	**114**	**43.0**	**124**	**54.6**	**342**	**41.8**
6C	0		1	0.5	3	1.1	10	4.4	14	1.7
8	0		2	1.0	2	0.8	2	0.9	6	0.7
9N	0		1	0.5	1	0.4	1	0.4	3	0.4
10	0		7	3.3	4	1.5	4	1.8	15	1.8
11	1	0.9	9	4.3	9	3.4	8	3.5	27	3.3
12	0		0		1	0.4	3	1.3	4	0.5
15A	0		0		3	1.1	3	1.3	6	0.7
15B	0		4	1.9	15	5.7	6	2.6	25	3.1
16F	1	0.9	3	1.4	7	2.6	6	2.6	17	2.1
21	1	0.9	2	1.0	10	3.8	4	1.8	17	2.1
22F	1	0.9	4	1.9	6	2.3	3	1.3	14	1.7
23A	1	0.9	2	1.0	4	1.5	2	0.9	9	1.1
23B	0		2	1.0	3	1.1	3	1.3	8	1.0
31	0		0		1	0.4	5	2.2	6	0.7
33	1	0.9	3	1.4	3	1.1	4	1.8	11	1.3
35	4	3.4	0		3	1.1	7	3.1	14	1.7
38	0		0		1	0.4	0		1	0.1
Other[4]	0		9	4.3	9	3.4	6	2.6	24	2.9
NT	3	2.6	2	1.0	4	1.5	0		9	1.1
Non PCV13	**13**	**11.1**	**51**	**24.4**	**89**	**33.6**	**77**	**33.9**	**230**	**28.1**
Total episodes	117		209		265		227		818	

[1]PCV7: number of isolates of serotypes included in the PCV7: serotypes 4, 6B, 9V, 14, 18C, 19F and 23F.
[2]PCV10: number of isolates of serotypes 1, 5, and 7F, included in the PCV10 but not in the PCV7.
[3]PCV13: number of isolates of serotypes 3, 6A, and 19A, included in the PCV13 but not in the PCV10.
[4]Non-PCV13 serotype (2, 7A, 13, 17F, 18F, 19B, 24, 25, 28, 29, 34, 36, 39,41,47) who total number was less than 4 were grouped as "Others".

reinfection, 13 had two, four had three, and one child had four episodes, making a total 110 episodes of reinfection (196 episodes of infection). PCV7 serotypes produced 26 episodes of reinfection in 24 children, of which only 8 children (9 episodes) were vaccinated at the time of the reinfection episode. Reinfections were more common in children under 24 months than in older children. Thirty infants younger than 1 year old (30/229, 13.1%) and 39 one-year-old children (39/270, 14.4%) acquired a second episode of infection versus 10 children aged 2 years old (10/105, 9.5%), five children aged 3 years old (5/63, 7.9%) and only one child aged 4 years old (1/41, 2.4%).

Reinfections were caused by an isolate with a different serotype than that causing the first infection in 69 children and by an isolate of the same serotype (RI-SS) in 17 children. Of these 17 children

Table 3. Relapses. Patients with a second episode or more of infection in an interval of between 7 and 90 days caused by isolates with the same serotype and genotype.

Patient	Age	Gender	Date (year/month/day)	Isolation interval (in days)	PCV7	Serotype	MLST	Resistance pattern[1]
RL_1	1 year	Male	1999/01/19	43	None	19F	ST63	PEN,ERY,CLI,TET,SXT
			1999/03/08					
RL_2	2 years	Male	1999/04/30	7	None	14	ST156	PEN,SXT
			1999/05/07					
RL_3	1 year	Male	2000/03/01	14	None	14	ST1964	PEN,ERY,CLI,TET,SXT,CHL
			2000/03/15					
RL_4	1 year	Male	2000/05/25	27	None	14	ST156	PEN,SXT
			2000/6/21					
RL _5	8 months	Male	2001/11/23	19	None	6B	ST1624	PEN,ERY,CLI,TET,SXT
			2001/12/12					
RL _6	2 years	Male	2002/01/22	10	None	11	ST42	-
			2002/02/01					
RL _7	<1 month	Male	2002/12/17	20	None	19F	ST88	PEN, TET, SXT,CHL
			2003/01/06					
RL _8	7 months	Female	2003/05/02	17	None	23F	ST81	PEN,ERY,CLI,TET,SXT,CHL
			2003/05/19					
RL _9	10 months	Male	2003/05/19	11	None	19A	ST199	-
			2003/05/30					
RL _10	2 months	Female	2003/12/12	18	None	19F	ST63	PEN,ERY,CLI,TET
			2003/12/30					
RL _11	8 months	Male	2004/03/30	13	None	14	Slv1964	PEN,ERY,CLI,SXT
			2004/04/12					
RL _12	1 year	Female	2004/08/03	21	None	19F	ST424	-
			2004/08/24					
RL _13	6 months	Male	2007/04/19	27	Yes	19A	ST320	PEN,ERY,CLI,TET,SXT
			2007/05/16	23				
			2007/06/08	29				
			2007/07/07					
RL _14	7 months	Female	2007/06/07	25	Yes	19A	ST193	ERY,CLI,TET
			2007/07/02					
RL _15	4 months	Male	2008/10/11	10	None	19A	ST320	PEN,ERY,CLI,TET,SXT
			2008/10/21					
RL _16	1 year	Male	2009/05/15	9	Yes	19A	ST320	PEN,ERY,CLI,TET,SXT
			2009/05/24					
RL _17	7 months	Male	2009/11/19	30	Yes	19A	ST320	PEN,ERY,CLI,TET,SXT
			2009/12/19					
RL _18	5 months	Male	2009/11/24	18	Yes	19A	ST320	PEN,ERY,CLI,TET,SXT
			2009/12/12					
RL _19	11 months	Female	2009/12/10	12	None	19A	ST276	PEN,ERY,CLI,TET,SXT
			2009/12/22					
RL _20	6 months	Male	2010/02/16	30	Yes	19A	ST193	ERY,CLI,TET
			2010/03/18					
RL _21	11 months	Male	2010/05/26	7	Yes	19A	ST276	PEN,ERY,CLI,TET
			2010/06/02					

[1]PEN = penicillin, ERY = erythromycin, CLI = clindamycin, TET = tetracycline, SXT = trimethoprim-sulfamethoxazole, CHL = chloramphenicol.

with RI-SS (Table 4) only three (17.6%) were unvaccinated and two of the reinfections were caused by serotype 19F. Serotype 19A was the most frequent serotype causing RI-SS (n = 9, 52.9%) while serotypes 3, 6C, 15A, 15B, 22F and 23A, caused one each.

Table 4. Patients with reinfections caused by the same serotype as the initial infection.

Patient	Age	Gender	Date (year/month/day)	Isolation interval (in days)	PCV7[a]	Serotype	PFGE pattern [b]	MLST
RI_1	1 year	Male	1999/12/11	128	None	19F	K	ST202
			2000/04/17		None	19F	B	ST276
RI _2	8 months	Female	2004/03/02	154	None	19F	E	ST424
			2004/08/03		None	19F	E	ST424
RI _3	1 year	Male	2005/02/07	746	Yes	3	D	ST180
			2007/02/23		Yes	3	D	ST180
RI _4	5 months	Female	2006/12/09	444	Yes	19A	C	ST199
			2008/02/26		Yes	19A	B	ST276
RI _5	10 months	Male	2007/02/05	1199	Yes	15A	O	ST2613
			2010/05/19		Yes	15A	P	NEW SLV193
RI _6	7 months	Male	2007/03/01	692	Yes	22F	H	ST30
			2009/01/21		Yes	22F	Q	ST433
RI _7	6 months	Male	2007/04/19	236	Yes	19A	A	ST320
			2007/12/11		Yes	19A	A	ST320
RI _8	1 year	Male	2007/06/03	145	Yes	19A	M	ST994
			2007/10/26		Yes	19A	C	ST199
RI _9	7 months	Female	2007/06/07	45	Yes	19A	J	ST193
			2007/07/22		Yes	19A	B	ST276
RI _10	1 year	Female	2008/01/23	365	Yes	23A	C	ST2829
			2009/01/22		Yes	23A	C	ST2829
RI _11	9 months	Female	2008/05/21	118	Yes	19A	B	ST276
			2008/09/16		Yes	19A	A	ST320
RI _12	1 year	Female	2008/07/08	400	Yes	15B	R	NEW SLV5216
			2009/08/12		Yes	15B	R	NEW SLV5216
RI _13	2 years	Female	2008/10/14	213	Yes	6C	N	ST1692
			2009/05/15		Yes	6C	L	ST386
RI _14	1 year	Male	2009/06/10	167	Yes	19A	A	ST320
			2009/11/24		Yes	19A	A	ST320
RI _15	1 year	Male	2009/10/13	267	Yes	19A	I	ST62
			2010/07/07		Yes	19A	C	ST199
RI _16	1year	Female	2009/12/10	111	Yes	19A	A	ST320
			2010/03/31		Yes	19A	A	ST320
RI_17	4 years	Male	2010/04/06	18	None	19A	C	ST199
			2010/04/24		None	19A	B	ST276

[a]PCV7:7-valent pneumococcal conjugate vaccination (PCV7 included serotypes: 4, 6B, 9V, 14, 18C, 19F and 23F).
[b]Pulse-field gel electrophoresis pattern, arbitrary named MLST = multilocus sequence typing.

After PFGE and MLST analysis, we observed that 10 (58.8%) of the 17 RI-SS had a different genotype, giving a total of 79 children with reinfections caused by a different strain and 7 with reinfections caused by isolates with the same genotype but with an interval of more than 90 days between the first episode and the reinfection. Among these 7 children with reinfections caused by the same genotype (same strain), three reinfections were caused by serotype 19A, all of which were ST320. None of these children showed anatomical lesions, chromosome anomalies, immunodeficiency, or any other apparent risk factor.

By age, no differences were found in the frequency of RI-SS when we grouped children into those aged younger or older than 2 years old (15/499 *versus* 2/209; $p = 0.2$) and into those younger than 1 year (7/229), those aged 1 to 3 years (8/438), and those aged more than 3 years (1/41) ($p = 0.6$).

Discussion

AOM is probably the most common infectious disease in young children treated by physicians and produces frequent recurrences [13]. Compared with other bacteria causing AOM, *S. pneumoniae* otitis has been associated with more severe signs and symptoms and more complications [14].

In this study, we analyzed the dynamics of *S. pneumoniae* clones causing AOM between 1999 and 2010 in a region of northern Spain and their involvement in recurrences. Despite the large number of studies of invasive pneumococcal disease (IPD) in the last few years, there is little information on pneumococcal AOM with full characterization of isolates from a single region over a broad time period. All capsulated isolates were serotyped, and only 9 of 818 isolates were unencapsulated, the uniqueness of this finding being well known [15].

One limitation of this study is that the number of isolates included in each period depended on physician demand. Considering that many patients with mild AOM never attend their physician and spontaneously cure, we could not determine changes or real incidence of AOM in our region. Unlike the diagnostic and therapeutic procedures performed in other regions, the tympanic membrane puncture was an infrequent practice in our region, for this reason all episodes in the present study were diagnosed after spontaneous middle-ear drainage, although sampling was not always performed when the perforation of the ear-drum was visually evident.

AOM is most prevalent in children under 2 years of age, with a peak incidence in children aged between 6 and 18 months [16]. In the present series, 69.1% of episodes occurred before the second year of age (70.5% of children had their first episode at this young age and 54.9% of them were boys).

Mixed infections were common and the most frequent accompanying bacterium was non-encapsulated *H. influenzae*. The association of these two otopathogens in AOM has been largely demonstrated [17,18]. Several studies suggested the possibility of an increase of *H. influenzae* AOM after the introduction of PCV7 [19]. In our experience, the number of AOM caused by *H. influenzae* increased (data not shown) but mixed infections with pneumococcus and *H. influenzae* were similar in the four study periods. Mixed infections were also similar in children under and over 2 years old. Serotypes 1, 3 and 19A were mainly found as single etiology infection, which could suggest a higher invasive disease potential.

As the number of colonies selected for serotyping as well as the methodology used may influence the number or diversity of serotypes found in the samples, in the present work we selected 3 or 4 isolated colonies from the primary culture plate to perform the initial serotype characterization. The frequency of the different serotypes causing pneumococcal diseases depends mainly on two factors: the capacity to spread and the disease potential for each site of infection [20]. As pneumococcal diseases start with nasopharynx colonization, a reduction in the number of infections caused by vaccine serotypes could be expected, since PCV7 has been demonstrated to reduce vaccine serotype carriage, decreasing the circulation of these serotypes [21]. It is well known that the introduction of the PCV7 has been accompanied by changes in the distribution of serotypes causing AOM [2,5,6]. In the present study, we observed a dramatic reduction in the proportion of PCV7 serotypes causing AOM, from 62.4% in the pre-vaccine period to 2.2% in 2008–2010. A similar reduction was observed in another Spanish study: from 70.7% in 1997–2000 to 10.6% in 2009 [22].

Among PCV7 serotypes, 19F was the most common, being especially prevalent in the first two periods. This association of 19F with AOM has also been observed in other studies [20,23]. The initial data suggested that the protection of PCV7 against serotype 19F infections, especially AOM, was lower than that against other serotypes included in the PCV7 [6,24]. However, we found that 19F was the PCV7 serotype with the largest drop in percentage across the four study periods (from 20.5% in the pre-PCV7 period to 1.3% in the last period), a decrease that seems not to be consistent with a questionable protective effect against serotype 19F of the PCV7. Serotype 19F was also common in the present work among unvaccinated children with recurrences.

There is currently some concern about the finding of discrepant results in the serotyping obtained by Quellung and PCR capsular typing in a few serotype 19F and 19A isolates [25]; however, in our series, serological and PCR results agreed for all 19F and 19A isolates.

The reduction in PCV7 serotypes causing AOM was accompanied by an increase in the rate of non-vaccine serotypes, especially of serotypes 19A and 3 and, to a lesser extent, of other less frequent serotypes or serogroups such as 6C, 15B, 11, 16F and 21. Serotype 6C was the third most frequent serotype from 2008–2010, a serotype recently described and detected for the first time in 2002 in the present study, although it was not detected in any IPD in children in our region until 2012 [26].

Serotype 19A was the most prevalent serotype in the three post-PCV7 periods and showed a similar prevalence in the pre-PCV7 period to serotype 19F, the most prevalent PCV7 serotype. The increased presence of serotypes 19A and 3 in AOM has also been found in other works [6,20,22]. In a study of IPD in children in our region in the same years, we found a decrease of infections due to PCV7 serotypes and an increase of serotype 19A similar to those observed for AOM [27]. However, there was no increase in the incidence of serotype 3 invasive infections in children, confirming the stronger association of serotype 3 with respiratory infections, both in the lower respiratory tract of older adults [28,29] and AOM in children [6,22,30]. Genotyping analysis of serotypes 19A and 3 isolates also showed a different distribution: while serotype 3 isolates belonged to only three well-known clones (ST180, ST260, and ST1220), serotype 19A isolates showed greater heterogeneity.

Phenotypic and genotypic analysis showed major changes in the dynamics of infection over the 12-year period. Genetic studies identified several apparently identical isolates as different strains. Two isolates of the same serotype, consecutively isolated from the same children, were frequently found to have different genotypes. Indeed, among 19 episodes of reinfection with the same serotype, the same strain (same genotype) was only found in 9.

Among serotype 19A isolates, ST276 was the most prevalent throughout the study. Furthermore, ST276 was the major clone circulating in the periods 1999–2001, 2002–2004 and 2005–2007, and was second only to the predominant ST320 from 2008–2010. In 2004–2005, we performed a study of carriers in healthy children attending a daycare center in this same region and observed that 19A was also the most prevalent serotype [31]. However, in that study of carriers, the most prevalent genotypes of serotype 19A were ST193 and ST199, and no ST276 or ST320 isolates were found in the sample studied [31]. In Asia and the USA, ST320 has been described as a highly prevalent clone showing a worldwide distribution and rapid and broad spread among children. To date, ST320 has had limited diffusion among the adult Spanish population [32].

The diversity of a community depends on the richness (number of species) and relative abundance of each species. The Simpson diversity index, used in this study to analyze the serotype diversity in distinct periods, takes into account the number of serotypes present, as well as the abundance of each serotype. In the present work, the serotype diversity increased from the first period (pre-vaccine) to the following post-vaccine periods. The increase was not only a consequence of the removal of competitive PCV7 types because excluding PCV7 serotypes, the difference between the first and remaining periods persisted. The fall in the diversity in the fourth period was not significant despite the disproportionate presence of serotype 19A isolates. Antimicrobial resistance decreased from 1999–2001 to 2005–2007, but in 2008–2010, resistance rates again increased due to the spread of multiresistant serotype 19A isolates [33].

Recurrent AOM is associated with several factors, including early onset of the disease [34]. Relapses in the present work occurred mainly among male infants that were unvaccinated or infected by isolates of serotypes not included in the PCV7 and were very often caused by antimicrobial resistant isolates. In the first 6 years (1999–2004) of the study, more than 80% of relapses were caused by serotypes included in the PCV7, while in the second 6-year period (2005–2010) 100% were caused by serotype 19A. We did not find any relapses caused by a PCV7 serotype in vaccinated children, once again, underscoring the protective effect of the vaccine. Reinfections or new episodes of AOM caused by a different strain from the original infection or by the same strain but after a long period of time were detected in 12.1% of children and 13.4% of episodes. Episodes of reinfections were more frequent in younger children. The number of episodes of reinfection in both genders was similar (48.8% in boys). If reinfection was due to the persistence of factors predisposing to infection, RI-SS could indicate a lack of adaptive immunological response. Serotype 19A caused 9/17 (52.9%) RI-SS, a ratio higher than that corresponding to the representation of serotype 19A in the whole sample ($p = 0.03$). Apparently, these children had no predisposing factors for these RI-SS, although a specific immunological study of these children was not performed. A less robust adaptive immune response to several *S. pneumoniae* proteins has been observed in children with relapses and reinfections [35]. Because the immune response depends not only on the host but also on the antigen, we speculate that 19A serotype isolates or any of its clones may have been the cause of a less adaptive immune response of the host. All together, the high number of total AOM cases caused by serotype 19A and the high percentage of relapses and RI-SS found in the present study seem to suggest an immunological hyporesponsiveness to previous colonization or infection with serotype 19A isolates that should be taken into account in future studies. The high burden of serotype 19A in AOM recurrences has also been previously reported [36].

In the present study, the criterion for considering a recurrence caused by the same strain as a relapse or reinfection was arbitrarily chosen because the length of time a pneumococcus stays in the middle ear is unknown. Some episodes of reinfection could probably have been a very late relapse, as occurred with relapsing child number 13, who had four recurrences with a serotype 19A ST320 between the ages of 6 and 14 months.

The two most prevalent serotypes causing AOM in the last time period in the present and in other similar studies were serotypes 19A and 3. Since both serotypes are included in the new PCV13, it will be interesting to measure the impact of PCV13 in the epidemiology of these two as well as in that of the other serotypes included in the vaccine. Assuming that in the next few years a drop in AOM caused by serotypes 19A and 3 might occur, continued surveillance is required because, in the absence of the competitive effect of these prevalent serotypes, other serotypes not present or poorly represented in the pre-vaccination period such as serotypes 6C, 15B, 11, 16F or 21 could become predominant.

Author Contributions

Conceived and designed the experiments: JMM EPT. Performed the experiments: MA ME JMM. Analyzed the data: MA ME JMM EGPY EPT. Contributed reagents/materials/analysis tools: MA ME EPT EGPY. Wrote the paper: JMM EPT.

References

1. Teele DW, Klein JO, Rosner B (1989) Epidemiology of otitis media during the first seven years of life in children in greater Boston: a prospective, cohort study. J Infect Dis 160: 83–94.
2. Eskola J, Kilpi T, Palmu A, Jokinen J, Haapakoski J, et al. (2001) Efficacy of a pneumococcal conjugate vaccine against acute otitis media. N Engl J Med 344: 403–409.
3. Fischer T, Singer AJ, Lee C, Thode HC Jr (2007) National trends in emergency department antibiotic prescribing for children with acute otitis media, 1996 2005. Acad Emerg Med 14: 1172–1175.
4. Chonmaitree T, Revai K, Grady JJ, Clos A, Patel JA, et al. (2008) Viral upper respiratory tract infection and otitis media complication in young children. Clin Infect Dis 46: 815–823.
5. Block SL, Hedrick J, Harrison CJ, Tyler R, Smith A, et al. (2004) Community-wide vaccination with the heptavalent pneumococcal conjugate significantly alters the microbiology of acute otitis media. Pediatr Infect Dis J 23: 829–833.
6. McEllistrem MC, Adams JM, Patel K, Mendelsohn AB, Kaplan SL, et al. (2005) Acute otitis media due to penicillin-nonsusceptible *Streptococcus pneumoniae* before and after the introduction of the pneumococcal conjugate vaccine. Clin Infect Dis 40: 1738–1744.
7. Marimon JM, Monasterio A, Ercibengoa M, Pascual J, Prieto I, et al. (2010) Antibody microarray typing, a novel technique for *Streptococcus pneumoniae* serotyping. J Microbiol Methods 80: 274–280.
8. Pai R, Gertz RE, Beall B (2006) Sequential multiplex PCR approach for determining capsular serotypes of *Streptococcus pneumoniae* isolates. J Clin Microbiol 44: 124–131.
9. Brito DA, Ramirez M, de Lencastre H (2003) Serotyping *Streptococcus pneumoniae* by multiplex PCR. J Clin Microbiol 41: 2378–2384.
10. Mintegi S, Benito J, González M, Astobiza E, Sánchez J, et al. (2006) Impact of the pneumococcal conjugate vaccine in the management of highly febrile children aged 6 to 24 months in an emergency department. Pediatr Emerg Care 22: 566–569.
11. Clinical and Laboratory Standards Institute (CLSI) (2010) Performance standards for antimicrobial susceptibility testing; 20th informational supplement. M 100-S20. Wayne, PA.
12. Marimón JM, Iglesias L, Vicente D, Pérez-Trallero E (2003) Molecular characterization of erythromycin-resistant clinical isolates of the four major antimicrobial-resistant Spanish clones of *Streptococcus pneumoniae* (Spain^{23F}-1, Spain^{6B}-2, Spain^{9V}-3, and Spain^{14}-5). Microb Drug Resist 9: 133–137.
13. Arguedas A, Kvaerner K, Liese J, Schilder AG, Pelton SI (2010) Otitis media across nine countries: disease burden and management. Int J Pediatr Otorhinolaryngol 74: 1419–1424.
14. Palmu AA, Herva E, Savolainen H, Karma P, Mäkelä PH, et al. (2004) Association of clinical signs and symptoms with bacterial findings in acute otitis media. Clin Infect Dis 38: 234–242.
15. Xu Q, Kaur R, Casey JR, Sabharwal V, Pelton S, et al. (2011) Nontypeable *Streptococcus pneumoniae* as an otopathogen. Diagn Microbiol Infect Dis 69: 200–204.
16. Kilpi T, Schuerman L (2008) Acute otitis media and its sequelae. In: Siber GR, Klugman KP, Mäkelä PH, editors. Pneumococcal vaccines: the impact of conjugated vaccine. Washington D.C: ASM Press. 301–315.
17. Leibovitz E, Serebro M, Givon-Lavi N, Greenberg D, Broides A, et al. (2009) Epidemiologic and microbiologic characteristics of culture-positive spontaneous otorrhea in children with acute otitis media. Pediatr Infect Dis J 28: 381–384.
18. Hausdorff WP, Yothers G, Dagan R, Kilpi T, Pelton SI, et al. (2002) Multinational study of pneumococcal serotypes causing acute otitis media in children. Pediatr Infect Dis J 21: 1008–1016.
19. Leibovitz E, Jacobs MR, Dagan R (2004) *Haemophilus influenzae*: a significant pathogen in acute otitis media. Pediatr Infect Dis J 23: 1142–1152.
20. Shouval DS, Greenberg D, Givon-Lavi N, Porat N, Dagan R (2006) Site-specific disease potential of individual *Streptococcus pneumoniae* serotypes in pediatric invasive disease, acute otitis media and acute conjunctivitis. Pediatr Infect Dis J 25: 602–607.
21. Hammitt LL, Bruden DL, Butler JC, Baggett HC, Hurlburt DA, et al. (2006) Indirect effect of conjugate vaccine on adult carriage of *Streptococcus pneumoniae*: an explanation of trends in invasive pneumococcal disease. J Infect Dis 193: 1487–1494.
22. Fenoll A, Aguilar L, Vicioso MD, Gimenez MJ, Robledo O, et al. (2011) Increase in serotype 19A prevalence and amoxicillin non-susceptibility among paediatric *Streptococcus pneumoniae* isolates from middle ear fluid in a passive laboratory-based surveillance in Spain, 1997–2009. BMC Infect Dis 11: 239.
23. Hanage WP, Auranen K, Syrjänen R, Herva E, Mäkelä PH, et al. (2004) Ability of pneumococcal serotypes and clones to cause acute otitis media: implications for the prevention of otitis media by conjugate vaccines. Infect Immun 72: 76–81.
24. Whitney CG, Farley MM, Hadler J, Harrison LH, Bennett NM, et al. (2003) Active bacterial core surveillance of the Emerging Infections Program Network.

Decline in invasive pneumococcal disease after the introduction of protein-polysaccharide conjugate vaccine. N Engl J Med 348: 1737–1746.

25. Pimenta FC, Gertz RE Jr, Roundtree A, Yu J, Nahm MH, et al. (2009) Rarely occurring 19A-like cps locus from a serotype 19F Pneumococcal isolate indicates continued need of serology-based quality control for PCR-based serotype determinations. J Clin Microbiol 47: 2353–2354.
26. Marimon JM, Ercibengoa M, Alonso M, García-Medina G, Pérez-Trallero E (2010) Prevalence and molecular characterization of *Streptococcus pneumoniae* serotype 6C causing invasive disease in Gipuzkoa, northern Spain, 1990–2009. Eur J Clin Microbiol Infect Dis 29: 1035–1038.
27. Pérez-Trallero E, Marimon JM, Ercibengoa M, Vicente D, Pérez-Yarza EG (2009) Invasive *Streptococcus pneumoniae* infections in children and older adults in the north of Spain before and after the introduction of the heptavalent pneumococcal conjugate vaccine. Eur J Clin Microbiol Infect Dis 28: 731–738.
28. Pérez-Trallero E, Marimón JM, Larruskain J, Alonso M, Ercibengoa M (2011) Antimicrobial susceptibilities and serotypes of *Streptococcus pneumoniae* isolates from elderly patients with pneumonia and acute exacerbation of chronic obstructive pulmonary disease. Antimicrob Agents Chemother 55: 2729–2734.
29. Luján M, Gallego M, Belmonte Y, Fontanals D, Vallès J, et al. (2010) Influence of pneumococcal serotype group on outcome in adults with bacteraemic pneumonia. Eur Respir J 36: 1073–1079.
30. Guevara S, Abdelnour A, Soley C, Porat N, Dagan R, et al. (2012) *Streptococcus pneumoniae* serotypes isolated from the middle ear fluid of Costa Rican children following introduction of the heptavalent pneumococcal conjugate vaccine into a limited population. Vaccine 19: In press.
31. Ercibengoa M, Arostegi N, Marimon JM, Alonso M, Perez-Trallero E (2012) Dynamics of pneumococcal nasopharyngeal carriage in healthy children attending a day care center in northern Spain. Influence of detection techniques on the results. BMC Infect Dis 12: 69.
32. Marimón JM, Alonso M, Rolo D, Ardanuy C, Liñares J, et al. (2012) Molecular characterization of *Streptococcus pneumoniae* invasive serotype 19A isolates from adults in two Spanish regions (1994–2009). Eur J Clin Microbiol Infect Dis 31: 1009–1013.
33. Pérez-Trallero E, Marimón JM, Alonso M, Ercibengoa M, García-Arenzana JM (2012) Decline and rise of the antimicrobial susceptibility of *Streptococcus pneumoniae* isolated from middle ear fluid in children. Influence of changes in circulating serotypes. Antimicrob Agents Chemother 30: In press.
34. Pelton SI, Leibovitz E (2009) Recent advances in otitis media. Pediatr Infect Dis J 28 (10 Suppl): S133–S137.
35. Kaur R, Casey JR, Pichichero ME (2011) Serum antibody response to five *Streptococcus pneumoniae* proteins during acute otitis media in otitis-prone and non-otitis-prone children. Pediatr Infect Dis J 30: 645–650.
36. Couloigner V, Levy C, François M, Bidet P, Hausdorff WP, et al. (2012) Pathogens implicated in acute otitis media failures after 7-valent pneumococcal conjugate vaccine implementation in France: distribution, serotypes, and resistance levels. Pediatr Infect Dis J. 2012; 31: 154–158.

9

Age-Specific Sex-Related Differences in Infections: A Statistical Analysis of National Surveillance Data in Japan

Nobuoki Eshima[1], Osamu Tokumaru[2]*, Shohei Hara[3], Kira Bacal[4], Seigo Korematsu[5], Shigeru Karukaya[6], Kiyo Uruma[1], Nobuhiko Okabe[7], Toyojiro Matsuishi[6]

1 Department of Biostatistics, Faculty of Medicine, Oita University, Yufu, Oita, Japan, 2 Department of Neurophysiology, Faculty of Medicine, Oita University, Yufu, Oita, Japan, 3 Editorial Bureau, The Yomiuri Shimbun Osaka (newspaper), Osaka, Japan, 4 Medical Programme Directorate, Faculty of Medical and Health Sciences, University of Auckland, Auckland, New Zealand, 5 Department of Pediatrics and Child Neurology, Faculty of Medicine, Oita University, Yufu, Oita, Japan, 6 Department of Pediatrics and Child Health, Kurume University School of Medicine, Kurume, Fukuoka, Japan, 7 Infectious Disease Surveillance Center, National Institute of Infectious Diseases, Shinjuku, Tokyo, Japan

Abstract

Background: To prevent and control infectious diseases, it is important to understand how sex and age influence morbidity rates, but consistent clear descriptions of differences in the reported incidence of infectious diseases in terms of sex and age are sparse.

Methods and Findings: Data from the Japanese surveillance system for infectious diseases from 2000 to 2009 were used in the analysis of seven viral and four bacterial infectious diseases with relatively large impact on the Japanese community. The male-to-female morbidity (MFM) ratios in different age groups were estimated to compare incidence rates of symptomatic reported infection between the sexes at different ages. MFM ratios were >1 for five viral infections out of seven in childhood, i.e. male children were more frequently reported as infected than females with pharyngoconjunctival fever, herpangina, hand-foot-and-mouth disease, mumps, and varicella. More males were also reported to be infected with erythema infectiosum and exanthema subitum, but only in children 1 year of age. By contrast, in adulthood the MFM ratios decreased to <1 for all of the viral infections above except varicella, i.e. adult women were more frequently reported to be infected than men. Sex- and age-related differences in reported morbidity were also documented for bacterial infections. Reported morbidity for enterohemorrhagic *Escherichia coli* infection was higher in adult females and females were reportedly more infected with mycoplasma pneumonia than males in all age groups up to 70 years.

Conclusions: Sex-related differences in reported morbidity for viral and bacterial infections were documented among different age groups. Changes in MFM ratios with age may reflect differences between the sexes in underlying development processes, including those affecting the immune, endocrine, and reproductive systems, or differences in reporting rates.

Editor: Lawrence Kazembe, Chancellor College, University of Malawi, Malawi

Funding: This work was supported in part by a Grant-in-Aid for Scientific Research (C) #22500260 to NE from the Japan Ministry of Education, Culture, Sports, Science and Technology. The funders had no role in study design, data collection and analysis, decision to publish, or preparation of the manuscript. No additional external funding was received for this study.

Competing Interests: The authors have declared that no competing interests exist.

* E-mail: ostokuma@oita-u.ac.jp

Introduction

Manifestation and morbidity of infections differ between the sexes and among different ages. For example, among viral infections, commonly accepted risk factors for enterovirus infections such as herpangina and hand-foot-and-mouth disease (HFMD) include age younger than 1 year and male sex, suggesting a predominance in male infants [1]. Further support for this idea came from a study on HFMD outbreaks in China [2], which demonstrated that boys were more susceptible than girls with the odds ratio of 1.56 (95% confidence interval [95%CI] 1.56–1.57). Although the major bulk of patients with erythema infectiosum (EI) are school-aged children, mothers are more infected than fathers, suggesting a female predominance in adulthood [1]. In addition, more patients with arthropathy, a major complication of EI in adults, are female than male [1,3]. More girls than boys also acquired human herpesvirus (HHV-6), the pathogen of exanthema subitum (ES), in childhood; the acquisition of the virus was associated with female sex with the adjusted hazard ratio of 1.7 (95%CI 1.2–2.4) [4]. By contrast, more males contracted mumps in a large outbreak in Bosnia and Herzegovina in 2010–2011, a pattern which was also seen in the 2010 outbreak of rubella in Bosnia and Herzegovina [5].

With regards to bacterial infections, there was a reported male predominance in the incidence of tuberculosis across all age groups except for 15–24 year olds [6]. In contrast to that, the morbidity of pertussis is slightly higher in adult females [7], and during a recent German outbreak of *Escherichia coli* O104 in 2011, the majority of infected people were adults, and women were infected at about twice the rate as men [8,9].

There are several studies describing age-specific sex-related differences in morbidity. The authors recently demonstrated that for influenza (H1N1) 2009 and seasonal influenza, the reported morbidity rate for males under twenty years old was statistically higher than that for females, while the relationship was reversed in adulthood [10]. Similar male predominance early in life and reversal at later ages were observed in human T-cell leukemia virus type I (HTLV-I) infection from blood donor data [11]. Thomas and Hall described age-specific sex-related differences in the morbidity of herpes zoster in the US [12], while Wu showed the annual incidence rates of chickenpox by age-group and sex, as well as the relative risks between sexes, using a large-scale database in Taiwan [13].

But studies which describe both age-specific and sex-related differences in morbidity are exceptional; the phenomenon is poorly documented in the literature as a recent review by the authors demonstrated. For example, one study reported that boys were more likely to be infected with adenovirus than girls, but no age-specific incidences were given by sex [14]. Reports by Zerr et al. [4] and Hukic et al. [5] described differences in morbidity for HHV-6 and mumps infections between the sexes, but did not mention age-specificity at all. In an analysis of serological surveys of the age-specific distribution of antibody to parvovirus B19, the pathogen of EI, no sex-related difference was described [15]. No sex-related age-specific difference in morbidity was mentioned in a survey on mumps in US [16]. Tan reported a thorough review on pertussis with international burden, but no description was given regarding sex-related difference in morbidity [17]. In a review on morbidity and mortality for vaccine-preventable diseases in the US, no description was given of sex-related differences in morbidity and mortality [18].

Even in a standard textbook of pediatrics [1] or handbook of communicable diseases [7], many infectious diseases are described with no information given about age-specific sex-related differences in their epidemiological profiles. Although peak ages of incidence or prevalence are detailed for many diseases, there is rarely any description of sex-based differences, including when such difference by sex occurs, until what age it continues, and what mechanism(s) might account for this effect. These shortcomings in knowledge can potentially hinder our understanding and control of infectious diseases.

The authors have developed a mathematical model based on nationwide data which enables the comparison of symptomatic reported morbidity rates of males and females by age groups [10]. The aim of the present study is to describe age-specific sex-related differences in infections using the Japanese nationwide infectious disease database and to consider sex- and age-related differences in viral and bacterial infections.

Methods

Ethics statement

Ethical approval and signed patient consent forms were not required for our study according to the Guideline for Epidemiological Studies [19], which was established by the Ministry of Health, Labor and Welfare and the Ministry of Education, Culture, Sports, Science and Technology of Japan in accordance with the World Medical Association's Declaration of Helsinki and Japan's Act on the Protection of Personal Information and other related acts. Specifically, (1) all individual data were collected by law and authorized to be utilized for academic purposes [20], and (2) patients could not be identified, as all data were de-identified; i.e., stripped of personal identifiers.

Study population and data sources

Japan has an active infectious disease surveillance system. Since 1999, the National Institute of Infectious Disease (NIID; Tokyo, Japan) has collected reports of patients with various infectious diseases, and the data have been reported in sex and age groups (National Epidemiological Surveillance of Infectious Diseases, NESID) [21]. Diseases of interest in the present study were selected from those reported in NESID.

Viral infectious diseases without availability of vaccination reported from the pediatric sentinel points. Five major viral diseases are reported from the pediatric sentinel points of NESID: pharyngoconjunctival fever (PCF), herpangina, hand-foot-and-mouth disease (HFMD), EI, and ES. No vaccinations are available for these diseases in Japan. Data were collected from approximately 3000 pediatric sentinel points all over Japan between 2000 and 2009 (Table 1). The number of the sentinel points represents approximately 10% of the pediatric facilities in Japan, and the average number of sentinel points in 2009 was 3,022. As shown in Table 1, the numbers of male and female cases from the sentinel points were reported across 13 age groups, and adult cases were also reported.

Vaccine-preventable viral infectious diseases reported from the pediatric sentinel points. Two vaccine-preventable viral infectious diseases, mumps and varicella, were studied using reports from the pediatric sentinel points of NESID. Vaccinations for mumps and varicella are optional for children older than 1 year under the Japanese law with vaccination rates being 23.2% and 21.3% against mumps and varicella, respectively [22]. The vaccination rates for those two infections are only available for combined males and females - vaccination rates for males and females were not available separately. However, it is assumed that there are no differences in the vaccination rates between the sexes, based on data from vaccination rates for the measles-rubella combination vaccine in Japan where rates are available for each sex, and there is no difference in the vaccination rates between the sexes [10,23].

Bacterial infectious diseases. Data for four bacterial infections were available from NESID for the present study (Table 2); Group A streptococcal pharyngitis (GAS), pertussis, enterohemorrhagic *Escherichia coli* (EHEC), and Mycoplasma pneumonia (MP). GAS and pertussis were reported from the pediatric sentinel points. EHEC cases must, by law, be reported by all clinical facilities in Japan and archived in NESID, while the data for MP were collected from approximately 470 NESID sentinel points. Of these, only pertussis is vaccine-preventable; the vaccine is generally provided four times between 3 months and 7·5 years as a component of the diphtheria, tetanus and pertussis combined vaccine which is recommended under Japanese law with a vaccination rate of 95.8% [22].

Statistical model and data analysis

Male-to-female morbidity ratios of infectious diseases without vaccine availability. Morbidities of males and females in each age group were compared through the male-to-female morbidity (MFM) ratios [10], statistics similar to ones used by Green [24] and Reller et al [25]. Since the present sampling is based on the data reported from the sentinel points, the sampling is viewed as a Poisson sampling. The morbidities (symptomatic incidence) at a current time, p_M and p_F, cannot be estimated from the observational patient data. Let π_M and π_F be the probabilities that male and female patients in the age group visit the sentinel points, respectively. From the present sampling from the sentinel points, the ratio $\gamma = \frac{\pi_M p_M}{\pi_F p_F}$ can be estimated by maximum

Table 1. Numbers of cases and male-to-female morbidity ratios of viral infections reported from the pediatric sentinel points from 2000 to 2009 in Japan.

		Age	0	1	2	3	4	5	6	7	8	9	10–14	15–19	≥20
Infection without vaccination available	Pharyngo-conjunctival fever	Male	12767	42019	35164	39772	38487	30997	18169	10849	7224	4736	7718	674	2710
		Female	9828	31158	28769	32303	32039	25289	15768	9704	6495	4205	6290	623	6159
		M/F (95%CI)	1.23 (1.19–1.28)	1.28 (1.25–1.31	1.16 (1.14–1.19)	1.17 (1.15–1.20)	1.14 (1.11–1.16)	1.17 (1.14–1.20)	1.10 (1.06–1.13)	1.06 (1.02–1.11)	1.06 (1.01–1.11)	1.07 (1.01–1.14)	1.17 (1.11–1.23)	1.03 (0.88–1.21)	0.47 (0.44–0.50)
	herpangina	Male	59707	156797	124871	102487	78634	52619	26410	14268	8337	5118	7668	943	2378
		Female	50588	136847	116722	95002	74895	48590	25267	14051	8228	5196	6677	925	4751
		M/F (95%CI)	1.12 (1.10–1.14	1.09 (1.08–1.10)	1.02 (1.01–1.03)	1.03 (1.01–1.04)	1.00 (0.99–1.01)	1.03 (1.01–1.05)	0.99 (0.97–1.02)	0.97 (0.93–1.00)	0.96 (0.92–1.01)	0.94 (0.89–0.99)	1.09 (1.04–1.15)	0.97 (0.85–1.11)	0.54 (0.50–0.58)
	hand-foot-and-mouth disease	Male	36820	148707	132150	108946	87667	61360	30191	15216	9401	5635	8159	528	2025
		Female	30282	118713	109409	88077	72002	48905	25046	13271	8256	5076	7319	678	7496
		M/F (95%CI)	1.15 (1.13–1.18)	1.19 (1.18–1.20)	1.15 (1.14–1.16)	1.18 (1.16–1.19)	1.16 (1.14–1.18)	1.19 (1.17–1.22)	1.15 (1.12–1.18)	1.09 (1.05–1.13)	1.08 (1.04–1.13)	1.06 (0.999–1.11)	1.06 (1.01–1.11)	0.74 (0.63–0.88)	0.29 (0.27–0.31)
	erythema infectiosum	Male	8592	12927	14981	24210	33013	36941	29507	23196	16828	11233	14160	286	1152
		Female	8308	11159	13856	22502	32320	35788	30213	24800	18581	12220	13923	729	8287
		M/F (95%CI)	0.98 (0.94–1.03)	1.10 (1.06–1.14)	1.03 (0.99–1.06)	1.02 (0.998–1.05)	0.97 (0.95–0.995)	0.98 (0.96–1.004)	0.93 (0.91–0.95)	0.89 (0.87–0.91)	0.86 (0.84–0.89)	0.87 (0.84–0.91)	0.97 (0.94–1.002)	0.37 (0.30–0.46)	0.15 (0.14–0.16)
	exanthema subitum	Male	373434	179507	13653	1909	658	436	342	291	209	157	199	30	58
		Female	358470	164154	12857	1837	601	378	309	224	207	130	158	14	116
		M/F (95%CI)	0.99 (0.98–1.00)	1.04 (1.03–1.05)	1.01 (0.98–1.05)	0.99 (0.90–1.09)	1.04 (0.89–1.23)	1.10 (0.90–1.35)	1.05 (0.84–1.32)	1.24 (0.96–1.60)	0.96 (0.72–1.28)	1.15 (0.82–1.62)	1.20 (0.88–1.63)	2.04 (0.80–5.19	0.54 (0.34–0.85)
Infection with vaccination available	mumps	Male	4594	36580	69515	108637	137520	130210	92099	60145	37935	24507	40165	3353	8123
		Female	3293	27218	57281	91629	118793	109838	79821	53468	34277	21889	35995	3952	16112
		M/F (95%CI)	1.32 (1.24–1.42)	1.28 (1.25–1.31)	1.15 (1.14–1.17)	1.13 (1.11–1.14)	1.10 (1.09–1.12)	1.13 (1.12–1.14)	1.10 (1.08–1.11)	1.07 (1.05–1.09)	1.05 (1.03–1.08)	1.07 (1.04–1.09)	1.06 (1.04–1.08)	0.81 (0.75–0.86)	0.54 (0.52–0.56)
	varicella	Male	109643	241632	234577	225454	196204	131974	66813	32708	19237	11455	18494	2108	7036
		Female	104740	218016	216904	204682	179400	117473	61408	30851	18679	11308	17515	1918	7222
		M/F (95%CI)	0.99 (0.98–1.01)	1.05 (1.04–1.06)	1.03 (1.02–1.04)	1.05 (1.04–1.06)	1.04 (1.03–1.05)	1.07 (1.06–1.08)	1.03 (1.02–1.05)	1.01 (0.99–1.03)	0.98 (0.95–1.01)	0.96 (0.93–1.001)	1.00 (0.97–1.04)	1.05 (0.95–1.14)	1.05 (0.996–1.10)
Male-to-female population ratio (2000–2009)			1.053	1.052	1.051	1.50	1.50	1.50	1.051	1.051	1.051	1.051	1.051	1.052	1.042

Table 2. Numbers of cases and male-to-female morbidity ratios of bacterial infections reported from the sentinel points from 2000 to 2009 in Japan.

	Age	0	1	2	3	4	5	6	7	8	9	10–14	15–19	≥20
group A streptococcal pharyngitis	Male	6932	30523	57869	111793	171059	191417	156717	113858	80190	54206	92088	7300	1101947
	Female	5865	24300	46038	85565	133386		147536	101195	74156	51505	80950	7361	954360
	M/F (95%CI)	1.12 (1.07–1.18)	1.19 (1.16–1.22)	1.20 (1.17–1.22)	1.24 (1.23–1.26)	1.22 (1.21–1.23)		1.14 (1.13–1.16)	1.07 (1.06–1.08)	1.03 (1.01–1.04)	1.00 (0.98–1.02)	1.08 (1.07–1.10)	0.94 (0.90–0.99)	0.45 (0.45–0.46)
pertussis	Male	4095	1505	654	683	578	501	357	356	366	382	1239	280	13080
	Female	3737	1384	750	733	683	468	399	347	361	343	1380	376	15430
	M/F (95%CI)	1.04 (0.97–1.11)	1.03 (0.93–1.15)	0.83 (0.71–0.97)	0.89 (0.76–1.03)	0.81 (0.68–0.95)	1.02 (0.85–1.23)	0.85 (0.69–1.05)	0.98 (0.78–1.21)	0.96 (0.78–1.20)	1.06 (0.85–1.31)	0.85 (0.76–0.96)	0.71 (0.56–0.89)	0.50 (0.46–0.54)
Male-to-female population ratio*		1.053	1.052	1.051	1.050	1.050	1.050	1.051	1.051	1.051	1.051	1.051	1.052	1.042

	Age	0	1–4	5–9	10–14	15–19	20–29	30–39	40–49	50–59	60–69	70≤
enterohemorrhagic *Escherichia coli*	Male	339	5344	3309	1645	1355	2698	1672	937	904	778	728
	Female	278	4344	2657	1280	1280	3064	2232	1299	1699	1122	1345
	M/F (95%CI)	1.16 (0.92–1.46)	1.17 (1.10–1.24)	1.19 (1.10–1.28)	1.22 (1.10–1.36)	1.01 (0.90–1.13)	0.85 (0.78–0.91)	0.73 (0.67–0.81)	0.71 (0.63–0.81)	0.54 (0.48–0.61)	0.75 (0.65–0.86)	0.81 (0.71–0.92)
mycoplasma pneumonia	Male	624	12013	9691	4358	731	784	720	347	273	354	813
	Female	836	13244	10170	4782	968	1842	1760	649	525	451	755
	M/F (95%CI)	0.71 (0.64–0.79)	0.86 (0.84–0.88)	0.91 (0.88–0.93)	0.87 (0.83–0.90)	0.72 (0.65–0.79)	0.41 (0.38–0.44)	0.40 (0.37–0.44)	0.53 (0.46–0.60)	0.53 (0.46–0.61)	0.85 (0.74–0.97)	1.60 (1.45–1.77)
Male-to-female population ratio		1.053	1.051	1.051	1.051	1.052	1.042	1.022	1.010	0.985	0.928	0.671

*identical to the bottom row of the Table 1.

likelihood estimator $\hat{\gamma} = \frac{n_M/N_M}{n_F/N_F} = \frac{n_M}{n_F}\frac{N_F}{N_M}$, where N_M and N_F are the subpopulations of males and females in an age group in Japanese population; i.e. fixed values, and n_M, and n_F are the random variables that describe the numbers of male and female patients. The ratio is referred to as the apparent MFM ratio. If $\frac{\pi_M}{\pi_F} = 1$, then, $\gamma = \frac{p_M}{p_F}$ is the true MFM ratio. For large n_M and n_F, $\log\hat{\gamma}$ is asymptotically normally distributed with mean $\log\gamma$ and variance $\frac{1}{n_M} + \frac{1}{n_F}$. In order to make multiple tests of MFM ratios in age groups, the Bonferroni method [26] is employed, and the Bonferroni 95% joint confidence intervals of MFM ratios are constructed.

In order to estimate MFM ratios, ratios of male and female population sizes in age groups should be paid attention, as explained above. The male-to-female population ratios in age were almost constant from 2000 to 2009. Ratios of average subpopulations of males and females from 2000 to 2009 were used in this study (Table 1).

Male-to-female morbidity ratios of vaccine-preventable pediatric infectious diseases. Let ω_{vM} and ω_{vF} be the probabilities that male and female patients in the age group get vaccinated and let ω_{iM} and ω_{iF} be the probabilities that vaccinated male and female patients in the age group get immunized, respectively. From the present sampling from sentinel points, the ratio $\gamma = \frac{(1-\omega_{vM}\omega_{iM})\pi_M p_M}{(1-\omega_{vF}\omega_{iF})\pi_F p_F}$ can be estimated by maximum likelihood estimator $\hat{\gamma} = \frac{n_M/N_M}{n_F/N_F} = \frac{n_M}{n_F}\frac{N_F}{N_M}$. If $\frac{\omega_{vM}}{\omega_{vF}} = \frac{\omega_{iM}}{\omega_{iF}} = 1$ and $\frac{\pi_M}{\pi_F} = 1$, then, $\gamma = \frac{p_M}{p_F}$ is the true MFM ratio.

Results

MFM ratios of viral infections

Viral infectious diseases without availability of vaccine. MFM ratios of five viral infectious diseases from NESID for which vaccination is not available are shown in Figure 1A–E. In this study, "children" refers to those aged younger than 15 years of age; "adolescence" 15–19 years of age and "adult" 20 years of age. In two diseases, MFM ratios of children under 15 years old were >1, i.e. male children under 15 years old were significantly more likely to be reported as infected with PCF, and HFMD ($p<0.05$, Figure 1A, C). The MFM ratios for reported cases of herpangina were >1 in 0–3, 5 and 10–14 years old ($p<0.05$, Figure 1B). The MFM ratios for reported EI was >1 only in children 1 year of age (MFM ratio 1.10, 95% confidence interval [95%CI] 1.06–1.14; Figure 1D). Of interest, MFM ratios for the above four diseases decreased to <1 by adulthood; i.e., by adolescence (15–19 years old), females were more frequently reported to be infected than males with HFMD (MFM ratio 0.74, 95%CI 0.63–0.88; Figure 1C), and by adulthood (≥20 year old) women were more affected than men by PCF (MFM ratio 0.47, 95%CI 0.44–0.50; Figure 1A) and herpangina (MFM ratio 0.54, 95%CI 0.50–0.58; Figure 1B). For EI, MFM ratios were <1 in 4, 6–9, and older than 15 years for age (Figure 1D). The MFM ratios for ES were 0.99 (95%CI 0.98–1.00) in 0 year and 1.04 (95%CI 1.03–1.05) in 1 year. In age groups over 4 years of age, the number of cases reported as "ES" were unreliable because ES is clinically unlikely in this group [1,7]. Thus the data are not plotted in age groups ≥ 4 years of age in Figure 1E.

Vaccine-preventable viral infectious diseases. MFM ratios for reported cases of mumps were >1 from 0 to 14 years of age ($p<0.05$) and <1 thereafter (MFM ratio 0.82, 95%CI 0.76–0.87 in 15–19 years of age, Figure 1F). For reported cases of varicella, MFM ratios were >1 in 1–6 year old ($p<0.05$) and not different from 1 in newborns and those older than 7 years (Figure 1G).

MFM ratios of bacterial infections

MFM ratios for reported cases of GAS were >1 in children under 15 years old (except 9 year olds) and <1 after adolescence (≥15 years of age, $p<0.05$); i.e. male children were reported significantly more often as infected than girls, but by adolescence, females were more frequently reported to be infected with GAS than males (MFM ratio 0.93, 95%CI 0.89–0.98 in 15–19 years of age; Figure 2A). In pertussis, the MFM ratios were <1 for children 2 years old, 4 years old, and over 10 years old ($p<0.05$, Figure 2B).

MFM ratios for EHEC were statistically >1 in 1–14 years old ($p<0.05$) and <1 in ages older than 15 years (MFM ratio 0.85, 95%CI 0.76–0.96 in 15–19 years of age; Figure 2C); i.e. boys under 14 years old were more frequently reported to be infected with EHEC than girls, whereas adult females were more reported to be infected with EHEC than males. The age category from 1 to 4 years old had the highest number of reported cases (Table 2).

As shown in Figure 2D, females are statistically more likely to be reported as infected with MP than males, except in elderly people above 70 years old. MFM ratios were the smallest in the age category from 30 to 39 years old (MFM ratio 0.40, 95%CI 0.37–0.44), while the highest number of reported cases is in those aged 1 to 4 years old (Table 2).

Discussion

Viral infections

The present study used the data of NESID, the national surveillance data of Japan, to demonstrate differences by sex and age in the symptomatic incidence of selected viral infections. The estimated incidence rates in Japan are as follows; PCF 22.2 per 1,000 population aged 0–14 years (95%CI 18.4–26.0), herpangina 51.7 (95%CI 47.8–55.6), HFMD 36.7 (95%CI 34.1–39.3), EI 15.2 (95%CI 13.9–16.6), ES 38.5 (95%CI 36.0–41.0), mumps 73.0 (95%CI 68.5–77.6), varicella 86.1 (95%CI 81.8–90.4) [27]. Statistical analysis of seven viral infectious diseases documented that male children are more likely to be reported as symptomatically infected than females in five out of the seven diseases (Figure 1A–C, F–G). Of these five diseases, the MFM ratios decrease to <1 by adulthood for PCF and herpangina, while those for HFMD and mumps were reversed to <1 in adolescence. For EI, the MFM ratio was 1.10 (95%CI 1.06–1.14) at 1 year of age, and ratios were <1 thereafter with smaller ratios ≥15 years of age. This might imply that there are age-specific sex-related differences in the immune response to viruses between childhood and adolescence/adulthood. However, every rule has its exception, and in this case the MFM ratio of varicella did not reverse to <1 in adults. MFM ratio for ES were <1 in infants and >1 at 1 year of age ($p<0.05$).

It is possible that the observed pattern is due to differences in social roles between the sexes; e.g. women may be more likely to take care of sick family members and thus are more likely to be affected by the disease [28]. Information about these diseases was obtained from ~3,000 pediatric sentinel points; adult cases were also reported, probably because some accompanying parents might have consulted the pediatricians about their own health during their children's visit. Hence, there is a possibility that

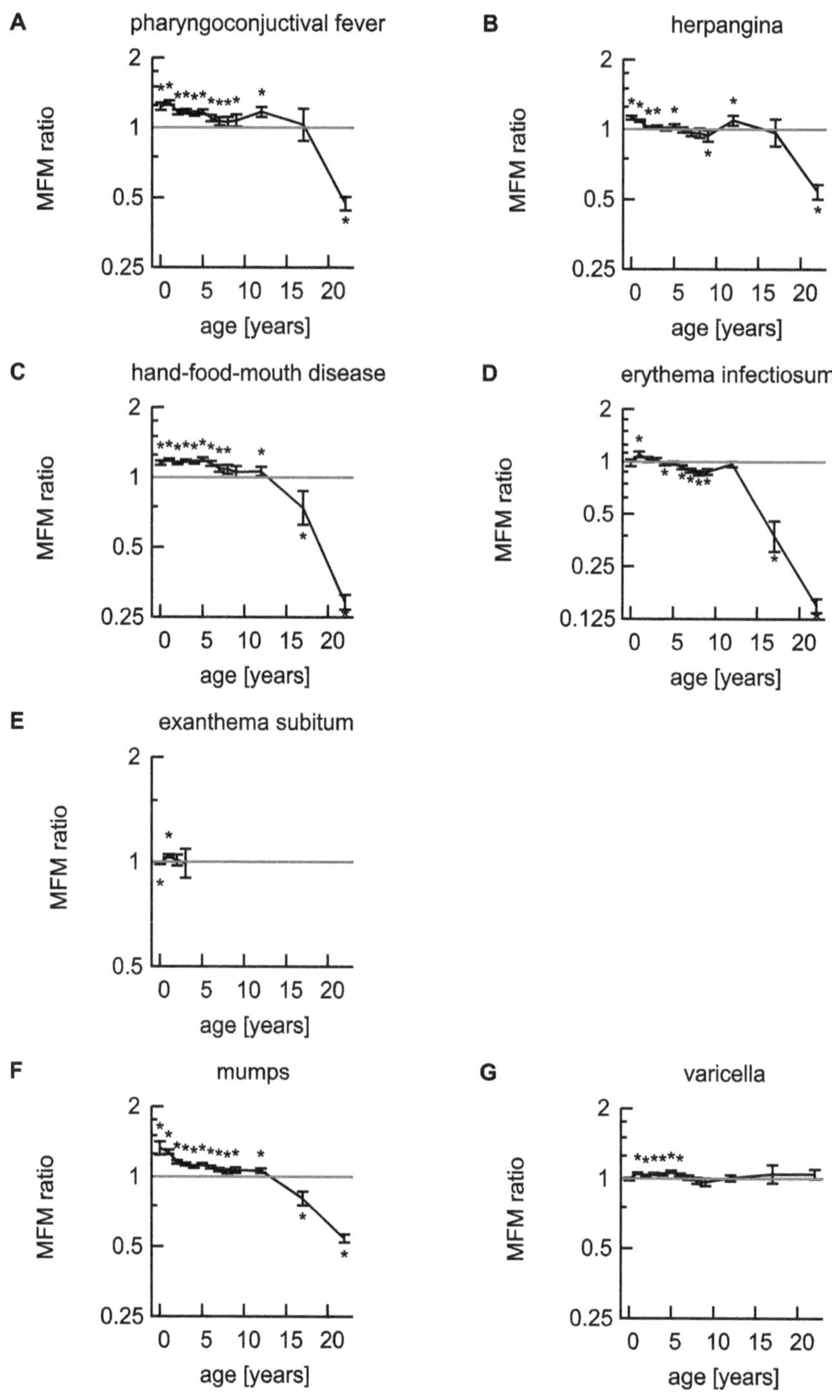

Figure 1. MFM ratios of viral infectious diseases reported from the pediatric sentinel points in Japan; pharyngoconjunctival fever (A), herpangina (B), hand-foot-mouth disease (C), erythema infectiosum (D) and exanthema subitum (E) for infections without availability of vaccination, and mumps (F) and varicella (G) for vaccine-preventable infections in Japan. 95% confidence intervals for MFM ratios are indicated by error bars. Red solid lines indicate MFM ratio of 1. *: Significant with the Bonferroni's correction ($p<0{\cdot}05/13$) [26].

reported data for adults might have been gender-biased as it is more likely in Japan that mothers would be the accompanying parent. However, considering that MFM ratio was not different from 1 for varicella in adults (Figure 1G) and that the decreases of MFM ratios of some other diseases were observed from adolescence onwards (≥15 years of age; Figure 1C, D, and F), it is unlikely that the reversal of the MFM ratios was simply due to over-reporting by mothers from the pediatric sentinel points. Further evidence to the contrary comes from epidemic kerato-conjunctivitis (EKC). The reported numbers of patients with EKC from the ophthalmological sentinel points of NESID (per 100,000) had two peaks at ages 1–4 and 30–39 years of age (Figure 3A), which may imply household transmission. However, MFM ratio was >1 (MFM ratio 1.12, 95%CI 1.11–1.14) in the age group 30–39 years old (Figure 3B), indicating that a bias due to accompanying parent gender would be unlikely.

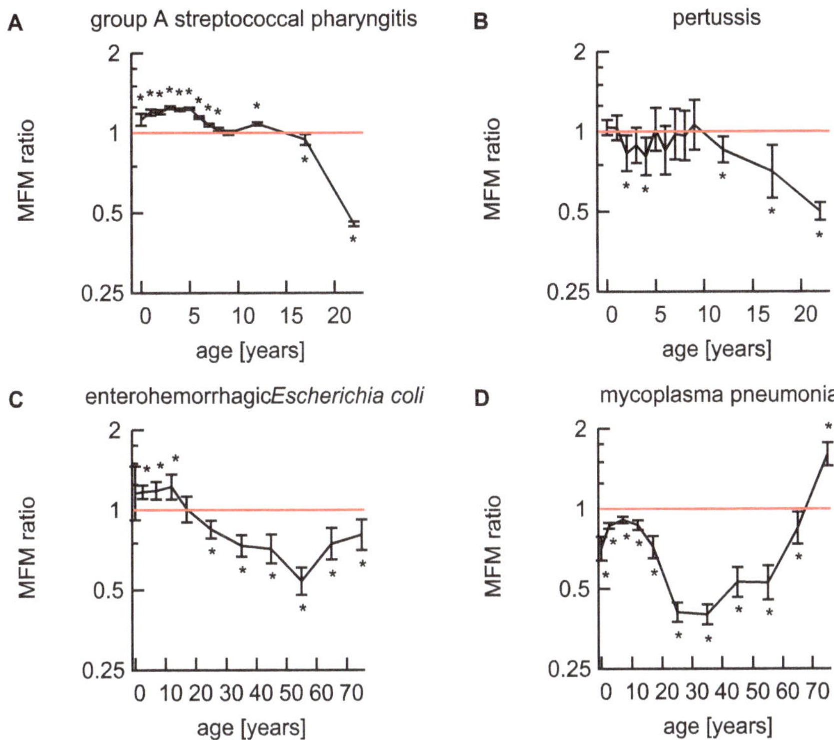

Figure 2. MFM ratios of bacterial infections; group A streptococcal pharyngitis (A), pertussis (B), enterohemorrhagic *Escherichia coli* (C) and mycoplasma pneumonia (D) reported from the sentinel points in Japan. 95% confidence intervals for MFM ratios are indicated by error bars. Horizontal red solid lines indicate MFM ratio of 1. *: Significant with the Bonferroni's correction (p<0.05/13 in A and B; p<0·05/11 in C and D) [26].

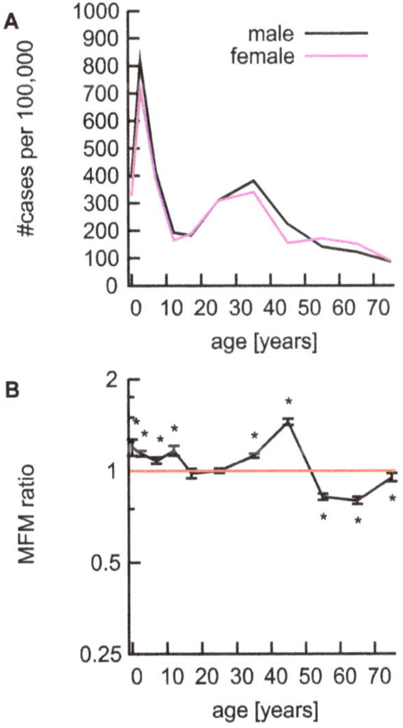

Figure 3. Epidemic keratoconjunctivitis (EKC) reported from the ophthalmological sentinel points in Japan. A: The number of reported cases of EKC (per 100,000 population) are illustrated for male (black) and female (red) separately. B: MFM ratios of EKC. 95% confidence intervals for MFM ratios are indicated by error bars, and horizontal red solid lines indicate MFM ratio of 1. *: Significant with the Bonferroni's correction (p<0·05/11) [26].

Bacterial infections

GAS with an estimated incidence of 66.6 per 1,000 (95%CI 60.5–72.6) [27] showed male predominance in childhood and the reversal in adolescence and adulthood. Morbidity of pertussis was never >1 in children or adults, indicating a female predominance at all ages as described elsewhere [7]. MFM ratios for EHEC were >1 in age groups 1–14 years of age and reversed to <1 in 15 year olds and older, i.e. boys were more likely to be reported as infected with EHEC than girls in childhood, while in adulthood, women were more likely to be reported as infected with EHEC than men. Total numbers of female and male cases with EHEC were 20,600 and 19,709, respectively, including 10,761 female and 7,717 male adult (≥20 years of age) cases (Table 2). Adults comprised 46% of the total cases, and 61% of the adult cases were in females. This is in accordance with the female adult preponderance in the 2011 outbreak of *Escherichia coli* O104 in Germany, where 87% of cases were adults and 68% of those adults were female [9].

Mycoplasma pneumoniae is the pathogen of MP with the second largest incidence rate of community-acquired pneumonia [29]. MP is unique among the bacterial infections examined in this study in that it showed a female preponderance in symptomatic infection at all ages except those over 70 years old (Figure 2D). In a population-based study on incidence of community-acquired pneumonia, it was reported that the incidence for *Mycoplasma pneumoniae* infection was not different in young and elderly people, and it was identical in males and females [29]. But the population size surveyed was ~200,000 and it is possible that the test power was not sufficient.

Strengths and weaknesses of the study

Several limitations of the present study should be noted. In general, observational studies do not verify the causality, because exposures to pathogens cannot be controlled. Covariates such as sex and age are confounded by human behavior, cultural influences, and other factors. The data used in the present study has a very large sample size collected through the official nationwide surveillance system in Japan [21]. Conservative 95% Bonferroni joint confidence intervals [26] of MFM ratios (Figures 1, 2 and 3) and assured precision of the estimates made it possible to demonstrate sex- and age-related differences in reported symptomatic infections.

It is possible that reporting rates are influenced by age and sex. In the model of the present analysis, the authors postulate that male and female patients consult physicians at the same rate. We further assume that parents seek health care equally for their sons and daughters. The latter assumption was based on the similar levels of immunization rates for boys and girls [23]. In 2008, male to female immunization ratios of measles-rubella combination vaccine were virtually 1 in children, indicating equality in vaccination rate [10,23]. Identical medical care-seeking was reported in both sexes for salmonellosis in US [25]. Thus, we suggest a sex-based bias in the probability of seeking medical care during childhood is unlikely [10]. The authors believe that any bias in estimates of the MFM ratios introduced by age- and/or sex-based difference in reporting is minimal.

Accurate and precise estimate of morbidity rates depends on complete observation on the number of cases. Incomplete reporting of the number of infected individuals makes it difficult to accurately estimate morbidity rates [30]. The present study analyzed only data of symptomatic cases. The omission of asymptomatic cases might lead to biased results between males and females; it would also be possible that symptomatic to asymptomatic infection ratios differ by sex and age. In this study, the morbidities P_M and P_F are considered to be products of probability of transmission and probability of developing symptomatic disease, neither of which can be estimated separately.

The pathogens of the analyzed infections include both viruses and bacteria. Immunological responses against viruses and bacteria are different. It is therefore worth separately documenting sex- and age-related differences in the reported morbidity of viral and bacterial infectious diseases in order to understand differences in their respective immune responses.

Putting research into context

This study documented examples of age-specific sex- related differences in morbidity for common infections. It also suggested a hypothesis that male children may be more susceptible to many of the common infectious diseases than female children, while this relationship is reversed by adulthood.

An apparent increased susceptibility of male children to selected infectious diseases has been frequently described [24]. But, with the exception of a limited number of studies [10–13], this increased susceptibility has been infrequently described in terms of sex and age as in the present study. In fact, some studies report no differences by sex for some diseases [15–18], for which significant differences were observed in this study. The merit of the methodology of the present study [10] is to show differences in morbidity by sex and age using observational data.

Genetic explanation for male-preponderance of infection in children has been proposed [31,32]. As children grow, their body systems develop, including immune, endocrine and reproductive systems. Both innate and acquired immunity are influenced by reproductive hormones [33–39]. Changes in MFM ratios by age might reflect differences in the relative physiological development of immune, endocrine, and reproductive systems between male and female children as they grow.

Male-to-female differences in response to vaccination (including non-targeted effects) were reported from epidemiological cohort data [40–45], appreciating that the sex differences in immune responses could lead to more efficient vaccination programs [46,47]. Despite data supporting an effect of sex in the response to vaccines, most studies do not document age-specific effects in vaccine efficacy or induced immune responses [47]. It is vital to understand sex- and age-related differences in the morbidity of infectious diseases in order to more efficiently prepare for and control outbreaks, investigate immune responses, and optimize disease-specific vaccine programs [47].

Population-based serological surveys studying antibodies (IgM and IgG) against pathogens or detecting pathogen DNA by polymerase chain reaction [4] would be more ideal in estimating accurate and precise infection rate. However, the cost of such investigations could pose a limiting factor in conducting a study using these methods. Another approach would be a large database where all cases of selected infections in a population are obligated to register, but the possibility of incomplete reporting (deliberate or unintentional) would still exist. The present study analyzed the data of NESID [21]. The sentinel points represent about 10% of all medical facilities in Japan, and the number of sentinel points in public health center areas are approximately proportional to their population size. Since reporting from the sentinel points is mandatory, the authors speculate that data from the sentinel points would proportionately represent the nation-wide trends.

In summary, this study provides evidence through the analysis of national data and calculation of MFM ratios that morbidity for viral and bacterial infections are sex- and age-dependent. Since our method uses observational data, we cannot avoid the possibility of under reporting which might confound the results [30]. However, under the proper circumstances, the methodology presented here may provide a powerful tool to study age-specific sex-related differences in the reported morbidities of selected diseases. These considerations have been poorly documented previously but have lately attracted more attention [48].

Author Contributions

Conceived and designed the experiments: NE OT SH. Analyzed the data: NE OT SH. Contributed reagents/materials/analysis tools: NE SH. Wrote the paper: NE OT KB S. Korematsu. Interpretation of the findings and the statistical assessment: NE OT KB S. Korematsu S. Karukaya KU NO TM.

References

1. Infections diseases. In: Kliegman RM, Behrman RE, Jenson HB, Stanton, ed. (2007) Nelson textbook of pediatrics 18th edition. Philadelphia: Saunders Elsevier. pp.1053–1519.
2. Wang Y, Feng Z, Yang Y, Self S, Gao Y, et al. (2011) Hand, foot, and mouth disease in China: patterns of spread and transmissibility. Epidemiol 22:781–792.
3. Frydenberg A, Starr M (2003) Slapped cheek disease: How it affects children and pregnant women. Aus Fam Physician 32: 589–592.
4. Zerr DM, Meier AS, Selke SS, Frenkel LM, Huang ML, et al. (2005) A population-based study of primary human herpesvirus 6 infection. N Engl J Med 352: 768–76
5. Hukic M, Ravlija J, Dedeic Ljubovic A, Moro A, Arapcic S, et al. (2010) Ongoing large mumps outbreak in the Federation of Bosnia and Herzegovina, Bosnia and Herzegovina, December 2010 to July 2011. Euro Surveill 16:pii = 19959. Available online: http://www.eurosurveillance.org/ViewArticle.aspx?ArticleId = 19959

6. Hamid Salim MA, Declercq E, Van Deun A, Saki KAR (2004) Gender differences in tuberculosis: a prevalence survey done in Bangladesh. Int J Tuberc Lung D 8: 952–957.
7. Heymann DL, ed. (2008) Control of communicable diseases manual 19th edition. Washington D.C.: American Public Health Association.
8. ECDC rapid risk assessment report (2011) Outbreak of Shiga toxin-producing *E. coli* (STEC) in Germany, 27 May 2011, European Centre for Disease Prevention and Control.
9. Frank C, Werber D, Cramer JP, et al. (2011) Epidemic profile of Shiga-toxin-producing *Escherichia coli* O104:H4 Outbreak in Germany-preliminary report. New Engl J Med 365: 1771–1780.
10. Eshima N, Tokumaru O, Hara S, Bacal K, Korematsu S, et al. (2011) Sex- and age-related differences in risks of infection by 2009 pandemic influenza A H1N1 virus of swine origin in Japan. PLoS ONE 6: e19409.
11. Eshima N, Iwata O, Iwata S, Tabata M, Higuchi Y, et al. (2009) Age and gender specific prevalence of HTLV-1. J Clin Virol 45: 135–138.
12. Thomas SL, Hall AJ (2004) What does epidemiology tell us about risk factors for herpes zoster? Lancet Infect Dis 4: 26–33.
13. Wu PY, Li YC, Wu HDI (2007) Risk factors for chickenpox incidence in Taiwan from a large-scale computerized database. Int J Dermatol 46: 362–366.
14. Cheng CC, Huang LM, Kao CL, Lee PI, Chen JM, et al. (2008) Molecular and clinical characteristics of adenoviral infections in Taiwanese children in 2004–2005. Eur J Pediatr 167: 633–640.
15. Gay NJ (1996) Analysis of serological surveys using mixture models: application to a survey of parvovirus B19. Stat Med 15: 1567–1573.
16. Barskey AE, Glasser JW, LeBaron CW (2009) Mumps resurgences in the United States: a historical perspective on unexpected elements. Vaccine 27: 6186–6195.
17. Tan T, Trindade E, Skowronski D (2005) Epidemiology of pertussis. Pediatr Infect Dis J 24: S10–S18.
18. Roush SW, Murphy TV, the Vaccine-Preventable Disease Table Working Group (2007) Historical comparisons of morbidity and mortality for vaccine-preventable diseases in the United States. JAMA 298: 2155–2163
19. Ministry of Education, Culture, Sports, Science and Technology, Ministry of Health, Labour and Welfare (2002) Ethical guidelines for epidemiological research. Available: http://www.niph.go.jp/wadai/ekigakurinri/guidelines.pdf. Accessed May 23, 2012.
20. Policy pertaining to quoting and setting links to the website of the Infectious Disease Surveillance Center, National Institute of Infectious Diseases. Available: http://idsc.nih.go.jp/about/idschp.html. Accessed May 23, 2012.
21. Infectious Disease Surveillance Center. Available: http://idsc.nih.go.jp/idwr/ydata/report-E.html.. Accessed Jan. 29, 2012.
22. Baba K, Okuno Y, Tanaka-Taya K, Okabe N (2011) Immunization coverage and natural infection rates of vaccine-preventable diseases among children by questionnaire survey in 2005 in Japan. Vaccine 29:3089–3092
23. Portal site of official Statistics of Japan website (in Japanese). Available: http://www.e-stat.go.jp/SG1/estat/eStatTopPortalE.do. Accessed Jan. 29, 2012.
24. Green MS (1992) The male predominance in the incidence of infectious diseases in children: a postulated explanation for disparities in the literature. Int J Epidemiol 21: 381–386.
25. Reller ME, Tauxe RV, Kalish LA, Mølbak K (2008) Excess salmonellosis in women in the United States: 1968–2000. Epidemiol Infect 136: 1109–1117.
26. Alt FB (1982) Bonferroni inequalities and intervals. In: Kotz S, Johnson NL, editors-in-chief. Encyclopedia of statistical sciences volume 1. New York: John Wiley & Sons. pp. 294–300.
27. Kawado M, Hashimoto S, Murakami Y, Izumida M, Ohta A, et al. (2007) Annual and weekly incidence rates of influenza and pediatric diseases estimated from infectious disease surveillance data in Japan, 2002–2005. J Epidemiol 17: S32–S41.
28. Departments of Gender, Women and Health, and Epidemic and Pandemic Alert and Response, WHO (2007) Addressing sex and gender in epidemic-prone infectious diseases. Geneva: WHO Press.
29. Gutiérrez F, Masiá M, Mirete C, Soldán B, Rodríguez JC, et al. (2006) The influence of age and gender on the population-based incidence of community-acquired pneumonia caused by different microbial pathogens. J Infect 53:166e174
30. Reich NG, Lessler J, Cummings DAT, Brookmeyer R (2012) Estimating absolute and relative case fatality ratios from infectious disease surveillance data. Biometrics DOI: 10.1111/j.1541-0420.2011.01709.x
31. Washburn TC, Medearis Jr DN, Childs B (1965) Sex differences in susceptibility to infections. Pediatrics 35: 57–64.
32. Schlegel RJ, Bellanti JA (1969) Increased susceptibility of males to infection. Lancet 294: 826–827.
33. Mariott I, Bost KL, Huet-Hudson YM (2006) Sex dimorphism in expression of receptors for bacterial lipopolysaccharides in murine macrophages: a possible mechanism for gender-based differences in endotoxic shock susceptibility. J Reprod Immunol 71: 12–27.
34. Rettew JA, Huet-Hudson YM, Mariott I (2009) Estrogens augment cell surface TLR4 expression on murine macrophages and regulate sepsis susceptibility in vivo. Endocrinology 150: 3877–3884.
35. Rettew JA, Huet-Hudson YM, Mariott I (2008) Testosterone reduces macrophage expression in the mouse of toll-like receptor 4, a trigger for inflammation and innate immunity. Biol Reprod 78: 432–437.
36. Pinzan CF, Ruas LP, Casabona-Fortunato AS, Carvalho FC, Roque-Barreira MC (2010) Immunological basis for the gender differences in murine *Paracoccidioides brasiliensis* infection. PLoS ONE 5: e10757.
37. Klein SL (2000) The effects of hormones on sex differences in infection: from genes to behavior. Neurosci Biobehav Rev 24: 627–638.
38. Klein SL, Marson AL, Scott AL, Ketner G, Glass GE (2002) Neonatal sex steroids affect responses to Seoul virus infection in male but not female Norway rats. Brain Behav Immun 16: 736–746.
39. Robinson DP, Lorenzo ME, Jian W, Klein SL (2011) Elevated 17β -estradiol protects females from influenza A virus pathogenesis by suppressing inflammatory responses. PLoS Pathog 7: e1002149.
40. Rodrigues A, Fischer TK, Valentiner-Branth P, Nielsen J, Steinsland H, et al. (2006) Community cohort study of rotavirus and other enteropathogens: are routine vaccinations associated with sex-differential incidence rates? Vaccine 24:4737–4746
41. Valentiner-Branth P, Perch M, Nielsen J, Steinsland H, Garly ML, et al. (2007) Community cohort study of Cryptosporidium parvum infections: sex-differential incidences associated with BCG and diphtheria-tetanus-pertussis vaccinations. Vaccine 25: 2733–2741.
42. Aaby P, Jensen H, Rodrigues A, Garly ML, Benn CS, et al. (2004) Divergent female-male mortality ratios associated with different routine vaccinations among female-male twin pairs. Int J Epidemiol 33: 367–373.
43. Aaby P, Jensen H, Walraven G (2006) Age specific changes in female-male mortality ratio related to the pattern of vaccinations: an observational study from rural Gambia. Vaccine 24: 4701–4708.
44. Aaby P, Vessari H, Nielsen J, Maleta K, Benn CS, et al. (2006) Sex differential effects of routine immunizations and childhood survival in rural Malawi. Pediatric Infect Dis J 25: 721–727.
45. Aaby P, Jensen H, Samb B, Cisse B, Sodemann M, et al. (2003) Differences in female-male mortality after high-titre measles vaccine and association with subsequent vaccination with diphtheria-tenanus-pertussis and inactivated poliovirus: reanalysis of West African studies. Lancet 361: 2183–2188.
46. Flanagan KL, Klein SL, Skakkebaek NE, Marriott I, Marchant A, et al. (2011) Sex differences in the vaccine-specific and non-targeted effects of vaccines. Vaccine 29: 2349–2354.
47. Klein SL, Jedlicka A, and Pekosz A (2010) The Xs and Y of immune responses to viral vaccines. Lancet Infect Dis 10: 338–349.
48. Editorial (2011) Taking sex into account in medicine. Lancet 378: 1826.

10

Mycobacterium tuberculosis Infection in Young Children: Analyzing the Performance of the Diagnostic Tests

Tomàs M. Pérez-Porcuna[1,2,3]*, Carlos Ascaso[2,4], Adriana Malheiro[5,6], Rosa Abellana[2], Marilaine Martins[7], José Felipe Jardim Sardinha[7], Patricia Quincó[1], Irineide Assumpção Antunes[8], Marlucia da Silva Garrido[1,9], Samira Bührer-Sékula[1,10], Flor Ernestina Martinez-Espinosa[1,11]

1 Pós-Graduação em Medicina Tropical, Universidade do Estado do Amazonas/Fundação de Medicina Tropical Dr. Heitor Vieira Dourado, Manaus, Amazonas, Brazil, **2** Departament de Salut Pública, Facultat de Medicina, Universitat de Barcelona, Barcelona, Catalunya, Spain, **3** Servei de Pediatria, CAP Valldoreix, Unitat de Investigació Fundació Mútua Terrassa, Hospital Universitari Mútua Terrassa, Terrassa, Catalunya, Spain, **4** Institut d'Investigacions Biomèdiques August Pi i Sunyer, Barcelona, Catalunya, Spain, **5** Laboratório de Imunologia Básica e Aplicada, Fundação de Hematologia e Hemoterapia do Amazonas, Manaus, Amazonas, Brazil, **6** Universidade Federal do Amazonas. Manaus, Amazonas, Brazil, **7** Fundação de Medicina Tropical Dr. Heitor Vieira Dourado, Manaus, Amazonas, Brazil, **8** Centro de Referência da Tuberculose, Policlínica Cardoso Fontes, Manaus, Amazonas, Brazil, **9** Programa de Controle da Tuberculose, Departamento de Vigilância Epidemiológica, Fundação de Vigilância em Saúde do Estado do Amazonas, Manaus, Amazonas, Brazil, **10** Instituto de Patologia Tropical e Saúde Pública, Universidade Federal de Goiás, Goiânia, Goiás, Brazil, **11** Instituto Leônidas e Maria Deane - Fiocruz Amazônia, Fundação Oswaldo Cruz, Manaus, Amazonas, Brazil

Abstract

Objective: This study evaluated the performance of the Tuberculin Skin Test (TST) and Quantiferon-TB Gold in-Tube (QFT) and the possible association of factors which may modify their results in young children (0–6 years) with recent contact with an index tuberculosis case.

Materials and Methods: A cross-sectional study including 135 children was conducted in Manaus, Amazonas-Brazil. The TST and QFT were performed and the tests results were analyzed in relation to the personal characteristics of the children studied and their relationship with the index case.

Results: The rates of positivity were 34.8% (TST) and 26.7% (QFT), with 14.1% of indeterminations by the QFT. Concordance between tests was fair (Kappa = 0.35 $P<0.001$). Both the TST and QFT were associated with the intensity of exposure (Linear OR = 1.286, $P=0.005$; Linear OR = 1.161, $P=0.035$ respectively) with only the TST being associated with the time of exposure (Linear OR = 1.149, $P=0.009$). The presence of intestinal helminths in the TST+ group was associated with negative QFT results (OR = 0.064, $P=0.049$). In the TST− group lower levels of ferritin were associated with QFT+ results (Linear OR = 0.956, $P=0.036$).

Conclusions: Concordance between the TST and QFT was lower than expected. The factors associated with the discordant results were intestinal helminths, ferritin levels and exposure time to the index tuberculosis case. In TST+ group, helminths were associated with negative QFT results suggesting impaired cell-mediated immunity. The TST−&QFT+ group had a shorter exposure time and lower ferritin levels, suggesting that QFT is faster and ferritin may be a potential biomarker of early stages of tuberculosis infection.

Editor: Pere-Joan Cardona, Fundació Institut d'Investigació en Ciències de la Salut Germans Trias i Pujol. Universitat Autònoma de Barcelona. CIBERES, Spain

Funding: This work was financially supported by the Brazilian National Counsel of Technological and Scientific Development (CNPq), the Foundation of Research Support of the State of Amazonas (FAPEAM), and the University of Barcelona. Cellestis Ltd. donated QuantiFERON test kits. The funders had no role in study design, data collection and analysis, decision to publish, or preparation of the manuscript.

Competing Interests: This work was financially supported by the Brazilian National Counsel of Technological and Scientific Development (CNPq), the Foundation of Research Support of the State of Amazonas (FAPEAM), and the University of Barcelona. Cellestis Ltd. donated QuantiFERON test kits. This does not alter adherence to all PLOS ONE policies on sharing data and materials.

* E-mail: tomas.perez.porcuna@gmail.com

Introduction

Tuberculosis (TB) is one of the infectious diseases producing the greatest morbidity and mortality worldwide [1]. Children represent 5 to 15% of the cases around the world and are more frequently infected and more easily affected and have the most severe forms of the disease [2].

Young children are mainly infected in the domiciliary setting by a household-sharing adult patient [3]. The main strategy of control of TB at a pediatric level is the detection of cases in the study of contacts and early treatment of the infection or disease. Diagnosis of infection is fundamental to implement this strategy [4].

The diagnosis of *Mycobacterium tuberculosis* (*Mtb*) infection is complex due to the lack of a gold standard [5]. The study of infection is based on the evaluation of immune response to the exposure of typical antigens of *Mtb* [5]. For decades the Tuberculin Skin Test (TST) has been the main diagnostic method of *Mtb* infection. It is based on the measurement of cell-mediated immunity expressed through delayed-type hypersensitivity response after subepidermic administration of purified protein derivatives (PPD) of *Mtb* [6]. The interpretation of the TST has been questioned especially because of the possibility of false positives in populations with high Calmette-Guérin bacillus vaccine (BCG) coverage and non-tuberculous mycobacteria (NTM) exposure [7]. In the last years new diagnostic techniques such as Interferon Gamma Release Assays (IGRAs) have been developed to improve the diagnosis of *Mtb* infection. The IGRAs are based on *in vitro* measurement of interferon gamma (IFN-γ) in the response of T lymphocytes versus the *Mtb*-specific region of difference 1 (RD1) antigens, which are very specific, albeit not exclusive, of *Mtb* [8]. Numerous studies have been performed to analyze these techniques but relatively few have assessed the performance of these tests in small children [9].

The aim of this study was to evaluate the response of the IGRA QuantiFERON-TB Gold In-Tube (QFT) and TST tests in young children with recent exposure to an index case. In addition, we evaluated the factors which may modify test results, with special emphasis on those which alter the immunity of children in a population systematically vaccinated with BCG in the perinatal period.

Materials and Methods

Ethics Statement

The study was approved by the Ethical Committee in Investigation of the Fundação de Medicina Tropical Dr. Heitor Vieira Dourado (FMT-HVD), October 26, 2007 (Protocol 2865-07). All legal guardians of participants provided written informed consent for inclusion in the study. All the individuals included in the studied received adequate treatment according to their clinical status.

Setting and Study Population

We conducted a cross-sectional study of comparison of diagnostic tests.

Case recruitment was performed in the Policlínica Cardoso Fontes (regional reference center for TB) and in the FMT-HVD, Manaus, Amazonas, Brazil from March 2009 to February 2010. The adults (greater than 12 years of age) diagnosed with tuberculosis in both centers were questioned about contact with children from 0 to 6 years of age. Those responding affirmatively were invited to bring the children to the center for evaluation and to be invited to participate in the study. All the adult index cases were sputum smear and/or culture positive.

We included children from 0–6 years of age with recent contact with an adult symptomatic TB index case within the last 12 months. Subjects receiving treatment or prophylaxis for TB were excluded. The study was undertaken at an outpatient level.

A sample size of 97 individuals was calculated for the study of concordance between diagnostic tests with a confidence level of 95%, precision of 15%, an expected kappa coefficient of 0.7 and with an expected proportion of positive classified by the diagnostic tests of 35%. These calculations were performed with the EPIDAT 3.1 program (Consellería de Sanidade, Xunta de Galicia, Spain and Pan American Health Organization, Washington D.C., USA).

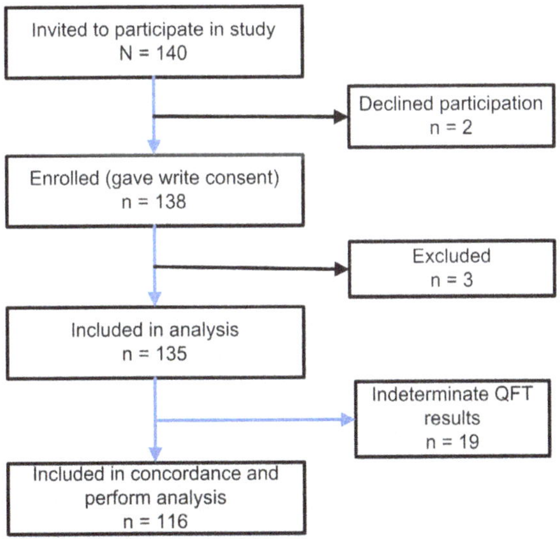

Figure 1. Flow diagram of enrolment (QFT: QuantiFERON-TB Gold In-Tube).

Data Collection

Demographic data, epidemiologic history of exposure to an index case of TB, the clinical history of the patient and physical examination were recorded. Chest X-ray, TST, stool and blood analysis (prior to the TST) were performed. The human immunodeficiency virus (HIV) test was not obligatory but was recommended to all the participants.

The *Mycobacterium tuberculosis* contact score (MTC-score) was used to evaluate the intensity of exposure [10]. The MTC-score is from 0 to 15 and is based on the assumption that the gradient of *Mtb* exposure is a composite function of the infectivity of the index case (0–4), the duration of exposure hours per day (0–4), the relationship to the index case (0–4) and the type of exposure (0–3) [10].

The time (month) from symptom onset to the time of initiation of treatment of the index case was calculated to measure the total exposure time (contagion) of the child to the index case.

Nutritional evaluation: The weight of all the study subjects was obtained and the standard deviation (SD) of the weight was calculated based on age and sex with the Anthro programme (WHO, version 3.2.2, January 2011). The risk of malnutrition was defined as gender-specific weight-for-age less than 1 SD and malnutrition was determined as less than 2 SDs [11].

Procedures

The TST was performed with an intradermic injection of 2 tuberculin units (TU) of PPD RT23 (Statens Serum Institut, Copenhagen, Denmark) and read 72 hours thereafter. A strong TST reaction (TST+) was defined when induration was $\geq$10 mm according to the protocols of the World Health Organization (WHO) [4].

Diagnostic Laboratory Tests

Blood tests. The QFT (Cellestis, Carnegie, Australia) was carried out and interpreted according to the manufacturer's instructions by experienced laboratory technicians who were unaware of the data of the study subjects. The result of the test was considered positive (QFT+) if the net value of IFN-γ to the TB antigens (after subtracting the negative control) was $\geq$0.35 IU/mL and $\geq$25% of the value of the negative control, independently of the response of the mitogen. The result of the test was considered negative (QFT−) if the net value of the IFN-γ was <0.35 IU/mL and mitogen response was sufficient ($\geq$0.50 IU/mL). A test result was considered indeterminate if there was excessive IFN-γ production with the negative control tube $\geq$8.0 IU/mL (indeter-

Table 1. Baseline demographic and clinical data of the study participants.

	Individuals evaluated	All Results#
Age (months)	135	46 (28.0; 64.5)
Less than 24 months		31 (23.0%)
Gender	135	
Male		61 (45.2%)
Female		74 (54.8%)
BCG scar	130	118 (90.8%)
BCG vaccination card	133	130 (97.7%)
Household contact	135	105 (77.8%)
Adult smear positive	135	61 (45.2%)
Time of exposure (months)	135	1.5 (0.2–3.7)
MTC-score	135	11 (6.3; 13.0)
Passive Smokers	130	44 (33.8%)
Previous viral infection[a]	135	28 (20.7%)
Previous vaccination (not BCG)[a]	135	71 (52.6%)
Previous corticoid therapy[a]	135	12 (8.9%)
Helminth infection	105	30 (28.6%)
Z scores forweight-for-age and gender	129	−0.13 (−0.9; 0.5)
Nutrition Status	129	
Risk of malnutrition[b]		19 (14.7%)
Malnutrition[b]		11 (8.5%)
Ferritin level (ng/mL)	135	31.9 (21.6; 45.9)
Vitamin D level (ng/mL)	135	38.1 (24.6; 48.8)
TST	135	
Strong reaction (≥10 mm)		47 (34.8%)
Weak reaction (5–9 mm)		0 (0.0%)
No reaction (0–4 mm)		88 (65.2%)
QFT result	135	
Positive		36 (26.7%)
Negative		80 (59.3%)
Hyperactivity of the negative control		10 (7.4%)
No reactivity of the positive control		9 (6.7%)

TST: Tuberculin Skin Test, QFT: QuantiFERON-TB Gold In-Tube, MTC-score: *Mycobacterium tuberculosis* contact score, BCG: Bacillus Calmette-Guérin.
#Categorical variables expressed as number of subjects (n) and percentage (%) compared to those evaluated with the characteristic studied. Quantitative variables expressed as mean and interquartile range (IQR).
[a]In the 12 weeks prior to the study.
[b]Risk of malnutrition was defined as a Z score for weight less than −1 SDs for age and gender; malnutrition was defined −2 SDs for age and gender.

Table 2. Comparison of the TST and QFT results.

		QFT results				
		Positive	Negative	Indeterminate	Indeterminate	Total
				Hyporeactive	Hyperreactive	n (%)
TST results	Positive	21	18	2	6	47 (34.8%)
	Negative	15	62	7	4	88 (65.2%)
	Total n (%)	36 (26.7%)	80 (59.3%)	9 (6.7%)	10 (7.4%)	135 (100.0%)

TST: Tuberculin Skin Test, QFT: QuantiFERON-TB Gold In-Tube, n: number of subjects.

Table 3. Bivariate analysis and Multivariate logistic regression for TST results and QFT results.

	TST results					QFT results				
	Bivariate			Multivariate		Bivariate			Multivariate	
	Positive[#]	Negative[#]	*P* value	*P* value	Odds Ratio	Positive[#]	Negative[#]	*P* value	*P* value	Odds Ratio
	N=39	N=77			(95% CI)	N=36	N=80			(95% CI)
Age (months)	45.0	46.0	0.863	0.729	-	47.5	44.0	0.241	0.412	-
	(26.0, 60.0)	(24.0, 65.0)				(32.0, 66.5)	(23.0, 62.0)			
Gender (male)	46.2%	40.3%	0.544	0.906	-	41.7%	43.2%	0.876	0.665	-
BCG scar	94.9%	90.5%	0.418	0.244	-	97.2%	89.7%	0.169	0.560	-
Time of exposure (months)	4.0	1.0	<0.001	0.009	1.15[b]	2.0	1.0	0.024	0.537	-
	(1.0, 10.0)	(0.0, 3.0)			(1.04; 1.27)	(1.0–5.2)	(0.0–3.0)			
MTC-score	12.0	10	<0.001	0.005	1.29[b]	12.0	10.0	0.021	0.035	1.16[b]
	(8.2, 14.0)	(0.0,12,0)			(1.08; 1.54)	(8.0, 14.0)	(0.0, 12.0)			(1.01; 1.33)
Passive Smokers	50.0%	27.4%	0.017	0.323	-	41.7%	32.9%	0.365	0.728	-
Previous infection[a]	15.4%	26.0%	0.196	0.203	-	16.7%	24.7%	0.335	0.836	-
Previous vaccination[a]	59.0%	49.4%	0.327	0.078	-	55.6%	50.6%	0.622	0.631	-
Previous corticoid therapy[a]	15.4%	6.5%	0.123	0.199	-	11.1%	8.6%	0.673	0.801	-
Helminth infection	42.9%	25.0%	0.091	0.252	-	21.4%	36.1%	0.167	0.324	-
Z scores for weight-for-age and gender	−0.1	−0.3	0.800	0.990	-	−0.3	−0.1	0.317	0.858	-
	(−1.0, 0.3)	(−0.9, 0.5)				(−1.0, 0.3)	(−0.9, 0.5)			
Ferritin level (ng/mL)	35.2%	30.6	0.243	0.767	-	29.9	35.4	0.323	0.705	-
	(26.4, 48.4)	(20.8, 44.7)				(22.3, 40.8)	(21.6, 49.9)			
Vitamin D level (ng/mL)	40	35.5	0.097	0.963	-	37.7	35.7	0.736	0.227	-
	(26.8, 59.8)	(23.8, 46.3)				(26.0, 49.1)	(24.4, 48.9)			

TST: Tuberculin Skin Test, QFT: QuantiFERON-TB Gold In-Tube, MTC-score: *Mycobacterium tuberculosis* contact score, BCG: Bacillus Calmette-Guérin.

[#]Categorical variables expressed as percentage (%) and quantitative variables expressed as mean and interquartile range (IQR).

[a]In the 12 weeks prior to the study.

[b]Linear odds ratio.

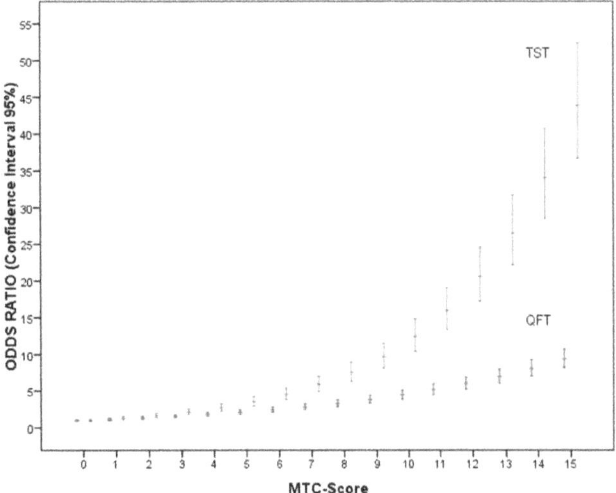

Figure 2. Odds ratio and confidence interval of 95% for the Tuberculin Skin Test -TST− (blue) and QuantiFERON-TB Gold in-Tube -QFT− (red) positive results according to the intensity of exposure to index case by *Mycobacterium tuberculosis* contact score (MTC-score). The MTC-score is from 0 to 15 and is based on the assumption that the gradient of *Mtb* exposure is a composite function of the infectivity of the index case (0–4), the duration of exposure - hours per day- (0–4), the relationship to index case (0–4) and the type of exposure (0–3).

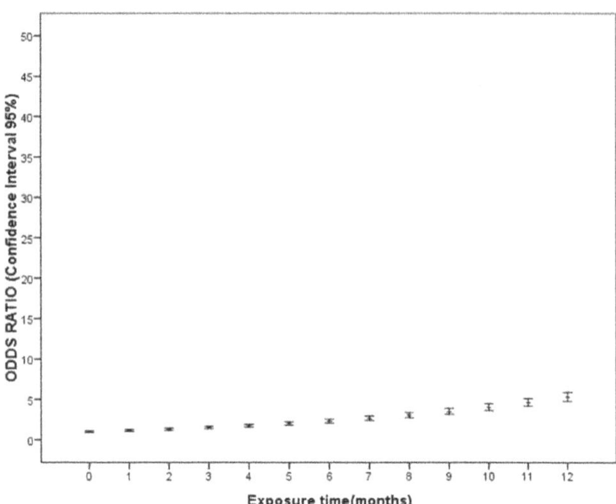

Figure 3. Odds ratio and confidence interal of 95% for the Tuberculosis Skin Test positive results according to time of exposure (months) to index case.

minate hypereactive) or with insufficient net mitogen response < 0.50 IU/mL plus insufficient net response of the TB antigen < 0.35 IU/mL (indeterminate hyporeactive). When the QFT result was indeterminate the test was repeated to confirm the result. Quantitative determination of 25-OH vitamin D and ferritin was made by immunoassay kits (LIAISON 25 OH Vitamin D Total and LIAISON Ferritin, DiaSorin, Saluggia, Italy).

Stool collection and examination. Three stool samples were collected from each child on three consecutive days in containers with a wide mouth screw-cap containing 10% formalin. Detection of eggs was made by the spontaneous sedimentation method [12].

Statistical Analysis

Description of categorical variables was performed using frequency tables, and quantitative variables were determined using medians, means, and interquartile range (IQR). To identify variables associated with the results of the tests bivariate analysis was first performed with the Fisher exact or Chi-square tests for categorical variables, and the Mann Whitney U test was used for quantitative variables followed by multiple logistic regression analysis. The independent variables analyzed were: sex, age, weight by age and sex, corticotherapy or vaccination within the previous 3 months, BCG, passive smoking, characteristics of the index case, characteristics of the child and vitamin D and ferritin levels and the presence of intestinal helminths.

To analyze the discordances between the TST and QFT results multivariate logistic regression was carried out and stratified on the basis of the results of the TST to know the differential behavior of the QFT. Associations between categorical independent variables and the test result are expressed as odds ratio and otherwise as linear odds ratios. The linear odds ratio quantifies the magnitude of the association between the positive response of the test and the change that occurs to a unit increase/decrease in the quantitative variable of interest. To show this effect, a plot of the odds ratio and its confidence interval for each value of levels of the variable was created. The y axis scaled is the same for all the plots.

Concordance between tests was measured using the Kappa index [13]. The receiver operating characteristic (ROC) curve was used in the TST negative (TST−) group to determine a cut-off of ferritin diagnosis between the QFT positive and negative (QFT+ and QFT−) populations. The type I error was set at 5%. The analyses were performed using the statistical package PASW Statistics 18 (SPSS Inc., Chicago, IL, USA).

Results

Descriptive

We evaluated 140 children for the study of the comparison of the TST and QFT results. Of these, 2 children refused to participate and 3 dropped out and thus, 135 were finally included in the study (Figure 1).

The median age of the participants was 46 months (IQR: 28.0–64.5), with 23.0% being of less than 24 months; 54.8% (74/135) were girls and 90.8% (118/130) presented the BCG scar. Contact with an intrahousehold index TB case occurred in 77.8% (105/135) of the children. The adult source case was smear positive in 45.2% (61/135) and the median MTC-score was 11 (IQR: 6.3–13.0) and the median time of exposure was 1.5 months (IQR: 0.2–3.7). The median ferritin level of the participants was 31.9 ng/mL (IQR: 21.6–45.9). Risk of malnutrition or status of malnutrition was presented by 23.3% (30/129) of the children, intestinal helminths (*Ascaris lumbricoides* and/or *Trichuris trichiura*) were present in 28.6% (30/105) and 33.8% (44/130) were passive smokers (Table 1).

The TST showed a strong reaction (≥10 mm) in 34.8% (47/135) of the children, a weak reaction (5–9 mm) in 0% (0/135) and no reaction (0–4 mm) in 65.2% (88/135). The QFT was positive in 26.7% (36/135) of the children, negative in 59.3% (80/135) and indeterminate in 14.1% (19/135) by hyperactivity of the negative control in 7.4% (10/135) [excessive background IFN-γ production] and no reactivity of the positive control in 6.7% (9/135) [insufficient IFN-γ response to mitogen]. Concordance between the TST and QFT (discarding the indeterminate cases) was fair, with a Kappa index of 0.350 ($P<0.001$) (Tables 1, 2).

Table 4. Multivariate logistic regression according to factors for positive QFT results stratified by TST results.

	TST+			TST−		
	P value	Regression Coefficient	Odds Ratio (95% CI)	*P* value	Regression Coefficient	Odds Ratio (95% CI)
Time of exposure (months)	0.667		-	0.593		-
MTC-score	0.020	0.547[a] (0.234)	1.727[b] (1.091; 2.735)	0.288		-
Helminth infection	0.049	−2.752 (1.395)	0.064 (0.004; 0.983)	0.895		-
Ferritin level	0.143		-	0.036	−0.045[a] (0.021)	0.956[b] (0.916; 0.997)

TST: Tuberculin Skin Test, QFT: QuantiFERON-TB Gold In-Tube, MTC-score: *Mycobacterium tuberculosis* contact score, BCG: Bacillus Calmette-Guérin.
[a]logistic regression coefficient related to quantitative variable.
[b]Linear odds ratio; exponential to the regression coefficient.

The samples required to perform the analysis of intestinal helminths were not available in 24.1% of the children. These missing data were not associated with the results of either the TST or the QFT (chi-squared = 1.055 and *P* = 0.788), and the missing data percentages for the four combinations of the test results ranged between 20% and 33%.

General Concordance and Analysis of the Test Responses

The results of each test were analyzed taking into account the different demographic, epidemiologic and clinical variables of the children included in the study.

Bivariate analysis of the TST+ respect to TST− results showed an association with a greater level of exposure -MTC-score- (U = 796.0 *P*<0.001), greater time of exposure (U = 581.0 *P*< 0.001) and with being a passive smoker (chi-square = 5.6 *P* = 0.017). The multivariate logistic regression model indicated that the TST depended on the time of exposure (Linear OR = 1.149; [95% Confidence Interval (CI): 1.036–1.274]) and the MTC-score (Linear OR = 1.286; CI: 1.077–1.536) (Table 3 and Figures 2, 3).

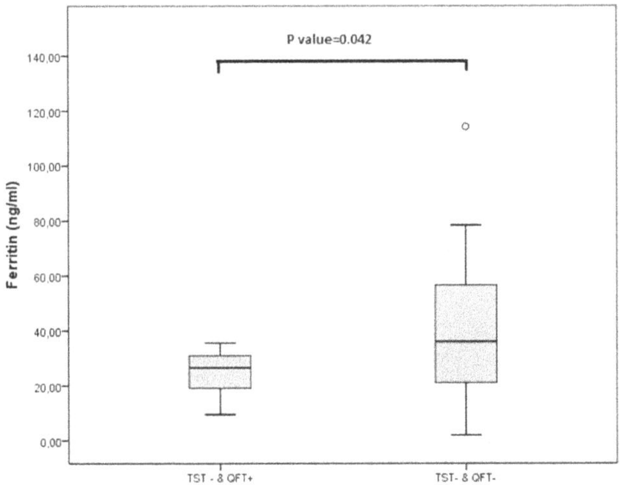

Figure 4. Box-plot of ferritin levels (ng/mL) according to TST−&QFT+ (n = 15) and TST−&QFT− (n = 62) groups. Tuberculin Skin Test (TST) and QuantiFERON-TB Gold in-Tube (QFT).

On analysis at a bivariate level, QFT+ respect to QFT− results showed an association with the MTC-score (U = 984.0, *P* = 0.021) and time of exposure (U = 894.5 *P* = 0.024). The logistic regression model showed that the QFT results only depended on the MTC-score (Linear OR = 1.161; CI: 1.010–1.333) (Table 3 and Figure 2).

Discordant Study Results

The discordance between the tests was analyzed based on the TST results to identify the possible factors that may explain the QFT results.

TST+ patients. In the TST+ patients the presence of greater exposure showed a greater possibility of QFT+ results (Linear OR = 1.727; CI: 1.091–2.735) while the presence of intestinal helminthiasis determined a greater possibility of QFT− results (OR = 0.064; CI: 0.004–0.983) (Table 4).

Among the TST+ individuals with intestinal heminths, 66.7% were QFT− (Table 5). However, among those who were TST+ but without helminths only 25.0% were QFT−. On analyzing the concordances between the tests according to the presence of intestinal helminths we found an absence of concordance with the presence of helminths with a Kappa index of 0.211 (*P* = 0.214), showing moderate concordance with a Kappa index of 0.471 (*P*< 0.001) when there were no helminths.

TST− patients. In the TST− patients the QFT results were related to the blood ferritin levels; specifically, the lower the level of ferritin the greater the possibility of being QFT+ (Linear OR = 0.956; CI: 0.916–0.997) (Table 4).

Of the TST− and QFT+ individuals, 86.7% (13/15) showed ferritin levels lower than 31.9 ng/mL (median of all children studied) (Figure 4). A cut-off point of 37.5 ng/mL was calculated for ferritin with a ROC curve which allowed differentiating the QFT+ from the QFT− individuals in this group, showing a sensitivity of 100% and a specificity of 51%.

Discussion

The diagnosis of infection by *Mtb* in children is of fundamental importance, especially in regions with a high incidence where BCG vaccination is common. In our study in small children the QFT and TST results were mainly related to the level of exposure to an index case of TB. The discordant results, and thus, the performance of the TST and QFT tests were associated with the

Table 5. Comparison of the main variables according to TST and QFT results.

Test results	N_1	MTC-score		Time of exposure		Ferritin		Helminths
		Median	IQR	Median	IQR	Median	IQR	% (n/N_2)
TST+&QFT+	21	12.50	10.25–14.75	4.00	1.00–12.00	34.35	24.15–65.60	25.0 (4/16)
TST+&QFT−	18	11.50	8.00–13.75	6.71	1.00–7.50	35.40	27.15–41.50	66.7 (8/12)
TST−&QFT+	15	10.00	7.00–12.00	2.00	1.00–4.00	26.60	17.10–31.90	16.7 (2/12)
TST−&QFT−	62	9.50	0.00–12.00	1.00	0.00–3.00	31.00	21.00–57.70	27.1 (13/48)

IQR: interquartile range,
N_1: number of subjects, TST: Tuberculin Skin Test, QFT: QuantiFERON-TB Gold In-Tube, MTC-score: *Mycobacterium tuberculosis* contact score, n: number of subjects with intestinal helminths;
N_2: number of subjects studied for helminths.

presence of intestinal helminths, the length of exposure to an index case and blood ferritin levels.

Although several studies have compared these two diagnostic techniques, the concordances vary widely especially based on the prevalence of TB in the region [14]. Few studies in young children have evaluated the discordant results between the tests [9] and the interpretation of the two tests according to the factors associated with the characteristics of contagion and those which may alter immune response.

General Concordance and Analysis of the Test Responses

In this study the percentage of positives for TST was 34.8%, being 26.7% for QFT, with fair concordance between the two tests (Kappa = 0.35). We observed that the results of both tests were related to the intensity of exposure, although, as previously reported, the TST was more strongly influenced by exposure than QFT [10,15]. Another factor we observed was that TST+ results were related to a greater time of exposure while the same was not observed for QFT. This finding is fundamental since young children have probably not been previously exposed to *Mtb* [6] thereby suggesting that in our study two different situations may be found, one with short exposure in which we find an early phase of primary infection by *Mtb* and another with a longer time of exposure showing latent tuberculosis infection (LTBI) secondary to primary infection. This may explain the behavior of the different tests according to the time of exposure [16] due to different immune response in relation to the time of infection observed.

Likewise, we did not observe any association between the TST results and age or the presence of a BCG scar. Thus, previous BCG vaccination or environmental exposure to NTM (in which the probability of weak or strong TST reactions should increase with age due to the greater probability of exposure to NTM) does not, *a priori*, seem to play an important role in TST behavior, similar to what other authors have reported [17,18], especially in tropical regions [19]. In addition, on analyzing our data the higher rate of TST+ results could be explained; at least in part, by a greater sensitivity or stability over time [20] versus the QFT which may be affected by reversion phenomenon (negativization of the test after positivity) during latent infection [21].

Discordant Test Results

On analyzing the discordant test results in our study the TST+ group was found to have a greater probability of presenting QFT− results in association with the presence of intestinal helminths. Intestinal helminths may explain up to two thirds of the discordant test results in this group, probably due to an ineffective Th1 immune response leading to a lower secretion of IFN-γ [22] and, thus, a false negativization of the QFT. On quantitative analysis of the values of IFN-γ in the individuals of this group we observed all presented values lower than 0.18 IU/mL. Thus, a lower threshold of positivity for QFT in this population, as suggested by some authors [23,24], would not explain the discordant results in this group. To our knowledge the association of intestinal helminths and QFT− results has not been previously described. The involvement of the presence of helminths on QFT performance has been previously reported, being associated with a greater percentage of indeterminate results secondary to no reactivity of the mitogen control [25,26]. This phenomenon may be explained by the immunomodulating capacity of infection by intestinal helminths, producing a strong Th2 immune response and thus, significant suppression of Th1 response [22]. Human and animal studies have shown that individuals with TB and helminthiasis have a reduction in IFN-γ secretion and the number of T CD4 lymphocytes compared to subjects with TB alone [22].

Effective immune response to *Mtb* requires complete Th1 response [27]. Some studies have reported that helminthic infections may facilitate the progression of *Mtb* [28,29].

This special immunological situation with the presence of helminths may also explain, in part, the QFT reversion phenomena. These reversion phenomena have, to date, been basically related to the clearance of *Mtb* [30], the intermittent expression of the antigens of the RD1 region of *Mtb* during the latent phase [31], variability in laboratory procedures [32] and non-specific variations in IFN-γ levels when the test is repeated in the same individual [21].

On analyzing the discordant test results in the TST− group we observed that low ferritin levels were associated with QFT+ results. Likewise, we found that the TST− group presented lower exposure times (mean = 2.11, median = 1) than the TST+ individuals (mean = 7.32, median = 4). These two facts together, in addition to the fact that small children had probably not been previously exposed to *Mtb*, suggest that these individuals may be in an early phase of primary infection by *Mtb*. It has previously been reported that the antigens used in the Interferon-γ Release Assays ESAT-6 and CPF-10 are secreted mainly in early infection [16,33,34] and some studies in animals have related the initial response of primary infection to *Mtb* to a rapid rise in IFN-γ and a fall in ferritin values [35] suggesting a true positivization of the QFT.

Iron (Fe) regulation requires a delicate balance between preventing an excess of Fe favoring survival, multiplication and virulence of *Mtb* [36] and providing sufficient Fe to ensure effective immune response [37]. Mycobacteria competes for the sources of Fe with the host, thus, one strategy of immune response would be to decrease the availability of Fe to the mycobacteria [37,38]. Ferritin is a fundamental protein for the regulation of Fe, acting as a storage protein and managing the intracellular distribution of this element [39]. The clinical evolution of TB is reportedly worse in humans with both high and low ferritin levels [40].

The results of animal studies have indicated that a decrease in ferritin levels in primary infection is mainly mediated by IFN-γ [35]. This phenomenon is not exclusive of subjects vaccinated with BCG but is more prolonged and more intense over time. Some authors have reported that strong regulation of Fe metabolism could explain, in part, the protector effect of the BCG vaccine against TB [35,37].

Analysis of our data supports the contention that QFT probably undergoes more rapid conversion (step from negative to positive) after primary infection than the TST and would explain most of the discordant test results in this group as well as reinforce the importance of iron metabolism in the immune response against *Mtb* [41]. This is, to our knowledge, one of the first studies to explain this discordance related to time of exposure, ferritin levels and relating the metabolism of Fe with the initial immune response to primary infection in humans [26,42].

Indeterminate QFT Results

The 14% of indeterminate results for QFT in this study suggests a limitation of the usefulness of IGRA in the pediatric TB setting. The proportion of indeterminate results varies greatly in studies in children [43–45] and may be associated with technical problems and probably also factors which alter Th1 immune response [46] such as age, the presence of helminths, and immunosuppression [25]. We found no association with any of the variables analyzed in this study or with the results of the TST, probably due to a lack of statistical power.

Conclusions

The results of the present study strongly suggest the utility of the systematic study of household pediatric contacts for early detection of infection by *Mtb*.

Despite observing a lower concordance than expected, we observed that the main variable which may explain the results of the TST and QFT tests was the level of exposure to an index case. Likewise, the time of exposure was critical in the evaluation and reading of the test results.

On studying the discordant results between the tests we found that the presence of intestinal helminths and a short exposure time explained a large part of these results. For the interpretation of the discordant test results we recommend the study of intestinal helminthiasis (especially in settings of high prevalence) and estimation of the time of exposure and measurement of ferritin levels.

In the case of TST+&QFT− results, the presence of intestinal helminths may produce false negative QFT results due to the negative impact of the helminths on Th1 immune response. In the case of TST−&QFT+ results, low ferritin levels (<37.5 ng/mL) and short time of exposure (<2 months) could indicate initial stages of infection by *Mtb* with possible false negative TST results.

This study suggests the important role of iron metabolism in human immune response in primary infection by *Mtb* and the possibility that ferritin may be a biomarker in this phase [42,47].

Acknowledgments

The authors would like to thank the Policilinica Cardoso Fontes team and Fundação de Medicina Tropical Dr. Heitor Vieira Dourado for overall support.

Author Contributions

Conceived and designed the experiments: TPP CA AM SBS FEME. Performed the experiments: TPP AM MM JFJS PQ. Analyzed the data: TPP CA RA. Contributed reagents/materials/analysis tools: TPP CA AM MM JFJS PQ IA MG SBS FEME. Wrote the paper: TPP CA RA. Data interpretation: TPP CA AM RA MM JFJS PQ SBS FEME. Reviewed and revised the manuscript: CA AM RA MM JFJS PQ IA MG SBS FEME.

References

1. World Health Organization (2011) Global tuberculosis control 2011. Geneve: WHO. Available: http://www.who.int/tb/publications/global_report/en/index.html. Accessed 2012 July 22.
2. Marais BJ, Gie RP, Schaaf HS, Hesseling AC, Obihara CC, et al. (2004) The natural history of childhood intra-thoracic tuberculosis: a critical review of literature from the pre-chemotherapy era. Int J Tuberc Lung Dis 8: 392–402.
3. Starke JR (2003) Pediatric tuberculosis: time for a new approach. Tuberculosis (Edinb) 83: 208–212.
4. Guidance for National Tuberculosis Programmes on the management of tuberculosis in children. Chapter 1: introduction and diagnosis of tuberculosis in children (2006). Int J Tuberc Lung Dis 10: 1091–1097.
5. Pai M, Riley LW, Colford JM (2004) Interferon-gamma assays in the immunodiagnosis of tuberculosis: a systematic review. Lancet InfectDis 4: 761–776.
6. Comstock GW, Livesay VT, Woolpert SF (1974) The prognosis of a positive tuberculin reaction in childhood and adolescence. Am J Epidemiol 99: 131–138.
7. Farhat M, Greenaway C, Pai M, Menzies D (2006) False-positive tuberculin skin tests: what is the absolute effect of BCG and non-tuberculous mycobacteria? Int J Tuberc Lung Dis 10: 1192–1204.
8. Pai M, Riley LW, Colford JM Jr (2004) Interferon-gamma assays in the immunodiagnosis of tuberculosis: a systematic review. Lancet Infect Dis 4: 761–776. doi:10.1016/S1473-3099(04)01206-X.
9. Machingaidze S, Wiysonge CS, Gonzalez-Angulo Y, Hatherill M, Moyo S, et al. (2011) The utility of an interferon gamma release assay for diagnosis of latent tuberculosis infection and disease in children: a systematic review and meta-analysis. Pediatr Infect Dis J 30: 694–700. doi:10.1097/INF.0b013e318214b915.

10. Hesseling AC, Mandalakas AM, Kirchner HL, Chegou NN, Marais BJ, et al. (2009) Highly discordant T cell responses in individuals with recent exposure to household tuberculosis. Thorax 64: 840–846. doi:10.1136/thx.2007.085340.
11. World Health Organization. The WHO Child Growth Standards. WHO. Available: http://www.who.int/childgrowth/standards/en/. Accessed 2012 May 1.
12. Lutz A (1919) *Schistosomum mansoni* and Schistosomatosis observed in Brazil. Mem Inst Oswaldo Cruz: 121–155.
13. Landis JR, Koch GG (1977) The measurement of observer agreement for categorical data. Biometrics 33: 159–174.
14. Powell DA (2009) Interferon Gamma Release Assays in the Evaluation of Children With Possible *Mycobacterium tuberculosis* Infection: A View to Caution. Pediatr Infect Dis J 28: 676–677.
15. Dheda K, van Zyl Smit R, Badri M, Pai M (2009) T-cell interferon-gamma release assays for the rapid immunodiagnosis of tuberculosis: clinical utility in high-burden vs. low-burden settings. Curr Opin Pulm Med 15: 188–200. doi:10.1097/MCP.0b013e32832a0adc.
16. Hill PC, Brookes RH, Adetifa IM, Fox A, Jackson-Sillah D, et al. (2006) Comparison of enzyme-linked immunospot assay and tuberculin skin test in healthy children exposed to *Mycobacterium tuberculosis*. Pediatrics 117: 1542–1548.
17. Almeida LM, Barbieri MA, Da Paixão AC, Cuevas LE (2001) Use of purified protein derivative to assess the risk of infection in children in close contact with adults with tuberculosis in a population with high Calmette-Guérin bacillus coverage. Pediatr Infect Dis J 20: 1061–1065.
18. Raharimanga V, Ratovoson R, Ratsitorahina M, Ramarokoto H, Rasolofo V, et al. (2012) Tuberculin reactivity in first-year schoolchildren in Madagascar. Trop Med Int Health 17: 871–876. doi:10.1111/j.1365-3156.2012.03013.x.
19. Hill PC, Ota MOC (2010) Tuberculosis case-contact research in endemic tropical settings: design, conduct, and relevance to other infectious diseases. Lancet Infect Dis 10: 723–732. doi:10.1016/S1473-3099(10)70164-X.
20. Shanaube K, Hargreaves J, Fielding K, Schaap A, Lawrence K-A, et al. (2011) Risk factors associated with positive QuantiFERON-TB Gold In-Tube and tuberculin skin tests results in Zambia and South Africa. PLoS ONE 6: e18206. doi:10.1371/journal.pone.0018206.
21. Pai M, Joshi R, Dogra S, Zwerling AA, Gajalakshmi D, et al. (2009) T-cell assay conversions and reversions among household contacts of tuberculosis patients in rural India. Int J Tuberc Lung Dis 13: 84–92.
22. Resende CT, Hirsch CS, Toossi Z, Dietze R, Ribeiro-Rodrigues R (2007) Intestinal helminth co-infection has a negative impact on both anti-*Mycobacterium tuberculosis* immunity and clinical response to tuberculosis therapy. Clin Exp Immunol 147: 45–52.
23. Pai M, Kalantri S, Menzies D (2006) Discordance between tuberculin skin test and interferon-gamma assays. Int J Tuberc Lung Dis 10: 942–943.
24. Mandalakas AM, Detjen AK, Hesseling AC, Benedetti A, Menzies D (2011) Interferon-gamma release assays and childhood tuberculosis: systematic review and meta-analysis. Int J Tuberc Lung Dis 15: 1018–1032. doi:10.5588/ijtld.10.0631.
25. Thomas TA, Mondal D, Noor Z, Liu L, Alam M, et al. (2010) Malnutrition and helminth infection affect performance of an interferon gamma-release assay. Pediatrics 126: e1522–1529. doi:10.1542/peds.2010-0885.
26. Banfield S, Pascoe E, Thambiran A, Siafarikas A, Burgner D (2012) Factors Associated with the Performance of a Blood-Based Interferon-γ Release Assay in Diagnosing Tuberculosis. PLoS ONE 7: e38556. doi:10.1371/journal.-pone.0038556.
27. Lewinsohn DA, Lewinsohn DM (2008) Immunologic susceptibility of young children to *Mycobacterium tuberculosis*. PediatrRes 63: 115.
28. Borkow G, Leng Q, Weisman Z, Stein M, Galai N, et al. (2000) Chronic immune activation associated with intestinal helminth infections results in impaired signal transduction and anergy. J Clin Invest 106: 1053–1060. doi:10.1172/JCI10182.
29. Tristao-Sa R, Ribeiro-Rodrigues R, Johnson LT, Pereira FE, Dietze R (2002) Intestinal nematodes and pulmonary tuberculosis. Rev Soc Bras Med Trop 35: 533–535.
30. Pai M, O'Brien R (2007) Serial testing for tuberculosis: can we make sense of T cell assay conversions and reversions? PLoS Med 4: e208. doi:10.1371/journal.pmed.0040208.
31. Hill PC, Brookes RH, Fox A, Jackson-Sillah D, Jeffries DJ, et al. (2007) Longitudinal assessment of an ELISPOT test for *Mycobacterium tuberculosis* infection. PLoS Med 4: e192. doi:10.1371/journal.pmed.0040192.
32. Veerapathran A, Joshi R, Goswami K, Dogra S, Moodie EEM, et al. (2008) T-cell assays for tuberculosis infection: deriving cut-offs for conversions using reproducibility data. PLoS ONE 3: e1850. doi:10.1371/journal.pone.0001850.
33. Andersen P, Askgaard D, Ljungqvist L, Bennedsen J, Heron I (1991) Proteins released from *Mycobacterium tuberculosis* during growth. Infect Immun 59: 1905–1910.
34. Haile Y, Bjune G, Wiker HG (2002) Expression of the mceA, esat-6 and hspX genes in *Mycobacterium tuberculosis* and their responses to aerobic conditions and to restricted oxygen supply. Microbiology (Reading, Engl) 148: 3881–3886.
35. Thom RE, Elmore MJ, Williams A, Andrews SC, Drobniewski F, et al. (2012) The expression of ferritin, lactoferrin, transferrin receptor and solute carrier family 11A1 in the host response to BCG-vaccination and *Mycobacterium tuberculosis* challenge. Vaccine 30: 3159–3168. doi:10.1016/j.vac-cine.2012.03.008.
36. Manabe YC, Saviola BJ, Sun L, Murphy JR, Bishai WR (1999) Attenuation of virulence in *Mycobacterium tuberculosis* expressing a constitutively active iron repressor. Proc Natl Acad Sci USA 96: 12844–12848.
37. Basaraba RJ, Bielefeldt-Ohmann H, Eschelbach EK, Reisenhauer C, Tolnay AE, et al. (2008) Increased expression of host iron-binding proteins precedes iron accumulation and calcification of primary lung lesions in experimental tuberculosis in the guinea pig. Tuberculosis (Edinb) 88: 69–79. doi:10.1016/j.tube.2007.09.002.
38. Ratledge C (2004) Iron, mycobacteria and tuberculosis. Tuberculosis(Edinb) 84: 110–130.
39. Harrison PM, Arosio P (1996) The ferritins: molecular properties, iron storage function and cellular regulation. Biochim Biophys Acta 1275: 161–203.
40. Isanaka S, Aboud S, Mugusi F, Bosch RJ, Willett WC, et al. (2012) Iron status predicts treatment failure and mortality in tuberculosis patients: a prospective cohort study from Dar es Salaam, Tanzania. PLoS ONE 7: e37350. doi:10.1371/journal.pone.0037350.
41. Reddy PV, Puri RV, Khera A, Tyagi AK (2012) Iron storage proteins are essential for the survival and pathogenesis of *Mycobacterium tuberculosis* in THP-1 macrophages and the guinea pig model of infection. J Bacteriol 194: 567–575. doi:10.1128/JB.05553-11.
42. Friis H, Range N, Braendgaard KC, Kaestel P, Changalucha J, et al. (2009) Acute- phase response and iron status markers among pulmonary tuberculosis patients: a cross-sectional study in Mwanza, Tanzania. BrJNutr 102: 310–317.
43. Bergamini BM, Losi M, Vaienti F, D'Amico R, Meccugni B, et al. (2009) Performance of commercial blood tests for the diagnosis of latent tuberculosis infection in children and adolescents. Pediatrics 123: e419–424. doi:10.1542/peds.2008-1722.
44. Connell TG, Ritz N, Paxton GA, Buttery JP, Curtis N, et al. (2008) A three-way comparison of tuberculin skin testing, QuantiFERON-TB gold and T-SPOT.TB in children. PLoSONE 3: e2624.
45. Haustein T, Ridout DA, Hartley JC, Thaker U, Shingadia D, et al. (2009) The likelihood of an indeterminate test result from a whole-blood interferon-gamma release assay for the diagnosis of *Mycobacterium tuberculosis* infection in children correlates with age and immune status. Pediatr Infect Dis J 28: 669–673. doi:10.1097/INF.0b013e3181a16394.
46. Grare M, Derelle J, Dailloux M, Laurain C (2010) QuantiFERON-TB Gold In-Tube as help for the diagnosis of tuberculosis in a French pediatric hospital. Diagn Microbiol Infect Dis 66: 366–372. doi:10.1016/j.diagmicro-bio.2009.11.002.
47. Jacobsen M, Repsilber D, Gutschmidt A, Neher A, Feldmann K, et al. (2007) Candidate biomarkers for discrimination between infection and disease caused by *Mycobacterium tuberculosis*. J Mol Med 85: 613–621. doi:10.1007/s00109-007-0157-6.

11

Identification of a Novel Human Polyomavirus in Organs of the Gastrointestinal Tract

Sarah Korup[1¶], Janita Rietscher[1¶], Sébastien Calvignac-Spencer[2], Franziska Trusch[1], Jörg Hofmann[3], Ugo Moens[4], Igor Sauer[5], Sebastian Voigt[1], Rosa Schmuck[5], Bernhard Ehlers[1]*

1 Division of Viral Infections, Robert Koch Institute, Berlin, Germany, **2** Research Group Emerging Zoonoses, Robert Koch Institute, Berlin, Germany, **3** Institute of Virology, Charité - Universitätsmedizin Berlin, Berlin, Germany, **4** Department of Medical Biology, University of Tromsø, Tromsø, Norway, **5** General, Visceral, and Transplantation Surgery, Experimental Surgery and Regenerative Medicine, Charité-Campus Virchow, Charité Universitätsmedizin Berlin, Germany

Abstract

Polyomaviruses are small, non-enveloped viruses with a circular double-stranded DNA genome. Using a generic polyomavirus PCR targeting the VP1 major structural protein gene, a novel polyomavirus was initially identified in resected human liver tissue and provisionally named Human Polyomavirus 12 (HPyV12). Its 5033 bp genome is predicted to encode large and small T antigens and the 3 structural proteins VP1, VP2 and VP3. Phylogenetic analyses did not reveal a close relationship to any known human or animal polyomavirus. Investigation of organs, body fluids and excretions of diseased individuals and healthy subjects with both HPyV12-specific nested PCR and quantitative real-time PCR revealed additional virus-positive samples of resected liver, cecum and rectum tissues and a positive fecal sample. A capsomer-based IgG ELISA was established using the major capsid protein VP1 of HPyV12. Seroprevalences of 23% and 17%, respectively, were determined in sera from healthy adults and adolescents and a pediatric group of children. These data indicate that the virus naturally infects humans and that primary infection may already occur in childhood.

Editor: Jianming Qiu, University of Kansas Medical Center, United States of America

Funding: These authors have no support or funding to report.

Competing Interests: The authors have declared that no competing interests exist.

* E-mail: EhlersB@rki.de

¶ These authors contributed equally to this work.

Introduction

Polyomaviruses are small non-enveloped viruses with a circular double-stranded DNA genome. They usually cause asymptomatic primary infections, and persist in the body throughout life [1]. Seroprevalence studies have revealed that most primary infections occur in childhood and that the majority of healthy adults had contact to one or more polyomaviruses [2–5]. In immunocompromised individuals, polyomavirus reactivation can be associated with clinical disease, i.e., JCPyV with progressive multifocal leukoencephalopathy, BKPyV with nephropathy and cystitis (both reviewed in: [6,7]), MCPyV with Merkel cell carcinoma [8], and TSPyV with *Trichodysplasia spinulosa* [9]. For the other human polyomaviruses known to date (KIPyV, WUPyV, HPyV6, HPyV7, HPyV9, MWPyV/HPyV10/MXPyV and STLPyV [10–17]) no associations with pathologic conditions have been found. BKPyV and JCPyV persist in the kidney [1], and MCPyV, HPyV6, HPyV7 and TSPyV are members of the skin microbiome and/or are detected in skin diseases ([8,9,12,15,18]; reviewed in: [19]). The tropism of the other human polyomaviruses is largely unknown.

Most human polyomaviruses were discovered by examining body fluids, se- and excretions [10–14,16,20]. In the present study we performed a search for yet unknown human polyomaviruses with generic PCR and focused on organs of the gastrointestinal tract since a number of human polyomaviruses had been detected in feces and sewage water [10,16,21–29]. In addition, spleens and lymph nodes were tested, since JCPyV, MCPyV, and MCPyV-related chimpanzee polyomaviruses had been reported to be present in these organs [30–32]. Of the known human polyomaviruses, only MCPyV and TSPyV were detected in the investigated organs. However, in resected liver, a novel polyomavirus was discovered.

Methods

Ethic statement

The study protocol for collection of gastrointestinal organ samples was approved by the local ethics committee of the Charité - Universitätsmedizin Berlin. Written informed consent was obtained from study participants. The ethics committee approved this consent procedure. Residual anonymized material from spleen and lymph node samples was collected from deceased individuals who donated organs for transplantation. Informed verbal consent for organ donation was obtained from the next of kin and documented by the responsible physician. The anonymized collection of residual materials was approved by the local ethics committee of the Charité - Universitätsmedizin Berlin. All samples of body fluids and excretions were residual materials from anonymized specimens originally submitted for routine diagnostics. Additionally, retain samples from anonymized blood donors collected after the retention period were used in this study. All procedures were in accordance with the ethical standards of the responsible committee on human experimentation and with the Helsinki Declaration.

Sample collection

For PCR purposes, spleen (n = 61) and lymph node (n = 22) specimens were provided by the German Foundation for Organ Transplants (Deutsche Stiftung Organtransplantation, DSO), Frankfurt am Main, Germany. Liver (n = 124), gall bladder (n = 21), esophagus (n = 2), stomach (cardia; n = 2), colon (n = 4) and rectum specimens (n = 6) were collected at the clinic of general, visceral and transplantation surgery of the Charité, Berlin, Germany. Serum, plasma, urine, fecal, bronchoalveolar lavage and cerebrospinal fluid samples were taken from the panel that had been previously collected in Germany and analyzed for the presence of HPyV9 [11]. Oral fluids (n = 30) were collected from patients with suspected but not confirmed measles virus infection in Germany. Native tissue samples were kept frozen at −80°C and liquid samples at −20°C.

For ELISA, serum samples from healthy adolescents and adults (age 16 to 72 years; n = 299) and from pediatric patients (age 2–11 years; n = 74) were used that had been collected previously for the determination of HPyV9 seroprevalence [33].

DNA extraction and PCR methods

DNA was extracted, purified and generic polyomavirus PCR was carried out as described previously [11,32]. To obtain additional sequence information of the novel polyomavirus, a 950 bp genome fragment was amplified with nested PCR using two degenerate sense primers targeting the VP3 gene of polyomaviruses [11] and two virus-specific antisense primers derived from the novel VP1 sequence (primers listed in Table S1; PCR conditions in Table S2). From the resulting sequence, tail-to-tail primers were derived and used in nested long-distance (LD) PCR for the amplification and sequencing of the remaining part of the virus genome (Tables S1 and S2). For diagnostic detection of the novel polyomavirus, specific nested PCR primers were selected (Table S1) and used under the conditions described in Table S2.

For specific quantitative PCR (qPCR), targeting a 139 bp sequence of the VP1 gene, a sense primer (5′- GTG-GGAAGCTGTCAGTGTGA), an antisense primer (5′- CCACC-TACTGCAAACATGTG) and a TaqMan probe (*FAM*-ACTA-CAGGATGGCCTACCCCATTGTCAGTC-*TAMRA*) were selected. Five µl of DNA from fluid samples and 250 ng of DNA from tissue samples were analyzed in a 96-well plate format. The PCR was performed in a total volume of 25 µl with 2 U Platinum Taq DNA polymerase (Life Technologies, Darmstadt, Germany), 400 nM of each primer, 150 nM probe, 800 µM dNTP PCR Mix (Metabion, Martinsried, Germany) and 4.5 mM $MgCl_2$. An MX 3000P (Stratagene, Waldbronn, Germany) was used with the following cycling conditions: 95°C for 5 min and 45 cycles of 95°C for 15 sec, followed by 59°C for 30 sec. Analysis was performed using the MXPro3000P V 4.10 software (Stratagene).

Genome annotation

Open reading frames (ORFs) were predicted using Geneious Pro 5.5.7 software. The region encoding the large T and small T antigens (LTAg; STAg) was scanned for splice sites using MacVector 12 software. Conserved motifs in all ORFs were identified using the EMBOSS Needle-Pairwise Sequence Alignment (Rice et al., 2000). Putative binding sites of transcription factors were predicted using Alggen PROMO software [34,35]. Amino acid percentage identities were calculated, and palindromes in the NCCR were identified using the EMBOSS Needle-Pairwise Sequence Alignment [36].

Phylogenetic analysis

VP1, VP2 and LTAg protein alignments comprising representative sequences from all polyomaviruses currently recognized as species by the International Committee on Taxonomy of Viruses (ICTV; [37]) or recently reported to likely account for novel species (e.g., MWPyV; [10]) were computed and used for phylogenetic analyses (Table S3). These datasets notably included 10 non-human polyomaviruses whose genomes were recently sequenced in our laboratory and which will be the subject of a separate publication. Phylogenetic analyses were performed using a workflow described previously [32], which ended up with maximum likelihood (ML) and Bayesian tree reconstruction. The three coding sequences were processed and analyzed individually.

It should be noted that during the revision process of this manuscript, novel polyomaviruses were identified (e.g. STLPyV). None, however, was closely related to the novel human polyomavirus described in this study (data not shown). It is therefore not expected that their inclusion would affect its phylogenetic placement.

Expression and purification of recombinant VP1 proteins

The major capsid proteins VP1 genes of HPyV12 and the avian polyomavirus APyV (former name: BFDPyV) were expressed as described previously [33]. In brief, the VP1 sequences were codon-optimized, commercially synthesized (MrGene GmbH, Regensburg, Germany) and inserted into a pTriEx-1.1 plasmid that generates VP1 constructs tagged with a 6x His-tag at the N-terminus. After transformation and expression in *E. coli* Rosetta (DE3)pLacITM cells (Novagen, San Diego, USA), insoluble recombinant proteins were obtained in inclusion bodies and purified with BugBuster Protein Extraction Reagent (Novagen) after lysis of cells and inclusion bodies with rLysozyme™ (Novagen). Purification of VP1 from other *E. coli* proteins was done under denaturing conditions with 8 M urea (Roth, Karlsruhe, Germany) using HIS-Select® Nickel Affinity Gel (Sigma-Aldrich, St. Louis, USA). Native conformation of the VP1 proteins was reconstituted by removing urea by dialysis. Purity of proteins was analyzed with SDS–PAGE and Western Blot using an anti-His monoclonal antibody (Sigma-Aldrich, St. Louis, USA). Protein concentration was determined with a Pierce BCA Protein Assay Kit (Thermo Scientific, Rockford, USA).

ELISA and statistical analysis

To detect antibodies with reactivity to HPyV12 VP1, an ELISA was performed as described earlier [33]. F96 maxisorp immuno plates (Nunc, Roskilde, Denmark) were incubated with purified VP1 (50 ng per well) in PBS (pH 7.2) for 1 h at 37°C. Plates were washed 3x with 800 µl PBS/0.05% Tween (PBS-T). To inhibit non-specific binding 200 µl blocking buffer (PBS-T with 5% milk powder) per well was added and incubated for 2 h at 37°C. Human sera were diluted 1:200 and allowed to react with the antigen-coated wells for 1 h at 37°C. Plates were washed 3x with 800 µl PBS-T and a HRPO-conjugated, secondary rabbit anti-human IgG antibody (Dianova, Hamburg, Germany), diluted 1:10,000, was added to detect IgG antibodies. After an additional washing step (3x with 800 µl PBS-T), peroxidase substrate TMB (tetramethylbenzidene, Taastrup, Denmark) was added for 10 min at room temperature in the dark. The reactions were stopped with 2 N H_2SO_4. Optical density was measured on a microplate spectrometer (BMG Labtech, Offenburg, Germany) at $\lambda = 450$ nm. All blank wells had absorbance values <0.1. The data were analyzed with the $X2$-test to estimate significance of differences among independent groups of individuals. For each ELISA plate, a fixed set of sera was used to control for interserial

Table 1. Detection of polyomaviruses in gastrointestinal and lymphoid organs with generic PCR.

Sample type	Source	No. of samples tested	Polyomaviruses[a] (no. of specimens)
Gastro-intestinal tract	Patients with malignant diseases	159	
Liver		124	HPyV12 (4), MCPyV (3)
Gall bladder		21	(0)
Esophagus		2	(0)
Stomach (Cardia)		2	(0)
Colon		4	(0)
Rectum		6	(0)
Spleen	Donors for transplantation	61	MCPyV (3)
Lymph node	Donors for transplantation	22	MCPyV (2), TSPyV (1)
Σ		242	(13)

[a]Detected with generic PCR.

variations. The cut-off value (COV) for the ELISA was determined experimentally. The background reactivities detected in wells without antigen coating and those without both antigen and serum (blanks) were subtracted from the ODs measured in VP1-coated wells. The COV defining a positive serologic response was defined as the mean of all negative ODs plus standard deviation (COV HPyV12: $OD_{450} = 0.086$). To further ensure that the final OD_{450} values for HPyV12 VP1 were not in part derived from unspecific antibody binding, reactivity of the sera to VP1 of an avian polyomavirus (APyV) was measured (Mean $OD_{450} = 0.07$), and the values obtained for each serum were subtracted from the ODs measured for HPyV12 VP1.

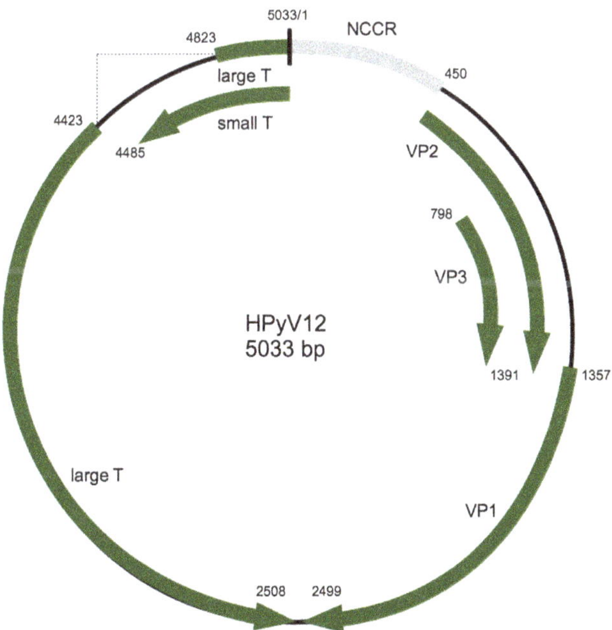

Figure 1. Genome organization of HPyV12. Putative coding regions for VP1 to VP3, STAg antigen, and LTAg antigen are marked by arrows.

Nucleotides sequence accession numbers

The annotated, complete genome sequence of HPyV12 has been submitted to GenBank (accession number JX308829). The Genbank accession numbers of PyV genomes that were used in phylogenetic analysis are listed in Table S3.

Results

Identification of HPyV12 and complete genome sequencing

Organs of the gastrointestinal tract (liver, gall bladder, esophagus, stomach, colon, rectum; n = 159) as well as spleen (n = 61) and lymph node (n = 22) specimens were tested with generic polyomavirus PCR targeting the VP1 gene (Table 1). In 13/242 PCR assays, fragments of the expected size were obtained, purified and sequenced. BLAST analysis [38] revealed that 8 of the 13 sequences originated from MCPyV (detected in 3 livers, 3 spleens, and 2 lymph nodes) and 1 from TSPyV (detected in a lymph node). Most importantly, an unknown polyomavirus sequence was amplified from liver specimens of 4 individuals, revealing a relatively low level of identity to all human and nonhuman polyomaviruses (pairwise amino acid identities: 51–67%). The complete genome sequence was then generated from a liver specimen with VP3/VP1-PCR and LD-PCR as described in the *Methods* section. After sequencing all products, a final circular genome of 5033 bp was obtained. Since 11 phylogenetically distinct polyomaviruses of human origin are known at present, the virus from which the sequence originated was tentatively named Human Polyomavirus 12 (HPyV12).

Analysis of the HPyV12 genome

Analysis of the HPyV12 genome for putative open reading frames (ORFs) revealed a genome structure typical for polyomaviruses. It includes an early region encoding regulatory proteins (STAg and LTAg) and a late region encoding structural proteins (VP1, VP2 and VP3) that are separated by a non-coding control region (NCCR) (Figure 1). An ORF encoding for the auxiliary agnoprotein [39] was not identified. The ORF locations on the viral genome, the encoded proteins and their percentages of identity to other human polyomaviruses are listed in Table 2.

HPyV12 LTAg and STAg share 71 amino acid residues that are encoded at the N-terminus. This region contains the DnaJ domain HPDKGG which is fully conserved between all known human

Table 2. Putative proteins encoded by HPyV12 and amino acid identities between HPyV12 and other polyomaviruses.

			Amino acid sequence identity (%)[a]						
Protein	Putative coding region	Amino acids[b]	TSPyV[c]	MCPyV	BKPyV	HPyV9	BatPyV	OraPyV	GHPyV
VP1	1357:2499	380	60	57	54	59	61	63	62
VP2	450:1391	313	42	31	31	36	36	42	35
VP3	798:1391	197	40	24	28	37	37	38	32
ST Ag	5033–4485	182	30	34	30	33	29	30	26
LTAg exon 1	5033–4823	708	46	52	38	41	39	46	31
LTAg exon 2	4423–2508								

[a]Determined with blastX (pairwise).
[b]Number of amino acids.
[c]Accession numbers for TSPyV to GHPyV: GU989205; HM355825; NC_001538; NC_015150; JQ958892; FN356901; NC_004800.

polyomaviruses identified so far [40]. However, HPyV12 LTAg lacks the retinoblastoma binding motif LxCxE which is present in LTAg sequences of all known human polyomaviruses. There is a putative ATPase domain in the C-terminal part of the protein. This domain consists of the conserved GPxxxGKT (GPINSGKT; residues 498–505 in HPyV12 LTAg) and GxxxVNLE (GSVTVNLE; residues 576–583 in HPyV12 LTAg). HPyV12 LTAg also has a Lys-rich sequence (PKSKKAK; residues 205–211) which may act as a nuclear localization signal. A Cys-rich sequence ($Cx_7CxCX_2Cx_{22}CxCx_2Cx_3WFG$) which has been shown to be required for binding of protein phosphatase PP2A by STAgs of other polyomaviruses, is conserved in HPyV12 STAg

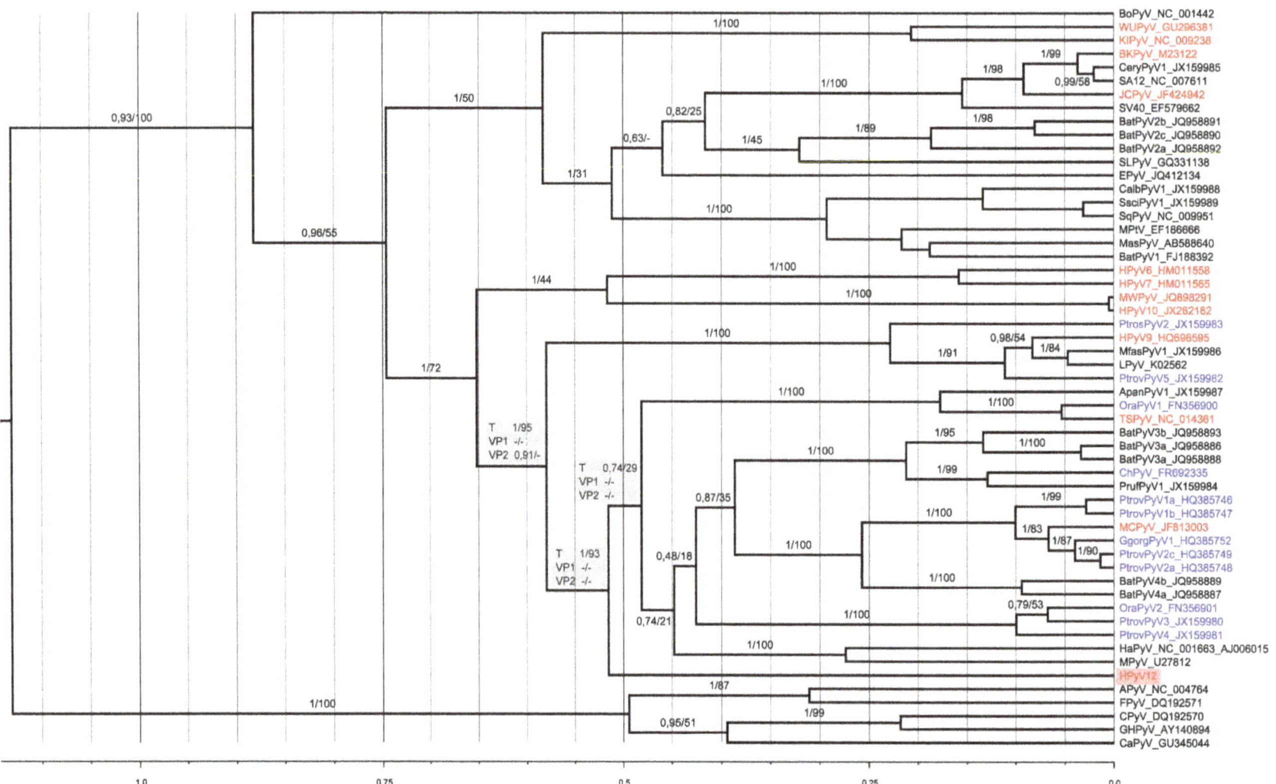

Figure 2. Phylogenetic analysis of HPyV12. A Bayesian chronogram was deduced from the analysis of a 488 amino acid alignment of LTAg sequences. Polyomaviruses identified from human hosts are in red, from apes in blue. The human polyomaviruses MXPyV and the US strain of MWPyV have the same phylogenetic position as HPyV10 and are not shown. The sequence of the very recently discovered human STLPyV which is most closely related to HPyV10, MWPyV and MXPyV, became only available at the end of the revision process of this manuscript; it was therefore not included in the datasets put together for the present study. Statistical support for branches is given as posterior probability/bootstrap. For three branches defining potentially meaningful bipartitions (with respect to the question of the phylogenetic placement of HPyV12), statistical support observed for the corresponding bipartitions in the VP2 and VP1 analyses is also shown (grey panels). Hyphen indicates that bipartition was not observed in the ML or Bayesian tree. The scale axis is in amino acid substitution per site. This chronogram was rooted using a relaxed clock. A maximum likelihood analysis of the same dataset concluded to a similar topology and is thus not shown here.

Table 3. Detection of HPyV12 with PCR.

Sample type	Source(s)	No. of samples tested	No. of samples PCR-positive for HPyV12[e]
Gastro-intestinal tract	Patients with malignant diseases	159	16
Liver		124	14
Gall bladder		21	0
Esophagus		2	0
Stomach (Cardia)		2	0
Colon		4	1
Rectum		6	1
Lymph node	Donors for transplantation	22	0
Spleen	Donors for transplantation	61	0
Feces	Patients with diarrhea	56	1
Plasma	Kidney transplant recipients[a]	54	0
Serum	Liver transplant recipients	45	0
Urine	Kidney transplant recipients[a]	12	0
	Stem cell transplant recipients[a]	14	0
	Patients with multiple sclerosis[b]	9	0
	Immunocompromised patients with malignant disease[a]	76	0
	Other[a]	41	0
Oral fluid	From measles diagnostics	30	0
Bronchoalveolar lavage fluid	Patients with pneumonia[c]	22	0
Cerebrospinal fluid	Patients with leukoencephalopathy[d]	35	0
Σ		636	17

[a]Samples collected for BKPyV infection diagnosis.
[b]From patients under natalizumab (Tysabri) therapy.
[c]Samples collected for herpesvirus infection diagnosis.
[d]Samples collected for JCPyV infection diagnosis.
[e]Combined results of specific nested PCR and real-time PCR; samples were considered as positive if the result could be independently reproduced on different days.

(residues 100–147). The NCCR contains 4 repeats of the putative GAGGC LTAg binding site and AT-rich palindromic sequences. The NCCR possesses potential binding sites for numerous cellular transcription factors, but the functional importance of these sites remains to be proven (Figure S4).

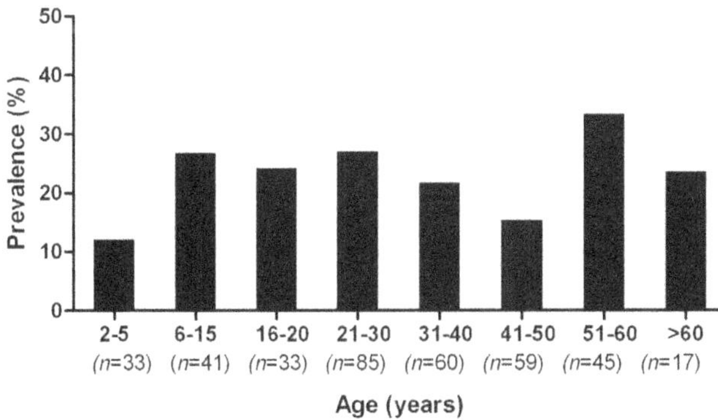

Figure 3. Reactivity of human sera to VP1 of HPyV12. The percentage of seroreactivity of pediatric sera (n = 74; 2–11 years) and sera of healthy adolescents and adults (n = 299; age: 16–72 years) in ELISA is shown. The results were stratified by age.

Phylogenetic analysis of HPyV12

Three alignments consisting of 98, 259, and 488 amino acids were generated from HPyV12 VP2, VP1 and LTAg sequences, respectively, and those of other polyomaviruses for which complete genomes were available (Table S3). On this basis, ML and Bayesian analyses of the individual coding sequences were performed. Only the analyses of LTAg sequences did support a clear placement of HPyV12, which was neither contradicted nor supported by VP2 and VP1 analyses (Figure 2). In the LTAg phylogeny, HPyV12 appeared as the earliest offshoot of a large clade comprising (by decreasing order of frequency) ape, bat, monkey, rodent and human PyVs (i.e., MCPyV and TSPyV). The branching order of the main lineages comprised within this clade could not be determined as most internal branches only received moderate statistical support. On the other hand, the clade comprising HPyV12 appeared quite clearly as the sister clade to a group of primate polyomaviruses including HPyV9.

Prevalence of HPyV12 in clinical samples

The 242 samples from gastrointestinal organs, spleens and lymph nodes were re-evaluated with diagnostic nested PCR and qPCR. The presence of HPyV12 sequences was confirmed in the samples that were originally HPyV12-positive in the initial generic PCR. In addition, 10 liver samples tested positive that had been negative in the generic PCR. In total, 14/124 liver samples (11%) were HPyV12-positive (Table 3). One positive sample each was also identified among rectum (n = 6) and colon (n = 4) samples. Analysis of gall bladder (n = 21), esophagus and stomach (cardia) (each n = 2) yielded negative results (Table 3). Spleens (n = 61) and lymph nodes (n = 22) were also HPyV12-negative (Table 3). To further elucidate the prevalence of HPyV12, body fluids and excretions were analyzed. Testing of feces (n = 56) revealed one HPyV12-positive sample. Plasma (n = 54), serum (n = 45), urine (n = 152), oral fluids (n = 30), bronchoalveolar lavage fluids (n = 22) and cerebrospinal fluids (n = 35) were negative (Table 3). In qPCR, the HPyV12-positive DNA samples revealed genome copy numbers of up to 133/PCR reaction (equivalent to 27 copies/µl DNA from fluid samples; 532 copies/ µg DNA from tissue samples). In summary, analysis of 636 clinical samples revealed the presence of HPyV12 only in organs of the gastrointestinal tract and in feces.

Seroprevalence of HPyV12

To detect antibodies against HPyV12 VP1, a capsomer-based ELISA was performed. A pediatric population of 74 subjects and 299 healthy adults and adolescents were tested, and the data were stratified by age. The seroprevalence of HPyV12 was 12% in children of age 2–5 and rose to 26% in the group of age 6–11. In young adults of age 21–30, a prevalence of 27% was determined. In older adults the prevalence ranged between 15% and 33% (Figure 3). A difference in HPyV12 seroprevalence between male and female adults was not observed (data not shown).

Discussion

The present study reports on the discovery of a hitherto unknown polyomavirus (HPyV12) in humans. The novel polyomavirus was detected by generic PCR, real-time PCR and conventional nested PCR in liver specimens of 14 individuals as well as in the colon, rectum and feces of single individuals (Tables 1 and 2). To study the seroprevalence of HPyV12, ELISA was performed that was considered to specifically detect VP1 antibodies against HPyV12. The assay revealed that healthy individuals are frequently infected with HPyV12 before the age of twenty (Figure 3). We believe that cross-reaction with antibodies raised against other known human polyomaviruses is unlikely to explain these results as none of their VP1 proteins displays more than 60% identity to HPyV12 VP1. Cross-reactions of VP1 proteins in serological assays have only been observed when the proteins revealed more than 75% identity [2,4,5,11,41], and no cross-reactivity between VP1 antibodies from the known human polyomaviruses has been detected [2,4,5,11,41–44]. We cannot, however, exclude cross-reactivity between HPyV12 VP1 and antibodies directed against not yet identified human polyomaviruses. The seroprevalence reported here should therefore be regarded as a first estimate. Taken together, HPyV12 can be regarded as a virus that naturally infects humans at young age and resides in the gastrointestinal tract.

It is remarkable that - besides the novel HPyV12 - only MCPyV was detected in liver and other organs of the gastrointestinal tract. It is unlikely that this would be the result of a failure of the applied PCR system to detect other polyomaviruses since this system allowed for the recovery of a number of polyomaviruses across the entire phylogeny [11,32]. Therefore, this may indicate that the other human polyomaviruses were at least not present in high copy numbers in the gastrointestinal tract. The multiple detection of MCPyV in livers is in line with a previous study that reported detection of MCPyV in livers and other sites of the gastrointestinal tract [25]. Since liver specimens were highly overrepresented in our panel of gastrointestinal tract specimens (124/159), it could be concluded that polyomaviruses other than HPyV12 and MCPyV do not reside regularly in the liver. A prediction on the other organs of the gastrointestinal tract studied here (gall bladder, stomach, colon, rectum) was not possible since sample numbers were too small. A similarly low abundance of polyomaviruses was observed in lymphoid organs (Table 1). This is in contrast to the frequent presence of polyomaviruses in lymphoid organs of the closest relative of humans, the chimpanzee [32], and indicates a major difference in polyomavirus tropism between these closely related hominine hosts.

Human polyomaviruses, such as BKPyV and JCPyV, induce tumors in animal models. However, their role in human cancer remains a matter of debate [45-47]. The recently identified MCPyV is the first polyomavirus that is etiologically associated with a human tumor [8,19,48]. It is noteworthy that HPyV12 is the first human polyomavirus whose LTAg lacks any LxCxE motif. As this motif is essential to the retinoblastoma protein-dependent transforming activity of other polyomaviruses, HPyV12 may exhibit a reduced transforming potential. It is clear that, in addition to continued efforts aimed at completing our view of the diversity of the human polyomavirome, efforts should also be made to characterize the biology and the possible impact on human health of novel human polyomaviruses.

Acknowledgments

The authors are grateful for the excellent technical assistance by Sonja Liebmann, Cornelia Walter and Nezlisah Yasmum. The supply of clinical samples by Annette Mankertz, Marina Höhne, and Joachim Kühn is kindly acknowledged.

Author Contributions

Conceived and designed the experiments: SK JR SCS FT JH IS SV RS UM BE. Performed the experiments: SK JR SCS FT JH SV RS. Analyzed the data: SK JR SCS FT JH UM IS SV RS BE. Contributed reagents/materials/analysis tools: JH SV RS BE. Wrote the paper: SK JR SCS FT JH UM SV RS BE.

References

1. Imperiale MJ, Major EO (2007) Polyomaviruses. In: Knipe DM, Howley PM, Griffin DE, Lamb RA, Martin MA et al., editors. Fields Virology. .Philadelphia: Lippincott Williams and Wilkins. pp. 2263–2298.
2. Kean JM, Rao S, Wang M, Garcea RL (2009) Seroepidemiology of human polyomaviruses. PLoS Pathog 5: e1000363.
3. Knowles WA, Pipkin P, Andrews N, Vyse A, Minor P, et al. (2003) Population-based study of antibody to the human polyomaviruses BKV and JCV and the simian polyomavirus SV40. J Med Virol 71: 115–123.
4. Stolt A, Sasnauskas K, Koskela P, Lehtinen M, Dillner J (2003) Seroepidemiology of the human polyomaviruses. J Gen Virol 84: 1499–1504.
5. Viscidi RP, Rollison DE, Sondak VK, Silver B, Messina JL, et al. (2011) Age-specific seroprevalence of Merkel cell polyomavirus, BK virus, and JC virus. Clin Vaccine Immunol 18: 1737–1743.
6. Jiang M, Abend JR, Johnson SF, Imperiale MJ (2009) The role of polyomaviruses in human disease. Virology 384: 266–273.
7. Imperiale MJ (2000) The human polyomaviruses, BKV and JCV: molecular pathogenesis of acute disease and potential role in cancer. Virology 267: 1–7.
8. Feng H, Shuda M, Chang Y, Moore PS (2008) Clonal integration of a polyomavirus in human Merkel cell carcinoma. Science 319: 1096–1100.
9. van der Meijden E, Janssens RW, Lauber C, Bouwes Bavinck JN, Gorbalenya AE, et al. (2010) Discovery of a new human polyomavirus associated with trichodysplasia spinulosa in an immunocompromized patient. PLoS Pathog 6: e1001024.
10. Siebrasse EA, Reyes A, Lim ES, Zhao G, Mkakosya RS, et al. (2012) Identification of MW polyomavirus, a novel polyomavirus in human stool. J Virol 86: 10321–10326.
11. Scuda N, Hofmann J, Calvignac-Spencer S, Ruprecht K, Liman P, et al. (2011) A novel human polyomavirus closely related to the african green monkey-derived lymphotropic polyomavirus. J Virol 85: 4586–4590.
12. Schowalter RM, Pastrana DV, Pumphrey KA, Moyer AL, Buck CB (2010) Merkel cell polyomavirus and two previously unknown polyomaviruses are chronically shed from human skin. Cell Host Microbe 7: 509–515.
13. Gaynor AM, Nissen MD, Whiley DM, Mackay IM, Lambert SB, et al. (2007) Identification of a novel polyomavirus from patients with acute respiratory tract infections. PLoS Pathog 3: e64.
14. Allander T, Andreasson K, Gupta S, Bjerkner A, Bogdanovic G, et al. (2007) Identification of a third human polyomavirus. J Virol 81: 4130–4136.
15. Buck CB, Phan GQ, Raiji MT, Murphy PM, McDermott DH, et al. (2012) Complete genome sequence of a tenth human polyomavirus. J Virol 86: 10887.
16. Yu G, Greninger AL, Isa P, Phan TG, Martinez MA, et al. (2012) Discovery of a Novel Polyomavirus in Acute Diarrheal Samples from Children. PLoS One 7: e49449.
17. Lim ES, Reyes A, Antonio M, Saha D, Ikumapayi UN, et al. (2012) Discovery of STL polyomavirus, a polyomavirus of ancestral recombinant origin that encodes a unique T antigen by alternative splicing. Virology.
18. Foulongne V, Sauvage V, Hebert C, Dereure O, Cheval J, et al. (2012) Human skin microbiota: high diversity of DNA viruses identified on the human skin by high throughput sequencing. PLoS One 7: e38499.
19. Moens U, Ludvigsen M, Van Ghelue M (2011) Human polyomaviruses in skin diseases. Patholog Res Int 2011: 123491.
20. Gardner SD, Field AM, Coleman DV, Hulme B (1971) New human papovavirus (B.K.) isolated from urine after renal transplantation. Lancet 1: 1253–1257.
21. Babakir-Mina M, Ciccozzi M, Alteri C, Polchi P, Picardi A, et al. (2009) Excretion of the novel polyomaviruses KI and WU in the stool of patients with hematological disorders. J Med Virol 81: 1668–1673.
22. Bergallo M, Terlizzi ME, Astegiano S, Ciotti M, Babakir-Mina M, et al. (2009) Real time PCR TaqMan assays for detection of polyomaviruses KIV and WUV in clinical samples. J Virol Methods 162: 69–74.
23. Bialasiewicz S, Whiley DM, Lambert SB, Nissen MD, Sloots TP (2009) Detection of BK, JC, WU, or KI polyomaviruses in faecal, urine, blood, cerebrospinal fluid and respiratory samples. J Clin Virol 45: 249–254.
24. Bofill-Mas S, Formiga-Cruz M, Clemente-Casares P, Calafell F, Girones R (2001) Potential transmission of human polyomaviruses through the gastrointestinal tract after exposure to virions or viral DNA. J Virol 75: 10290–10299.
25. Loyo M, Guerrero-Preston R, Brait M, Hoque MO, Chuang A, et al. (2010) Quantitative detection of Merkel cell virus in human tissues and possible mode of transmission. Int J Cancer 126: 2991–2996.
26. Neske F, Blessing K, Prottel A, Ullrich F, Kreth HW, et al. (2009) Detection of WU polyomavirus DNA by real-time PCR in nasopharyngeal aspirates, serum, and stool samples. J Clin Virol 44: 115–118.
27. Ren L, Gonzalez R, Xu X, Li J, Zhang J, et al. (2009) WU polyomavirus in fecal specimens of children with acute gastroenteritis, China. Emerg Infect Dis 15: 134–135.
28. Ricciardiello L, Laghi L, Ramamirtham P, Chang CL, Chang DK, et al. (2000) JC virus DNA sequences are frequently present in the human upper and lower gastrointestinal tract. Gastroenterology 119: 1228–1235.
29. Vanchiere JA, Nicome RK, Greer JM, Demmler GJ, Butel JS (2005) Frequent detection of polyomaviruses in stool samples from hospitalized children. J Infect Dis 192: 658–664.
30. Toracchio S, Foyle A, Sroller V, Reed JA, Wu J, et al. (2010) Lymphotropism of Merkel cell polyomavirus infection, Nova Scotia, Canada. Emerg Infect Dis 16: 1702–1709.
31. Tan CS, Ellis LC, Wuthrich C, Ngo L, Broge TA, Jr., et al. (2010) JC virus latency in the brain and extraneural organs of patients with and without progressive multifocal leukoencephalopathy. J Virol 84: 9200–9209.
32. Leendertz FH, Scuda N, Cameron KN, Kidega T, Zuberbuhler K, et al. (2011) African great apes are naturally infected with polyomaviruses closely related to Merkel cell polyomavirus. J Virol 85: 916–924.
33. Trusch F, Klein M, Finsterbusch T, Kuhn J, Hofmann J, et al. (2012) Seroprevalence of human polyomavirus 9 and cross-reactivity to African green monkey-derived lymphotropic polyomavirus. J Gen Virol 93: 698–705.
34. Messeguer X, Escudero R, Farre D, Nunez O, Martinez J, et al. (2002) PROMO: detection of known transcription regulatory elements using species-tailored searches. Bioinformatics 18: 333–334.
35. Farre D, Roset R, Huerta M, Adsuara JE, Rosello L, et al. (2003) Identification of patterns in biological sequences at the ALGGEN server: PROMO and MALGEN. Nucleic Acids Res 31: 3651–3653.
36. Rice P, Longden I, Bleasby A (2000) EMBOSS: the European Molecular Biology Open Software Suite. Trends Genet 16: 276–277.
37. Johne R, Buck CB, Allander T, Atwood WJ, Garcea RL, et al. (2011) Taxonomical developments in the family Polyomaviridae. Arch Virol 156: 1627–1634.
38. Altschul SF, Gish W, Miller W, Myers EW, Lipman DJ (1990) Basic local alignment search tool. J Mol Biol 215: 403–410.
39. Gerits N, Moens U (2012) Agnoprotein of mammalian polyomaviruses. Virology 432: 316–326.
40. Van Ghelue M, Khan MT, Ehlers B, Moens U (2012) Genome analysis of the new human polyomaviruses. Rev Med Virol 22: 354–377.
41. Chen T, Mattila PS, Jartti T, Ruuskanen O, Soderlund-Venermo M, et al. (2011) Seroepidemiology of the newly found trichodysplasia spinulosa-associated polyomavirus. J Infect Dis 204: 1523–1526.
42. Viscidi RP, Clayman B (2006) Serological cross reactivity between polyomavirus capsids. Adv Exp Med Biol 577: 73–84.
43. Touze A, Gaitan J, Arnold F, Cazal R, Fleury MJ, et al. (2010) Generation of Merkel cell polyomavirus (MCV)-like particles and their application to detection of MCV antibodies. J Clin Microbiol 48: 1767–1770.
44. Tolstov YL, Pastrana DV, Feng H, Becker JC, Jenkins FJ, et al. (2009) Human Merkel cell polyomavirus infection II. MCV is a common human infection that can be detected by conformational capsid epitope immunoassays. Int J Cancer 125: 1250–1256.
45. Abend JR, Jiang M, Imperiale MJ (2009) BK virus and human cancer: innocent until proven guilty. Semin Cancer Biol 19: 252–260.
46. Maginnis MS, Atwood WJ (2009) JC virus: an oncogenic virus in animals and humans? Semin Cancer Biol 19: 261–269.
47. Moens U, Johannessen M (2008) Human polyomaviruses and cancer: expanding repertoire. J Dtsch Dermatol Ges 6: 704–708.
48. Donepudi S, DeConti RC, Samlowski WE (2012) Recent advances in the understanding of the genetics, etiology, and treatment of Merkel cell carcinoma. Semin Oncol 39: 163–172.

12

Molecular Epidemiology and Disease Severity of Human Respiratory Syncytial Virus in Vietnam

Dinh Nguyen Tran[1,2,3], Thi Minh Hong Pham[2], Manh Tuan Ha[3], Thi Thu Loan Tran[3], Thi Kim Huyen Dang[3], Lay-Myint Yoshida[4], Shoko Okitsu[1,5], Satoshi Hayakawa[5], Masashi Mizuguchi[1], Hiroshi Ushijima[1,5]*

1 Department of Developmental Medical Sciences, School of International Health, Graduate School of Medicine, The University of Tokyo, Tokyo, Japan, **2** Department of Pediatrics, University of Medicine and Pharmacy at Ho Chi Minh City, Ho Chi Minh City, Vietnam, **3** Children's Hospital 2, Ho Chi Minh City, Vietnam, **4** Institute of Tropical Medicine, Nagasaki University, Nagasaki, Japan, **5** Division of Microbiology, Department of Pathology and Microbiology, Nihon University, School of Medicine, Tokyo, Japan

Abstract

Respiratory syncytial virus (RSV) is a major cause of acute respiratory infections (ARIs) in children worldwide and can cause high mortality, especially in developing countries. However, information on the clinical and molecular characteristics of RSV infection in developing countries is limited. From April 2010 to May 2011, 1,082 nasopharyngeal swabs were collected from children with ARI admitted to the Children's Hospital 2, Ho Chi Minh City, Vietnam. Samples were screened for RSV and genotyped by reverse transcription-PCR and sequencing. Demographic and clinical data was also recorded. RSV was found in 23.8% (257/1,082) of samples. RSV A was the dominant subgroup, accounting for 91.4% (235/257), followed by RSV B, 5.1% (13/257), and 9 cases (3.5%) were mixed infection of these subgroups. The phylogenetic analysis revealed that all group A strains belonged to the GA2 genotype. All group B strains belonged to the recently identified BA genotype, and further clustered into 2 recently described subgenotypes BA9 and BA10. One GA2 genotype strain had a premature stop codon which shortened the G protein length. RSV infection was significantly associated with younger age and higher severity score than those without. Co-infection with other viruses did not affect disease severity. RSV A caused more severe disease than RSV B. The results from this study will not only contribute to the growing database on the molecular diversity of RSV circulating worldwide but may be also useful in clinical management and vaccine development.

Editor: Steven M. Varga, University of Iowa, United States of America

Funding: This study was supported by Grants-in-Aid from the Ministry of Education and Sciences and the Ministry of Health, Labor and Welfare, Japan. The funders had no role in study design, data collection and analysis, decision to publish, or preparation of the manuscript.

Competing Interests: The authors have declared that no competing interests exist.

* E-mail: ushijima-hiroshi@jcom.home.ne.jp

Introduction

Respiratory syncytial virus (RSV) is the major cause of acute respiratory infections (ARIs) among infants and young children worldwide [1]. The clinical presentations can vary from mild upper respiratory tract infections (URTIs) to life threatening bronchiolitis and pneumonia which result in significant pediatric hospitalization and economic burden [2]. Primary RSV infections occur during the first year of life in more than 50% of infants, and by 2 years of age, almost all children have been infected at least once [3]. RSV can cause re-infections throughout life with milder disease, indicating that either RSV infection induces an inadequate immune response or genetic variability of RSV is extensive [4]. RSV is a negative-sense single-stranded RNA virus that belongs to the *Paramyxoviridae* family. RSV is divided into two major groups, A and B, initially based on the reaction of the virus with monoclonal antibodies against the major structural glycoproteins G and F [5] and later by genetic analysis [6]. Each group can be further subdivided into genotypes by nucleotide sequence variability. The attachment glycoprotein G is the most divergent viral protein, both between and within the two groups, and a major target for neutralizing and protective antibody responses [7].

Along with the F protein, the second variable region at the C-terminal of the G protein that contains much of the G gene variability is commonly used in molecular epidemiological studies [8]. So far, RSV group A is divided into 8 genotypes (GA1 to GA7, and SAA1), and so is RSV group B (GB1 to GB4, SAB1 to SAB3, and BA) [9]. BA, which was first isolated in Buenos Aires in 1999, is a new genotype of group B with a 60-nucleotide duplication in the second variable region of the G protein gene [10]. The two groups circulate independently, but often at the same time, although group A viruses tend to predominate [3,11]. The presence of two groups has led to the speculation that there might be a relationship between the RSV-group infections and clinical severity. A number of studies were carried out but such a relationship has not been fully elucidated [12].

Although RSV has been recognized as an important pathogen in childhood, there is no published information regarding the molecular epidemiology and clinical characteristics of RSV infections in Vietnam. The aims of this study were to investigate the molecular epidemiology of RSV infections, as well as to compare the clinical characteristics of diseases caused by group A and B strains in hospitalized children in Ho Chi Minh City, Vietnam.

Materials and Methods

Patients and samples

The study was conducted from April 2010 to May 2011 at the Respiratory Ward, the Children's Hospital 2, in Ho Chi Minh City, Vietnam. The Children's Hospital 2 is a 1,000-bed tertiary referral and university-affiliated hospital, receiving pediatric patients from most parts of the city as well as other provinces in the south of Vietnam. This area has a tropical climate with two distinct seasons: rainy season (May–October) and dry season (November–April). The daily temperature does not change much during the year conducting this study.

Under 15-year-old children admitted for an ARI condition with an onset of illness less than 7 days were enrolled. The study was approved by the Scientific and Ethical Committee of the Children's Hospital 2. The written consent was obtained from the parent or legal guardian of the participants. An ARI case was defined as any child presenting with cough and/or difficult breathing [13]. Patients who had underlying chronic diseases (e.g. cystic fibrosis, bronchopulmonary dysplasia, congenital heart disease, immunodeficiency) or who were discharged from the hospital within the previous 7 days, or who had coexisting acute systemic illnesses (e.g. sepsis), or proven or suspected non-infectious respiratory symptoms (e.g. asthma), were all excluded from the study.

Demographic and clinical data were recorded on a standardized questionnaire. The diagnosis was made on the basis of clinical findings and chest X-ray (CXR). ARI patients with the presence of an infiltrate on CXR were categorized as pneumonia. Bronchiolitis was defined as ARI patient under 2 years old presenting with wheezing and hyperaeration, atelectasis, or peribronchial thickening on CXR. Croup was characterized by hoarseness, cough, and stridor. URTI was defined as ARI with no abnormalities on CXR. The disease severity was assessed by using the previously published severity score [14,15].

Nasopharyngeal flocked swabs (MicroRheologics, Brescia, Italy) were obtained by trained personnel on 2 fixed days each week from all enrolled children within 24 hr after admission. The specimens were immediately placed in tubes containing 2 ml sterile physiological saline fluid and stored at −20°C until further analysis at the laboratory.

Virus detection

Viral genomes were extracted directly from the specimens by using the QIAamp Viral RNA Mini Kit (Qiagen, Hilden, Germany) according to the manufacturer's instructions and stored at −80°C.

All specimens were screened for RSV and other respiratory viruses such as influenza virus A and B, human metapneumovirus, parainfluenza virus types 1 to 4, human rhinoviruses (HRV), human coronaviruses (229E and OC43), adenovirus and human bocavirus by using multiplex hemi-nested (RT)-PCR as described previously [16]. The detection primers were targeted to the conserved region of nucleoprotein gene of RSV.

Genotyping of RSV

All samples positive for RSV by screening test were then subjected to grouping and genotyping by a hemi-nested PCR as described previously [8]. The second hypervariable region of the G protein gene of RSV was the target for the outer and inner PCRs. The final product sizes were possible for differentiating RSV group A, group B, and genotype BA with each other. The genotypes within each group were further identified by sequence analysis.

The products of nested PCR were sequenced bi-directionally by the commercial company (Macrogen Japan Corp., Tokyo, Japan). The nucleotide sequences were analyzed and compared with the reference strains available in the GenBank database. The sequence data and the phylogenesis were analyzed using BioEdit v.7.0.5 [17]. A parsimony analysis was also conducted using MEGA version 3.1 [18]. The method was performed using close-neighbor interchange with a random option and with 1,000 bootstrap repetitions.

The sequences of RSVs detected in this study have been submitted to GenBank and assigned accession numbers JX079948–JX079993.

Statistical analysis

Values were given as percentages for categorical variables, and as median with range for continuous variables. Categorical variables were compared by using χ^2 test or Fisher's exact test, and continuous variables were compared by using the Mann-Whitney *U* test. A two sided value of $p<0.05$ was considered statistically significant. All analyses were conducted using the Statistical Package for Social Sciences version 16.0 (SPSS, Inc., Chicago, IL, USA).

Results

From April 2010 to May 2011, 1,082 cases of ARI were enrolled in this study. The median age was 9 months (ranged from 0 to 161 months), 86% of patients were under 2 years old. The boy to girl ratio was 1.8:1, indicating that boys were more commonly affected than girls.

RSV detection and seasonal pattern

One or more respiratory viruses were identified in 63.8% (690/1,082) of patients, including 23.8% (257/1,082) that were positive for RSV. RSV was the second most common virus following HRV. Additionally, 23% (59/257) of all RSV positive samples contained at least one other respiratory virus. Co-infection between RSV and HRV was the most frequent (51 cases). RSV A was the dominant subgroup with 91.4% (235/257). RSV subgroup B had 5.1% (13/257). Interestingly, 9 cases (3.5%) contained both subgroup A and B RSV. The RSV epidemic occurred during the rainy season, from May to October (Figure 1).

Molecular epidemiology of RSV

Twenty-seven RSV A and 19 RSV B samples were selected randomly for sequencing. Twenty-seven of the group A strains clustered into one genotype, GA2 (Figure 2). Of these, 9 sequences were found only once. Of the remaining 18 sequences, 5 sequence groups were found, with 2 to 9 isolates per group. The rates of divergence between prototype strain A2 and the Vietnamese strains were 12.2% to 14% at the nucleotide level and 24.2% to 28.8% at the amino acid level. Differences of up to 3.2% at the nucleotide level and 7.6% at the amino acid level were observed among the group A Vietnamese strains. The nucleotide and amino acid distances between the Vietnamese strains and the GA2 reference strains were up to 9% and 21.2%, respectively. The G protein gene of one of these strains, 1310-HCM/05.11-A, was identical to three sequences in GenBank, from Brazil (EU625712-SPIAL 1401/2006), Thailand (FJ489656-1359/BKK/07), and Scotland (HQ731741-R9061/07-08).

All 19 of the group B strains belonged to the recently identified BA genotype, with a 60-nucleotide duplication in the second variable region of the G protein gene [10]. These BA genotype strains were further clustered into 2 recently described subgeno-

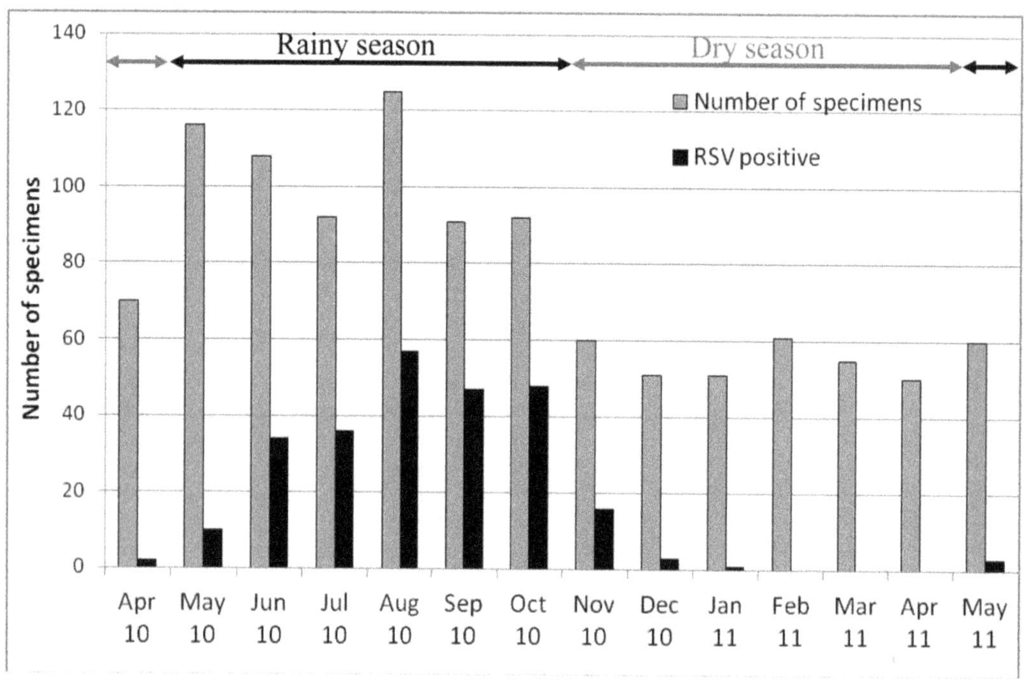

Figure 1. Monthly distribution of RSV infections from April 2010 to May 2011.

types BA9 and BA10 [19] (Figure 3). The nucleotide and amino acid variations among the Vietnamese BA genotype strains were up to 7% and 12.9%, respectively. There was 2.5% to 6% divergence at the nucleotide level and 4.8% to 11.3% divergence at the amino acid level between the Vietnamese strains and the prototype genotype BA. Regarding the BA9 subgenotype, differences of up to 6% at the nucleotide level and 8.1% at the amino acid level were observed when comparing Vietnamese strains with reference strains. The nucleotide and amino acid distances between Vietnamese BA10 strains and BA10 reference strains were up to 5.5% and 11.2%, respectively.

The deduced amino acid sequences of the group A and group B isolates were compared to those of the prototype A2 and BA strains, respectively (Figure 4). Twenty-seven of the Vietnamese group A viruses exhibited changes in the stop codon position compared with that of prototype strain A2, which had 298 amino acids in the deduced G-protein sequence. Among these, 26 Vietnamese group A strains had a predicted G protein of 297 amino acids, while 1 strain (763-HCM/09.10-A) had a premature stop codon that shortened the G polypeptide to 286 amino acids.

The G protein genes of the BA genotype were predicted to encode proteins of 2 different lengths, 312 (16/19 isolates) and 319 (3/19 isolates) amino acids. A serine (S) to proline (P) substitution was found within the 20-amino acid duplicated region at position 247 in all the Vietnamese BA strains. In addition, 14 of the 15 BA9 strains had a V271A substitution relative to the BA prototype strain, whereas all 4 BA10 strains had an E292G change. The majority (11/15) of the BA9 isolates also had amino acid substitutions at positions 270 (T270I) and 287 (H287Y).

The G protein is heavily glycosylated with both N-linked and O-linked sugars. Two putative N-glycosylation sites (NXT, where X is not proline) were identified in the second variable region of the G protein among the majority of the RSV A strains. The amino acid substitutions at some positions made these strains gain or lose the N-glycosylation sites. Similarly, two N-glycosylation sites were found to be conserved in all BA strains examined. Two of the BA10 isolates, 960-HCM/11.10-BA10 and 566-HCM/07.10-BA10, each acquired an additional N-glycosylation site as a result of amino acid substitutions at P231S and K258N, respectively.

Disease severity of RSV infections

To examine the disease severity in the RSV positive and negative groups, clinical and demographic data were compared (Table 1). With regard to age, RSV positive children were significantly younger than RSV negative ones (7 vs. 11 months, $p<0.001$). RSV positive patients were admitted to the hospital earlier in the course of their disease than RSV negative patients (2 vs. 3 days, $p=0.017$). They also had higher rates of fever (72.8 vs. 65.5%, $p=0.033$), runny nose (82.5 vs. 70.5%, $p<0.001$), and lower chest indrawing (68.5 vs. 51.0%, $p<0.001$). Most importantly, the clinical severity score of the RSV positive children was significantly higher (12 vs. 11, $p=0.003$) than the RSV negative group. Regarding the diagnosis, RSV positive patients were more likely to have bronchiolitis (47.1 vs. 28.8%, $p<0.001$).

To address the question of whether children with RSV co-infection have different characteristics to those with RSV mono-infection, attempts were made to compare these two groups (Table 1). However, differences were not statistically significant.

To assess the relationship between clinical severity and RSV subgroup, subjects that were co-infected with other viruses were excluded. The 177 cases with RSV A, 12 cases with RSV B, and 9 cases with mixed infection of both RSV A and B were compared (Table 1). No significant differences were found with respect to the presence of fever, cough, runny nose, tachypnea, lower chest indrawing, and hypoxemia among the three groups. However, both wheezing and the clinical severity scores were greater in patients with group A and mixed A and B infection than those with group B infection ($p<0.05$).

In multivariate analysis adjusted for age, sex, prematurity, malnutrition and infection with other viruses, the difference on days before hospitalization and on the clinical severity score

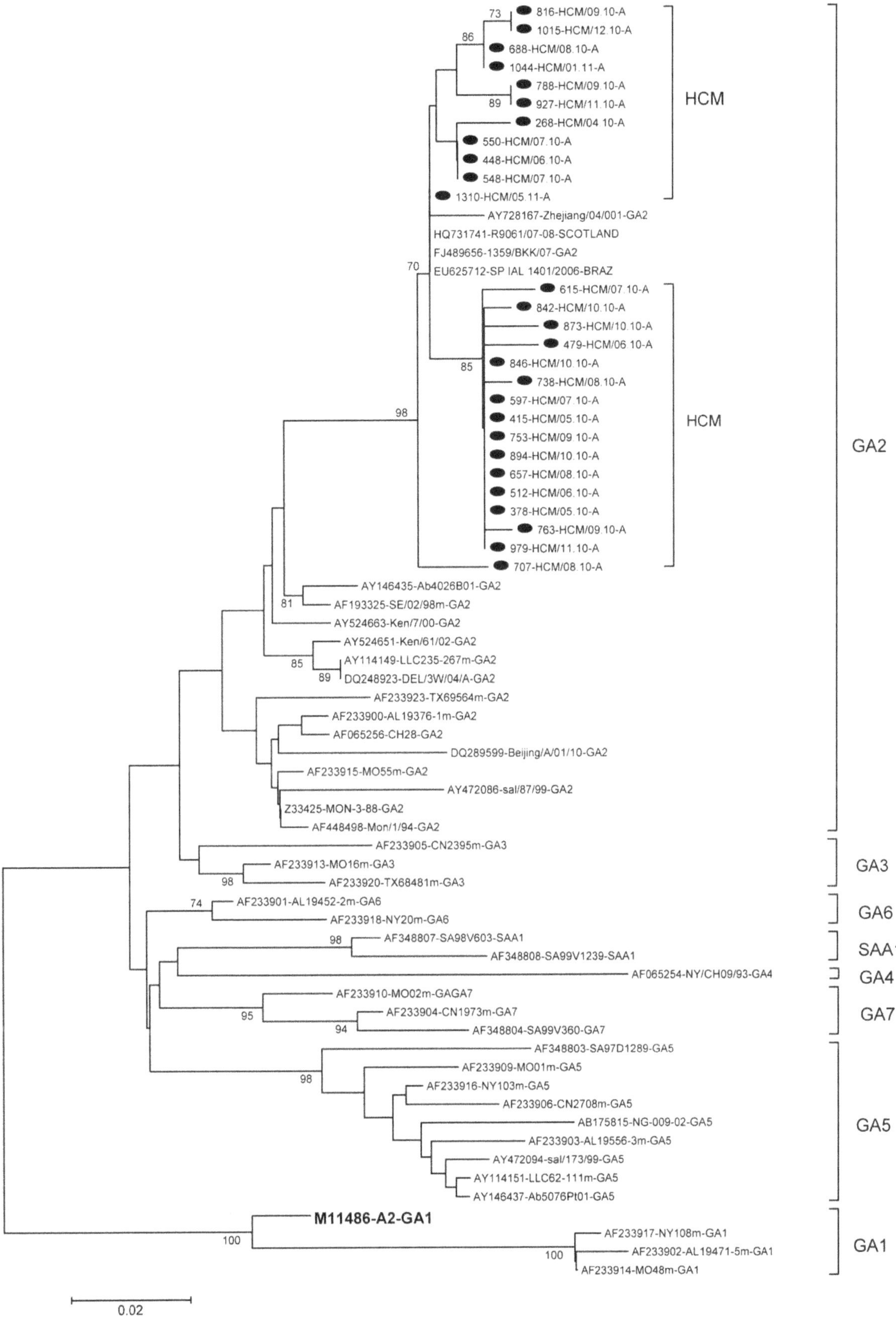

Figure 2. Phylogenetic tree for RSV-A nucleotide sequences based on 2nd variable region of G gene. Phylogenetic tree was constructed with MEGA 3.1 software using the neighbor-joining method. Bootstrap values of greater than 70% are shown at the branch nodes. The RSV strains in this study are marked with solid round. Prototype strain A2 (in bold face) for group A was also included. The genotype assignment is indicated by the brackets on the right.

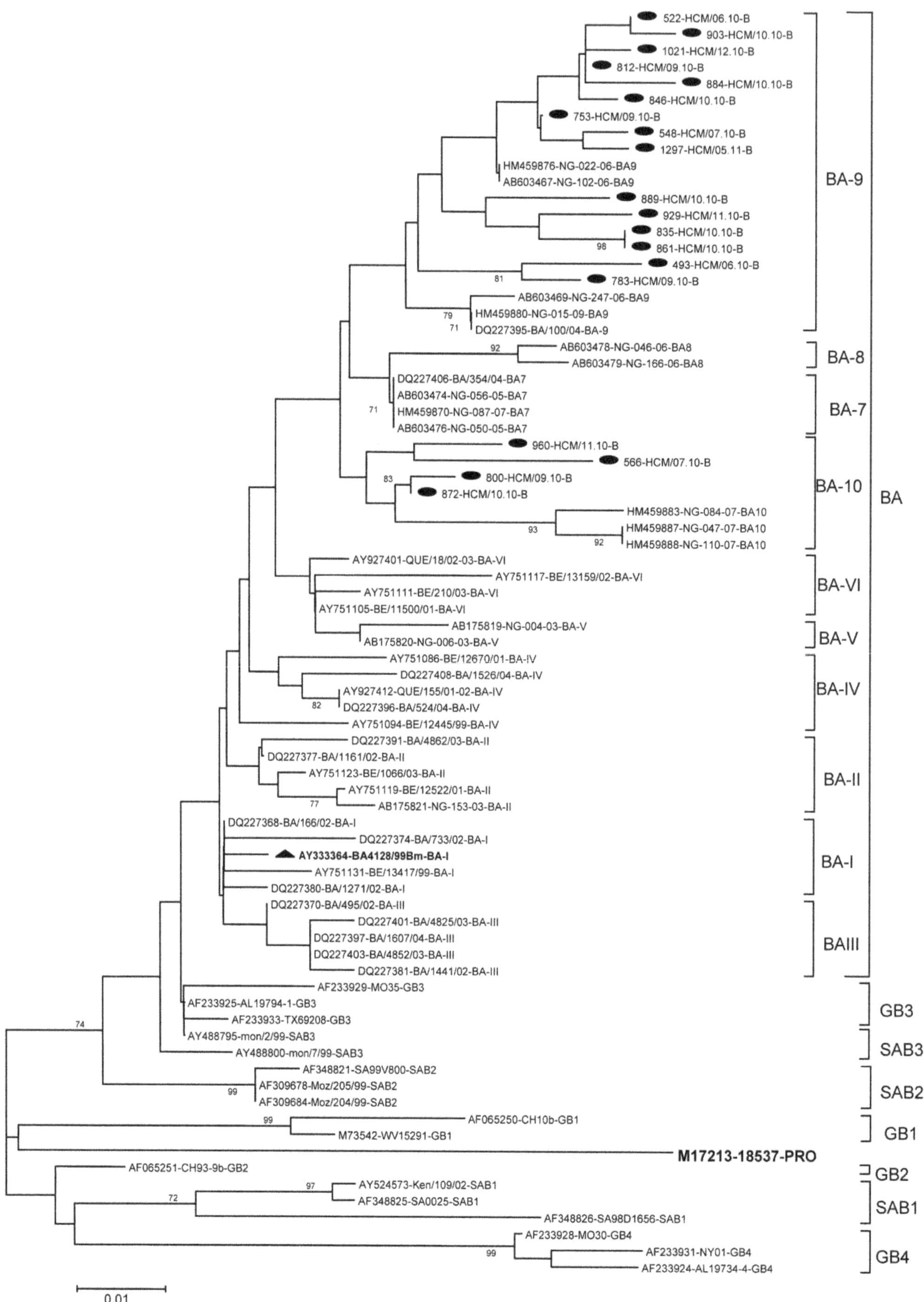
522-HCM/06.10-B
903-HCM/10.10-B
1021-HCM/12.10-B
812-HCM/09.10-B
884-HCM/10.10-B
846-HCM/10.10-B
753-HCM/09.10-B
548-HCM/07.10-B
1297-HCM/05.11-B
HM459876-NG-022-06-BA9
AB603467-NG-102-06-BA9
889-HCM/10.10-B
929-HCM/11.10-B
835-HCM/10.10-B
98
861-HCM/10.10-B
493-HCM/06.10-B
81
783-HCM/09.10-B
AB603469-NG-247-06-BA9
79
HM459880-NG-015-09-BA9
71
DQ227395-BA/100/04-BA-9
BA-9
92
AB603478-NG-046-06-BA8
AB603479-NG-166-06-BA8
BA-8
DQ227406-BA/354/04-BA7
AB603474-NG-056-05-BA7
71
HM459870-NG-087-07-BA7
AB603476-NG-050-05-BA7
BA-7
960-HCM/11.10-B
566-HCM/07.10-B
83
800-HCM/09.10-B
872-HCM/10.10-B
HM459883-NG-084-07-BA10
93
HM459887-NG-047-07-BA10
92
HM459888-NG-110-07-BA10
BA-10
BA
AY927401-QUE/18/02-03-BA-VI
AY751117-BE/13159/02-BA-VI
AY751111-BE/210/03-BA-VI
AY751105-BE/11500/01-BA-VI
BA-VI
AB175819-NG-004-03-BA-V
AB175820-NG-006-03-BA-V
BA-V
AY751086-BE/12670/01-BA-IV
DQ227408-BA/1526/04-BA-IV
AY927412-QUE/155/01-02-BA-IV
82
DQ227396-BA/524/04-BA-IV
AY751094-BE/12445/99-BA-IV
BA-IV
DQ227391-BA/4862/03-BA-II
DQ227377-BA/1161/02-BA-II
AY751123-BE/1066/03-BA-II
AY751119-BE/12522/01-BA-II
77
AB175821-NG-153-03-BA-II
BA-II
DQ227368-BA/166/02-BA-I
DQ227374-BA/733/02-BA-I
AY333364-BA4128/99Bm-BA-I
AY751131-BE/13417/99-BA-I
DQ227380-BA/1271/02-BA-I
BA-I
DQ227370-BA/495/02-BA-III
DQ227401-BA/4825/03-BA-III
DQ227397-BA/1607/04-BA-III
DQ227403-BA/4852/03-BA-III
DQ227381-BA/1441/02-BA-III
BAIII
AF233929-MO35-GB3
AF233925-AL19794-1-GB3
AF233933-TX69208-GB3
GB3
74
AY488795-mon/2/99-SAB3
AY488800-mon/7/99-SAB3
SAB3
AF348821-SA99V800-SAB2
AF309678-Moz/205/99-SAB2
99
AF309684-Moz/204/99-SAB2
SAB2
99
AF065250-CH10b-GB1
M73542-WV15291-GB1
GB1
M17213-18537-PRO
AF065251-CH93-9b-GB2
GB2
97
AY524573-Ken/109/02-SAB1
72
AF348825-SA0025-SAB1
AF348826-SA98D1656-SAB1
SAB1
AF233928-MO30-GB4
99
AF233931-NY01-GB4
AF233924-AL19734-4-GB4
GB4
0.01

Figure 3. Phylogenetic tree for RSV-B nucleotide sequences based on 2nd variable region of G gene. Phylogenetic tree was constructed with MEGA 3.1 software using the neighbor-joining method. Bootstrap values of greater than 70% are shown at the branch nodes. The RSV strains in this study are marked with solid round. Prototype strain of BA genotype is marked with solid triangle. Prototype strain 18537 for group B was also included. The genotype assignment is indicated by the brackets on the right.

remained significant between the RSV positive and negative group ($p<0.001$ and <0.001, respectively). Children infected with group A virus still had a significantly higher clinical severity score than those infected with group B ($p=0.049$) but those with mixed infection of both groups did not ($p=0.064$).

Discussion

RSV is one of the most important respiratory pathogens among infants worldwide. The identification of RSV in about one fourth of cases in this study confirmed that this virus is a dominant agent of respiratory disease in children. This finding is in line with previous reports from Vietnam and other countries [16,20,21,22,23,24].

Regarding the seasonality in this study, the RSV epidemic peaked during the rainy season. Interestingly, RSV activity was completely absent for the 3 months of the dry season (February to April, 2011). The presence of RSV infection seasonality in relation to rainfall has been observed in India [25], Hong Kong [26], Thailand [27], the Philippines [27], Colombia [28], and Kenya [29]. In tropical regions, children tend to be kept indoors during the rainy season, and the resultant crowding may account for the increased incidence of RSV infection. Another reason that has been suggested is that high humidity may help to prevent the virus from desiccation and loss of infectivity.

RSV is the most common viral pathogen causing lower respiratory tract infections (LRTIs) among infants and young children. However, there has been no information about the molecular epidemiology of RSV in Vietnam. This report provides data on the molecular characteristics of RSV from hospitalized children in Ho Chi Minh City and represents the first such study in Vietnam. Information from this study will contribute to the growing database on the molecular diversity of RSV circulating worldwide. The results of this study indicated that RSV subgroup A and B co-existed in one epidemic and cases of RSV subgroup A infection predominated over those of subgroup B. These findings are in agreement with majority of studies in many countries around the world including Germany [30], Belgium [31], Argentina [2], Kenya [32], Japan [33], and India [8], with various patterns of subgroup predominance.

The identification of the GA2 as the predominant genotype in this study was consistent with the results of other reports. GA2 was the most common genotype of RSV group A found around the world and has persisted for many years [8,30,31,33,34]. On the other hand, the G protein gene variable region of one Vietnamese strain was identical to strains from different parts of the world, including Thailand, Scotland, and Brazil.

In this study, 26/27 of GA2 genotype strains were predicted to encode a G protein of 297 amino acids in length, while one strain was shorter, of 286 amino acids. This mutant strain was sequenced directly from the clinical sample. To our knowledge, there has been one previous report of such a mutant strain, by Cane and Pringle [35]. In that report, an isolate with the G protein of 289 amino acids was obtained from virus culture. Our strain was genotype GA2. The previously reported strain was genotype GA1 (data not shown).

Surprisingly, all Vietnamese subgroup B viruses fell into a new genotype BA, which was first detected in Buenos Aires, Argentina during 1999 [10]. The major characteristic of genotype BA is that the G protein gene contains a 60-nucleotide duplication in the second variable region. The BA genotype strains in this study were further clustered into 2 recently described subgenotypes, BA9 and BA10. These subgenotypes were first described from RSV isolates in Japan in 2006 [19] but have not been reported elsewhere until now.

The Vietnamese BA strains had two different G protein lengths, 312 and 319 amino acids, which were reported in previous studies [36]. In addition, alterations had occurred so that the duplicated region was no longer identical to the original one. Since its first appearance, the BA genotype has spread globally and was reported from many regions around the world. Some recent reports also showed that genotype BA has gradually replaced the other group B genotypes [10]. It is possible that these changes in the G protein enhance the attachment of the virus to the host cell, or result in the antigenic modification which allows this virus to escape the immune response.

Potential N-glycosylation sites are thought to play an important role in helping viruses escape from the host immune response [37]. The number and distribution pattern of glycosylation sites identified in this study were different between the 2 RSV subgroups. Our group A strains had 2 N-glycosylation sites within the second variable region of G protein while group B had 4 (Figure 4). Variations in the number and location of these sites can inhibit the recognition of RSV by antibodies to particular epitope [38].

The demographic and clinical information is important to put the results into a practical context and allow them to be applied in clinical practice. In the current study, statistical significance was achieved for the detection of RSV and its association with clinical severity. The RSV-positive patients tended to have more severe symptoms and a higher severity score that probably led them to seek hospital care earlier than the RSV-negative patients.

The fact that nearly half of the RSV infections (42.8%) occurred in children under 6 months showed that patients in this age group are the most vulnerable to RSV infections, despite the presence of maternal antibodies. Maternal antibodies are able to protect against severe RSV in children, however relatively high tilters are required [39]. Unfortunately, with a half-life of 26 days antibodies received at birth quickly drop to unprotective levels within the first month of life [39]. The finding that RSV infections were mainly associated with bronchiolitis and pneumonia (47.1 and 36.2% of the cases, respectively), in which the diagnosis of bronchiolitis was significantly related to RSV, confirmed that this agent is an important cause of LRTIs, as have other studies [40,41].

The detection of co-infection has led to the speculation that the presence of several types of virus in one respiratory specimen may affect the clinical presentation of ARIs. Viruses might interact indirectly or directly, and the effect may depend upon which viruses are co-infecting. The combination of hMPV and RSV has been associated with increased disease severity requiring the use of mechanical ventilation [42,43]. No additional effect of mixed infection of HRV and RSV on disease severity was observed [41]. In the present study, no relationship between RSV co-infections and increased disease severity was established.

Regarding clinical manifestation of each group, by using a composite severity score, we found that infections involving RSV group A (alone or mixed with RSV group B) were associated with

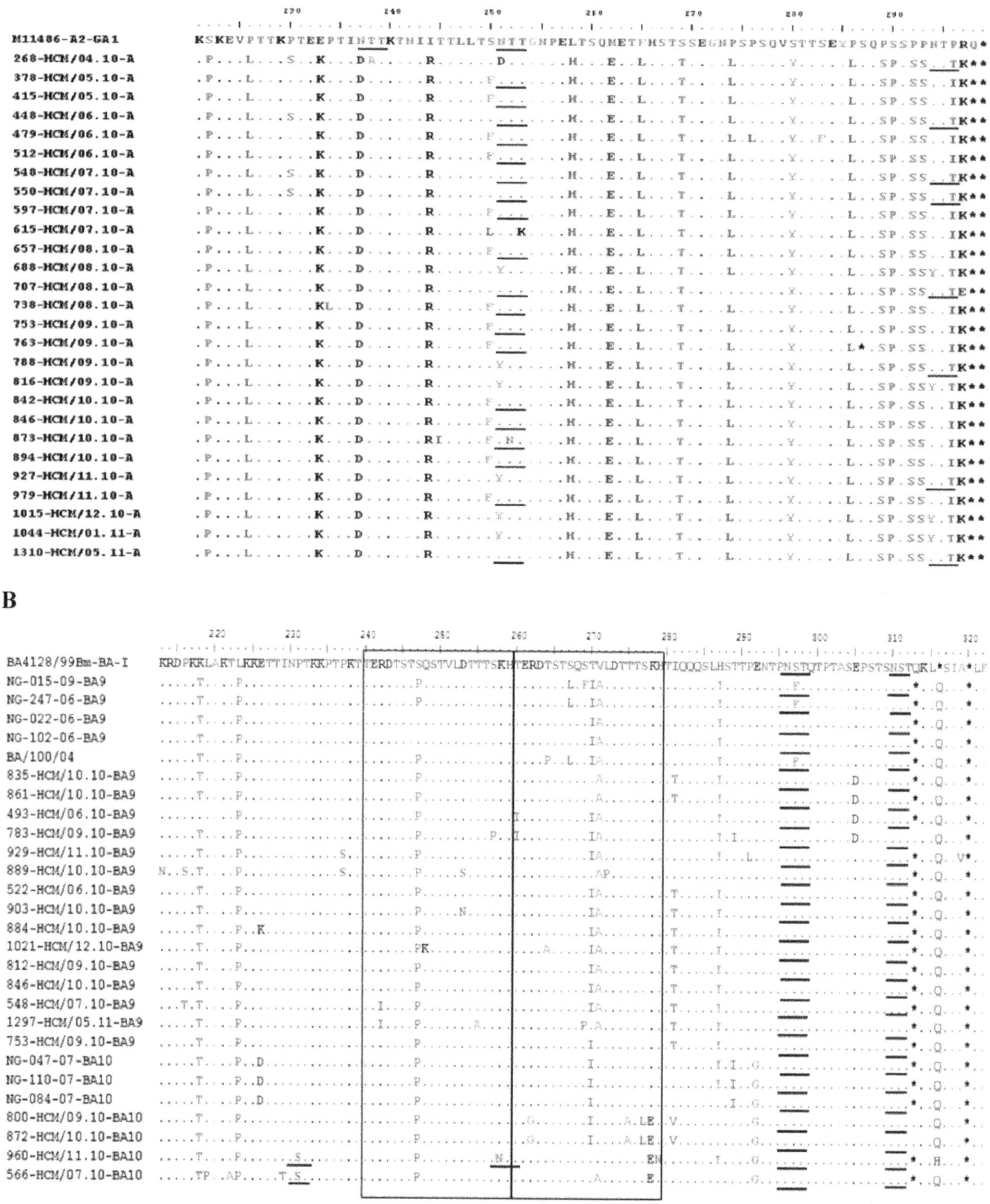

```
                      230       240       250       260       270       280       290
M11486-A2-GA1       KSKEVPTTKPTEEPTINTTKTNIITTLLTSNTTGNPELTSQMETFHSTSSEGNPSPSQVSTTSEYPSQPSSPPNTPRQ*
268-HCM/04.10-A     .P...L...S..K...DA.....R......D......H...E..L...T....L.....Y.....L..SP.SS..TK**
378-HCM/05.10-A     .P...L......K...D......R.....F.......H...E..L...T....L.....Y.....L..SP.SS..IK**
415-HCM/05.10-A     .P...L......K...D......R.....F.......H...E..L...T....L.....Y.....L..SP.SS..IK**
448-HCM/06.10-A     .P...L...S..K...D......R.............H...E..L...T....L.....Y.....L..SP.SS..TK**
479-HCM/06.10-A     .P...L......K...D......R.....F.......H...E..L...T....L.L...Y..F..L..SP.SS..IK**
512-HCM/06.10-A     .P...L......K...D......R.....F.......H...E..L...T....L.....Y.....L..SP.SS..IK**
548-HCM/07.10-A     .P...L...S..K...D......R.............H...E..L...T....L.....Y.....L..SP.SS..TK**
550-HCM/07.10-A     .P...L...S..K...D......R.............H...E..L...T....L.....Y.....L..SP.SS..TK**
597-HCM/07.10-A     .P...L......K...D......R.....F.......H...E..L...T....L.....Y.....L..SP.SS..IK**
615-HCM/07.10-A     .P...L......K...D......R.....L..K....H...E..L...T....L.....Y.....L..SP.SS..IK**
657-HCM/08.10-A     .P...L......K...D......R.....F.......H...E..L...T....L.....Y.....L..SP.SS..IK**
688-HCM/08.10-A     .P...L......K...D......R......Y......H...E..L...T....L.....Y.....L..SP.SSY.TK**
707-HCM/08.10-A     .P...L......K...D......R.............H...E..L...T..........Y.....L..SP.SS..TE**
738-HCM/08.10-A     .P...L......KL..D......R.....F.......H...E..L...T....L.....Y.....L..SP.SS..IK**
753-HCM/09.10-A     .P...L......K...D......R.....F.......H...E..L...T....L.....Y.....L..SP.SS..IK**
763-HCM/09.10-A     .P...L......K...D......R.....F.......H...E..L...T....L.....Y.....L*.SP.SS..IK**
788-HCM/09.10-A     .P...L......K...D......R......Y......H...E..L...T....L.....Y.....L..SP.SS..TK**
816-HCM/09.10-A     .P...L......K...D......R......Y......H...E..L...T....L.....Y.....L..SP.SSY.TK**
842-HCM/10.10-A     .P...L......K...D......R.....F.......H...E..L...T....L.....Y.....L..SP.SS..IK**
846-HCM/10.10-A     .P...L......K...D......R.....F.......H...E..L...T....L.....Y.....L..SP.SS..IK**
873-HCM/10.10-A     .P...L......K...D......RI....F.N.....H...E..L...T....L.....Y.....L..SP.SS..IK**
894-HCM/10.10-A     .P...L......K...D......R.....F.......H...E..L...T....L.....Y.....L..SP.SS..IK**
927-HCM/11.10-A     .P...L......K...D......R......Y......H...E..L...T....L.....Y.....L..SP.SS..TK**
979-HCM/11.10-A     .P...L......K...D......R.....F.......H...E..L...T....L.....Y.....L..SP.SS..IK**
1015-HCM/12.10-A    .P...L......K...D......R......Y......H...E..L...T....L.....Y.....L..SP.SSY.TK**
1044-HCM/01.11-A    .P...L......K...D......R......Y......H...E..L...T....L.....Y.....L..SP.SSY.TK**
1310-HCM/05.11-A    .P...L......K...D......R.............H...E..L...T....L.....Y.....L..SP.SS..TK**
```

B

```
                           220       230       240       250       260       270       280       290       300       310       320
BA4128/99Bm-BA-I     KRDPKKLAKTLKKETTINPTKKPTPKTTERDTSTSQSTVLDTTTSKHTERDTSTSQSTVLDTTTSKHTIQQQSLHSTTPENTPNSTQTPTASEPSTSNSTQKL*SIA*LF
NG-015-09-BA9        .....T....P.......................P...................L.FIA...............I.........F...............*..Q...*..
NG-247-06-BA9        .....T....P.......................P...................L..IA...............I.........F...............*..Q...*..
NG-022-06-BA9        .....T....P..............................................IA...............I.........................*..Q...*..
NG-102-06-BA9        .....T....P..............................................IA...............I.........................*..Q...*..
BA/100/04            .....T....P.......................P................P..L..IA...............I.........F...............*..Q...*..
835-HCM/10.10-BA9    .....T....P.......................P.......................A.........T.....I.................D.......*..Q...*..
861-HCM/10.10-BA9    .....T....P.......................P.......................A.........T.....I.................D.......*..Q...*..
493-HCM/06.10-BA9    ..........P.......................P............I.........IA...............I.................D.......*..Q...*..
783-HCM/09.10-BA9    .....T....P.......................P.........P..I.........IA...............I.I...............D..........Q...*..
929-HCM/11.10-BA9    .....T....P.............S.........P......................IA...............I...L.....................*..Q..V*..
889-HCM/10.10-BA9    N..S.T....P.............S.........P.....S.................AP..............................................*..Q...*..
522-HCM/06.10-BA9    .....T....P.......................P......................IA.........T.....I.........................*..Q...*..
903-HCM/10.10-BA9    .....T....P.......................P.....N................IA.........T.....I.........................*..Q...*..
884-HCM/10.10-BA9    .....T....P..K....................P......................IA.........T.....I.........................*..Q...*..
1021-HCM/12.10-BA9   .....T....P.......................PK...............A.....IA.........T.....I.........................*..Q...*..
812-HCM/09.10-BA9    .....T....P.......................P......................IA.........T.....I.........................*..Q...*..
846-HCM/10.10-BA9    .....T....P.......................P......................IA.........T.....I.........................*..Q...*..
548-HCM/07.10-BA9    ...T.T....P..................I....P......................IA.........T.....I.........................*..Q...*..
1297-HCM/05.11-BA9   .....T....P..................I....P.......A.............P.A.........T.....I.........................*..Q...*..
753-HCM/09.10-BA9    .....T....P.......................P......................I..........T.....I.........................*..Q...*..
NG-047-07-BA10       .....T....P..D....................P......................I...............I.I..G.....................*..Q...*..
NG-110-07-BA10       .....T....P..D....................P......................I...............I.I..G.....................*..Q...*..
NG-084-07-BA10       .....T....P..D....................P......................I.................I..G.....................*..Q...*..
800-HCM/09.10-BA10   .....T....P.......................P..............G.......I....A.LE..V..........G.........................Q...*..
872-HCM/10.10-BA10   .....T....P.......................P..............G.......I....A.LE..V..........G.........................Q...*..
960-HCM/11.10-BA10   .....T....P.......S...............P..........N...................EN.......I....G.....................*..H...*..
566-HCM/07.10-BA10   .....TP..AP.....T.S...............P.......................A......E.............G.....................*..Q...*..
```

Figure 4. Amino acid alignments of 2nd variable region of G protein from RSV-A (A) and RSV-B (B). Alignments are shown relative to the sequences of prototype strain A2 (GenBank accession number M11486) (A) and genotype BA strain BA4128/99B (GenBank accession number AY333364) (B). The amino acids shown correspond to strain A2 G protein positions 221 to 299 for the group A viruses or to strain BA4128/99B G protein positions 213 to 320 for the group B viruses. Identical residues are indicated by dashes. The two copies of the duplicated 20-amino-acid region in group B viruses are indicated by rectangles. Stop codons are indicated by asterisks. Potential N-glycosylation sites (NXT, where X is not proline) are underlined.

Table 1. Demographic and clinical characteristics associated with RSV-positive, negative, mono-, co-infection and subgroups.

Characteristics (%)	RSV pos N = 257	RSV neg N = 825	p	RSV mono N = 198	RSV co N = 59	p	RSV A N = 177	RSV B N = 12	RSV A&B N = 9	p
Male	63	65.2	NS	63.6	61	NS	64.4	50	66.7	NS
Age (m)[a]	7(3–14)	11(4.5–19)	**<0.001**[c]	7.5(3–14)	6(2–13.5)	NS	7 (3–14.5)	7.5 (3–13.5)	8 (2–11)	NS
Age group										
<6 m	42.8	29.9	**<0.001**[b]	41.4	47.5	NS	41.7	41.7	44.4	NS
6–<12 m	26.5	23.2	NS	28.3	20.3	NS	27.8	16.7	44.4	NS
12–<24 m	20.2	29.6	**0.003**[b]	19.7	22.0	NS	18.9	41.7	11.1	NS
≥24 m	10.5	17.3	**0.008**[b]	10.6	10.2	NS	11.7	0	0	NS
Prematurity (<37 weeks)	10.9	8.6	NS	10.7	11.9	NS	10.6	16.7	0	NS
Malnutrition	6.2	10.5	**0.039**[b]	7.1	3.4	NS	6.1	25	0	RSV A v RSV B p = 0.046[b]
Infection with other viruses	23.0	52.5	**<0.001**[b]	NA	NA		NA	NA	NA	
Days before hos.[a]	2(2–4)	3(2–5)	**0.017**[c]	2(2–4)	3(2–4)	NS	2 (2–4)	2 (1–2.5)	3 (3–5)	RSV B v RSV AB p = 0.023[c]
Fever	72.8	65.5	**0.033**[b]	74.7	66.1	NS	73.3	83.3	100	NS
Cough	93.8	89.9	NS	93.4	94.9	NS	92.8	100	100	NS
Runny nose	82.5	70.5	**<0.001**[b]	84.3	76.3	NS	83.9	83.3	100	NS
$SpO_2 \leq 92\%$	5.8	9.3	NS	4.5	10.2	NS	4.4	8.3	0	NS
Tachypnea	41.6	45.5	NS	42.9	37.3	NS	44.4	41.7	11.1	NS
Lower chest indrawing	68.5	51.0	**<0.001**[b]	69.2	66.1	NS	70	50	77.8	NS
Wheezing[d]	59.9	58.5	NS	59.6	61	NS	60.6	25	88.9	RSV A v RSV B p = 0.03[b]; RSV B v RSV AB p = 0.014[b];
Clinical Severity Score[a]	12(8–13)	11(7–13)	**0.003**[c]	12(8–13)	12(8–13)	NS	12 (8–13)	8 (7.5–12)	13 (8–14)	RSV A v RSV B p = 0.031[c]; RSV B v RSV AB p = 0.028[c];
Diagnosis										
URTIs	16.0	23.4	**0.012**[b]	17.7	10.2	NS	18.9	8.3	0	NS
Croup	0.8	7.8	**<0.001**[b]	1	0	NS	1.1	0	0	NS
Bronchiolitis	47.1	28.8	**<0.001**[b]	44.9	54.2	NS	42.8	66.7	66.7	NS
Pneumonia	36.2	40.0	NS	36.4	35.6	NS	37.2	25	33.3	NS
Hos. duration[a]	6(4–8)	5(4–8)	NS	6(4–8)	6(4–7.5)	NS	6 (4–8)	7 (5–8)	6 (3–6)	NS

Abbreviation: d, day; m, month; hos, hospitalization; URTI, upper respiratory infection; RSV, respiratory syncytial virus; NA, not applicable; NS, not significant; pos, positive; neg, negative; mono, mono-infection; co, co-infection.
Note: All results are expressed in percentages except for ([a]) in median with interquartile range between brackets.
[b]Chi-squared test.
[c]Mann-Whitney-*U* test.

more severe disease than infection with RSV group B. Besides virus factors, the clinical severity of RSV infection is also associated with epidemiological and host factors, which include socioeconomic status, age, prematurity, and underlying heart and/ or lung disease. To exclude these confounding factors, patients with underlying diseases or having co-infection with other viruses were not included.

Subgroup B infected children were admitted to the hospital less frequently than subgroup A infected children. Either subgroup B strains cause such a mild illness that there is no need to hospitalize the patient or the prevalence of subgroup B is truly low. However, in two studies, the proportions of subgroup A and subgroup B infected children in the hospital and in the community were similar [44,45].

Several studies have examined the relationship between clinical severity and RSV subgroups. In approximately half of these studies, group A seemed to be associated with more severe clinical disease [44,45,46,47,48,49,50], whereas no such difference was found in the others [11,51,52,53,54,55,56]. In only two studies have group B infections been reported to cause more severe disease [57,58]. This inconsistency could be attributed to difference in study design and population, definition of disease severity, the distribution of RSV subgroups, etc. In the recent study, Houben *et al.* reported that disease severity correlated positively with viral load during primary RSV infection [15].

The current study was limited to only one epidemic season. Because the predominant subgroups shift from year to year, the immunity against the previous circulating groups could have altered the severity of disease caused by specific subgroups. Therefore, continued observation and analysis of additional seasons is required to determine the association between subgroups and severity of disease.

In summary, RSV was found to be the viral pathogen most commonly and frequently associated with severe acute respiratory diseases in infants and children. Co-infections between RSV and other respiratory viruses did not lead to increased disease severity. The molecular characteristics of RSV were determined for the first time in Vietnam, and carried characteristics both similar to strains from other parts of the world and specific to Vietnam. Subgroup A and B of RSV were co-circulating and subgroup A caused more severe disease than subgroup B. Similar surveillance should be continued to follow the epidemiology of this virus. A better understanding of RSV epidemiology is essential to enable prediction of outbreaks and for planning preventive and therapeutic control measures.

Acknowledgments

We deeply thank Dr. Nguyen Tran Quynh Nhu and Ms. Pham Thi Ngoc Hue, Cardiovascular Department, Children's Hospital 2, Ho Chi Minh City for their help in patient counseling and sample collection. DNT is a recipient of the scholarship from the Honjo International Scholarship Foundation.

Author Contributions

Conceived and designed the experiments: DNT TMHP MTH LY MM HU. Performed the experiments: DNT. Analyzed the data: DNT TTLT TKHD. Contributed reagents/materials/analysis tools: SO SH MM HU. Wrote the paper: DNT HU.

References

1. Collins PL, and Crowe JE Jr (2007) Respiratory syncytial virus and Metapneumovirus. P. 1601–46. *In* Knipe DM, Howley PM, Griffin DE, Lamb RA, Martin MA, Roizman B, and Straus SE (ed.), Fields Virology, 5th ed. Lippincott Williams & Wilkins, Philadelphia, PA.
2. Viegas M, Barrero PR, Maffey AF, Mistchenko AS (2004) Respiratory viruses seasonality in children under five years of age in Buenos Aires, Argentina: a five-year analysis. J Infect 49:222–8.
3. Cane PA (2001) Molecular epidemiology of respiratory syncytial virus. Rev Med Virol 11:103–16.
4. Scott PD, Ochola R, Sande C, Ngama M, Okiro EA, et al. (2007) Comparison of strain-specific antibody responses during primary and secondary infections with respiratory syncytial virus. J Med Virol 79: 1943–50.
5. Mufson MA, Orvell C, Rafnar B, Norrby E (1985) Two distinctsubtypes of human respiratory syncytial virus. J Gen Virol 66:2111–24.
6. Sullender WM (2000) Respiratory syncytial virus genetic and antigenic diversity. Clin Microbiol Rev 13: 1–15.
7. Johnson PR, Spriggs MK, Olmsted RA, Collins PL (1987) The G glycoprotein of human respiratory syncytial viruses of subgroups A and B: extensive sequence divergence between antigenically related proteins. Proc Natl Acad Sci USA 84: 5625–9.
8. Parveen S, Sullender WM, Fowler K, Lefkowitz EJ, Kapoor SK, et al. (2006) Genetic variability in the G protein gene of group A and B respiratory syncytial viruses from India. J Clin Microbiol 44: 3055–64.
9. Shobugawa Y, Saito R, Sano Y, Zaraket H, Suzuki Y, et al. (2009) Emerging genotypes of human respiratory syncytial virus subgroup A among patients in Japan. J Clin Microbiol 47: 2475–82.
10. Trento A, Casas I, Calderon A, Garcia-Garcia ML, Calvo C, et al. (2010) Ten years of global evolution of the human respiratory syncytial virus BA genotype with a 60-nucleotide duplication in the G protein gene. J Virol 84: 7500–12.
11. Hendry RM, Talis AL, Godfrey E, Anderson LJ, Fernie BF, et al. (1986) Concurrent circulation of antigenically distinct strains of respiratory syncytial virus during community outbreaks. J Infect Dis 153: 291–7.
12. Brandenburg AH, van Beek R, Moll HA, Osterhaus AD, Claas EC (2000) G protein variation in respiratory syncytial virus group A does not correlate with clinical severity. J Clin Microbiol 38: 3849–52.
13. World Health Organization (2005) Pocket Book of Hospital Care for Children: Guidelines for the Management of Common Illnesses with Limited Resources. Geneva: WHO.
14. Gern JE, Martin MS, Anklam KA, Shen K, Roberg KA, et al. (2002) Relationships among specific viral pathogens, virus-induced interleukin-8, and respiratory symptoms in infancy. Pediatr Allergy Immunol 13: 386–93.
15. Houben ML, Coenjaerts FEJ, Rossen JWA, Belderbos ME, Hofland RW, et al. (2010) Disease Severity and Viral Load Are Correlated in Infants With Primary Respiratory Syncytial Virus Infection in the Community. J of Med Virol 82:1266–71.
16. Yoshida LM, Suzuki M, Yamamoto T, Nguyen HA, Nguyen CD, et al. (2010) Viral pathogens associated with acute respiratory infections in central Vietnamese children. Pediatr Infect Dis J 29: 75–7.
17. Hall TA (1999) BioEdit: a user-friendly biological sequence alignment editor and analysis program for Windows 95/98/NT. Nucl Acids Symp Ser 41:95–8.
18. Kumar S, Tamura K, Nei M (2004) MEGA3: Integrated software for Molecular Evolutionary Genetics Analysis and sequence alignment. Brief Bioinform 5:150–63.
19. Dapat CI, Shobugawa Y, Sano Y, Saito R, Sasaki A, et al. (2010) New genotypes within respiratory syncytial virus group B genotype BA in Nigata, Japan. J Clin Microbiol 48: 3423–7.
20. Berkley JA, Munywoki P, Ngama M, Kazungu S, Abwao J, et al. (2010) Viral etiology of severe pneumonia among Kenyan infants and children. JAMA 303:2051–7.
21. Choi EH, Lee HJ, Kim SJ, Eun BW, Kim NH, et al. (2006) The association of newly identified respiratory viruses with lower respiratory tract infections in Korean children, 2000–2005. Clin Infect Dis 43:585–92.
22. Do AHL, van Doorn HR, Nghiem MN, Bryant JE, Hoang THt, et al. (2011) Viral Etiologies of Acute Respiratory Infections among Hospitalized Vietnamese Children in Ho Chi Minh City, 2004–2008. PLoS ONE 6: e18176.
23. Ekalaksananan T, Pientong C, Kongyingyoes B, Pairojkul S, Teeratakulpisarn J, et al. (2001) Etiology of acute lower respiratory tract infection in children at Srinagarind Hospital, Khon Kaen, Thailand. Southeast Asian J Trop Med Public Health 32: 513–9.
24. Wang W, Cavailler P, Ren P, Zhang J, Dong W, et al. (2010) Molecular monitoring of causative viruses in child acute respiratory infection in endemo-epidemic situations in Shanghai. J Clin Virol 49:211–8.
25. Cherian T, Simoes EA, Steinhoff MC, Chitra K, John M, et al. (1990) Bronchiolitis in tropical south India. Am J Dis Child 144: 1026–30.
26. Chan PK, Sung RY, Fung KS, Hui M, Chik KW, et al. (1999) Epidemiology of respiratory syncytial virus infection among paediatric patients in Hong Kong: seasonality and disease impact. Epidemiol Infect 123: 257–62.
27. Weber MW, Mulholland EK, Greenwood BM (1998) Respiratory syncytial virus infection in tropical and developing countries. Trop Med Int Health 3:268–80.
28. Bedoya VI, Abad V, Trujillo H (1996) Frequency of respiratory syncytial virus in hospitalized infants with lower acute respiratory tract infection in Colombia. Pediatr Infect Dis J 15: 1123–4.

29. Hazlett DT, Bell TM, Tukei PM, Ademba GR, Ochieng WO, et al. (1988) Viral etiology and epidemiology of acute respiratory infections in children in Nairobi, Kenya. Am J Trop Med Hyg 39: 632–40.
30. Reiche J, Schweiger B (2009) Genetic variability of group A human respiratory syncytial virus strains circulating in Germany from 1998 to 2007. J Clin Microbiol 47:1800–10.
31. Zlateva KT, Vijgen L, Dekeersmaeker N, Naranjo C, Van Ranst M (2007) Subgroup prevalence and genotype circulation patterns of humanrespiratory syncytial virus in Belgium during ten successive epidemic seasons. J Clin Microbiol 45:3022–30.
32. Scott PD, Ochola R, Ngama M, Okiro EA, Nokes DJ, et al. (2004) Molecular epidemiology of respiratory syncytial virus in Kilifi district, Kenya. J Med Virol 74:344–54.
33. Sato M, Saito R, Sakai T, Sano Y, Nishikawa M, et al. (2005) Molecular epidemiology of respiratory syncytial virus infections among children with acute respiratory symptoms in a community over three seasons. J Clin Microbiol 43:36–40.
34. Boonyasuppayakorn S, Kowitdamrong E, Bhattarakosol P (2010) Molecular and demographic analysis of respiratory syncytial virus infection in King Chulalongkorn Memorial Hospital admitted patients, Thailand, 2007. Influenza and Other Respiratory Viruses 4: 313–23.
35. Cane PA, Pringle CR (1995) Evolution of subgroup A respiratory syncytial virus: evidence for progressive accumulation of amino acid changes in the attachment protein. J Virol 69:2918–25.
36. Zlateva KT, Lemey P, Moes E, Vandamme AM, Van Ranst M (2005) Genetic variability and molecular evolution of the human respiratory syncytial virus subgroup B attachment G protein. J Virol 79:9157–67.
37. Roca A, Loscertales MP, Quinto L, Perez-Brena P, Vaz N, et al. (2001) Genetic variability among group A and B respiratory syncytial viruses in Mozambique: Identification of a new cluster of group B isolates. J Gen Virol 82:103–11.
38. Palomo C, Cane PA, Melero JA (2000) Evaluation of the antibody specificities of human convalescent-phase sera against the attachment (G) protein of human respiratory syncytial virus: influence of strain variation and carbohydrate side chains. J Med Virol 60:468–74.
39. Brandenburg AH, Groen J, Steensel-Moll HA, Claas EC, Rothbarth PH, et al. (1997) Respiratory syncytial virus specific serum antibodies in infants under six months of age: limited serological response upon infection. J Med Virol 52:97–104.
40. Juvén T, Mertsola J, Waris M, Leinonen M, Meurman O, et al. (2000) Etiology of community-acquired pneumonia in 254 hospitalized children. Pediatr Infect Dis J 19: 293–8.
41. Marguet C, Lubrano M, Gueudin M, Le roux P, Deschildre A, et al. (2009) In very young infants severity of acute bronchiolitis depends on carried viruses. Plos one 4: e4596.
42. Richard N, Komurian-Pradel F, Javouhey E, Perret M, Rajoharison A, et al. (2008) The impact of dual viral infection in infants admitted to a pediatric intensive care unit associated with severe bronchiolitis. Pediatr Infect Dis J 27: 213–7.
43. Semple MG, Cowell A, Dove W, Greensill J, McNamara PS, et al. (2005) Dual infection of infants by human metapneumovirus and human respiratory syncytial virus is strongly associated with severe bronchiolitis. J Infect Dis 191:382–6.
44. Mufson MA, Belshe RB, Orvell C, Norrby E (1988) Respiratory syncytial virus epidemics: variable dominance of Subgroups A and B among children, 1981–1986. J Infect Dis 157:143–148.
45. Hall CB, Walsh EE, Schnabel KC, Long CE, McConnochie KM, et al. (1990) Occurrence of Groups A and B of respiratory syncytial virus over 15 years: associated epidemiologic and clinical characteristics in hospitalized and ambulatory children. J Infect Dis 162:1283–90.
46. Heikkinen T, Waris M, Ruuskanen O, Putto-Laurila O, Mertsola J (1995) Incidence of acute otitis media associated with group A and B respiratory syncytial virus infections. Acta Paediatr 84:419–23.
47. McConnochie KM, Hall CB, Walsh EE, Roghmann KJ (1990) Variation in severity of respiratory syncytial virus infections with subtype. J Pediatr 117:52–62.
48. Salomon HE, Avila MM, Cerqueiro MC, Orvell C, Weissenbacher M (1991) Clinical and epidemiologic aspects of respiratory syncytial virus antigenic variants in Argentinian children. (Letter.) J Infect Dis 163:1167.
49. Taylor CE, Morrow S, Scott M, Young B, Toms GL (1989) Comparative virulence of respiratory syncytial virus subgroups A and B. (Letter.) Lancet 1:777–8.
50. Walsh EE, McConnochie KM, Long CE, Hall CB (1997) Severity of respiratory syncytial virus infection is related to virus strain. J Infect Dis 175:814–20.
51. Kneyber MC, Brandenburg AH, Rothbarth PH, de Groot R, Ott A, et al. (1996) Relationship between clinical severity of respiratory syncytial virus infection and subtype. Arch Dis Child 75:137–40.
52. McIntosh ED, De Silva LM, Oates RK (1993) Clinical severity of respiratory syncytial virus group A and B infection in Sydney, Australia. Pediatr Infect Dis J 12:815–9.
53. Monto AS, Ohmit S (1990) Respiratory syncytial virus in a community population: circulation of subgroups A and B since 1965. J Infect Dis 161:781–3.
54. Russi JC, Chiparelli H, Montano A, Etorena P, Hortal M (1989) Respiratory syncytial virus subgroups and pneumonia in children. (Letter and comment.) Lancet 2:1039–40.
55. Tsutsumi H, Onuma M, Nagai K, Yamazaki H, Chiba S (1991) Clinical characteristics of respiratory syncytial virus (RSV) subgroup infections in Japan. Scand J Infect Dis 23:671–4.
56. Wang EE, Law BJ, Stephens D (1995) Pediatric Investigators Collaborative Network on Infections in Canada (PICNIC) prospective study of risk factors and outcomes in patients hospitalized with respiratory syncytial viral lower respiratory tract infection. J Pediatr 126:212–9.
57. Hornsleth A, Klug B, Nir M, Johansen J, Hansen KS, et al. (1998) Severity of respiratory syncytial virus disease related to type and genotype of virus and to cytokine values in nasopharyngeal secretions. Pediatr Infect Dis J 17:1114–21
58. Straliotto SM, Roitman B, Lima JB, Fischer GB, Siqueira MM (1994) Respiratory syncytial virus bronchiolitis: competitive study of RSV groups A and B infected children. Rev Soc Bras Med Trop 27: 1–4.

13

Assessment of Genetic Associations between Common Single Nucleotide Polymorphisms in RIG-I-Like Receptor and IL-4 Signaling Genes and Severe Respiratory Syncytial Virus Infection in Children: A Candidate Gene Case-Control Study

Nico Marr*, Aaron F. Hirschfeld, Angie Lam, Shirley Wang, Pascal M. Lavoie, Stuart E. Turvey*

Department of Pediatrics, University of British Columbia, Child and Family Research Institute, Vancouver, British Columbia, Canada

Abstract

The majority of cases of severe pediatric respiratory syncytial virus (RSV) infection occur in otherwise healthy infants who have no identifiable risk factors, suggesting that additional subclinical factors, such as population genetic variation, influence the course of RSV infection. The objective of this study was to test if common single nucleotide polymorphisms (SNPs) in genes encoding for immune signalling components of the RIG-I-like receptor (RLR) and IL-4-signalling pathways affect the outcome of RSV infection in early life. We genotyped 8 SNPs using allele-specific probes combined with real-time PCR. Each of the SNPs tested had previously been established to have a functional impact on immune responsiveness and two of the SNPs in the *IL4* and *IL4R* genes had previously been associated with severe RSV bronchiolitis. Association with susceptibility to severe RSV infection was tested by statistically comparing genotype and allele frequencies in infants and young children hospitalized with severe RSV bronchiolitis (n = 140) with two control groups—children who tested positive for RSV but did not require hospitalization (n = 100), and a general population control group (n = 285). Our study was designed with sufficient power (>80%) to detect clinically-relevant associations with effect sizes ≥1.5. However, we detected no statistically significant differences in allele and genotype frequencies of the investigated SNPs between the inpatient and control groups. To conclude, we could not replicate the previously reported association with SNPs in the *IL4* and *IL4R* genes in our independent cohort, nor did we find that common SNPs in genes encoding for RLRs and the downstream adapter MAVS were associated with susceptibility to severe RSV infections. Despite the existing evidence demonstrating a functional immunological impact of these SNPs, our data suggest that the biological effect of each individual SNP is unlikely to affect clinical outcomes of RSV infection.

Editor: Steven M. Varga, University of Iowa, United States of America

Funding: This study was funded by the British Columbia Lung Association (to N.M.), and the Canadian Institutes of Health Research (to S.E.T.). A.L. and S.W. were recipients of undergraduate summer studentships from AllerGen N.C.E., Canada and the Child and Family Research Institute. P.M.L. and S.E.T. acknowledge support from the Michael Smith Foundation for Health Research. The funders had no role in the study design, data collection and analysis, decision to publish, or preparation of the manuscript.

Competing Interests: Stuart E. Turvey and Pascal M. Lavoie are PLOS ONE Editorial Board members. This does not alter their adherence to PLOS ONE Editorial policies and criteria.

* Email: nmarr@cfri.ca (NM); sturvey@cw.bc.ca (SET)

Introduction

Human respiratory syncytial virus (RSV) is the most important respiratory pathogen of early life. In developed countries, RSV infection accounts for more than half of all cases of acute respiratory tract infections and influenza-like illnesses in infants and young children [1,2]. Recent estimates suggest that each year, up to 234,000 children under age 5 die from clinical complications due to RSV infections worldwide [3,4]. In addition, severe respiratory virus infection in early life is an important risk factor for the development of asthma [5].

A complex combination of environmental, pathogen and host genetic factors determines both susceptibility to pathogens and the course of infection. Nevertheless, infectious diseases have an inherited element and individuals with different genetic backgrounds respond differently to particular infections. Adoption studies, which effectively separate genetic and environmental confounders, have indicated a substantial genetic effect involved in susceptibility to infection. For example, the early death of a biological parent from infection increased the risk of death of the child from an infectious disease nearly six-fold. In contrast, the death of an adoptive parent from an infectious disease had no significant effect on the adoptees' risk of such a death [6,7].

A variety of clinical risk factors are associated with severe RSV infection—premature birth, bronchopulmonary dysplasia, congenital heart disease, and immunodeficiency [1]. Nevertheless, the majority of severe RSV infections occur in infants born at term who were previously healthy [8,9,10]. This strongly suggests that additional influences, such as genetic variability of the host, contribute to disease severity. The importance of the contribution of host genetics in RSV immunopathogenesis was further highlighted by twin studies, revealing that identical twin pairs had significantly higher concordance rates in the susceptibility to severe RSV infection when compared with fraternal twin pairs [11]. These findings are consistent with genetic association and case-control studies suggesting a role of familial susceptibility to severe viral respiratory infections in early life [12,13,14,15].

The goal of this study was to test if common single nucleotide polymorphisms (SNPs) in genes coding for immune signalling components of the RIG-I-like receptor (RLR) and IL-4-signalling pathways affect the outcome of RSV infection. We chose to employ this targeted candidate gene approach because there is strong evidence that both pathways play a critical role in RSV immunopathogenesis. The importance of the ubiquitously expressed cytosolic receptor, RIG-I, in the replication-dependent recognition of RSV in airway epithelial cells (AEC) has been well established [16] and we have recently demonstrated a role of RIG-I in the innate antiviral response to RSV in human plasmacytoid dendritic cells [8]. In addition, its structural homolog MDA5 appears to play a non-redundant role, at the least in AEC [16,17]. The innate antiviral response elicited through these cytosolic PRRs is critical in restricting RSV replication in the respiratory tract [18,19]. Similarly, IL-4-mediated signaling appears to play a pathological role later during RSV infection [20]. RSV infection in early life has been shown to be associated with Th2-biased immune responses following RSV infection [21,22]. This is likely due to increased IL-4Rα expression levels in neonatal CD4+T cells, which triggers increased immunopathology and perhaps also long-term changes in normal immune function (e.g. asthma development) following neonatal RSV infection [20,23].

We investigated the role of common, non-synonymous coding SNPs and one promoter SNP in the genes encoding RIG-I and MDA5, its specific adaptor protein MAVS, as well as the genes encoding IL-4 and the IL-4 receptor alpha (IL-4Rα) (Table 1). All SNPs that we analyzed in this present study have been reported to play a functional role in immune signalling in cell models *in vitro*, in antibody responses to vaccination, and/or in the manifestation of a variety of human illnesses *in vivo*, ranging from infections with other RNA viruses to non-communicable diseases such as type 1 diabetes or systemic lupus (for details see Table 1). The *IL4* promoter and *IL4R* gene SNPs examined in this study have been reported to be associated with severe RSV bronchiolitis in children in Korea and the Netherlands, respectively [24,25]. However, another independent study of a cohort of children in Germany [26] did not find an association between this *IL4* promoter SNP and outcomes of pediatric RSV infection thus warranting further confirmation using our cohort of children in Canada.

Materials and Methods

DNA sample collection and genotyping

We obtained de-identified genomic DNA samples from nasopharyngeal washes (NPW) of children (n = 240) visiting the Emergency Room at Children's & Women's Health Centre of British Columbia (Vancouver, Canada) and who tested positive for RSV infection by direct immunofluorescence assays as previously described [27]. We differentiated between children who required hospitalization due to severe RSV bronchiolitis (inpatients, n = 140) and children with confirmed RSV infection who did not require hospital admission (outpatients, n = 100). Moreover, we collected genomic DNA samples of a general population control group (n = 285) from umbilical cord blood of healthy term neonates born by scheduled Cesarean sections at the same institution. DNA collection was approved by the University of British Columbia's Clinical Research Ethics Board. Specifically, written parental consent was obtained for umbilical cord blood collections of healthy term neonates providing genomic DNA samples of the general population control group. For subjects who tested positive for RSV, DNA was isolated from de-identified NPW samples where an individual's identifying information had been removed, and in this specific circumstance consent was not obtained. Our institutional ethics committee has approved DNA collection from all subjects, including DNA collection from de-identified NPW samples where consent was not obtained. Genotyping was performed by real time PCR assays using allele-specific Taqman probes (Fig. 1) as previously described [27,28].

Statistical analysis

Genotype and allele frequencies in the outpatient group and the general population control group were compared separately to the inpatient group using Pearson Chi-Square tests, or when one of the genotype or allele counts in any given group was less than 5 we applied the Fisher Exact Probability tests. Allelic association was tested by comparing the allele counts in the case and control groups using 2×2 contingency tables. Genotypic association was tested by comparing the genotype counts using 2×3 contingency tables (general model with 2 degrees of freedom), as well as by comparing the genotype counts after combining the homozygous and heterozygous genotype counts carrying the minor allele and using 2×2 contingency tables (dominant model) [29]. P values ≤ 0.05 and odds ratios (OR) with a 95% confidence interval (CI) $\neq 1$ were considered statistically significant. Statistics were computed using utilities available at the VassarStats website for statistical computation (http://vassarstats.net). Power calculations were made using CaTS software [30].

Results

In the present study we used a targeted candidate gene approach and analyzed SNPs in genes encoding RIG-I and MDA-5, its downstream adapter MAVS, as well as IL-4 and IL-4Rα, since there is evidence that these immune signaling components play a pivotal role during RSV immunopathogenesis [8,16,20]. We chose to focus on common SNPs where a functional role had been reported in independent studies (Table 1). SNPs were considered common if they had a global minor allele frequency (MAF) of >5% (i.e. MAF reported in dbSNP from the current 1000Genome default population including 1094 world-wide individuals [31]). All synonymous SNPs as well as rare SNPs (i.e. SNPs with low or undetermined MAF, or rare mutations) were excluded from our analysis since they are less likely to play a biological role and/or are unlikely to affect outcomes at the population level, respectively. In the case of multiple variants in strong linkage disequilibrium (LD), only one SNP was analyzed.

Using these selection criteria, we analyzed 8 SNPs in total (Table 1). To test whether any of these SNPs may affect the outcome of RSV infection in children, we genotyped 140 children who were hospitalized with confirmed RSV infection (inpatients), 100 children who tested positive for RSV infection but had less severe disease manifestations and therefore did not require hospital admission (outpatients), as well as a general population control group (n = 285) of healthy term neonates. Genotyping was performed by real-time PCR assays using allele-specific TaqMan probes (Fig. 1). Based upon the sample size of our inpatient and

Table 1. SNPs analyzed in this study.

Gene name (protein)	SNP ID	Position	Nucleotide Change	Amino Acid Change	Evidence for functional role
DDX58 (RIG-I)	rs10813831	CDS	C→T	Arg7Cys	Increased *DDX58* and *IFNB1* transcription in Newcastle disease virus-infected primary DCs [44]; allele dose-related decrease of antibody levels after rubella vaccination [46]
	rs17217280	CDS	T→A	Asp580Glu	Reduced IFN-β-, IRF-3-, NF-κB-dependent reporter gene activation in HEK 293T or BEAS-2B cells at baseline and upon Influenza virus A challenge [45]
IFIH1 (MDA-5)	rs3747517	CDS	A→G	His843Arg	Type 1 diabetes [51]
	rs1990760	CDS	G→A	Ala946Thr	Type 1 diabetes [50]
MAVS (MAVS)	rs17857295	CDS	C→G	Gln93Glu	Subgroup of systematic lupus erythematoses patients with renal nephritis [47]
	rs7269320	CDS	C→T	Ser409Phe*	Subgroup of systematic lupus erythematosus patients with arthritis [47]
IL4 (IL-4)	rs2243250	promoter	C→T	N/A	Hospitalization due to RSV bronchiolitis [24,25]
IL4R (IL4-Rα)	rs1801275	CDS	A→G	Gln576Arg*	Hospitalization due to RSV bronchiolitis in children >6 months old [24]

CDS, coding sequence; *transcript variant 1.

population control group, we estimated that our study had ≥80% power to detect clinically-actionable associations; specifically, with relative risks of ≥1.9, ≥1.7, ≥1.6 and ≥1.5 for disease allele frequencies of 10–14%, 15–20%, 21–36%, and ≥37%, respectively (Fig. 2). All analyzed SNPs had a genotyping call rate between 96 and 100% (Table 2).

To test for associations in our candidate gene case-control study, we performed χ^2 tests or Fisher exact probability tests when appropriate, applying three standard models of disease penetrance. First we tested for allelic association by comparing the allele counts in the control groups with that in the inpatient group (multiplicative model). In addition, we assessed genotypic association, assuming that each of the genotypes has an independent association with disease (2 degrees of freedom). To account for an alternative model of disease penetrance, we also applied a dominant model by combining the homozygous and heterozygous genotype counts carrying the minor allele [29]. We separately compared the allele and genotype frequencies of each SNP in the inpatient group with that in our two control groups, namely (i) outpatients with confirmed RSV infection, or (ii) a population control group of term infants who were recruited at the same institution, and applied the three models of disease penetrance as outlined above for each comparison. As shown in Table 2, we found no statistically significant associations between a particular

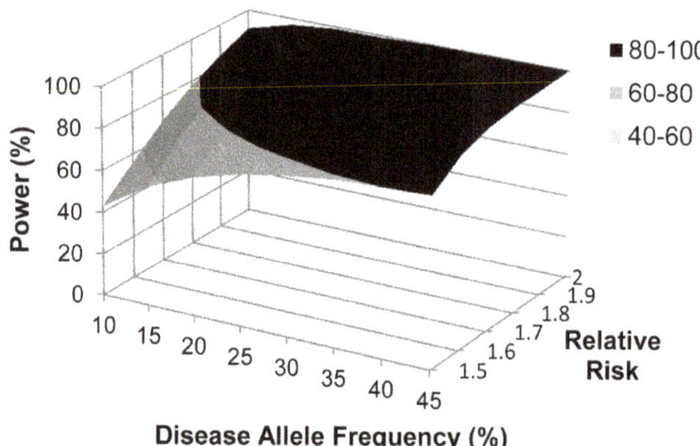

Figure 2. Statistical power to detect associations in our case-control study (n = 140 cases and 285 controls). Power calculations were done for combinations of disease allele frequencies between 10% and 45% (in increments of 5%) and relative risks between 1.5 and 2 (in increments of 0.1) using a multiplicative model of penetrance and a significance level of 0.05. Disease prevalence was set at 2%. Area shaded in black indicates ≥80 power.

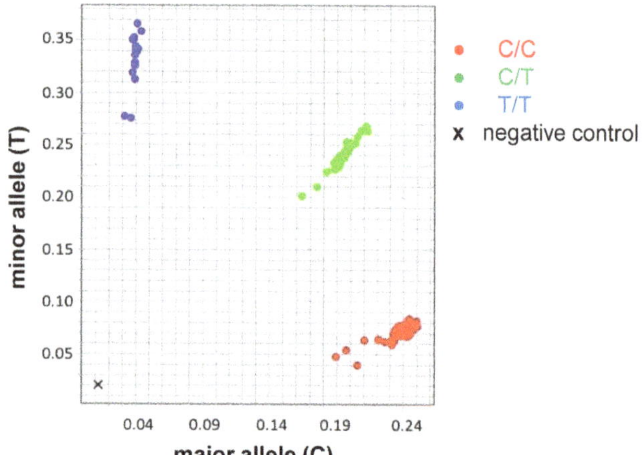

Figure 1. Representative data set (*IL4* C→T, rs2243250) analyzed by real-time PCR assay using allele-specific probes.

Table 2. Case-control association analysis between SNPs in RIG-like receptor and IL-4 signaling genes and severe RSV infection.

Gene and SNP ID	call rate % (n)	Allele Freq. % (n)		P_a	OR (95% CI)	Genotype Freq. % (n)			P_b	P_c	OR (95% CI)
DDX58											
rs10813831		C	T			CC	CT	TT			
Population Control	99 (281)	79 (444)	21 (118)	0.47	0.87 (0.61–1.26)	64 (179)	31 (86)	6 (16)	0.25	0.86	0.97 (0.63–1.48)
Outpatients	100 (100)	84 (167)	17 (33)	0.51	1.17 (0.73–1.90)	71 (71)	25 (25)	4 (4)	0.33*	0.29	1.35 (0.77–2.35)
Inpatients	99 (138)	81 (224)	19 (52)			64 (89)	33 (46)	2 (3)			
rs17217280		A	T			AA	AT	TT			
Population Control	99 (283)	89 (502)	11 (64)	0.68	0.91 (0.57–1.44)	78 (221)	21 (60)	1 (2)	0.57	0.53	0.85 (0.51–1.41)
Outpatients	100 (100)	90 (180)	10 (20)	0.89	1.04 (0.57–1.90)	80 (80)	20 (20)	0 (0)	0.58*	0.89	0.96 (0.50–1.82)
Inpatients	100 (140)	90 (251)	10 (29)			81 (113)	18 (25)	1 (2)			
IFIH1											
rs3747517		G	A			GG	GA	AA			
Population Control	98 (279)	57 (317)	43 (241)	0.40	0.88 (0.66–1.18)	34 (95)	46 (127)	20 (57)	0.42	0.22	0.77 (0.50–1.17)
Outpatients	98 (98)	59 (116)	41 (80)	0.89	0.97 (0.67–1.41)	43 (42)	33 (32)	24 (24)	0.54	0.68	1.12 (0.66–1.89)
Inpatients	98 (137)	60 (164)	40 (110)			40 (55)	39 (54)	20 (28)			
rs1990760		A	G			AA	AG	GG			
Population Control	98 (278)	45 (252)	55 (304)	0.21	0.83 (0.62–1.11)	26 (72)	39 (108)	35 (98)	0.43	0.52	0.86 (0.54–1.36)
Outpatients	98 (98)	52 (101)	48 (95)	0.74	1.06 (0.74–1.54)	34 (33)	36 (35)	31 (30)	0.58	0.43	1.25 (0.71–2.19)
Inpatients	96 (135)	50 (135)	50 (135)			29 (39)	42 (57)	29 (39)			
MAVS											
rs17857295		C	G			CC	CG	GG			
Population Control	99 (283)	67 (382)	33 (184)	0.81	1.04 (0.76–1.41)	49 (139)	37 (104)	14 (40)	0.96	0.92	1.02 (0.68–1.54)
Outpatients	100 (100)	66 (132)	34 (68)	0.89	0.97 (0.66–1.43)	45 (45)	42 (42)	13 (13)	0.65	0.59	0.87 (0.52–1.45)
Inpatients	99 (138)	67 (184)	33 (92)			49 (67)	36 (50)	15 (21)			
rs7269320		C	T			CC	CT	TT			
Population Control	99 (283)	85 (480)	15 (86)	0.79	0.95 (0.63–1.42)	72 (205)	25 (70)	3 (8)	0.74	0.63	0.89 (0.56–1.42)
Outpatients	100 (100)	86 (172)	14 (28)	0.89	1.04 (0.62–1.75)	76 (76)	20 (20)	4 (4)	0.97*	0.81	1.08 (0.59–1.96)
Inpatients	99 (138)	86 (236)	14 (40)			75 (103)	22 (30)	4 (5)			
IL4											
rs2243250		C	T			CC	CT	TT			
Population Control	100 (284)	65 (368)	35 (200)	0.36	0.87 (0.64–1.18)	46 (130)	38 (108)	16 (46)	0.69	0.42	0.84 (0.54–1.27)
Outpatients	100 (100)	64 (128)	36 (72)	0.36	0.84 (0.57–1.23)	48 (48)	32 (32)	20 (20)	0.45	0.76	0.92 (0.55–1.55)
Inpatients	96 (136)	68 (185)	32 (87)			50 (68)	36 (49)	14 (19)			
IL4R											
rs1801275		A	G			AA	AG	GG			
Population Control	99 (283)	77 (434)	23 (132)	**0.05**	0.69 (0.48–1.00)	59 (168)	35 (98)	6 (17)	0.12	0.11	0.71 (0.46–1.08)
Outpatients	100 (100)	76 (151)	25 (49)	0.06	0.65 (0.41–1.02)	57 (57)	37 (37)	6 (6)	0.14*	0.10	0.64 (0.38–1.09)
Inpatients	99 (138)	83 (228)	17 (48)			67 (93)	30 (42)	2 (3)			

P_a: uncorrected P values vs. inpatient group for allelic association;
P_b: uncorrected P values vs. inpatient group for genotypic association (2 degrees of freedom);
P_c: uncorrected P values vs. inpatient group for genotypic association after combining the homozygous and heterozygous genotype counts carrying the minor allele (dominant model);
*Indicates P values computed by Fisher exact probability tests; OR: Odds Ratios; 95%CI: 95% confidence intervals.

genotype or allele frequency and hospitalization due to RSV bronchiolitis, regardless of the genetic model, and whether the inpatient group was compared to the outpatient group, or the general population control group. Our analysis only revealed a modest overrepresentation of the minor allele of the IL-4Rα SNP among the general population control group (uncorrected *P* value = 0.05; OR 0.69; 95%CI 0.48–1.00), which was not statistically significant after correction for multiple comparisons. Of note, Hoebee *et al.* [24] had previously reported an association between the *IL4* SNP tested in our study and severe RSV infection, which appeared to be more robust when children <6 month of age, or those with recurrent wheezing, cardiac or lung disease were excluded. However, comparison of our inpatient group with our outpatient group using the three standard models of disease penetrance as outlined above did not reveal a statistically significant association between any of the SNPs tested here and severe RSV infection after stratification of the RSV-infected inpatients and outpatients in a group ≤6 month of age and a group >6 months of age (Tables S1A and S1B). DNA samples of our population control group were obtained from cord blood (i.e. at birth) and were therefore not used to separately assess the effect of age as a co-variable. In our study, we did not collect additional clinical data, thus precluding inclusion of other risk factors as co-variables in our analysis. De-identified genotype data and related metadata (i.e. ages, study group) are listed in Table S2. Further inquiries for additional data should be made to either SET or NM.

Discussion

Today the only effective option to reduce the risk for severe RSV disease in infants is passive immunization with palivizumab (commonly referred to as RSV immunoprophylaxis), which is given by monthly intramuscular injections during the RSV season. However, the high costs of this therapy and the lack of useful indicators restricts its use to relatively few high-risk children, such as infants with congenital abnormalities or those born very early in gestation [32,33]. There is a pressing need to establish novel indicators for the identification of children at high risk of developing severe RSV infections who do not meet the current criteria for RSV immunoprophylaxis. Genetic variants, such as common SNPs in genes coding for pattern recognition receptors or other crucial immune signalling and defence components, are an attractive target [34]. Gene SNPs have been shown to play a role in the clinical manifestations and outcome of a variety of infectious and immune-mediated human diseases; most notable examples include hepatitis C virus infections, Crohn's disease, and type 1 diabetes [35,36,37]. However, there is only limited information available about the role of SNPs and the risk of developing severe RSV infection in early life. Candidate gene association studies have largely focused on SNPs in the genes encoding Toll-like receptor (TLR) 4 or surfactant proteins A and D (SP-A, SP-D) and outcome of RSV infection [34]. However, independent studies assessing associations between *TLR4* SNPs and susceptibility to RSV infection have led to contradictory results [27,38,39,40], and the role of this pattern recognition receptor (PRR) in RSV pathogenesis remains controversial [16]. Moreover, reported relative risks associated with SP-A and SP-D variants [34,41] are not robust enough to justify their clinical use for the identification of at-risk children who may benefit from, but currently do not qualify for, RSV immunoprophylaxis.

Our results suggest that none of the common SNPs in the *IL4* and *IL4R* genes tested in this study appear to play a clinically-significant biological role in the outcome of pediatric RSV infection on its own. Although we found a modest overrepresentation of the minor allele for the *IL4R* SNP (rs1801275) among the general population control, this was not statistically significant after correcting for multiple testing. In addition, this modest overrepresentation of the *IL4R* SNP among the control group was in the opposite direction compared to a previous genetic association study by Hoebee *et al.* [24], who found this SNP to be associated with severe RSV infection in a subpopulation of children hospitalized at >6 month of age. The *IL4* promoter SNP tested in our study was associated with severe RSV infection in two association studies of children in Korea and the Netherlands, respectively [24,25]. However, the lack of an association in our Canadian cohort is consistent with the finding of a previous study in a German cohort of children with severe RSV infection, who also showed no significant difference in the minor allele frequency in comparison to control subjects [26]. This is despite evidence of a functional role of this SNP in atopic disorders by contributing to enhanced IgE synthesis [42,43]. The discrepancy between the results of genetic association studies focused on the *IL4* promoter SNP and severe RSV infection could have various reasons, including ethnic diversity, choice of control groups, differences in study design and statistical analysis. For example, Hoebee *et al.* [24] obtained DNA samples from children hospitalized with RSV and their parents, thereby combining a case-control study with a transmission/disequilibrium test. It should be noted that p-values reported by Hoebee *et al.* [24] and Choi *et al.* [25] were not corrected for multiple testing. If conservative correction for multiple testing of 3 or more SNPs in the same cohort is applied, associations reported in both studies become marginal.

Similarly, although there is evidence for a functional role of non-synonymous SNPs in genes encoding for RIG-I, MDA5, and its downstream adapter MAVS, we did not find an association of these SNPs with severe RSV infection. The two *DDX58* (*RIG-I*) SNPs analyzed in our study have been shown to cause modest changes in the innate antiviral response of human dendritic cells [44], HEK 293T or BEAS-2B cells [45]. One of the SNPs (rs10813831, Arg7Cys) in the gene encoding RIG-I was also found to be associated with an allele dose-related decrease in rubella antibody levels, further supporting a functional role of this variant [46]. The SNPs in the gene coding for MAVS appeared to be associated with systemic lupus erythematosus in the Chinese population, albeit only in patients with renal nephritis and arthritis, respectively [47]. Another study did not find an association between either of the SNPs in the genes coding for RIG-I and MAVS and outcome of hepatitis C virus infections [48]. Other variants with more deleterious effects on RIG-I [45] and MAVS [49] expression or function are rare, and therefore are unlikely to play a significant role in the outcome of RSV infection at the population level. Genome-wide association studies suggested a role of common variants in the gene encoding MDA5 in type I diabetes, which was later validated in independent cohorts [37,50,51]. Association studies linking SNPs in the gene encoding MDA5 with the outcome of viral infection are largely lacking. This is perhaps because MDA5 was initially believed to play a role in innate immune recognition of only a subset of RNA viruses [52]. However, more recent reports suggest that several viruses, including ssRNA viruses, are sensed by both RIG-I and MDA5, thereby engaging non-redundant signaling pathways [16,53,54].

It is important to point out strengths and limitations of our study. In our candidate gene case-control study, we applied three different models of disease penetrance and separately compared genotype and allele frequencies in our inpatient group with severe RSV disease (i.e. case group) with two different control groups, namely (i) a general population control group of term infants born at the same institution and (ii) a group of outpatients who visited the Children's & Women's Health Centre of British Columbia and were tested positive for acute RSV infection but did not require hospitalization (i.e. had less severe RSV disease). Comparison to each control group bears advantages and limitations over the other. Although our general population control group of term infants is characterized as a "low risk" group when considering all known clinical risk factors for severe RSV infection, this group likely includes some individuals who will go on to develop severe RSV infection requiring hospitalization. This is because even some previously healthy infants and young children develop severe RSV infection for reasons that remain unknown [8]. Nevertheless, the number of these individuals in our control group is expected to be very small and therefore, unlikely to skew the results of our genetic association study. Specifically, all individuals of our population control group were born by scheduled Cesarean section at term. Clinical conditions that are known to increase the risk factors for severe RSV disease among term infants, such as cardiac or lung disease, are relatively rare. Consequently, we estimate the rate of hospitalization due to RSV among our general population control group to be ≤2%, as reported for similar pediatric cohorts in other geographical regions [55]. The outpatient group which we used as a second control group lacks any children that required hospital admission. Nonetheless, one may consider this group as a medium rather than a low risk group, because all these children had symptomatic respiratory infection that prompted their caregivers and/or general physicians to bring them/to refer them to the Children's & Women's Health Centre of British Columbia.

In summary, our findings suggest that the SNPs analyzed in the present study are unlikely to significantly increase the risk of children developing severe RSV infection. These variants may still have minor effects on the outcome of RSV infection in infants and young children (RR≤1.4), a possibility that would require larger cohort size to prove. Nevertheless, the fact that various previously reported relative risks associated with common variants in host defense genes (e.g. *TLR4*, *IL4R*) and severe outcomes of pediatric RSV infection are generally low and that reported associations are often not reproducible in independent studies [34] highlights the need for more robust approaches for genetic susceptibility testing in the context of RSV infection and prophylaxis. Importantly, genetic variants exerting larger biological effects are generally too rare to justify clinical use. Future research is needed to test whether assessment of a combination of multiple common variants, rather than single risk alleles, may justify the use of genetic susceptibility testing to aid clinical decision-making for the purpose of selecting at-risk children for RSV immunoprophylaxis.

Author Contributions

Conceived and designed the experiments: NM SET. Performed the experiments: AFH AL SW. Analyzed the data: NM AFH AL. Contributed to the writing of the manuscript: NM PML SET.

References

1. Welliver RC (2003) Review of epidemiology and clinical risk factors for severe respiratory syncytial virus (RSV) infection. J Pediatr 143: S112–117.
2. Simoes EA, Carbonell-Estrany X (2003) Impact of severe disease caused by respiratory syncytial virus in children living in developed countries. Pediatr Infect Dis J 22: S13–18; discussion S18–20.
3. Nair H, Nokes DJ, Gessner BD, Dherani M, Madhi SA, et al. (2010) Global burden of acute lower respiratory infections due to respiratory syncytial virus in young children: a systematic review and meta-analysis. Lancet 375: 1545–1555.
4. Lozano R, Naghavi M, Foreman K, Lim S, Shibuya K, et al. (2012) Global and regional mortality from 235 causes of death for 20 age groups in 1990 and 2010: a systematic analysis for the Global Burden of Disease Study 2010. Lancet 380: 2095–2128.
5. Hashimoto S, Matsumoto K, Gon Y, Ichiwata T, Takahashi N, et al. (2008) Viral infection in asthma. Allergol Int 57: 21–31.
6. Sorensen TI, Nielsen GG, Andersen PK, Teasdale TW (1988) Genetic and environmental influences on premature death in adult adoptees. N Engl J Med 318: 727–732.
7. Petersen L, Andersen PK, Sorensen TI (2010) Genetic influences on incidence and case-fatality of infectious disease. PLoS One 5: e10603.
8. Marr N, Wang TI, Kam SH, Hu YS, Sharma AA, et al. (2014) Attenuation of Respiratory Syncytial Virus-Induced and RIG-I-Dependent Type I IFN Responses in Human Neonates and Very Young Children. J Immunol 192: 948–957.
9. Garcia CG, Bhore R, Soriano-Fallas A, Trost M, Chason R, et al. (2010) Risk factors in children hospitalized with RSV bronchiolitis versus non-RSV bronchiolitis. Pediatrics 126: e1453–1460.
10. Hall CB, Weinberg GA, Iwane MK, Blumkin AK, Edwards KM, et al. (2009) The burden of respiratory syncytial virus infection in young children. N Engl J Med 360: 588–598.
11. Thomsen SF, Stensballe LG, Skytthe A, Kyvik KO, Backer V, et al. (2008) Increased concordance of severe respiratory syncytial virus infection in identical twins. Pediatrics 121: 493–496.
12. Goetghebuer T, Kwiatkowski D, Thomson A, Hull J (2004) Familial susceptibility to severe respiratory infection in early life. Pediatr Pulmonol 38: 321–328.
13. Kwiatkowski D (2000) Science, medicine, and the future: susceptibility to infection. BMJ 321: 1061–1065.
14. Siezen CL, Bont L, Hodemaekers HM, Ermers MJ, Doornbos G, et al. (2009) Genetic susceptibility to respiratory syncytial virus bronchiolitis in preterm children is associated with airway remodeling genes and innate immune genes. Pediatr Infect Dis J 28: 333–335.
15. Amanatidou V, Apostolakis S, Spandidos DA (2009) Genetic diversity of the host and severe respiratory syncytial virus-induced lower respiratory tract infection. Pediatr Infect Dis J 28: 135–140.
16. Marr N, Turvey SE, Grandvaux N (2013) Pathogen recognition receptor crosstalk in respiratory syncytial virus sensing: a host and cell type perspective. Trends Microbiol 21: 568–574.
17. Soucy-Faulkner A, Mukawera E, Fink K, Martel A, Jouan L, et al. (2010) Requirement of NOX2 and reactive oxygen species for efficient RIG-I-mediated antiviral response through regulation of MAVS expression. PLoS Pathog 6: e1000930.
18. Demoor T, Petersen BC, Morris S, Mukherjee S, Ptaschinski C, et al. (2012) IPS-1 signaling has a nonredundant role in mediating antiviral responses and the clearance of respiratory syncytial virus. J Immunol 189: 5942–5953.
19. Bhoj VG, Sun Q, Bhoj EJ, Somers C, Chen X, et al. (2008) MAVS and MyD88 are essential for innate immunity but not cytotoxic T lymphocyte response against respiratory syncytial virus. Proc Natl Acad Sci U S A 105: 14046–14051.
20. You D, Marr N, Saravia J, Shrestha B, Lee GI, et al. (2013) IL-4Ralpha on CD4+T cells plays a pathogenic role in respiratory syncytial virus reinfection in mice infected initially as neonates. J Leukoc Biol 93: 933–942.
21. Culley FJ, Pollott J, Openshaw PJ (2002) Age at first viral infection determines the pattern of T cell-mediated disease during reinfection in adulthood. J Exp Med 196: 1381–1386.
22. Bendelja K, Gagro A, Bace A, Lokar-Kolbas R, Krsulovic-Hresic V, et al. (2000) Predominant type-2 response in infants with respiratory syncytial virus (RSV) infection demonstrated by cytokine flow cytometry. Clin Exp Immunol 121: 332–338.
23. Ripple MJ, You D, Honnegowda S, Giaimo JD, Sewell AB, et al. (2010) Immunomodulation with IL-4R alpha antisense oligonucleotide prevents respiratory syncytial virus-mediated pulmonary disease. J Immunol 185: 4804–4811.
24. Hoebee B, Rietveld E, Bont L, Oosten M, Hodemaekers HM, et al. (2003) Association of severe respiratory syncytial virus bronchiolitis with interleukin-4 and interleukin-4 receptor alpha polymorphisms. J Infect Dis 187: 2–11.
25. Choi EH, Lee HJ, Yoo T, Chanock SJ (2002) A common haplotype of interleukin-4 gene IL4 is associated with severe respiratory syncytial virus disease in Korean children. J Infect Dis 186: 1207–1211.

26. Puthothu B, Krueger M, Forster J, Heinzmann A (2006) Association between severe respiratory syncytial virus infection and IL13/IL4 haplotypes. J Infect Dis 193: 438–441.
27. Paulus SC, Hirschfeld AF, Victor RE, Brunstein J, Thomas E, et al. (2007) Common human Toll-like receptor 4 polymorphisms—role in susceptibility to respiratory syncytial virus infection and functional immunological relevance. Clin Immunol 123: 252–257.
28. Ali S, Hirschfeld AF, Mayer ML, Fortuno ES 3rd, Corbett N, et al. (2013) Functional genetic variation in NFKBIA and susceptibility to childhood asthma, bronchiolitis, and bronchopulmonary dysplasia. J Immunol 190: 3949–3958.
29. Clarke GM, Anderson CA, Pettersson FH, Cardon LR, Morris AP, et al. (2011) Basic statistical analysis in genetic case-control studies. Nat Protoc 6: 121–133.
30. Skol AD, Scott LJ, Abecasis GR, Boehnke M (2006) Joint analysis is more efficient than replication-based analysis for two-stage genome-wide association studies. Nat Genet 38: 209–213.
31. NCBI New SNP Attributes. Available: http://www.ncbi.nlm.nih.gov/projects/SNP/docs/rs_attributes.html. Accessed 1 Apr 2014.
32. Paes BA, Mitchell I, Banerji A, Lanctot KL, Langley JM (2011) A decade of respiratory syncytial virus epidemiology and prophylaxis: Translating evidence into everyday clinical practice. Can Respir J 18: e10–19.
33. American Academy of Pediatrics (2012). Respiratory Syncytial Virus. In: Pickering LK, editor. Red Book: 2012 Report of the Committee on Infectious Diseases. 29th ed: Elk Grove Village, IL, American Academy of Pediatrics. pp. 609–618.
34. Ramet M, Korppi M, Hallman M (2011) Pattern recognition receptors and genetic risk for rsv infection: value for clinical decision-making? Pediatr Pulmonol 46: 101–110.
35. Selvarajah S, Tobler LH, Simmons G, Busch MP (2010) Host genetic basis for hepatitis C virus clearance: a role for blood collection centers. Curr Opin Hematol 17: 550–557.
36. Parkes M, Cortes A, van Heel DA, Brown MA (2013) Genetic insights into common pathways and complex relationships among immune-mediated diseases. Nat Rev Genet 14: 661–673.
37. Hakonarson H, Grant SF (2009) Genome-wide association studies in type 1 diabetes, inflammatory bowel disease and other immune-mediated disorders. Semin Immunol 21: 355–362.
38. Awomoyi AA, Rallabhandi P, Pollin TI, Lorenz E, Sztein MB, et al. (2007) Association of TLR4 polymorphisms with symptomatic respiratory syncytial virus infection in high-risk infants and young children. J Immunol 179: 3171–3177.
39. Tal G, Mandelberg A, Dalal I, Cesar K, Somekh E, et al. (2004) Association between common Toll-like receptor 4 mutations and severe respiratory syncytial virus disease. J Infect Dis 189: 2057–2063.
40. Lofgren J, Marttila R, Renko M, Ramet M, Hallman M (2010) Toll-like receptor 4 Asp299Gly polymorphism in respiratory syncytial virus epidemics. Pediatr Pulmonol 45: 687–692.
41. Lahti M, Lofgren J, Marttila R, Renko M, Klaavuniemi T, et al. (2002) Surfactant protein D gene polymorphism associated with severe respiratory syncytial virus infection. Pediatr Res 51: 696–699.
42. Mitsuyasu H, Izuhara K, Mao XQ, Gao PS, Arinobu Y, et al. (1998) Ile50Val variant of IL4R alpha upregulates IgE synthesis and associates with atopic asthma. Nat Genet 19: 119–120.
43. Mitsuyasu H, Yanagihara Y, Mao XQ, Gao PS, Arinobu Y, et al. (1999) Cutting edge: dominant effect of Ile50Val variant of the human IL-4 receptor alpha-chain in IgE synthesis. J Immunol 162: 1227–1231.
44. Hu J, Nistal-Villan E, Voho A, Ganee A, Kumar M, et al. (2010) A common polymorphism in the caspase recruitment domain of RIG-I modifies the innate immune response of human dendritic cells. J Immunol 185: 424–432.
45. Pothlichet J, Burtey A, Kubarenko AV, Caignard G, Solhonne B, et al. (2009) Study of human RIG-I polymorphisms identifies two variants with an opposite impact on the antiviral immune response. PLoS One 4: e7582.
46. Ovsyannikova IG, Haralambieva IH, Dhiman N, O'Byrne MM, Pankratz VS, et al. (2010) Polymorphisms in the vitamin A receptor and innate immunity genes influence the antibody response to rubella vaccination. J Infect Dis 201: 207–213.
47. Liu X, Jiao Y, Wen X, Wang L, Ma C, et al. (2011) Possible association of VISA gene polymorphisms with susceptibility to systemic lupus erythematosus in Chinese population. Mol Biol Rep 38: 4583–4588.
48. Clausen LN, Ladelund S, Weis N, Bukh J, Benfield T (2013) Genetic variation in toll-like receptors and retinoic acid-inducible gene I and outcome of hepatitis C virus infection: a candidate gene association study. J Viral Hepat doi:10.1111/jvh.12188.
49. Pothlichet J, Niewold TB, Vitour D, Solhonne B, Crow MK, et al. (2011) A loss-of-function variant of the antiviral molecule MAVS is associated with a subset of systemic lupus patients. EMBO Mol Med 3: 142–152.
50. Smyth DJ, Cooper JD, Bailey R, Field S, Burren O, et al. (2006) A genome-wide association study of nonsynonymous SNPs identifies a type 1 diabetes locus in the interferon-induced helicase (IFIH1) region. Nat Genet 38: 617–619.
51. Yang H, Wang Z, Xu K, Gu R, Chen H, et al. (2012) IFIH1 gene polymorphisms in type 1 diabetes: genetic association analysis and genotype-phenotype correlation in Chinese Han population. Autoimmunity 45: 226–232.
52. Loo YM, Fornek J, Crochet N, Bajwa G, Perwitasari O, et al. (2008) Distinct RIG-I and MDA5 signaling by RNA viruses in innate immunity. J Virol 82: 335–345.
53. Yoboua F, Martel A, Duval A, Mukawera E, Grandvaux N (2010) Respiratory syncytial virus-mediated NF-kappa B p65 phosphorylation at serine 536 is dependent on RIG-I, TRAF6, and IKK beta. J Virol 84: 7267–7277.
54. Loo YM, Gale M Jr (2011) Immune signaling by RIG-I-like receptors. Immunity 34: 680–692.
55. Boyce TG, Mellen BG, Mitchel EF Jr, Wright PF, Griffin MR (2000) Rates of hospitalization for respiratory syncytial virus infection among children in medicaid. J Pediatr 137: 865–870.

14

POPI (Pediatrics: Omission of Prescriptions and Inappropriate Prescriptions): Development of a Tool to Identify Inappropriate Prescribing

Sonia Prot-Labarthe[1*¶], Thomas Weil[1,2¶], François Angoulvant[3], Rym Boulkedid[4,5], Corinne Alberti[4,5,6], Olivier Bourdon[1,2,7]

1 Pharmacie, AP-HP Hôpital Robert-Debré, Paris, France, **2** Pharmacie Clinique, Université Paris Descartes, Paris, France, **3** Service d'Accueil des Urgences, AP-HP Hôpital Robert-Debré, Paris, France, **4** Unité d'Epidémiologie Clinique, AP-HP Hôpital Robert Debré, Paris, France, **5** Inserm U 1123 et CIC 1426, Paris, France, **6** Sorbonne Paris Cité UMRS 1123, Université Paris Diderot, Paris, France, **7** Laboratoire Educations et Pratiques de Santé, Université Paris XIII, Bobigny, France

Abstract

Introduction: Rational prescribing for children is an issue for all countries and has been inadequately studied. Inappropriate prescriptions, including drug omissions, are one of the main causes of medication errors in this population. Our aim is to develop a screening tool to identify omissions and inappropriate prescriptions in pediatrics based on French and international guidelines.

Methods: A selection of diseases was included in the tool using data from social security and hospital statistics. A literature review was done to obtain criteria which could be included in the tool called POPI. A 2-round-Delphi consensus technique was used to establish the content validity of POPI; panelists were asked to rate their level of agreement with each proposition on a 9-point Likert scale and add suggestions if necessary.

Results: 108 explicit criteria (80 inappropriate prescriptions and 28 omissions) were obtained and submitted to a 16-member expert panel (8 pharmacists, 8 pediatricians hospital-based −50%- or working in community −50%-). Criteria were categorized according to the main physiological systems (gastroenterology, respiratory infections, pain, neurology, dermatology and miscellaneous). Each criterion was accompanied by a concise explanation as to why the practice is potentially inappropriate in pediatrics (including references). Two round of Delphi process were completed via an online questionnaire. 104 out of the 108 criteria submitted to experts were selected after 2 Delphi rounds (79 inappropriate prescriptions and 25 omissions).

Discussion Conclusion: POPI is the first screening-tool develop to detect inappropriate prescriptions and omissions in pediatrics based on explicit criteria. Inter-user reliability study is necessary before using the tool, and prospective study to assess the effectiveness of POPI is also necessary.

Editor: Imti Choonara, Nottingham University, United Kingdom

Funding: The authors have no support or funding to report.

Competing Interests: The authors have declared that no competing interests exist.

* Email: sonia.prot-labarthe@rdb.aphp.fr

¶ These authors are joint senior authors on this work

Introduction

Rational use of medicines refers to the correct, proper and appropriate use of medicines. The WHO estimates that over 50% of medications are prescribed, dispensed or sold inappropriately and that more than 50% of all countries do not implement basic policies to promote rational use of medicines [1]. In developing countries, less than 40% of patients in the public sector and 30% in the private sector are treated according to clinical guidelines [1]. The use of medication in pediatrics should be based on established recommendations from well-conducted clinical trials, however in the absence of such trials, recommendations are often based on clinical experience. Rational prescribing for children is an issue for all countries and has been inadequately studied [2,3].

The Medical Subject Headings (MeSH) tool is a thesaurus integrated into the PubMed search engine that allows access to the MEDLINE database. In 2011, it introduced the term '*Inappropriate Prescribing*' [4]. The use of a medication for which the associated risks outweigh the expected benefits can be considered as inappropriate, especially if an alternative treatment has been shown to be safer and more effective. According to a report published by the French National Authority for Health, both prescription of medication for excessively long periods and the failure to prescribe recommended medications can be classified as inappropriate prescribing [5]. In addition, the prescription of medications that have a high risk to interact with other drugs, or with the disease can also be considered as inappropriate. All of these examples will be herein described as inappropriate prescription (IP).

Many tools have been developed to detect IP in the elderly. This is largely due to the susceptibility of the elderly to disease and the prevalence of polypharmacy in this population. The *Beers Criteria for Potentially Inappropriate Medication Use in Older Adults* [6] were the first criteria to be proposed and are also the most well-known. However, one major disadvantage of this tool is that it includes many medications that are not sold in Europe. In 2008, Gallagher *et al.* developed a tool called STOPP/START (*Screening Tool of Older Person's Prescriptions/Screening Tool to Alert doctors to Right Treatment*) that comprises two medication lists [7]. The 'STOPP' list includes prescriptions that should be stopped and the 'START' list includes prescriptions that should be initiated, in the absence of any contra-indication. This system is particularly useful because it classifies drugs according to various medical conditions that are commonly found in the elderly. In a study in 2008, the use of the STOPP list identified IPs in 35% of a cohort of elderly patients and one third of these IPs were associated with an adverse drug event [8]. Another study involving randomized hospitalized patients showed that the occurrence of IP was 35% lower in patients who were prescribed drugs according to STOPP/START criteria than in patients for who usual pharmaceutical criteria were used [9]. However, so far no tool has been created to the pediatric population.

Our objective was to create the first IP tool in pediatrics, which we called POPI (Pediatrics: Omission of Prescriptions and Inappropriate prescriptions) [10]. Our objective was to raise awareness about this tool and to validate its content through a network of medical professionals working in pediatrics.

Materials and Methods

POPI should contain around 100 propositions that were classified according to biological system and classified according to whether they involve an omitted or an inappropriate prescription. The propositions were further divided within these two lists according to the major biological systems (as this was done for other geriatric tools [6,8]). We decided to include around 100 propositions: this was a good compromise between the number of major biological systems to explore, the number of items in the geriatric lists and the maximum number of items compatible with a tool easy use.

This project began in the Robert-Debré University Hospital, AP-HP (Assistance Publique-Hôpitaux de Paris) in Paris, France. POPI is comprised of a list of health problems frequently encountered in pediatrics. These problems were chosen in 2010 according to the following criteria, as concerns pediatrics: their frequency in the general population, the reasons for hospitalization (listed in the French hospital system's medico-administrative database in 2011 'programme de médicalisation des systèmes d'information' [PMSI] at the Robert-Debré University Hospital), and their prevalence according to data from the French National Health Insurance Fund for Employees (la caisse nationale de l'assurance maladie des travailleurs salariés [CNAMTS]) of long-term illnesses [11]. According to these criteria, we selected health problems requiring either drug intervention, or no pharmacological intervention whatsoever (i.e. treatment in such cases would be considered as inappropriate).

For each disease, we considered the recommended pharmacological treatments, the risks of errors, contra-indications, drug-drug interactions, drug-disease interactions, and issues associated with dose and route.

For each of the chosen themes (or diseases), we established a literature search strategy to retrieve management recommendations. We selected only recommendations that were both backed up by evidence and were published after 2000. Recommendations were weighted according to their publication date. Data was obtained from learned or professional societies or agencies in France, the United States, or Great Britain: the French Health Products Safety Agency (ANSM or *Agence Française de Sécurité Sanitaire des Produits de Santé*), the French National Authority for Health (*Haute Autorité de Santé Française*), the French Society for Pediatricians (*Société Française de Pédiatrie*), the American Academy of Pediatrics (National Guideline Clearing House), and finally the National Institute for Health and Clinical Evidence, Cochrane Library (UK). We used the following databases for the origin of pharmacological agents, the commercially available forms, and potential drug-drug interactions: Thériaque [12], Micromedex [13], Lexi-Comp's Pediatric & Neonatal Dosage Handbook [14], and the French medical journal 'La Revue Prescrire' [15]. We also used the MEDLINE database to search for examples of medication error and inappropriate prescription.

We validated the propositions included in POPI by a two round Delphi method [16,17]. The aim of the Delphi method is to achieve a convergence of opinion and a general consensus on a particular topic, by questioning experts through successive questionnaires. The experts were chosen according to their area of expertise, and included pediatricians most of who are members of the French Society of Pediatricians, and pharmacists mostly members of the French Society of Clinical Pharmacy. Each expert has disclosed his conflicts of interest.

The fisrt round questionnaire comprised all of the propositions included in POPI draft, which were graded according to a nine-point Likert scale for agreement. A score of 1 indicates 'total disagreement' whereas a score of 9 'total agreement', with intermediate values indicating degrees of agreement between these two extremes. The experts were also encouraged to make suggestions about the dose, the frequency, and the duration of treatment, provided that they could cite appropriate references to back up these suggestions. The experts could also comment on the propositions. The questionnaire was available online via the website 'SurveyMonkey', which is a tool designed to conduct web-based surveys [18].

Each of the panelists who had participated in the first round was sent the second-round questionnaire. These panelists were also given feedback on the results of the first round (their own previous individual ratings, median panel rating, and frequency distribution of the agreement rating). The panelists were then asked to re-rate each proposition based on both their own opinion and the group response to the previous round.

Only the propositions that obtained a median score in the upper tertile (between 7 and 9) with an agreement of more than 65% of participants in the first round of Delphi were retained. These propositions were modified according to the experts' comments, and were subjected to a second round of questioning. Only the propositions that obtained a median score between 7 and 9 with an agreement of more than 75% of participants in this second round were retained. The experts had two weeks to reply to the questionnaire. For both the first and second questionnaire, a reminder was sent out one and two weeks before the deadline.

Experts characteristics were also noted, including their age, their place of work, and their number of years of experience.

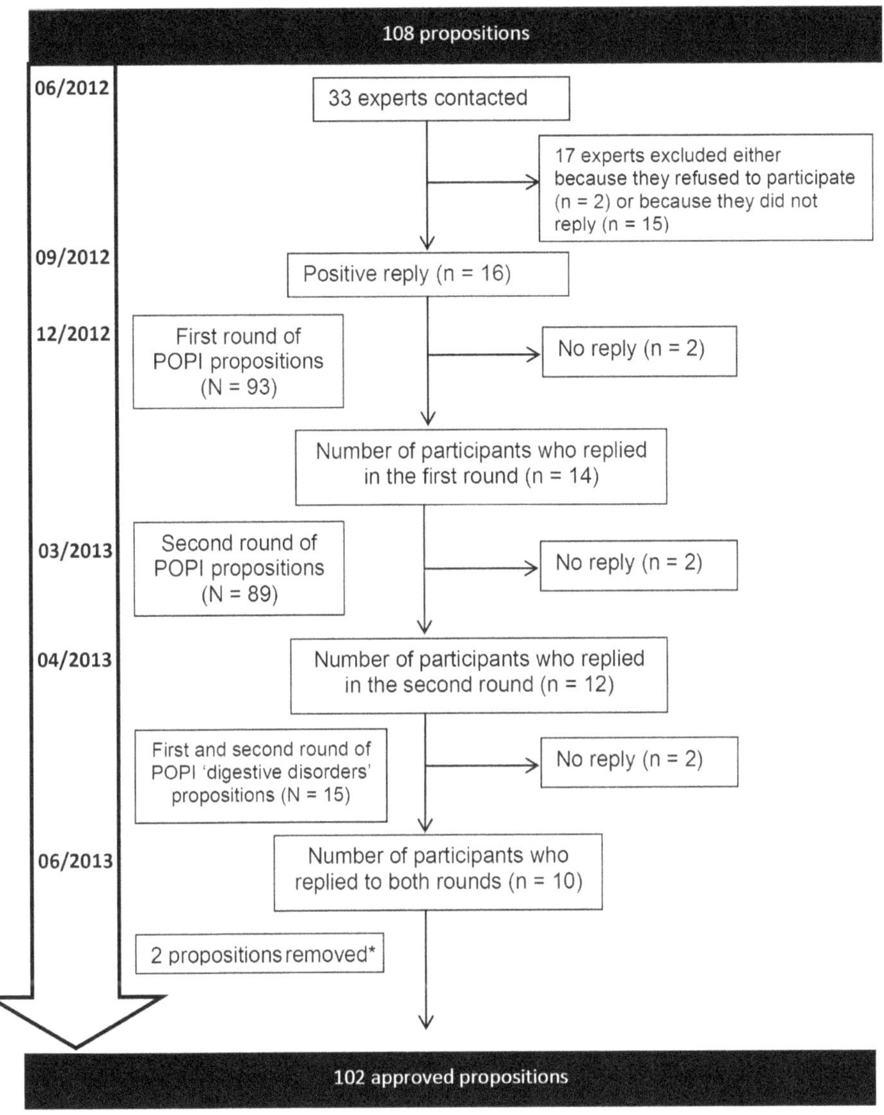

Figure 1. Workflow for the validation of POPI.*An item involving codeine was removed subsequent to the validation of the propositions included in POPI, following the revelation of new contraindications for this drug in children under 12 years old [22]. N: Number of items; n: number of panelists.

Qualitative data are expressed as numbers (percentages) and quantitative data as median (quartiles) and minima, maxima. SAS software (VERSION 9.3) was used for statistical analysis.

The study was reviewed and approved by the Robert-Debré institutional review board.

Results

The first draft of POPI contained 108 propositions: 80 propositions of Inappropriate Prescription (IP) and 28 propositions of Omission of Prescription (OP). These propositions were classified into five broad categories: digestive problems (n = 15); Ear, Nose and Throat (ENT) problems or pulmonary problems (n = 23); dermatological problems (n = 30); neuropsychiatric disorders (n = 16); and diverse illnesses (n = 24). Each category was further divided into several medical conditions. We contacted 33 experts between June and September 2012. Sixteen experts agreed to participate in the development of the POPI tool. The median expert age was 49 years, range [32–66 years] and their median number of years of experience was 25 years, range [3–40 years]. The ratio of pediatricians to pharmacists was 1:1. Half were working in a hospital environment and the other half were working in the community. Each physician working within a hospital environment was specialized in a particular medical domain: endocrinology, hematology, nephrology, cancerology, or pulmonology.

Figure 1 shows the workflow of the study. The first round questionnaire was sent to the 16 experts at the start of December 2012 and the replies were collected by the start of January 2013; 14 (14/16, 87.5%) participants responded to the first round of questions. Two propositions received 13 replies because one expert did not use the answer grid properly. More than 65% of the panelists gave top-tertile (7–9) agreement to 93 propositions. Ten propositions were modified according to the experts' comments during this first round of questions producing 93 propositions for the second round.

Table 1. Propositions validated for use in POPI.

DIVERSE ILLNESSES	**PAIN AND FEVER**
	Inappropriate prescriptions
	Prescription of two alternating antipyretics as a first-line treatment
	Prescription of a medication other than paracetamol as a first line treatment (except in the case of migraine)
	Rectal administration of paracetamol as a first-line treatment
	The combined use of two NSAIDs
	Oral solutions of ibuprofen administered in more than three doses per day using a graduated pipette of 10mg/kg (other than Advil)
	Opiates to treat migraine attacks
	Omissions
	Failure to give sugar solution to new-born babies and infants under four months old two minutes prior to venipuncture
	Failure to give an osmotic laxative to patients being treated with morphine for a period of more than 48 hours
	URINARY INFECTIONS
	Inappropriate prescriptions
	Nitrofurantoin used as a prophylactic
	Nitrofurantoin used as a curative agent in children under six years of age, or indeed any other antibiotic if avoidable
	Antibiotic prophylaxis following an initial infection without complications (except in the case of uropathy)
	Antibiotic prophylaxis in the case of asymptomatic bacterial infection (except in the case of uropathy)
	VITAMIN SUPPLEMENTS AND ANTIBIOTIC PROPHYLAXIS
	Inappropriate prescriptions
	Fluoride supplements prior to six months of age
	Omissions
	Insufficient intake of vitamin D. Minimum vitamin D intake: Breastfed baby = 1 000 to 1 200 IU/day; Infant <18 months of age (milk enriched in vitamin D) = 600 to 800 IU/day; Child aged between 18 months and five years, and adolescents aged between 10 and 18 years: two quarterly loading doses of 80 000 to 100 000 IU/day in winter (adolescents can take this dose in one go)
	Antibiotic prophylaxis with phenoxymethylpenicillin (Oracilline) starting from two months of age and lasting until five years of age for children with sickle-cell anemia: 100 000 IU/kg/day (in two doses) for children weighing 10kg or less and 50 000 IU/kg/day for children weighing over 10kg (also in two doses)
	MOSQUITOS
	Inappropriate prescriptions
	The use of skin repellents in infants less than six months old and picardin in children less than 24 months old
	Citronella (lemon grass) oil (essential oil)
	Anti-insect bracelets to protect against mosquitos and ticks
	Ultrasonic pest control devices, vitamin B1, homeopathy, electric bug zappers, sticky tapes without insecticide
	Omissions
	DEET: "30%" (max) before 12 years old; "50%" (max) after 12 years old
	IR3535: "20%" (max) before 24 months old; "35%" (max) after 24 months old
	Mosquito nets and clothes treated with pyrethroids
DIGESTIVE PROBLEMS	**NAUSEA, VOMITTING, OR GASTROESOPHAGEAL REFLUX**
	Inappropriate prescriptions
	Metoclopramide
	Domperidone
	Oral administration of an intravenous proton pump inhibitor (notably by nasogastric tube)
	Gastric antisecretory drugs to treat gastroesophageal reflux, dyspepsia, the crying of new-born babies (in the absence of any other signs or symptoms), as well as faintness in infants
	The combined use of proton pump inhibitors and NSAIDs, for a short period of time, in patients without risk factors
	The use of type H2 antihistamines for long periods of treatment
	Erythromycin as a prokinetic agent
	The use of setrons (5-HT3 antagonists) for chemotherapy-associated nausea and vomiting
	Omissions
	Oral rehydration solution
	DIARRHEA

Table 1. Cont.

	Inappropriate prescriptions
	Loperamide before 3 years of age
	Loperamide in the case of invasive diarrhea
	The use of Diosmectite (Smecta) in combination with another medication
	The use of Saccharomyces boulardii (Ultralevure) in powder form, or in a capsule that has to be opened prior to ingestion, to treat patients with a central venous catheter or an immunodeficiency
	Intestinal antiseptics
	Omissions
	Oral rehydration solution
-ENT-PULMONARY PROBLEMS	**COUGH**
	Inappropriate prescriptions
	Pholcodine
	Mucolytic drugs, mucokinetic drugs, or helicidine before two years of age
	Alimemazine (Theralene), oxomemazine (Toplexil), promethazine (Phenergan, and other types)
	Terpene-based suppositories
	Omissions
	Failure to propose a whooping cough booster vaccine for adults who are likely to become parents in the coming months or years (only applicable if the previous vaccination was more than 10 years ago). This booster vaccination should also be proposed to the family and entourage of expectant parents (parents, grand-parents, nannies/child minders)
	BRONCHIOLITIS IN INFANTS
	Inappropriate prescriptions
	Beta2 agonists, corticosteroids to treat an infant's first case of bronchiolitis
	H1-antagonists, cough suppressants, mucolytic drugs, or ribavirin to treat bronchiolitis
	Antibiotics in the absence of signs indicating a bacterial infection (acute otitis media, fever, etc.)
	Omissions
	0.9% NaCl to relieve nasal congestion (not applicable if nasal congestion is already being treated with 3% NaCl delivered by a nebulizer)
	Palivizumab in the following cases: (1) babies born both at less than 35 weeks of gestation and less than six months prior to the onset of a seasonal RSV epidemic; (2) children less than two years old who have received treatment for bronchopulmonary dysplasia in the past six months; (3) children less than two years old suffering from congenital heart disease with hemodynamic abnormalities
	ENT INFECTIONS
	Inappropriate prescriptions
	An antibiotic other than amoxicillin as a first-line treatment for acute otitis media, strep throat, or sinusitis (provided that the patient is not allergic to amoxicillin). An effective dose of amoxicillin for an pneumoncoccal infection is 80–90 mg/kg/day and an effective dose for a streptococcal infection is 50 mg/kg/day
	Antibiotic treatment for a sore throat, without a positive rapid diagnostic test result, in children less than three years old
	Antibiotics for nasopharyngitis, congestive otitis, sore throat before three years of age, or laryngitis; antibiotics as a first-line treatment for acute otitis media showing few symptoms, before two years of age
	Antibiotics to treat otitis media with effusion (OME), except in the case of hearing loss or if OME lasts for more than three months
	Corticosteroids to treat acute suppurative otitis media, nasopharyngitis, or strep throat
	Nasal or oral decongestant (oxymetazoline (Aturgyl), pseudoephedrine (Sudafed), naphazoline (Derinox), ephedrine (Rhinamide), tuaminoheptane (Rhinofluimicil), phenylephrine (Humoxal))
	H1-antagonists with sedative or atropine-like effects (pheniramine, chlorpheniramine), or camphor; inhalers, nasal sprays, or suppositories containing menthol (or any terpene derivatives) before 30 months of age
	Ethanolamine tenoate (Rhinotrophyl) and other nasal antiseptics
	Ear drops in the case of acute otitis media
	Omissions
	Doses in mg for drinkable (solutions of) amoxicillin or josamycin
	Paracetamol combined with antibiotic treatment for ear infections to relieve pain
	ASTHMA
	Inappropriate prescriptions
	Ketotifen and other H1-antagonists, sodium cromoglycate
	Cough suppressants
	Omissions

Table 1. Cont.

	Asthma inhaler appropriate for the child's age
	Preventative treatment (inhaled corticosteroids) in the case of persistent asthma
DERMATOLOGICAL PROBLEMS	**ACNE VULGARIS**
	Inappropriate prescriptions
	Minocycline
	Isotretinoin in combination with a member of the tetracycline family of antibiotics
	The combined use of an oral and a local antibiotic
	Oral or local antibiotics as a monotherapy (not in combination with another drug)
	Cyproterone+ethinylestradiol (Diane 35) as a contraceptive to allow isotretinoin per os
	Androgenic progestins (levonorgestrel, norgestrel, norethisterone, lynestrenol, dienogest, contraceptive implants or vaginal rings)
	Omissions
	Contraception (provided with a logbook/diary) for menstruating girls taking isotretinoin
	Topical treatment (benzoyl peroxide, retinoids, or both) in combination with antibiotic therapy
	SCABIES
	Inappropriate prescriptions
	The application of benzyl benzoate (Ascabiol) for periods longer than eight hours for infants and 12 hours for children or for pregnant girls
	Omissions
	A second dose of ivermectin two weeks after the first
	Decontamination of household linen and clothes and treatment for other family members
	LICE
	Inappropriate prescriptions
	The use of aerosols for infants, children with asthma, or children showing asthma-like symptoms such as dyspnea
	RINGWORM
	Inappropriate prescriptions
	Treatment other than griseofulvin for Microsporum
	Omissions
	Topical treatment combined with an orally-administered treatment
	Griseofulvin taken during a meal containing a moderate amount of fat
	IMPETIGO
	Inappropriate prescriptions
	The combination of locally applied and orally administered antibiotic
	Fewer than two applications per day for topical antibiotics
	Any antibiotic other than mupirocin as a first-line treatment (except in cases of hypersensitivity to mupirocin)
	HERPES SIMPLEX
	Inappropriate prescriptions
	Topical agents containing corticosteroids
	Topical agents containing acyclovir before six years of age
	Omissions
	Paracetamol during an outbreak of herpes
	Orally administered acyclovir to treat primary herpetic gingivostomatitis
	ATOPIC ECZEMA
	Inappropriate prescriptions
	A strong dermocorticoid (clobetasol propionate 0.05% Dermoval, betamethasone dipropionate Diprosone) applied to the face, the armpits or groin, and the backside of babies or young children
	More than one application per day of a dermocorticoid, except in cases of severe lichenification
	Local or systemic antihistamine during the treatment of outbreaks
	Topically applied 0.03% tacrolimus before two years of age
	Topically applied 0.1% tacrolimus before 16 years of age
	Oral corticosteroids to treat outbreaks

Table 1. Cont.

NEUROPSYCHIATRIC DISORDERS	**EPILEPSY**
	Inappropriate prescriptions
	Carbamazepine, gabapentin, oxcarbazepine, phenytoin, pregabalin, tiagabine, or vigabatrin in the case of myoclonic epilepsy
	Carbamazepine, gabapentin, oxcarbazepine, phenytoin, pregabaline, tiagabine, or vigabatrin in the case of epilepsy with absence seizures (especially for childhood absence epilepsy or juvenile absence epilepsy)
	Levetiracetam, oxcarbamazepine in mL or in mg without systematically writing XX mg per Y mL
	DEPRESSION
	Inappropriate prescriptions
	An SSRI antidepressant other than fluoxetine as a first-line treatment (in the case of pharmacotherapy)
	Tricyclic antidepressants to treat depression
	NOCTURNAL ENURESIS
	Inappropriate prescriptions
	Desmopressin administered by a nasal spray
	Desmopressin in the case of daytime symptoms
	An anticholinergic agent used as a monotherapy in the absence of daytime symptoms
	Tricyclic agents in combination with anticholinergic agents
	Tricyclic agents as a first-line treatment
	ANOREXIA
	Inappropriate prescriptions
	Cyproheptadine (Periactin), clonidine
	ATTENTION DEFICIT DISORDER WITH OR WITHOUT HYPERACTIVITY
	Inappropriate prescriptions
	Pharmacological treatment before age six (before school), except in severe cases
	Antipsychotic drugs to treat attention deficit disorder without hyperactivity
	Slow release methylphenidate as two doses per day, rather than only one dose
	Omissions
	Recording a growth chart (height and weight) if the patient is taking methylphenidate

The second questionnaire was submitted at the end of March 2013 and the replies were collected within one month. During this second round of questions, 85.5% (12/14) of participants replied. More than 75% of the panelists gave top-tertile agreement to all the 93 propositions submitted.

The propositions involving the category 'digestive problems' (n = 15) were submitted separately in April 2013 for 2 rounds rating. All of these propositions were unanimously accepted during two rounds of questions that took place between April and May 2013. Ten experts participated in these rounds of questions (i.e. 71.5% of the 14 experts who replied in the initial survey carried out between December 2012 and January 2013.

Table 1 shows the 102 propositions that were validated for use in POPI. A proposition involving codeine was removed subsequent to the validation of POPI, following the revelation of new contraindications for this drug in children under 12 years old [19]. Another proposition about the use of permethrin for lice was removed because of new recommendation to use dimeticone first (lack of resistance) [20]. Table 2 summarizes the references justification for each table 1 pathology.

Discussion

POPI (Pediatrics: Omission of Prescriptions and Inappropriate prescriptions) is the first tool that has been designed to detect the omission of prescriptions or inappropriate prescriptions specifically in pediatric patients [21]. If polymedication is unusual for children, there are however multiple health care professional who prescribe or counsel drug for children: general practitioner, paediatricians, pharmacists, nurses, midwives etc.

The POPI criteria are based on the same classification system as the STOPP/START criteria, (i.e. according to the major biological systems [8]). We selected this form because such lists have been successfully used to detect preventable adverse drug events [8,9,22]. The Beers criteria were updated in 2012 to incorporate this classification system [6]. Our tool, which was developed using a Delphi method, was validated by 14 health care professionals. The Delphi method is one of the main method used for the development of tools designed to detect inappropriate prescriptions in geriatric patients [6,8,22–26]. The number of experts to develop geriatric tools vary between 11 and 32 and their specialties include pharmacy, psychopharmacology, pharmacology, pharmacoepidemiology, internal medicine or geriatrics [6,7,23,24,26]. For the validation of POPI, the number of experts in each category was equal so as to ensure that hospital and community environments were equally represented. There is currently no consensus regarding the composition of such panels of experts; there are no recommendations about the numbers or qualifications of experts to be included. More pharmacists were involved in the validation of the POPI criteria than in the validation of similar criteria that were developed for geriatrics.

Table 2. References justification for each POPI statement.

Pain and Fever
Mise au point sur la prise en charge de la fièvre chez l'enfant – **AFSSAPS** -2005
Fever and Antipyretic use in children – American Academy of Pediatrics (AAP) -2011
Feverish illness in children – **NICE** -2007
Prise en charge médicamenteuse de la douleur aiguë et chronique chez l'enfant - **AFSSAPS** -2009
Prevention and Management of Pain in the Neonate - **AAP** -2006
Urinary Infections
Nitrofurantoïne et risque de survenue d'effets indésirables hépatiques et pulmonaires lors de traitements prolongés – **AFSSAPS** -2011
Urinary tract infection in children – **NICE** -2007
Vitamin Supplements and Antibiotic Prophylaxis
Utilisation du fluor dans la prévention de la carie dentaire avant l'âge de 18 ans – **AFSSAPS** -10/2008
Dents et fluor chez les enfants – **Idées-Forces Prescrire** – Novembre 2011
Alimentation du nourrisson et de l'enfant en bas âge. Réalisation pratique – **SFP** (Société Française de Pédiatrie) -2003
La Vitamine D : une vitamine toujours d'actualité chez l'enfant et l'adolescent. Mise au point par le Comité de nutrition de la Société française de pédiatrie – **SFP** -2012
Prise en charge de la drépanocytose chez l'enfant et l'adolescent – **HAS** -09/2005
Mosquitos
Protection Antivectorielle RBP – **Société Française de Parasitologie** -2010
BEH -29 mai 2012- n°20-21
Prévention des piqûres de moustiques ou des morsures de tiques – **Idées-Forces Prescrire** – Juin 2012
Nausea, Vomitting, or Gastroesophageal Reflux
Contre-indication des spécialités à base de métoclopramide (Primpéran et génériques) chez l'enfant et l'adolescent et renforcement des informations sur les risques neurologiques et cardiovasculaires – **AFSSAPS** - Lettre aux professionnels de santé -08/02/2012
Antisécrétoires gastriques chez l'enfant – **AFSSAPS** -06/2008
Pediatric Gastroesophageal Reflux Clinical Practice Guidelines – **NASPGHAN** -2009
Traitement médicamenteux des diarrhées aiguës infectieuses du nourrisson et de l'enfant - **SFP** -2002
Managing Acute Gastroenteritis Among Children: Oral Rehydration, Maintenance, and Nutritional Therapy - Centers for Disease Control and Prevention – **AAP** -2003
Diarrhoea and vomiting in children under 5– **NICE** -2009
Diarrhea
Diarrhoea and vomiting in children under 5– **NICE** -2009
Traitement médicamenteux des diarrhées aiguës infectieuses du nourrisson et de l'enfant – **SFP** -2002
Managing Acute Gastroenteritis Among Children: Oral Rehydration, Maintenance, and Nutritional Therapy - Centers for Disease Control and Prevention – **AAP** -2003
Cough
Pholcodine – **AFSSSAPS** -2011
Toux aiguë chez les enfants de moins de 2 ans – AFSSAPS -2010
BHE – Calendrier vaccinal -10 avril 2012- n°14-15
Bronchiolotis in Infants
Diagnosis and Management of Bronchiolitis – **AAP** -2006
Bronchiolite du nourrisson – Conférence de consensus – HAS -2000
Bronchiolite chez les nourrissons – Traitement – **Idées-Forces Prescrire** – Septembre 2011
Ear Infections
Antibiothérapie dans les infections respiratoires hautes – **SFP** -12/2011
Respiratory tract infections – **NICE** -2011
Rhume : traitements – **Idées-Forces Prescrire** – Avril 2011
Otite moyenne aiguë : traitement antibiotique – **Idées-Forces Prescrire** – Janvier 2011
Diagnosis and Management of Acute Otitis Media – **AAP** -2004
Asthma
Global Initiative for Asthma -2011
Asthme de l'enfant de moins de 36 mois : diagnostic, prise en charge et traitement en dehors des épisodes aigus – **HAS** – Mars 2009
Managing Asthma Long Term In Children 0-4 and 5-11 Years of Age – **NHLBI** -2007
Acne Vulgaris
Recommandations de bonne pratique – **AFSSAPS**-2007

Table 2. Cont.

Minocycline : restriction d'utilisation en raison d'un risque de syndromes d'hypersensibilité graves et d'atteintes auto-immunes – Lettre aux professionnels de santé – **ANSM** -2012

Isotrétinoïne orale – Renforcement du Programme de Prévention des Grossesses et rappel sur la survenue éventuelle de troubles psychiatriques – **AFSSAPS** -05/ 2009

Scabies

Sexually Transmitted Diseases Treatment Guidelines – **CDC** -2010

Gale – **Avis du conseil supérieur d'hygiène publique de France** -2003

Lice

Poux du cuir chevelu – **La Revue Prescrire N°365**-2014

Ringworm

Guidelines for the Management of Tinea Capitis in Children – **ESPD** -2010

Impetigo

Prescription des antibiotiques par voie locale dans les infections cutanées bactériennes primitives et secondaires – **AFSSAPS** -2004

Herpes Simplex

Prise en charge de l'herpès cutanéo-muqueux chez le sujet immunocompétent – **SFD** -2001

Atopic Eczema

Prise en charge de la dermatite atopique de l'enfant – **Société Française de Dermatologie** -2005

Atopic eczema in children – **NICE** -2007

Protopic – **HAS** – Commission transparence -2011

Epilepsy

Epilepsy – **NICE** -2012

Epilepsies graves – **HAS** -07/2007

Depression

Bon usage des antidépresseurs au cours de la dépression de l'enfant et de l'adolescent – **AFSSAPS** – Janvier 2008

Depression in children and young people – **NICE** -2009

Nocturnal Enuresis

Utilisation de la desmopressine (Minirin) dans l'énurésie nocturne isolée chez l'enfant – **AFSSAPS** -2006

Nocturnal enuresis – **NICE** -2010

Anorexia

Anorexie : recommandation pour la pratique clinique – **HAS** – Juin 2010

Attention Deficit Disorder with or withou Hyperactivity

Attention deficit hyperactivity disorder Diagnosis and management of ADHD in children, young people and adults – **NICE** -2008

ADHD : Clinical Practice Guideline for the Diagnosis, Evaluation, and Treatment of Attention-Deficit/Hyperactiviy Disorder in Children and Adolescents – **AAP** -2010

This strong representation is partly because the initial project was developed by hospital pharmacists. One limitation of our study in the absence of general practitioners from our panel of experts. Indeed, these doctors regularly deliver health care to children in the community and hence could greatly benefit from the use of POPI.

Few data about inappropriate prescriptions have been published in pediatric patients. Although studies have investigated medication errors [27–29], not one study has examined the link between the rate of medication errors and the rate of adverse drug events in pediatrics. In adults, it is estimated that around one adverse drug occurs for every 100 medication errors [30,31]. There is increasing recognition that rational prescribing is an important issue in children [2].

The different propositions included in POPI were based on recommendations from recognized learned and academic societies and were preselected by the initial working group. Of the 108 propositions, 104 were validated by experts in the first round of Delphi, and all of the propositions submitted in the second round were subsequently validated. The final version of the POPI criteria contains 79 examples of inappropriate prescription and 25 examples of omission of prescription. The modifications that were made during the first and second rounds of Delphi involved refinements in the phrasing and exact details of the propositions. Overall, the experts were very responsive, and we collected around 80% of replies within three weeks of sending the questionnaires. The feedback of the experts was very positive and many of them commented that they were very interested in the development of POPI. The STOPP/START criteria contained as many propositions to validate as the POPI criteria. For STOPP/START, a consensus was obtained for 77 out of 80 propositions that were submitted in the first round [7]. For the criteria developed by Laroche *et al.* a consensus was reached for 33 out of 37 criteria during the first round [26]. This illustrates the importance of preselecting the propositions prior to their submission to experts, to ensure that a consensus will be reached on the largest possible number of propositions. The time that experts were given to reply to questionnaires during the development of criteria similar to POPI is often not stated, with the exception of STOPP/START, in which all answers were obtained within two months [7]. We estimated that one month (a minimum of two weeks with two reminders) was a reasonable amount of time for the completion of the questionnaire. This time constraint was applied to both rounds of questions.

Our criteria contain more propositions than the STOPP/START criteria (83 propositions vs. 102 for POPI) and more than the updated 2012 Beers criteria (85 propositions). The classification of these propositions by biological system makes the POPI criteria fast to use, and POPI considers only those medical conditions that require prescriptions. The categories that we used are not the same as those in the STOPP/START criteria or the updated 2012 Beers criteria because diseases that affect children are not the same as those that affect the elderly. Indeed, in most criteria designed for use in geriatrics, psychiatry and cardiology constitute major categories [6,7,26], whereas the categories that contain the most propositions in POPI are respiratory problems, gastroenterology, and dermatology.

The POPI criteria have not yet been tested in the setting of routine prescriptions and needs validating clinically. Two studies will be carried out with this objective in mind. One study will examine the degree of inter-rater agreement of the various propositions of POPI, by assessing the percentage of concordance corrected for chance agreement, termed κ (Kappa). This will provide a measure of the precision of the POPI criteria. A second study will examine the capacity of the POPI criteria to identify medication errors and evaluate the safety of drug used (involved drugs, indication) prospectively.

Conclusion

We created the first set of criteria for the detection of inappropriate prescriptions and the omission of prescriptions in pediatrics. The resulting tool, named POPI, is available to all medical professionals (clinicians, pharmacists, in hospital or community working environment) liable to prescribe or dispense medication to children.

Acknowledgments

Thanks to our panelists: F Amouroux, R Assathiany, JP Blanc, V Breant, D Cau, L Cret, N Davoust, M Detavernier, N Duval-Ehrenfeld, A Lecoeur, F Netzer, L Priqueler, H Sarda, E Séror, B Virey, C Wehrle.

Thanks to the PMSI unit at the Robert-Debré University Hospital for the data concerning the patients' reasons for hospitalizations.

Thanks to S Auvin, E Bourrat, A Hubert, MF Le Heuzey, C Madre.

Author Contributions

Conceived and designed the experiments: SPL TW FA OB. Performed the experiments: SPL TW FA OB. Analyzed the data: TW RB CA. Contributed reagents/materials/analysis tools: SPL TW FA RB CA OB. Contributed to the writing of the manuscript: SPL TW FA RB CA OB.

References

1. WHO | Medicines: rational use of medicines (n.d.). WHO. Available: http://www.who.int/mediacentre/factsheets/fs338/en/. Accessed 2014 May 12.
2. Choonara I (2013) Rational prescribing is important in all settings. Arch Dis Child 98: 720–720. doi:10.1136/archdischild-2013-304559.
3. Risk R, Naismith H, Burnett A, Moore SE, Cham M, et al. (2013) Rational prescribing in paediatrics in a resource-limited setting. Arch Dis Child 98: 503–509. doi:10.1136/archdischild-2012-302987.
4. Inappropriate Prescribing - MeSH - NCBI (n.d.). Available: http://www.ncbi.nlm.nih.gov/mesh?term = inappropriate%20prescription. Accessed 2012 June 18.
5. Legrain S, others (2005) Consommation médicamenteuse chez le sujet âgé. Consomm Prescr Iatrogénie Obs. Available: http://has-sante.fr/portail/upload/docs/application/pdf/pmsa_synth_biblio_2006_08_28_16_44_51_580.pdf. Accessed 2012 June 17.
6. Fick D, Semla T, Beizer J, Brandt N (2012) American Geriatrics Society Updated Beers Criteria for Potentially Inappropriate Medication Use in Older Adults - J Am Geriatrics Society - 2012.pdf. J Am Geriatr Soc 60: 616–631. doi:10.1111/j.1532-5415.2012.03923.x.
7. Gallagher P, Ryan C, Kennedy J, O'Mahony D (2008) STOPP (Screening Tool of Older Person's Prescriptions) and START (Screening Tool to Alert doctors to Right Treatment). Consensus validation. Int J Clin Pharmacol Ther 46: 72–83.
8. Gallagher P, O'Mahony D (2008) STOPP (Screening Tool of Older Persons' potentially inappropriate Prescriptions): application to acutely ill elderly patients and comparison with Beers' criteria. Age Ageing 37: 673–679. doi:10.1093/ageing/afn197.
9. Gallagher P, O'Connor M, O'Mahony D (2011) Prevention of Potentially Inappropriate Prescribing for Elderly Patients: A Randomized Controlled Trial Using STOPP/START Criteria. Clin Pharmacol Ther 89: 845–854. doi:10.1038/clpt.2011.44.
10. Prot-Labarthe S, Vercheval C, Angoulvant F, Brion F, Bourdon O (2011) «POPI; pédiatrie: omissions et prescriptions inappropriées». Outil d'identification des prescriptions inappropriées chez l'enfant. Arch Pédiatrie Organe Off Sociéte Fr Pédiatrie 18: 1231–1232. doi:10.1016/j.arcped.2011.08.019.
11. ameli.fr - Affection de longue durée (ALD) (n.d.). Available: http://www.ameli.fr/l-assurance-maladie/statistiques-et-publications/donnees-statistiques/affection-de-longue-duree-ald/index.php. Accessed 2012 June 18.
12. Thériaque (n.d.). Available: http://www.theriaque.org. Accessed: 2012 July 3.
13. Thomson Healthcare Products (n.d.). Available: http://www.thomsonhc.com/home/dispatch. Accessed: 2012 July 3.
14. Taketomo CK, Hodding JH, Kraus DM (2011) Pediatric & neonatal dosage handbook: a comprehensive resource for all clinicians treating pediatric and neonatal patients. Hudson, Ohio; [United States]: Lexi-Comp; American Pharmacists Association.
15. La Revue Prescrire (n.d.). Rev Prescrire. Available: http://www.prescrire.org/fr/. Accessed Accessed: 2012 July 12.
16. Bourrée F, Michel P, Salmi LR (2008) Methodes de consensus: Revue des méthodes originales et de leurs grandes variantes utilisées en santé publique. Rev Epidémiologie Santé Publique 56.
17. Hsu CC, Sandford BA (2007) The Delphi technique: Making sense of consensus. Pract Assess Res Eval 12: 1–8.
18. SurveyMonkey (n.d.) SurveyMonkey. SurveyMonkey. Available: http://fr.surveymonkey.net/home/. Accessed: 2012 Sept 12.
19. ANSM (2013) Médicaments à base de tétrazépam, d'almitrine, de ranélate de strontium et de codéine (chez l'enfant) - Retour d'information sur le PRAC - ANSM. Médicam À Base Tétrazépam Almitrine Ranélate Strontium Codéine Chez Enfant - Retour Inf Sur Pr - ANSM. Available: http://ansm.sante.fr/S-informer/Du-cote-de-l-Agence-europeenne-des-medicaments-Retours-d-information-sur-le-PRAC/Medicaments-a-base-de-tetrazepam-d-almitrine-de-ranelate-de-strontium-et-de-codeine-chez-l-enfant-Retour-d-information-sur-le-PRAC/(language)/fre-FR. Accessed 2013 June 23.
20. La Revue Prescrire (2014) Poux du cuir chevelu - Diméticone, substance pédiculicide de premier choix. Rev Prescrire 34: 198–202.
21. Kaufmann CP, Tremp R, Hersberger KE, Lampert ML (2013) Inappropriate prescribing: a systematic overview of published assessment tools. Eur J Clin Pharmacol. Available: http://link.springer.com/10.1007/s00228-013-1575-8. Accessed 2013 Dec 16.
22. Levy HB, Marcus EL, Christen C (2010) Beyond the beers criteria: A comparative overview of explicit criteria. Ann Pharmacother 44: 1968–1975.
23. Beers MH, Ouslander JG, Rollingher I, Reuben DB, Brooks J, et al. (1991) Explicit Criteria for Determining Inappropriate Medication Use in Nursing Home Residents. Arch Intern Med 151: 18255–32.
24. McLeod PJ, Huang AR, Tamblyn RM, Gayton DC (1997) Defining inappropriate practices in prescribing for elderly people: a national consensus panel. Can Med Assoc J 156: 385.
25. Waller JL, Maclean JR (2003) Updating the Beers Criteria for potentially inappropriate medication use in older adults. Arch Intern Med 163: 2716–2724.
26. Laroche M-L, Charmes J-P, Merle L (2007) Potentially inappropriate medications in the elderly: a French consensus panel list. Eur J Clin Pharmacol 63: 725–731. doi:10.1007/s00228-007-0324-2.
27. Kaushal R, Bates DW, Landrigan C, McKenna KJ, Clapp MD, et al. (2001) Medication errors and adverse drug events in pediatric inpatients. JAMA J Am Med Assoc 285: 2114.
28. Kaushal R, Goldmann DA, Keohane CA, Abramson EL, Woolf S, et al. (2010) Medication errors in paediatric outpatients. Qual Saf Health Care 19: 1–6. doi:10.1136/qshc.2008.031179.
29. Davis T (2010) Paediatric prescribing errors. Arch Dis Child 96: 489–491. doi:10.1136/adc.2010.200295.
30. Bates DW, Boyle DL, Vliet MBV, Schneider J, Leape L (1995) Relationship between medication errors and adverse drug events. J Gen Intern Med 10: 199–205.
31. Schmitt E (1999) Le risque médicamenteux nosocomial: circuit hospitalier du médicament et qualité des soins. Masson. IX–287 p.

15

Genetic Polymorphisms in Toll-Like Receptors among Pediatric Patients with Renal Parenchymal Infections of Different Clinical Severities

Chi-Hui Cheng[1,2]*, Yun-Shien Lee[3,4], Chee-Jen Chang[5], Tzou-Yien Lin[2,6]

1 Division of Pediatric Nephrology, Department of Pediatrics, Chang Gung Children's Hospital, Chang Gung Memorial Hospital, Taoyuan, Taiwan, **2** College of Medicine, Chang Gung University, Taoyuan, Taiwan, **3** Genomic Medicine Research Core Laboratory (GMRCL), Chang Gung Memorial Hospital, Taoyuan, Taiwan, **4** Department of Biotechnology, Ming-Chuan University, Taoyuan, Taiwan, **5** Statistical Center for Clinical Research, Chang Gung Memorial Hospital, Taoyuan, Taiwan, **6** Division of Pediatric Infectious Diseases, Department of Pediatrics, Chang Gung Children's Hospital, Chang Gung Memorial Hospital, Taoyuan, Taiwan

Abstract

Background: Although several studies have suggested single gene defects or variations in the genes associated with host immune response could confer differences in susceptibility to urinary pathogen invasion, no studies have examined the genetic polymorphisms in various toll-like receptors (TLRs) that activate innate immune responses in pediatric renal parenchymal infections of different clinical severities, namely acute pyelonephritis and the clinically more severe disease, acute lobar nephronia.

Methodology: Patients who fulfilled the diagnostic criteria for acute pyelonephritis (APN) and acute lobar nephronia (ALN) without underlying diseases or structural anomalies, except for vesicoureteral reflux (VUR), were enrolled. Genotyping of the single nucleotide polymorphisms (SNPs) in the genes encoding TLR-1, TLR-2, TLR-4, TLR-5, and TLR-6 was performed by matrix-assisted laser desorption/ionization time-of-flight-based mini-sequencing analysis.

Principal Findings: A total of 16 SNPs were selected for genotyping. Analysis of 96 normal and 48 patients' samples revealed that only four SNPs had heterozygosity rates >0.01. These SNPs were selected for further investigation. Hardy-Weinberg equilibrium was satisfied for the observed genotype frequencies. Statistically significant differences in the genotype frequency of *TLR-2* (rs3804100, T1350C) between controls and ALN or (APN+ALN) combined group were identified using the recessive model with the correction for multiple-SNP testing. Further genotype pattern frequency analysis in *TLR-2* SNPs (rs3804099 and rs3804100) showed significantly reduced occurrence of the rare allele homozygote (CC+CC) in the no-VUR subgroup of APN and ALN cases.

Conclusions: As the inflammatory responses in ALN patients are more severe than those in APN patients (higher CRP levels, longer duration of fever after antibiotic treatment), these findings suggest that the genetic variant in *TLR-2* (rs3804100, T1350C) may protect the host from severe urinary tract infections as ALN.

Editor: Ashok Kumar, Wayne State University School of Medicine, United States of America

Funding: Financial support was provided by the National Science Council of Taiwan (98-2314-B-182A-007-MY3) and Chang Gung Memorial Hospital (CMRPG 470033, 4A0111). The funders had no role in study design, data collection and analysis, decision to publish, or preparation of the manuscript.

Competing Interests: The authors have declared that no competing interests exist.

* E-mail: pedneph.cheng@msa.hinet.net

Introduction

Urinary tract infections (UTIs) are among the most prevalent infectious bacterial diseases in infants and children. The morbidity risk was estimated to be approximately 3% in prepubertal girls, 1% in prepubertal boys, and 8% in girls [1]. The clinical severity of UTIs ranges from uncomplicated lower urinary tract infections to frank abscess formation. Among the UTIs, acute lobar nephronia (ALN), also known as acute focal bacterial nephritis, presents as a localized nonliquefactive inflammatory renal bacterial infection and has previously been identified as a complicated form of acute renal infection, representing progression of the inflammatory process of acute pyelonephritis (APN) [2]. ALN may also represent a relatively early stage in renal abscess development [3]. It is generally accepted that renal parenchymal infections, including APN, ALN, and intrarenal abscess formation, are the more serious forms of UTI and have a longer duration of antibiotic treatment. Moreover, in some cases, surgical procedures are recommended for proper management [2,4,5].

Complex host-pathogen interactions determine patient susceptibility to UTIs and clinical severity. A number of studies have demonstrated that certain virulence factors associated with the uropathogenic bacterium Escherichia coli, a common clinical isolate, are more prevalent in specific UTIs [4,6]. Nevertheless, intra-individual variation in clinical presentation has been noted among UTI patients. This indicates that host factors such as mechanistic dysfunction [e.g., vesicoureteral reflux (VUR)] and

Table 1. Primers used for the amplification and mini-sequencing analysis of the SNPs.

Position	Primer sequence (5′→3′)	PCR product size	Mini-sequencing primer sequence (5′→3′)	Molecular weight of mini-sequencing product
TLR-1 (rs4833095), C>T	Sense: tccagctgaccctgtagctt	157 bp	caatgttgtttaaggtaaga	Primer: 6,195.06
	Anti-sense: ttctggcgaaacttcaaaca			T allele: 6,483.25
				C allele: 6,772.43
TLR-2 (rs3804099), C>T	Sense: tgctggacttaccttccttga	182 bp	agtttgaagtcaattcagaa	Primer: 6,164.05
	Anti-sense: ctcgcagttccaaacattcc			T allele: 6,781.45
				C allele: 6,437.23
TLR-2 (rs3804100), T>C	Sense: aaccggagagactttgctca	226 bp	agcacacgaatacacag	Primer: 5,181.42
	Anti-sense: gagttgcggcaaattcaaag			C allele: 5,454.60
				T allele: 5,798.82
TLR-5 (rs5744168), C>T	Sense: acggacttgacaacctccaa	223 bp	tacagaccttggatctc	Primer: 5,145.36
	Anti-sense: tcgggtatgcttggaataaaa			T allele: 5,762.76
				C allele: 5,418.55

genetic variation in the susceptibility to bacterial invasion and infection should not be overlooked [7–9].

The innate immune system has been recognized as the first line of defense against invading pathogens and plays a primary role in acute host defense [10]. Variations in genes that modulate innate immune responses may result in distinct clinical presentations in UTIs. Among these genes are those encoding Toll-like receptors (TLRs), which recognize pathogen-associated molecular patterns (PAMPs), and those encoding chemokines and chemokine receptors, which facilitate the migration of neutrophils to the infected urinary tract. Single gene defects or variations in these genes could confer differences in susceptibility to urinary pathogen invasion [7–9,11–13].

Escherichia coli, the most common uropathogen in renal parenchymal infections [4,5], is recognized by various TLRs, including TLR-1, TLR-2, TLR-4, TLR-5, TLR-6 (in humans and mice), and TLR-11 (in mice) [7,11,14,15]. Previous studies have shown that single nucleotide polymorphisms (SNPs) in the TLR-2 and TLR-4 genes can affect host susceptibility to UTIs [7,11,13,16–19]. In contrast, we did not observe this association for TLR-4 in APN and ALN [12].

To extend our previous analysis of genetic polymorphisms in pediatric patients with renal parenchymal infections [12], this study explored the correlations between polymorphisms in UTI-related TLR genes (TLR-1, TLR-2, TLR-4, TLR-5, and TLR-6) and clinical severity among pediatric patients with UTIs of different severities (APN and the clinically more severe disease, ALN). In addition, as VUR is a well-known risk factor for severe parenchymal infectious disease [8,20], a subgroup of APN and ALN patients without VUR was also examined to exclude the possible effects of VUR.

Materials and Methods

Ethics Statement

This investigation was approved by the Institutional Review Board of Chang Gung Memorial Hospital, and following a full explanation of the study, written informed consent was obtained from the parents of all patients.

Study Setting and Patient Selection Criteria

This study is a part of our continuing analyses of the pathogenic host and bacterial urovirulence factors related to APN and ALN [4,5,12]. The participating patients were admitted to Chang Gung Children's Hospital, a tertiary medical center located in a suburb of Taipei in northern Taiwan, between January 2004 and December 2008. Patients who fulfilled the diagnostic criteria for APN and ALN caused by *E. coli* while lacking any of the exclusion

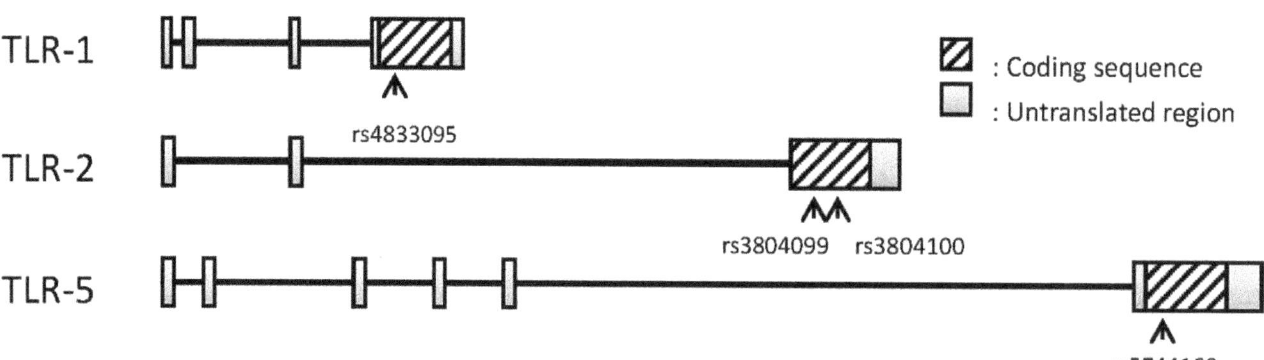

Figure 1. Position of the four SNPs that had heterozygosity rates >0.01 in each TLR sequence.

criteria were enrolled in the study. The controls were pediatric patients who presented to the outpatient clinic for reasons other than a UTI or severe infection and were interviewed to ensure that they did not have a history of UTI or severe infections as well as not having positive urine culture.

The diagnostic scheme for patients suspected of having APN or ALN was as described previously [2,4,5,12]. In brief, all patients with a suspected UTI because of the presence of pyuria (>5 white blood cells/high-power field) and fever with symptoms and signs related to UTIs (*e.g.*, pain, dysuria, and frequency of urination) or without focus underwent renal ultrasonography on the first or second day after admission. Computed tomography (CT) was performed immediately when the initial ultrasonographic findings met either of two criteria: evidence of unilateral or bilateral nephromegaly or a focal renal mass. For children who presented with borderline nephromegaly on ultrasonography, CT was performed when the child remained febrile for 72 h after the commencement of antibiotic therapy. A diagnosis of ALN was made on the basis of positive CT findings. Technetium 99m-dimercaptosuccinic acid scintigraphy (^{99m}Tc-DMSA) was performed within 3–7 days of admission in patients suspected of having a febrile UTI who did not satisfy the sonographic criteria for ALN. APN was defined as focal or diffuse areas of decreased ^{99m}Tc-DMSA uptake without evidence of cortical loss.

Patients with evidence of an underlying disease, including diabetes and immunodeficiency, or structural anomalies such as neurogenic bladder, posterior urethral valve, urinary diversion, bladder diverticulum, ureterocele, or urinary tract obstruction other than VUR were excluded.

Genotyping by Matrix-assisted Laser Desorption/ ionization Time-of-flight (MALDI-TOF)-based Mini-sequencing Analysis

SNPs in the genes encoding TLR-1, TLR-2, TLR-4, TLR-5, and TLR-6, as well as in their respective promoter regions, were identified in the NCBI dbSNP database [21]. A total of 16 SNPs (rs4833095, rs5743611, and rs5743618 for *TLR-1*; rs3804099, rs3804100, rs5743704, and rs5743708 for *TLR-2*; zA11547G, rs2149356, and rs5030710 for *TLR-4*; rs2072493, rs5744168, and rs5744174 for *TLR-5* and rs3821985, rs5743810 and rs5743815 for *TLR-6*) were selected for genotyping based on previous studies on Toll-like receptors polymorphisms on APN adult patients [7,11]. Analysis of 96 normal and 48 patients' samples revealed that only four SNPs had heterozygosity rates >0.01. These SNPs (Table 1, Figure 1) were used to analyze the control and patient genotypes by a MALDI-TOF-based mini-sequencing genotyping method.

Genomic DNA was extracted from peripheral blood lymphocytes using a Nucleospin® blood kit (Macherey-Nagel, Düren,

Table 2. Genotypic analysis of the SNPs.

SNP	Group	Genotype, *n* (%)			Log-additive model		Dominant model		Recessive model	
		00	01	11			(01, 11 *vs.* 00)		(11 *vs.* 00, 01)	
		CC	**CT**	**TT**	**OR (95% CI)**	***P*[a]**	**OR (95% CI)**	***P*[a]**	**OR (95% CI)**	***P*[a]**
TLR-1	Control	75 (34.1)	113 (51.4)	32 (14.5)			1.00		1.00	
(rs4833095)	APN	44 (40.7)	51 (47.2)	13 (12.0)	0.81 (0.57, 1.15)	0.243	0.75 (0.47, 1.21)	0.241	0.80 (0.40, 1.69)	0.531
	ALN	59 (35.1)	81 (48.2)	28 (16.7)	1.02 (0.76, 1.37)	0.876	0.96 (0.63, 1.46)	0.833	1.17 (0.68, 2.04)	0.568
	Combined[b]	103 (37.3)	132 (47.8)	41 (14.9)	0.94 (0.72, 1.22)	0.635	0.87 (0.60, 1.26)	0.456	1.02 (0.62, 1.69)	0.923
		TT	**TC**	**CC**	**OR (95% CI)**	***P***	**OR (95% CI)**	***P***	**OR (95% CI)**	***P***
TLR-2	Control	102 (46.8)	97 (44.5)	19 (8.7)			1.00		1.00	
(rs3804099)	APN	47 (43.5)	57 (52.8)	4 (3.7)	0.95 (0.66, 1.39)	0.810	1.14 (0.72, 1.82)	0.577	0.40 (0.13, 1.22)	0.080
	ALN	72 (43.4)	81 (48.8)	13 (7.8)	1.07 (0.77, 1.47)	0.698	1.15 (0.76, 1.72)	0.505	0.89 (0.43, 1.86)	0.756
	Combined	119 (43.4)	138 (50.4)	17 (6.2)	1.02 (0.77, 1.36)	0.880	1.15 (0.80, 1.64)	0.457	0.69 (0.35, 1.37)	0.290
		TT	**TC**	**CC**	**OR (95% CI)**	***P***	**OR (95% CI)**	***P***	**OR (95% CI)**	***P***
TLR-2	Control	112 (50.9)	92 (41.8)	16 (7.3)			1.00		1.00	
(rs3804100)	APN	53 (48.6)	54 (49.5)	2 (1.8)	0.91 (0.62, 1.35)	0.652	1.10 (0.69, 1.73)	0.696	0.24 (0.05, 1.06)	**0.026**
	ALN	83 (50.0)	80 (48.2)	3 (1.8)	0.88 (0.62, 1.24)	0.451	1.04 (0.69, 1.55)	0.860	0.23 (0.07, 0.82)	**0.009**[c]
	Combined	136 (49.5)	134 (48.7)	5 (1.8)	0.89 (0.65, 1.21)	0.444	1.06 (0.74, 1.51)	0.748	0.24 (0.09, 0.66)	**0.003**[c]
		CC	**CT**	**TT**	**OR (95% CI)**	***P***	**OR (95% CI)**	***P***	**OR (95% CI)**	***P***
TLR-5	Control	210 (95.5)	10 (4.5)	0 (0.0)						
(rs5744168)	APN	100 (92.6)	8 (7.4)	0 (0.0)	1.68 (0.64, 4.39)	0.296				
	ALN	153 (93.9)	10 (6.1)	0 (0.0)	1.37 (0.56, 3.38)	0.492				
	Combined	253 (93.4)	18 (6.6)	0 (0.0)	1.49 (0.68, 3.31)	0.315				

[a]*P* values <0.05 are shown in bold.
[b]APN+ALN.
[c]Statistical significance with correction for multiple-SNP testing ($P<0.0125$).

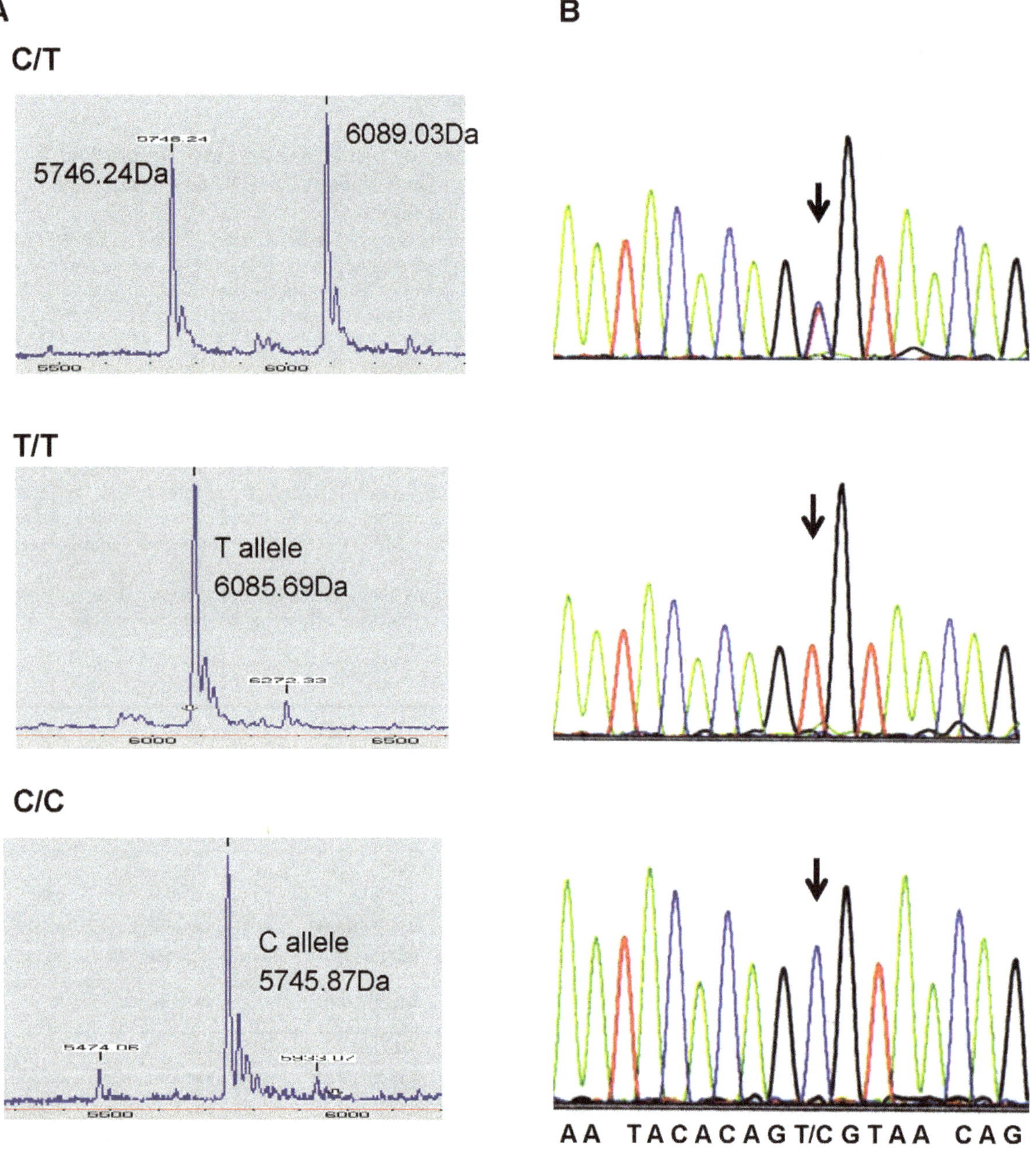

Figure 2. MALDI-TOF mass spectra from the genotyping of *TLR-2* (rs3804100) PCR product and its sequencing results. (A) The SNPs were genotyped by MALDI-TOF MS based on the molecular weights of the mini-sequencing products listed in Table 1. (B) Sequencing results for each of the PCR products from the C/T, T/T, and C/C genotypes of rs3804100. The SNPs are indicated by arrowheads.

Germany) according to the manufacturer's recommendations. The SNPs were genotyped as described previously [12] using the primers listed in Table 1. Briefly, PCR was performed in a total volume of 25 μL containing 200 ng of genomic DNA, primers (25 pM each), dNTPs (0.2 mM), 1× Fast-Start PCR buffer (50 mM Tris-HCl, 10 mM KCl, 5 mM $[NH_4]_2SO_4$, 2mM $MgCl_2$; pH 8.3), 1 M betaine, and 1 U of Fast-Start Taq Polymerase (Roche Diagnostics, Basel, Switzerland). The reaction comprised initiation at 95°C for 5 min, followed by 40 cycles of 95°C for 45 s, 50°C for 45 s, and 60°C for 45 s, with a final extension at 52°C for 10 min. Unincorporated dNTPs and primers were removed automatically by MAPIIA (GenePure PCR Purification System; Bruker, Bremen, Germany). The purified products were collected and mini-sequencing reactions were run using individual mini-sequencing primers (Table 1) in 20 μL of a solution containing 50 ng of the PCR product, 1 μL (10 pmol) of mini-sequencing primer, 0.5 μL of 1 mM ddNTP/dNTP mixture (for *TLR-1* rs4833095, dC ddT; for *TLR-2* rs3804099, dT ddC ddG; for *TLR-2* rs3804100, dT ddC ddG; and for *TLR-5* rs5744168, dT ddC ddG), 0.5 U of Thermo Sequenase DNA Polymerase (Amersham Biosciences, Piscataway, NJ), and 2 μL of the reaction buffer provided by the manufacturer. The reactions were carried out in a multiblock thermal cycler (Thermo Hybaid, Waltham, MA) with initial denaturation

Table 3. Allele frequency analysis of the SNPs using the logistic regression model.

SNP	T allele frequency (%)				APN *vs.* control		ALN *vs.* control		Combined[a] *vs.* control	
	Control	APN	ALN	Combined[a]	OR (95% CI)	*P*	OR (95% CI)	*P*	OR (95% CI)	*P*
TLR-1 (rs4833095)	40.23	35.65	40.77	38.77	0.82 (0.59, 1.15)	0.257	1.02 (0.77, 1.37)	0.878	0.94 (0.73, 1.22)	0.640
TLR-2 (rs3804099)	69.04	69.91	67.77	68.61	1.04 (0.73, 1.49)	0.820	0.94 (0.69, 1.28)	0.709	0.98 (0.75, 1.29)	0.887
TLR-2 (rs3804100)	71.82	73.39	74.10	73.82	1.08 (0.75, 1.56)	0.670	1.12 (0.81, 1.55)	0.481	1.11 (0.83, 1.47)	0.482
TLR-5 (rs5744168)	2.27	3.70	3.07	3.32	1.65 (0.64, 4.25)	0.303	1.36 (0.56, 3.31)	0.500	1.48 (0.67, 3.23)	0.322

[a]APN+ALN.

at 96°C for 1 min, followed by 50 cycles of 96°C for 15 s, 50°C for 15 s, 60°C for 100 s, and 96°C for 30 s. The reaction products were purified automatically by MAPIIA (Single-Strand DNA Binding Beads; Bruker) and analyzed by MALDI-TOF mass spectrometry (MS).

The samples were then mixed with 0.5 μL of matrix solution (50 mg/mL 3-hydropicolinic acid in a 4:5:1 mixture of water, acetonitrile, and 50 mg/mL diammonium citrate) and spotted onto 384-well Teflon sample plates (PerSeptive Biosystems, Framingham, MA). MALDI-TOF mass spectra were acquired with a Bruker Autoflex MALDI-TOF mass spectrometer (Bruker) and AutoXecute software (Bruker) to validate the genotype data. To confirm the MALDI-TOF analysis results, 10% of the PCR products were randomly selected for auto-sequencing analysis using an ABI 3730 autosequencer (Applied Biosystems, Foster City, CA).

Statistical Analysis

Hardy-Weinberg equilibrium was tested for goodness-of-fit using a χ^2 test with one degree of freedom, to compare the observed and expected genotype frequencies among the study subjects. The association of case-control status (outcome) and SNP genotype was analyzed using log-additive (or allelic-trend test), recessive, and dominant models [7,11]. In the log-additive model, common homozygous genotypes (00) were assigned a value of 0; heterozygotes (01), a value of 1; and minor homozygous genotypes (11), a value of 2. For the dominant model, the genotypes 01 and 11 were combined and compared with genotype 00. In a similar manner, the genotypes 00 and 01 were combined and compared with genotype 11 for recessive model analysis. Odds ratios and significance levels were assessed using a logistic regression model. Statistical comparisons of categorical variables or binominal results (*e.g.*, allele frequency) among the control, APN, and ALN groups were performed by χ^2 analysis or two-sided Fisher's exact test, as appropriate. Genotype pattern frequency analysis for the SNPs with heterozygosity rates >0.01 in *TLR-2* (i.e. rs3804099, rs3804100) was also performed using a similar method as described by Ragnarsdóttir et al [17]. All statistical analyses were performed using SPSS software (Version 16.0, IBM SPSS Statistics) or otherwise, the website tools as stated.

At first, 96 cases (48 APN and 48 ALN) and 96 control samples were analyzed for *TLR-2* (rs3804100) SNP. The prior data (192 samples) indicated that the probability of exposure among controls is 0.10417. With the recessive model, if the true odds ratio for disease in exposed subjects relative to unexposed subjects is 0.182979 as we noted among these 192 samples, we will need to study 154 patients and 154 control patients to be able to reject the null hypothesis that this odds ratio equals 1 with probability (power) of 0.8. The Type I error probability associated with this test of this null hypothesis is 0.05. The samples size estimate was performed with PS Power and Sample Size Calculations Version 3.0 (http://biostat.mc.vanderbilt.edu/PowerSampleSize) [22].

The demographic and clinical characteristics of the patients enrolled were described in a previous publication [12]. All cases are Taiwanese. The gender ratio and age were not significantly different (p>0.05) among the control patients (n = 222), APN patients (n = 113), and ALN patients (n = 172). In addition, patients with ALN (the clinically more severe UTI) presented with a significantly higher C-reactive protein (CRP) level than the APN patients. Moreover, the durations of fever prior to admission and after antibiotic treatment were longer in the ALN patients than in the APN patients. However, no statistically significant difference in white blood cell count was noted.

Results

Hardy-Weinberg equilibrium was satisfied in the observed genotype frequencies for all groups (Table 2). Auto-sequencing of randomly selected PCR products, for example, *TLR-2* (rs3804100) for three enrolled individuals, gave results that were identical to those derived from the MALDI-TOF mass spectra (Figure 2). This indicates the MALDI-TOF method was able to precisely determine the DNA sequences of the SNPs.

Statistical analyses revealed that only the *TLR-2* (rs3804100) SNP showed a significant difference in genotype frequency between the control group and the APN and ALN groups (and a combined APN+ALN group) using the recessive model [OR (95% CI): APN *vs.* control, 0.24 (0.05, 1.06); ALN *vs.* control, 0.23 (0.07, 0.82); APN+ALN *vs.* control, 0.24 (0.09, 0.66)] (Table 2). After correction for multiple-SNP testing (4 SNPs examined here), only ALN and (APN+ALN) groups showed significant difference *vs.* control in recessive model (P<0.0125). There were no statistically significant differences in the allele frequencies of the SNPs we examined (Table 3).

Because VUR has been suggested to be a significant host risk factor for upper UTIs [8,20], further genetic analysis was conducted in subgroups of APN and ALN patients with no VUR (APN, 50 patients; ALN, 108 patients). As a voiding cystourethrography was not medically indicated in the control patients, the number of patients with VUR in the control group was calculated based on a reported prevalence rate [23]. Given a 0.3% prevalence rate of VUR at the mean age of the control group (2.91±3.01 years), the number of individuals with VUR among the 222 control cases was assumed to be zero. The age and gender ratios remained not significantly different (p>0.05) between the control group and the APN and ALN subgroups with no VUR.

In comparison with the *TLR-2* (rs3804100) TT and TC genotype frequencies, the CC genotype frequency was significantly

Table 4. Genotypic analysis of the SNPs in the no-VUR patient subgroup.

SNP	Group	Genotype, *n* (%)			Log-additive model		Dominant model		Recessive model	
		00	01	11			(01, 11 *vs.* 00)		(11 *vs.* 00, 01)	
		CC	CT	TT	OR (95% CI)	P^a	OR (95% CI)	P^a	OR (95% CI)	P^a
TLR-1	Control	75 (34.1)	113 (51.4)	32 (14.5)			1.00		1.00	
(rs4833095)	APN	21 (42.0)	24 (48.0)	5 (10.0)	0.75 (0.47, 1.20)	0.230	0.71 (0.38, 1.34)	0.296	0.65 (0.24, 1.77)	0.383
	ALN	33 (30.6)	55 (50.9)	20 (18.5)	1.18 (0.84, 1.65)	0.346	1.18 (0.72, 1.93)	0.521	1.34 (0.72, 2.47)	0.360
	Combined[b]	54 (34.2)	79 (50.0)	25 (15.8)	1.03 (0.76, 1.39)	0.866	1.00 (0.65, 1.53)	0.986	1.10 (0.63, 1.95)	0.733
		TT	TC	CC	OR (95% CI)	*P*	OR (95% CI)	*P*	OR (95% CI)	*P*
TLR-2	Control	102 (46.8)	97 (44.5)	19 (8.7)			1.00		1.00	
(rs3804099)	APN	21 (42.0)	27 (54.0)	2 (4.0)	1.00 (0.61, 1.64)	0.994	1.21 (0.65, 2.26)	0.539	0.44 (0.10, 1.94)	0.228
	ALN	46 (42.6)	56 (51.9)	6 (5.6)	1.03 (0.71, 1.49)	0.888	1.19 (0.74, 1.89)	0.473	0.62 (0.24, 1.59)	0.300
	Combined	67 (42.4)	83 (52.5)	8 (5.1)	1.02 (0.73, 1.42)	0.909	1.19 (0.79, 1.80)	0.399	0.56 (0.24, 1.31)	0.168
		TT	TC	CC	OR (95% CI)	*P*	OR (95% CI)	*P*	OR (95% CI)	*P*
TLR-2	Control	112 (50.9)	92 (41.8)	16 (7.3)			1.00		1.00	
(rs3804100)	APN	25 (50.0)	23 (46.0)	2 (4.0)	0.94 (0.57, 1.55)	0.806	1.04 (0.56, 1.92)	0.908	0.53 (0.12, 2.39)	0.375
	ALN	54 (50.0)	52 (48.1)	2 (1.9)	0.88 (0.60, 1.30)	0.519	1.04 (0.65, 1.64)	0.877	0.24 (0.05, 1.07)	**0.027**[c]
	Combined	79 (50.0)	75 (47.5)	4 (2.5)	0.90 (0.64, 1.27)	0.536	1.04 (0.69, 1.56)	0.862	0.33 (0.11, 1.01)	**0.034**[c]
		CC	CT	TT	OR (95% CI)	*P*	OR (95% CI)	*P*	OR (95% CI)	*P*
TLR-5	Control	210 (95.5)	10 (4.5)	0 (0.0)						
(rs5744168)	APN	45 (93.8)	3 (6.2)	0 (0.0)	1.40 (0.37, 5.29)	0.630				
	ALN	99 (94.3)	6 (5.7)	0 (0.0)	1.27 (0.45, 3.60)	0.653				
	Combined	144 (94.1)	9 (5.9)	0 (0.0)	1.31 (0.52, 3.31)	0.566				

[a]*P* values <0.05 are shown in bold.
[b]APN+ALN.
[c]Statistical non-significance with correction for multiple-SNP testing ($P>0.0125$).

lower in the no-VUR ALN and APN+ALN patient subgroups [recessive model, OR (95% CI): ALN *vs.* control, 0.24 (0.05, 1.07); APN+ALN *vs.* control, 0.33 (0.11, 1.01)] (Table 4). With correction for multiple-SNP testing, no significant difference was noted between the control and the no-VUR disease subgroups. The allele frequency analyses showed no significant difference between the control group and the no-VUR APN, ALN, or APN+ALN patient subgroup (Table 5).

Genotype patterns in *TLR-2* were assigned by combining multiple SNPs that had heterozygosity rates >0.01 (i.e. rs3804099, rs3804100) in each individual (Figure 3) [17]. The frequency of genotype pattern IV (CC+CC) was significantly reduced in the APN+ALN combined group (Table 6). After the elimination of cases with VUR, genotype pattern IV can not even be noted in the no-VUR subgroup of APN and ALN (Table 7).

Discussion

Successful defense against bacterial infection requires well-integrated host innate and adaptive immune responses. The initial pathogen recognition process is mediated by the coordinated actions of various TLRs, which are located on the cell surface or

Table 5. Allele frequency analysis of the SNPs in the no-VUR patient subgroup using the logistic regression model.

SNP	T allele frequency (%)				APN *vs.* control		ALN *vs.* control		Combined[a] *vs.* control	
	Control	APN	ALN	Combined[a]	OR (95% CI)	*P*	OR (95% CI)	*P*	OR (95% CI)	*P*
TLR-1 (rs4833095)	40.23	34.00	43.98	40.82	0.77 (0.49, 1.21)	0.246	1.17 (0.84, 1.62)	0.360	1.03 (0.76, 1.38)	0.869
TLR-2 (rs3804099)	69.04	69.00	68.52	68.67	1.00 (0.62, 1.60)	0.994	0.98 (0.69, 1.39)	0.893	0.98 (0.72, 1.34)	0.915
TLR-2 (rs3804100)	71.82	73.00	74.07	73.73	1.06 (0.65, 1.73)	0.812	1.12 (0.78, 1.62)	0.542	1.10 (0.80, 1.53)	0.560
TLR-5 (rs5744168)	2.27	3.13	2.86	2.94	1.39 (0.37, 5.14)	0.634	1.26 (0.45, 3.53)	0.657	1.30 (0.52, 3.25)	0.571

[a]APN+ALN.

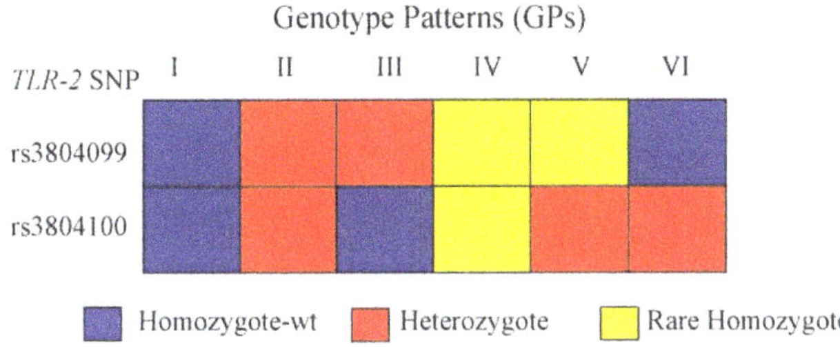

Figure 3. *TLR-2* genotype patterns of the SNPs with heterozygosity rates >0.01. Each column represents a genotype pattern and each row a SNP in *TLR-2*. Common allele homozygote (blue), heterozygote (red) and rare allele homozygote (yellow) are shown.

within organelles such as phagosomes, and PAMPs, including bacterial flagellin, lipopolysaccharide, and bacterial lipopeptides [7,10–12]. Following this microbe-sensing step, sequential activation of the immune system leads to cytokine release, recruitment of neutrophils to the site of infection, phagocytosis, and the release of free radicals [16]. The cytokines that are released play essential roles in the host innate immune response and activation of the adaptive immune system [24]. These responses determine the balance between health and disease severity [8]. Defective signal transmission in the immune response due to, for example, genetic polymorphisms in receptors and cytokines, influences an individual's risk for infectious diseases [7,9,11,12,16,19].

TLRs are crucial for the recognition of microbes by the innate immune system and for bridging the innate and acquired immune responses [16]. In addition to acting as critical sensors of microbial attack, TLRs also serve as effectors of TLR-dependent innate defense, which enables the host to eliminate pathogens that would otherwise cause disease morbidity or mortality [17]. Many studies have suggested that SNPs in TLR genes can affect an individual's ability to respond to TLR ligands, leading to altered susceptibility to infections or inflammation [25]. This altered susceptibility can be either a reduced inflammatory response, as occurs in asymptomatic bacteriuria, protection against pyelonephritis, and recurrent UTIs [11,17,19], or an exaggerated immune response that results in a severe infection, as occurs in tuberculosis and severe atopic dermatitis [26,27].

The APN and ALN patients in this study had a lower TLR-2 (rs3804100) CC genotype frequency compared with the controls. No differences in the other TLR SNPs examined were noted among the APN, ALN, and control groups. Furthermore, after the elimination of patients with VUR, a well-known risk factor for severe UTI, from the analysis, patients with ALN, but not those with APN, had a lower TLR-2 (rs3804100) CC genotype frequency. With the correction for multiple-SNP testing, only the ALN and (APN+ALN) combined group that include VUR diagnosis showed significant reduced TLR-2 (rs3804100) CC genotype frequency compared with the controls. Further, the genotype pattern frequency analysis for the TLR-2 has shown the genotype pattern of CC+CC (rs3804099+rs3804100) was not even noted in the no-VUR subgroup of patients with APN and ALN. As the inflammatory responses in ALN patients are more severe than those in APN patients (higher CRP levels, longer fever duration after antibiotic treatment), these findings suggest that the genetic variant in TLR-2 (rs3804100, T1350C) may protect the host from severe urinary tract infections as ALN.

Among the TLRs that have been described, TLR-2 was the first human TLR to be described in host defense against gram-negative bacteria [28] but subsequent studies have demonstrated that TLR-4 is the receptor for lipopolysaccharide [16,29]. TLR-2 polymorphisms have also been linked to various severe infections, including tuberculosis, leprosy, and septic shock [10,30,31]. A few studies have reported associations between UTIs and TLR-2 polymorphism at the TLR-2 (rs5743708; G2258A; Arg753Gln) site [11,16]. The current study found that another TLR-2 genetic variant, TLR-2 (rs3804100; T1350C; Ser450Ser), can also change the host risk to severe UTIs (APN vs. ALN).

The TLR-2 (rs3804100; T1350C; Ser450Ser) SNP described here did not induce an amino acid change, and the molecular mechanism by which this synonymous polymorphism affects host susceptibility to severe UTIs is not fully understood. Many studies have provided evidence that synonymous SNPs lead to changes in protein amount, structure, and/or function via alterations in mRNA structure and stability, kinetics of translation, and alternative splicing. Moreover, synonymous SNPs may be proxies for other polymorphisms that have not been examined [32]. Further investigations of phenotypes or functional assessment of synonymous SNPs, such as using the luciferase reporter assay or gene knock-out mice [9,17,19], are warranted to properly determine their effects on TLR-2 expression.

Table 6. Genotype pattern frequency analysis of the SNPs in *TLR-2* (rs3804099 and rs3804100) using the two-tailed Fisher's Exact Test[#].

Genotype pattern	Genotype pattern frequency (*n*)			APN *vs.* control	ALN *vs.* control	Combined[b] *vs.* Control
	Control (218)	APN (107)	ALN (166)	*P*[a]	*P*[a]	*P*[a]
I (TT+TT)	99	43	70	0.406	0.535	0.409
II (TC+TC)	83	49	70	0.189	0.462	0.231
III (TC+TT)	12	8	11	0.624	0.669	0.578
IV (CC+CC)	12	2	3	0.156	0.108	**0.044**
V (CC+TC)	7	2	8	0.723	0.438	0.810
VI (TT+TC)	1	3	2	0.106	0.581	0.234
Others	4	0	2	0.307	0.702	0.414

[a]*P* values <0.05 are shown in bold.
[b]APN+ALN.
[#]2×2 contingency table, http://www.vassarstats.net/tab2×2.html.

Table 7. Genotype pattern frequency analysis of the SNPs in *TLR-2* (rs3804099 and rs3804100) in the no-VUR patient subgroup using the two-tailed Fisher's Exact Test[#].

Genotype pattern	Genotype pattern frequency (*n*)			APN *vs.* control	ALN *vs.* control	Combined[b] *vs.* Control
	Control (218)	APN (50)	ALN (108)	*P*[a]	*P*[a]	*P*[a]
I (TT+TT)	99	19	42	0.350	0.286	0.206
II (TC+TC)	83	20	47	0.872	0.400	0.455
III (TC+TT)	12	6	9	0.116	0.344	0.159
IV (CC+CC)	12	0	0	0.131	**0.023**	**0.002**
V (CC+TC)	7	2	3	1.000	1.000	1.000
VI (TT+TC)	1	1	2	0.339	0.256	0.314
Others	4	2	5	0.597	0.164	0.214

[a]*P* values <0.05 are shown in bold.
[b]APN+ALN.
[#]2×2 contingency table, http://www.vassarstats.net/tab2×2.html.

As the statistical power to detect significant associations with rare genetic variants is determined based on sample size, the major limitation of this study is the small population of individuals with the CC genotype of TLR-2 (rs3804100, T1350C). A large cohort study is recommended to replicate and validate the associations of SNPs with the severe UTIs, APN and ALN.

Acknowledgments

The authors thank Mr. Yu-Jr Lin for his assistance with the statistical analyses.

Author Contributions

Conceived and designed the experiments: CHC YSL TYL. Performed the experiments: CHC YSL. Analyzed the data: CHC YSL CJC. Contributed reagents/materials/analysis tools: CHC YSL CJC. Wrote the paper: CHC.

References

1. Ma JF, Shortliffe LM (2004) Urinary tract infection in children: etiology and epidemiology. Urologic Clinics of North America 31: 517–526.
2. Cheng CH, Tsau YK, Lin TY (2006) Effective duration of antimicrobial therapy for the treatment of acute lobar nephronia. Pediatrics 117: e84–89.
3. Cheng CH, Tsau YK, Lin TY (2010) Is acute lobar nephronia the midpoint in the spectrum of upper urinary tract infections between acute pyelonephritis and renal abscess? Journal of Pediatrics 156: 82–86.
4. Cheng CH, Tsau YK, Su LH, Lin CL, Lin TY (2007) Comparison of urovirulence factors and genotypes for bacteria causing acute lobar nephronia and acute pyelonephritis. Pediatric Infectious Disease Journal 26: 228–232.
5. Cheng CH, Tsau YK, Kuo CY, Su LH, Lin TY (2010) Comparison of extended virulence genotypes for bacteria isolated from pediatric patients with urosepsis, acute pyelonephritis, and acute lobar nephronia. Pediatric Infectious Disease Journal 29: 736–740.
6. Tseng CC, Wu JJ, Liu HL, Sung JM, Huang JJ (2002) Roles of host and bacterial virulence factors in the development of upper urinary tract infection caused by Escherichia coli. Am J Kidney Dis 39: 744–752.
7. Hawn TR, Scholes D, Li SS, Wang H, Yang Y, et al. (2009) Toll-like receptor polymorphisms and susceptibility to urinary tract infections in adult women. PLoS ONE [Electronic Resource] 4: e5990.
8. Artifoni L, Negrisolo S, Montini G, Zucchetta P, Molinari PP, et al. (2007) Interleukin-8 and CXCR1 receptor functional polymorphisms and susceptibility to acute pyelonephritis. Journal of Urology 177: 1102–1106.
9. Lundstedt AC, McCarthy S, Gustafsson MC, Godaly G, Jodal U, et al. (2007) A genetic basis of susceptibility to acute pyelonephritis. PLoS ONE [Electronic Resource] 2: e825.
10. Texereau J, Chiche J-D, Taylor W, Choukroun G, Comba B, et al. (2005) The importance of Toll-like receptor 2 polymorphisms in severe infections. Clinical Infectious Diseases 41 Suppl 7: S408–415.
11. Hawn TR, Scholes D, Wang H, Li SS, Stapleton AE, et al. (2009) Genetic variation of the human urinary tract innate immune response and asymptomatic bacteriuria in women. PLoS ONE [Electronic Resource] 4: e8300.
12. Cheng CH, Lee YS, Tsau YK, Lin TY (2011) Genetic polymorphisms and susceptibility to parenchymal renal infection among pediatric patients. Pediatric Infectious Disease Journal 30: 309–314.
13. Yin X, Hou T, Liu Y, Chen J, Yao Z, et al. (2010) Association of Toll-like receptor 4 gene polymorphism and expression with urinary tract infection types in adults. PLoS ONE [Electronic Resource] 5: e14223.
14. Medzhitov R (2007) Recognition of microorganisms and activation of the immune response. Nature 449: 819–826.
15. Beutler B, Jiang Z, Georgel P, Crozat K, Croker B, et al. (2006) Genetic analysis of host resistance: Toll-like receptor signaling and immunity at large. Annual Review of Immunology 24: 353–389.
16. Tabel Y, Berdeli A, Mir S (2007) Association of TLR2 gene Arg753Gln polymorphism with urinary tract infection in children. International Journal of Immunogenetics 34: 399–405.
17. Ragnarsdottir B, Jonsson K, Urbano A, Gronberg-Hernandez J, Lutay N, et al. (2010) Toll-like receptor 4 promoter polymorphisms: common TLR4 variants may protect against severe urinary tract infection. PLoS ONE [Electronic Resource] 5: e10734.
18. Karoly E, Fekete A, Banki NF, Szebeni B, Vannay A, et al. (2007) Heat shock protein 72 (HSPA1B) gene polymorphism and Toll-like receptor (TLR) 4 mutation are associated with increased risk of urinary tract infection in children. Pediatr Res 61: 371–374.
19. Ragnarsdottir B, Lutay N, Gronberg-Hernandez J, Koves B, Svanborg C (2011) Genetics of innate immunity and UTI susceptibility. Nature Reviews Urology 8: 449–468.
20. Orellana P, Baquedano P, Rangarajan V, Zhao JH, Eng ND, et al. (2004) Relationship between acute pyelonephritis, renal scarring, and vesicoureteral reflux. Results of a coordinated research project. Pediatric Nephrology 19: 1122–1126.
21. Sayers EW, Barrett T, Benson DA, Bolton E, Bryant SH, et al. (2010) Database resources of the National Center for Biotechnology Information. Nucleic Acids Research 38: D5–16.
22. Dupont WD, Plummer WD Jr (1998) Power and sample size calculations for studies involving linear regression. Controlled Clinical Trials 19: 589–601.
23. American Academy of Pediatrics, Committee on Quality Improvement, Subcommittee on Urinary Tract Infection (1999) Practice parameter: the diagnosis, treatment, and evaluation of the initial urinary tract infection in febrile infants and young children. Pediatrics 103: 843–852.
24. Bochud P-Y, Hawn TR, Siddiqui MR, Saunderson P, Britton S, et al. (2008) Toll-like receptor 2 (TLR2) polymorphisms are associated with reversal reaction in leprosy. Journal of Infectious Diseases 197: 253–261.
25. Netea MG, Wijmenga C, O'Neill LA (2012) Genetic variation in Toll-like receptors and disease susceptibility. Nat Immunol 13: 535–542.
26. Ogus AC, Yoldas B, Ozdemir T, Uguz A, Olcen S, et al. (2004) The Arg753GLn polymorphism of the human toll-like receptor 2 gene in tuberculosis disease. European Respiratory Journal 23: 219–223.
27. Ahmad-Nejad P, Mrabet-Dahbi S, Breuer K, Klotz M, Werfel T, et al. (2004) The toll-like receptor 2 R753Q polymorphism defines a subgroup of patients

with atopic dermatitis having severe phenotype. Journal of Allergy & Clinical Immunology 113: 565–567.

28. Kirschning CJ, Wesche H, Merrill Ayres T, Rothe M (1998) Human toll-like receptor 2 confers responsiveness to bacterial lipopolysaccharide. Journal of Experimental Medicine 188: 2091–2097.
29. Beutler B, Du X, Poltorak A (2001) Identification of Toll-like receptor 4 (Tlr4) as the sole conduit for LPS signal transduction: genetic and evolutionary studies. Journal of Endotoxin Research 7: 277–280.
30. Abu-Maziad A, Schaa K, Bell EF, Dagle JM, Cooper M, et al. (2010) Role of polymorphic variants as genetic modulators of infection in neonatal sepsis. Pediatric Research 68: 323–329.
31. Chen Y-C, Hsiao C-C, Chen C-J, Chin C-H, Liu S-F, et al. (2010) Toll-like receptor 2 gene polymorphisms, pulmonary tuberculosis, and natural killer cell counts. BMC Medical Genetics 11: 17.
32. Junpee A, Tencomnao T, Sanprasert V, Nuchprayoon S (2010) Association between Toll-like receptor 2 (TLR2) polymorphisms and asymptomatic bancroftian filariasis. Parasitology Research 107: 807–816.

16

Novel Respiratory Syncytial Virus (RSV) Genotype ON1 Predominates in Germany during Winter Season 2012–13

Julia Tabatabai[1,2], Christiane Prifert[3], Johannes Pfeil[4,5], Jürgen Grulich-Henn[4], Paul Schnitzler[1]*

1 Department of Infectious Diseases, Virology, University of Heidelberg, Heidelberg, Germany, **2** London School of Hygiene and Tropical Medicine, London, United Kingdom, **3** Institute of Virology and Immunobiology, University of Würzburg, Würzburg, Germany, **4** Department of Pediatrics, University of Heidelberg, Heidelberg, Germany, **5** German Centre for Infectious Diseases (DZIF), Heidelberg, Germany

Abstract

Respiratory syncytial virus (RSV) is the leading cause of hospitalization especially in young children with respiratory tract infections (RTI). Patterns of circulating RSV genotypes can provide a better understanding of the molecular epidemiology of RSV infection. We retrospectively analyzed the genetic diversity of RSV infection in hospitalized children with acute RTI admitted to University Hospital Heidelberg/Germany between October 2012 and April 2013. Nasopharyngeal aspirates (NPA) were routinely obtained in 240 children younger than 2 years of age who presented with clinical symptoms of upper or lower RTI. We analyzed NPAs via PCR and sequence analysis of the second variable region of the RSV G gene coding for the attachment glycoprotein. We obtained medical records reviewing routine clinical data. RSV was detected in 134/240 children. In RSV-positive patients the most common diagnosis was bronchitis/bronchiolitis (75.4%). The mean duration of hospitalization was longer in RSV-positive compared to RSV-negative patients (3.5 vs. 5.1 days; $p<0.01$). RSV-A was detected in 82.1%, RSV-B in 17.9% of all samples. Phylogenetic analysis of 112 isolates revealed that the majority of RSV-A strains (65%) belonged to the novel ON1 genotype containing a 72-nucleotide duplication. However, genotype ON1 was not associated with a more severe course of illness when taking basic clinical/laboratory parameters into account. Molecular characterization of RSV confirms the co-circulation of multiple genotypes of subtype RSV-A and RSV-B. The duplication in the G gene of genotype ON1 might have an effect on the rapid spread of this emerging RSV strain.

Editor: Steven M. Varga, University of Iowa, United States of America

Funding: The authors have no support or funding to report.

Competing Interests: The authors have declared that no competing interests exist.

* Email: Paul_Schnitzler@med.uni-heidelberg.de

Introduction

Respiratory syncytial virus (RSV) is the major pathogen of lower respiratory tract infections (RTI) in infants and young children. By the age of 2 years, virtually all children have been infected at least once with RSV [1]. Re-infections are common throughout life; in older children and adults infections are associated with milder disease indicating that RSV induces only partial immunity [2]. Strain variation is thought to contribute to its ability to cause frequent re-infections [3] enabling RSV to remain present at high levels in the population [4]. Viral strains are separated into two major groups based on its genetic and antigenic variability. Several lineages within the subtypes RSV-A and RSV-B co-circulate simultaneously in the population [5] and their relative proportions may differ between epidemics, although RSV-A viruses tend to predominate [6]. The main differences between RSV-A and RSV-B are found in the attachment (G) glycoprotein [7]. The G protein is a type II surface glycoprotein of about 300 amino acids in length, consisting of a cytoplasmic domain, a transmembrane domain and an ectodomain. The G protein is heavily glycosylated with N-linked and O-linked sugars. However, the amino acid sequence positions of potential glycosylation sites are poorly conserved [8].

This protein is able to accommodate drastic changes with the emergence of new variants. Diversity occurs mainly in the two hypervariable regions of the ectodomain which are separated by a highly conserved 13-amino acid (aa) length domain [9]. Sequencing of the second hypervariable region at the C-terminal end of the G gene has been widely used to further subdivide RSV-A and RSV-B into genotypes and facilitated differentiation between RSV isolates. To date, 11 RSV-A genotypes, GA1-GA7, SAA1, NA1-NA2, and ON1 [10–12], and 23 RSV-B genotypes, GB1-GB4, SAB1-SAB3, SAB4, URU1, URU2, BAI - BAXII, and THB [10,13–21] have been described based on nucleotide sequence analysis.

RSV strains show an accumulation of translated amino acid changes over the years, suggesting antigenic drift-based immunity-mediated selection [22]. In 1999, a new RSV-B genotype BA emerged in Buenos Aires, Argentina, containing a 60-nucleotide (nt) duplication in the second hypervariable region of the G gene [23]. In the following ten years, the BA genotype spread worldwide and largely replaced previous described RSV-B genotypes [24]. During the 2010–11 winter season, a novel

RSV-A genotype ON1 with a 72-nt duplication has been reported in Canada [14]. In line with the gradual spread of the BA genotype making it the dominant circulating RSV-B genotype today, the nucleotide duplication of the ON1 genotype might likewise result in a similar selection advantage [25]. There is an increasing number of reports from across the world describing this novel genotype and the following seasons will show its impact on the evolution of RSV-A [6].

In Germany, there is only limited information regarding the molecular epidemiology of RSV, the emergence of novel viral strains and their impact on the course of RSV infection. In the present study, we evaluated hospitalized children below the age of 2 years presenting with acute RTI in the Pediatric Department in Heidelberg, Germany during the winter season 2012–13. We investigated the genetic diversity and patterns of the co-circulating genotypes of Heidelberg RSV-A and RSV-B strains in comparison with other RSV strains circulating worldwide. Furthermore we explored a possible association between individual RSV genotypes and the course of RSV infection by retrospectively analyzing basic clinical and laboratory data.

Materials and Methods

Patients and clinical samples

We retrospectively analyzed children under the age of 2 years admitted to the Pediatric Department at the Heidelberg University Hospital between October 2012 and April 2013 with clinical symptoms of upper or lower respiratory tract infection (RTI) as part of their admission diagnosis or as concomitant symptom. Prior to the transfer to the inpatient unit, nasopharyngeal aspirates (NPA) are obtained and these children are routinely screened for RSV infection using a rapid antigen test in order to inform for isolation strategies. All obtained NPAs (242 samples from 240 children) were collected and stored frozen for further molecular analysis by RSV PCR and phylogenetic analysis. Medical records were reviewed from all children to obtain routine clinical and laboratory data. Patient records were anonymized and de-identified prior to analysis. The Ethical Committee of the University of Heidelberg has approved this study (S-166/2014).

PCR and sequencing

For PCR analysis, RNA was extracted from NPAs using the QIAamp viral RNA mini kit (Qiagen, Hilden, Germany) according to the manufacturer's protocol. Amplification and detection of viral RNA was performed with the RealStar RSV real-time PCR kit (altona Diagnostics, Hamburg, Germany) on a LightCycler 480 instrument II (Roche, Mannheim, Germany). This assay differentiated RSV into subtypes A and B. For sequencing and identification of RSV genotypes, extracted RNA was initially reverse transcribed and cDNA was synthesized using random hexamer primers. Subsequently, PCR targeting the second hypervariable region of the G gene was performed using primer pairs as previously described by Peret et al. [11]. PCR products were sequenced with the same primer pairs previously used for amplification. Overlapping sequences were assembled and edited using the SEQMAN II software of the Lasergene package (DNAstar, Madsion, WI). Nucleotide sequences of the second hypervariable region of the G gene retrieved in this study were deposited in GenBank under accession numbers [KJ710364-KJ710420].

Phylogenetic and deduced amino acid sequence analysis

Multiple sequence alignments and phylogenetic analysis of the second hypervariable region of the G gene were conducted using the Clustal W 1.6 method of MEGA software version 6 [26]. Phylogenetic trees were generated using the maximum-likelihood method and bootstrap values with 1,000 replicates were calculated to evaluate confidence estimates. Reference strains representing known genotypes were retrieved from GenBank (http://www.ncbi.lm.nih.gov) and included in the tree. Pairwise nucleotide distances were calculated to compare the differences within and between genotypes of subgroup RSV-A and RSV-B using MEGA software version 6. Positive selected sites were estimated by use of the Datamonkey Web server (http://www.datamonkey.org) identifying the rates of non-synonymous and synonymous substitutions [27].

Deduced amino acid sequences were translated with the standard genetic code using MEGA software version 6. Alignments of the second hypervariable region of the G protein of Heidelberg RSV-A and RSV-B strains were compared to references strains from GenBank to identify amino acid substitutions. Putative N-glycosylation sites were predicted if the encoded amino acid sequence was Asn-Xaa-Thr/Ser, where Xaa was not a proline and accepted if the glycosylation potential was ≥ 0.5 in NetNGlyc 1.0 server [28]. O-glycosylation was determined using the NetOGlyc 3.1 server and sites were predicted using a G-score ≥ 0.5 [29].

Statistical analysis of epidemiological factors

To describe the temporal distribution of admitted RSV cases, we aggregated RSV results as obtained by PCR by calendar month and week. Demographic and clinical data in our study population was summarized. Group comparisons were performed using $\chi 2$ or Fisher's exact test for categorical variables and by Student's t-test or analysis of variance (ANOVA) for continuous variables, as appropriate. P-values <0.05 were considered statistically significant. Stata/IC13.0 (StataCorp. LP, College Station, TX, USA) was used for all statistical analysis.

Results

Detection of RSV

Between October 2012 and April 2013, a total of 242 samples from hospitalized infants and children were analyzed for RSV infection by PCR resulting in 134 (55.4%) RSV-positive samples. Among these RSV-positive samples, 110 (82.1%) were subgrouped as RSV-A and 24 (17.9%) as RSV-B, respectively. No co-infection for RSV-A and RSV-B was detected. Two children presented twice and were tested RSV-positive at their first admission and RSV-negative at the consecutive admission few weeks later. The distribution of RSV-A and RSV-B per calendar week and month is shown in Fig. 1.

Sequence alignments and phylogenetic analysis

Sequences of the second hypervariable region of the G gene from 97 (72.4%) RSV-A and 15 (11.2%) RSV-B samples were successfully obtained and aligned with representative GenBank sequences of previously published genotypes. Due to a low viral load some RSV-positive samples (n = 22; 16.4%) could not be sequenced. The phylogenetic trees of RSV-A and RSV-B sequences are shown in Figure 2. Heidelberg RSV_A and RSV-B strains clustered into three genotypes for RSV-A and two genotypes for RSV-B, respectively.

The majority of RSV-A strains (n = 73, 75.3%) clustered with strains that were previously assigned to the novel ON1 genotype with a 72-nt duplication, followed by strains clustering with genotype NA1 (n = 23, 31.5%) and one strain clustering with GA5 (Fig. 2A). Sequence homology between Heidelberg sequences and

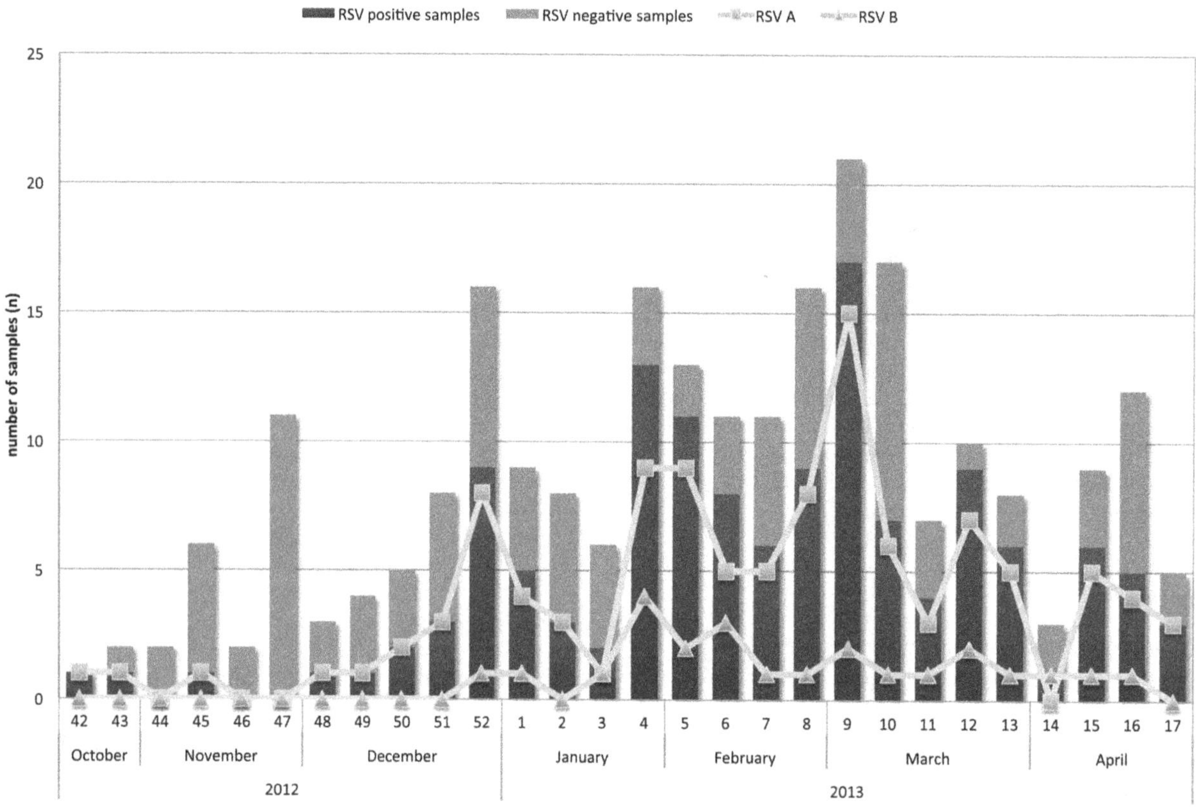

Figure 1. Weekly/monthly distribution of subgroup RSV A/RSV B in children ≤2 years with acute RTI in Heidelberg/Germany, winter season 2012/13.

the ON1 reference strain [JN257693] was ≥96.9% at the nucleotide level and ≥94.1% at the amino acid level. The intragenotypic p-distance was 1.9% for ON1 and 6.2% for NA1 for Heidelberg sequences. The intergenotypic p-distance for ON1 and NA1 was not comparable because of the 72-nt duplication.

All RSV-B strains (n = 15) clustered with strains that were previously assigned to the BA genotype with a 60-nt duplication. In addition, BA strains could be further differentiated into the previously designated genotypes BAIX (n = 10, 66.7%) and BAX (n = 5, 33.3%) (Fig. 2B). Sequence homology between Heidelberg sequences and the BA reference strain (AY333364) was 94.3%–96.6% at the nucleotide level and 87%–95% at the amino acid level. The intergenotypic p-distance for BAIX and BAX was 4.7% for Heidelberg sequences, with an intragenotypic p-distance of 3% for BAIX and 0.8% for BAX.

Deduced amino acid sequence analysis

We aligned and compared Heidelberg RSV-A genotype NA1 and GA5 strains with the A2 reference strain (M11486) (Fig. 3A). The majority of NA1 strains had three predicted N-glycosylation sites at amino acid (aa) positions 237, 251 and 294. However, HD12262 had an additional predicted N-glycosylation site at aa position 242 and HD12188 at aa position 273. A group of 11 isolates lost the N-glycosylation site at aa positions 237 due to a N237D/H substitution. Strain HD12055 lost all N-glycosylation site but the aa position 294. The N-glycosylation site at aa position 250 is characteristic for the GA5 genotype as found in one of the Heidelberg isolates. O-glycosylation patterns varied between Heidelberg isolates with 32±3 sites potentially O-glycosylated (G-score ≥0.5) in NA1 isolates and 23 sites in the one GA5 isolate.

As a consequence of the insertion in the G gene, ON1 genotype strains translate into a polypeptide with a length of 321 amino acids and are thereby lengthened by 24 aa when compared to the A2 reference strain (Fig. 3B). The insertion contains a 23 aa duplicated region. The comparison of Heidelberg ON1 strains with ON1 strains from other countries with reference to the original strain from Canada (JN257693) revealed that Heidelberg isolates can be divided into three sub-clusters: The first sub-cluster (n = 12) comprises isolates closely related to the primary Canadian strain (JN257693) with few mixed substitutions. This sub-cluster also includes one strain with an E308K substitution as previously described in South African strains [JX885730]. The second sub-cluster (n = 28) contained three characteristic substitutions, L274P, L298P and Y304H as previously described in strains from Wuerzburg, Germany [JX912364, JX12364], as well as in strains from Italy and Japan [KC858245, KC587959; AB808774, AB808757]. Furthermore, on group of 13 identical isolates showed a E287K substitution which was unique for Heidelberg strains. The third sub-cluster consists of 28 isolates with a L310P substitution in addition to the three substitutions found in the second sub-cluster and aligned with isolates from Japan, India and Kenya [AB808774, AB808757; KF246641, KF246640; KF587959]. A group of 19 identical strains additionally showed a V303A substitution, which was also seen in strains from Italy, Croatia and India [KC858245, KC587959; KF057865;

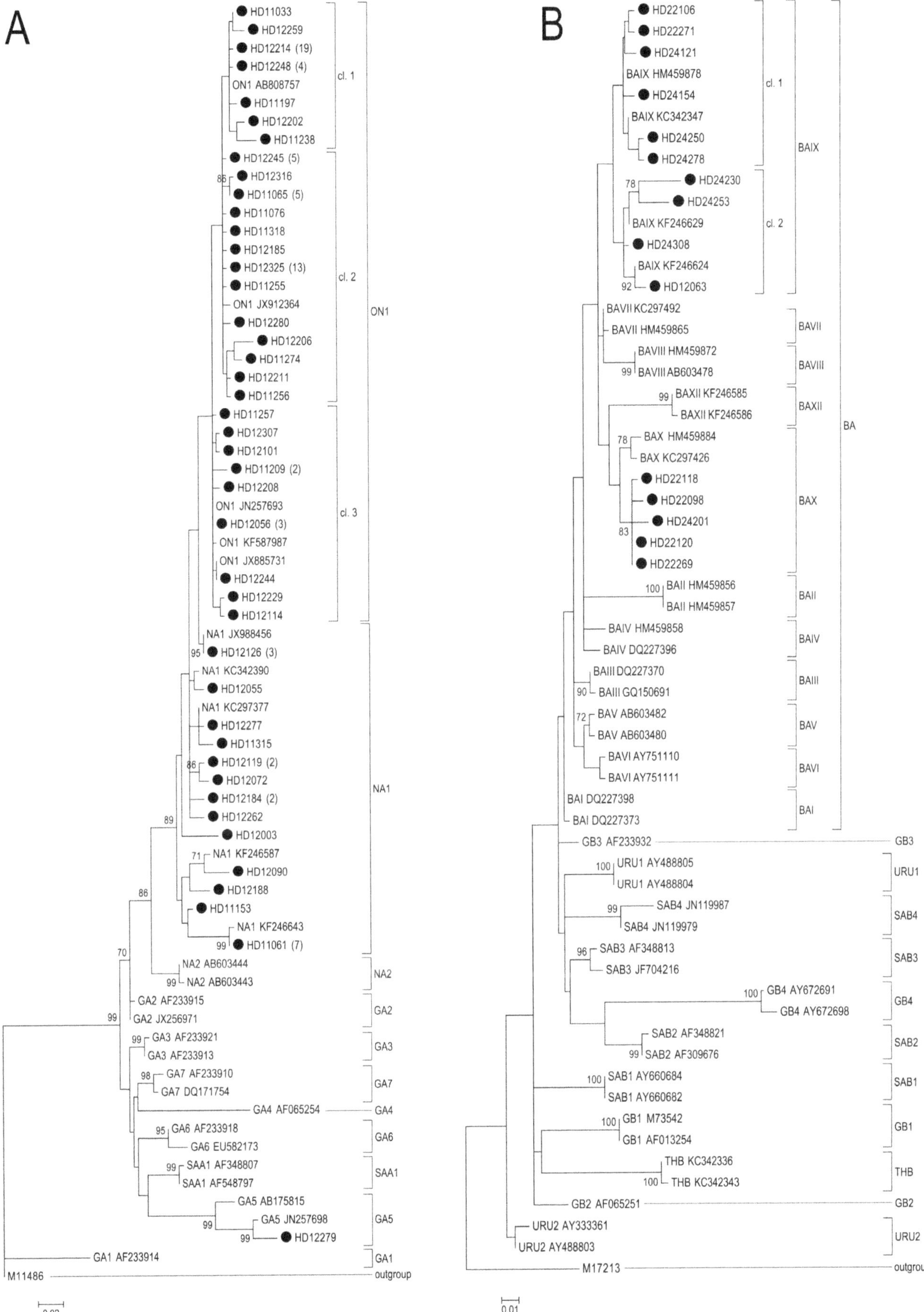
A
HD11033
HD12259
HD12214 (19)
HD12248 (4)
ON1 AB808757
HD11197
HD12202
HD11238
HD12245 (5)
86
HD12316
HD11065 (5)
HD11076
HD11318
HD12185
HD12325 (13)
HD11255
ON1 JX912364
HD12280
HD12206
HD11274
HD12211
HD11256
HD11257
HD12307
HD12101
HD11209 (2)
HD12208
ON1 JN257693
HD12056 (3)
ON1 KF587987
ON1 JX885731
HD12244
HD12229
HD12114
NA1 JX988456
95
HD12126 (3)
NA1 KC342390
HD12055
NA1 KC297377
HD12277
HD11315
86
HD12119 (2)
HD12072
HD12184 (2)
HD12262
89
HD12003
71
NA1 KF246587
HD12090
HD12188
86
HD11153
NA1 KF246643
99
HD11061 (7)
70
NA2 AB603444
99
NA2 AB603443
GA2 AF233915
99
GA2 JX256971
99
GA3 AF233921
GA3 AF233913
98
GA7 AF233910
GA7 DQ171754
GA4 AF065254
95
GA6 AF233918
GA6 EU582173
99
SAA1 AF348807
SAA1 AF548797
GA5 AB175815
99
GA5 JN257698
99
HD12279
GA1 AF233914
M11486
0.02
cl. 1
cl. 2
cl. 3
ON1
NA1
NA2
GA2
GA3
GA7
GA4
GA6
SAA1
GA5
GA1
outgroup
B
HD22106
HD22271
HD24121
BAIX HM459878
HD24154
BAIX KC342347
HD24250
HD24278
78
HD24230
HD24253
BAIX KF246629
HD24308
BAIX KF246624
92
HD12063
BAVII KC297492
BAVII HM459865
BAVIII HM459872
99
BAVIII AB603478
99
BAXII KF246585
BAXII KF246586
78
BAX HM459884
BAX KC297426
HD22118
HD22098
HD24201
83
HD22120
HD22269
100
BAII HM459856
BAII HM459857
BAIV HM459858
BAIV DQ227396
BAIII DQ227370
90
BAIII GQ150691
72
BAV AB603482
BAV AB603480
BAVI AY751110
BAVI AY751111
BAI DQ227398
BAI DQ227373
GB3 AF233932
100
URU1 AY488805
URU1 AY488804
99
SAB4 JN119987
SAB4 JN119979
96
SAB3 AF348813
SAB3 JF704216
100
GB4 AY672691
GB4 AY672698
SAB2 AF348821
99
SAB2 AF309676
100
SAB1 AY660684
SAB1 AY660682
100
GB1 M73542
GB1 AF013254
THB KC342336
100
THB KC342343
GB2 AF065251
URU2 AY333361
URU2 AY488803
M17213
0.01
cl. 1
cl. 2
BAIX
BAVII
BAVIII
BAXII
BA
BAX
BAII
BAIV
BAIII
BAV
BAVI
BAI
GB3
URU1
SAB4
SAB3
GB4
SAB2
SAB1
GB1
THB
GB2
URU2
outgroup

Figure 2. Phylogenetic tree of RSV A/RSV B strains and reference sequences of identified genotypes. Phylogenetic trees for RSV A (A) and RSV B (B) strains were constructed with maximum-likelihood method with 1,000 bootstrap replicates using MEGA 6 software. RSV strains from Heidelberg/Germany are indicated by "●HD" followed by their strain identification number. Number of identical strains is indicated in brackets after the strain identifier. Reference strains representing known genotypes were retrieved from GenBank and included in the tree (labels include accession number). The genotype assignment is shown on the right by brackets. Prototype strains (M11486 for subgroup A and M17213 for subgroup B) were used as an outgroup. Bootstrap values greater than 70% are indicated at the branch nodes. The scale bar represents the number of nucleotide substitutions per site. cl. = cluster.

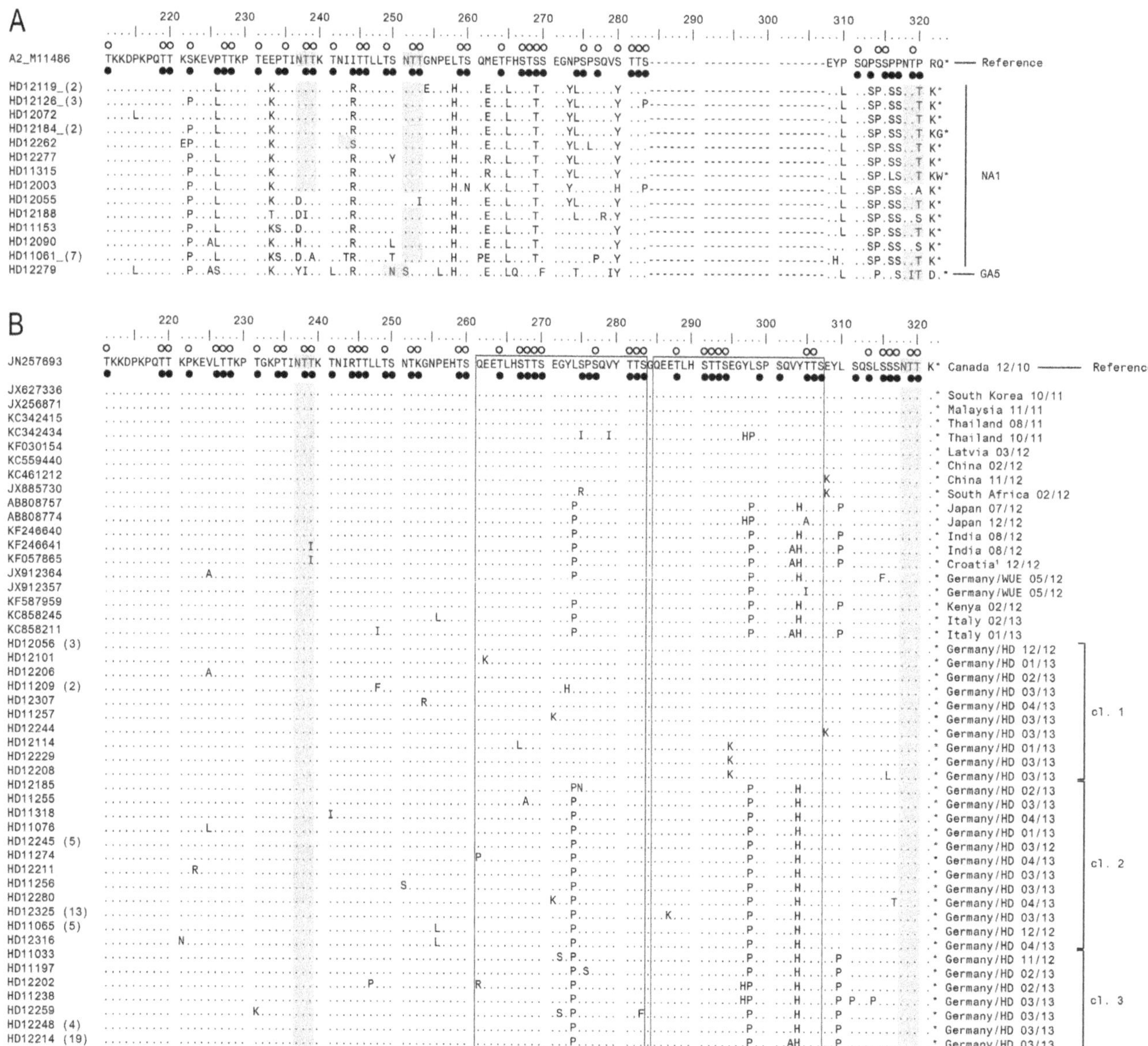

Figure 3. Alignment of deduced amino acid sequences of RSV-A strains. A) Alignment of RSV-A genotype NA1 and GA5 are shown relative to the sequence of prototype strain A2 (GenBank accession number M11486). Alignment of sequences was performed using the Clustal W 1.6 method via MEGA 6 software. The amino acid positions correspond to positions 210 to 298 of the G protein of strain A2. Identical residues are indicated by dots, asterisks indicate the position of stop codons. Number of identical strains is indicated in brackets after the strain identifier in the left column. Gray shading highlights predicted N-glycosylation sites. Unfilled circles indicate predicted O-glycosylation sites of the prototype strain A2; potential O-glycosylation sites of Heidelberg strains are indicated by black dots. The genotype assignment is shown on the right by brackets. B) Alignments are shown relative to the sequence of ON1 strain first described in Canada (GenBank accession number JN257693). Alignment of sequences was performed using the Clustal W 1.6 method via MEGA 6 software. The amino acid positions correspond to positions 210 to 298 of the G protein of the prototype strain A2. Identical residues are indicated by dots, asterisks indicate the position of stop codons. Boxes frame the 23 amino acid duplicated region of the 24 amino acid insertion. Gray shading highlights predicted N-glycosylation sites. Unfilled circles indicate predicted O-glycosylation sites of the Canadian reference ON1 strain; potential O-glycosylation sites of Heidelberg strains are indicated by black dots. On the right hand site, GenBank and Heidelberg strains are labeled with the country and time of occurrence (month/year).

[1] Sequences were published in GenBank only.

HD = Heidelberg; WUE = Wuerzburg, cl. = cluster.

KF246641, KF246640]. However, positive selection analysis of ON1 strains revealed no positive selected site.

All Heidelberg ON1 strains had two predicted N-glycosylation sites at aa positions 237 and 318 and lost the N-glycosylation sites at aa position 251 due to a T251K substitution. ON1 strains showed different patterns of O-glycosylation sites with 31 to 44 predicted sites and showed some new sites when compared to the Ontario reference strain. The 23-aa duplicated region contained a maximum of 10 glycosylation sites as observed in 17 ON1 isolates from Heidelberg.

Heidelberg RSV-B genotype BA strains were compared to BA reference strain from Buenos Aires [AF33364] (Fig. 4). Stop codons were either at aa position 320 for HD24308, HD24250 and HD24278 or at aa position 313 for the remaining BA strains. All BA strains had a K218P, L223P and S247P substitution. The BAIX genotype had a H287Y and a V271A substitution. Furthermore some BAIX strains (sub-cluster 1) had a P291L substitution whereas other BAIX strains (sub-cluster 2) had an I281T substitution. The BAX strains had a P291G substitution.

All Heidelberg RSV B strains had a predicted N-glycosylation site at aa positions 296. However the N-glycosylation site at aa position 310 only fulfilled the typical amino acid patterns but the glycosylation potential calculated by NetOGlyc 3.1 server was below 0.5 in isolates with a stop codon at aa position 313. HD24253 had an additional potential N-glycosylation site at aa position 230. O-glycosylation of BA strains varied between 40 and 47 predicted sites and showed an additional predicted site at aa position 317 in longer strains with a stop codon at aa position 320.

Basic and clinical characteristics of the study cohort

The mean age of the all screened children was 7.9 months and ranged in line with the inclusion criteria between 11 days and 23.8 months. RSV-positive patients were significantly younger compared to RSV-negative patients (t-test; $p<0.001$). The age group distribution showed that 62.7% RSV-positive children were below 6 months of age. All children had at least a concomitant acute RTI at time of admission; however, in some patients the main clinical diagnosis was non-respiratory (total 12.4%, RSV positive 4.5%). In RSV-positive patients the most common diagnosis was bronchitis/bronchiolitis (75.4%). The mean duration of hospitalization was longer in RSV-positive patients (3.5 vs. 5.1 days; $p<0.01$).

We performed a group comparison of the main three genotypes (RSV-A: ON1 and NA1; RSV-B: BA) using basic and clinical characteristics of RSV-positive infants and children (Table 1). There were no risk factors for one of the three groups of genotypes identified when looking at the demographic characteristics (age, gender, weight). Furthermore, we could not identify any association between a specific genotype and a more severe course of illness when taking the retrospectively available clinical and laboratory parameters into account.

Discussion

RSV accounts for a significant burden of acute respiratory tract infections particularly in infants and young children in need for hospital care [30]. Patterns of circulating RSV genotypes can provide a better understanding of the molecular epidemiology of RSV infection. In our study, we analyzed the genetic diversity and patterns of co-circulating genotypes of both, subtypes RSV-A and RSV-B, during the winter season 2012–13 in Heidelberg/Germany. RSV was detected in 134 out of 242 samples of which 110 (82.1%) were sub-grouped as RSV-A and 24 (17.9%) as RSV-B, respectively. Phylogenetic analysis revealed that the majority of RSV-A strains (n = 73, 75.3%) clustered with strains of the novel ON1 genotype with a 72-nt duplication first described by Eshaghi et al. in Ontario, Canada in 2010 [14]. In Germany, circulation of this genotype was reported for the first time in Wuerzburg in winter 2011–12 [31]. In line with another study in Europe, this study reports ON1 as the predominant genotype during the RSV epidemic season 2012–13, suggesting a rapid spread of this emerging RSV strain [32,33].

Most RSV cases were detected between December 2012 and April 2013, which is in line with the previously described seasonality of RSV infection in Germany [30]. However, the core season with more than half of all RSV-positive cases was from end-January to mid-March, which can be considered a late pattern of a RSV epidemic season in Germany [22]. Within our study population RSV was detectable in 55.4% of hospitalized children below the age of 2 years emphasizing the need for RSV screening on admission to assure proper management and to prevent nosocomial infections [34].

In our cohort, age group analysis revealed that infants below 6 months of age had the highest infection rates, as expected. Primary RSV infection commonly occurs within the first year of life [13]

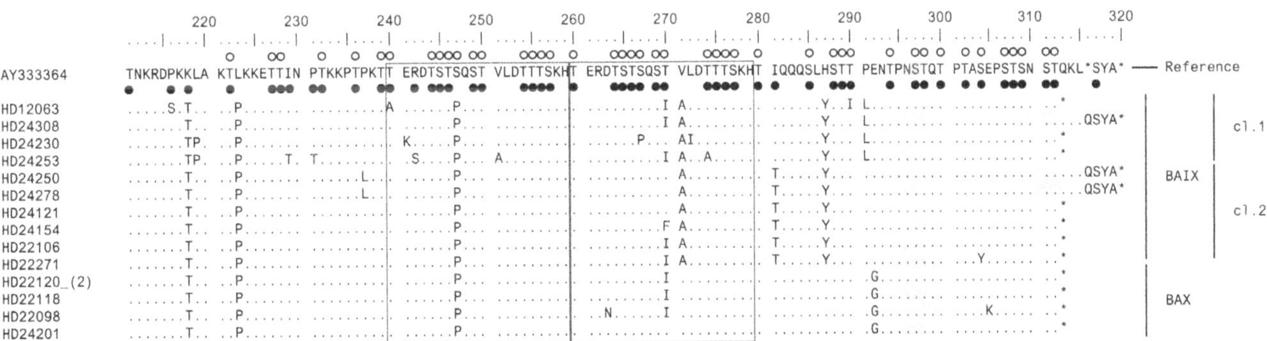

Figure 4. Alignment of deduced amino acid sequences of the second variable region of the G protein of RSV-B strains isolated in Heidelberg/Germany during 2012–2013 winter season. Alignments are shown relative to the sequence of a prototype BA strain (GenBank accession number AY333364). Alignment of sequences was performed using the Clustal W 1.6 method via MEGA 6 software. The amino acid positions correspond to positions 210 to 315 of the G protein of the BA strain. Identical residues are indicated by dots, asterisks indicate the position of stop codons. Number of identical strains is indicated in brackets after the strain identifier in the left column. Boxes frame the 20 amino acid duplication. Gray shading highlights predicted N-glycosylation sites. Open circles indicate predicted O-glycosylation sites of the prototype BA strain; potential O-glycosylation sites of Heidelberg strains are indicated by black dots. Genotypes are shown on the right by brackets.

Table 1. Basic and clinical characteristics of RSV positive children by genotype.

	RSV positive	RSV A*		RSV B	p-value
		ON1	NA1	BA	
	n = 134	n = 73	n = 23	n = 15	
Demographic characteristics					
Age in months, mean ±SD	6.5±6.2	6.4±6.2	5.7±5.6	4.8±5.1	0.63
Age group, n (%)					
0–6 months	84 (62.7)	48 (65.8)	15 (65.2)	10 (66.7)	0.18
>6–12 months	20 (14.9)	7 (9.6)	6 (26.1)	3 (20.0)	
>12–18 months	20 (14.9)	13(17.8)	0 (0.0)	2 (13.3)	
>18–24 months	10 (7.5)	15 (6.9)	2 (8.7)	0 (0.0)	
Gender, n (%)					
Male	83 (61.9)	44 (60.3)	18 (78.3)	9 (60.0)	0.28
Female	51 (38.1)	29 (39.7)	5 (21.7)	6 (40.0)	
Weight in kg, mean ±SD	6.2±2.3	5.9±2.1	7.0±2.7	5.8±2.3	0.11
Leading clinical diagnosis, n (%)					
Non-respiratory	6 (4.5)	4 (5.5)	0 (0.0)	1 (6.7)	0.49
Respiratory	128 (95.5)	69 (94.5)	23 (100.0)	14 (93.3)	
Upper RTI	4 (3.0)	1 (1.4)	1 (4.4)	0 (0.0)	0.61
Bronchitis/Bronchiolitis	101 (75.4)	54 (74.0)	20 (87.0)	12 (80.0)	
Pneumonia	23 (17.2)	14 (19.2)	2 (8.7)	2 (6.7)	
Course of disease					
Symptoms prior to hospitalization in days, mean ±SD	4.2±3.6	3.9±3.1	3.9±2.9	3.8±5.0	0.98
Hospital stay in days, mean ±SD#	5.3±3.9	5.3±3.8	5.5±2.8	4.5±2.1	0.68
Need for intensive care, n (%)	6 (4.5)	4 (5.5)	0 (0.0)	1 (6.7)	0.49
Laboratory parameters on admission					
Hemoglobin in g/dl, mean ±SD	11.7±1.7	11.4±1.5	11.9±1.9	11.7±2.0	0.45
Leucocytes/nl, mean ±SD	11.5±4.7	11.0±4.5	10.1±3.6	10.4±3.8	0.64
Thrombocytes/nl, mean ±SD	434.2±120.5	435.8±130.9	391.5±84.6	467.9±117.4	0.17
C-reactive protein in mg/L, mean ±SD	22.5±37.0	20.1±26.7	22.4±24.5	17.5±17.7	0.88
pCO2 in mmHg, mean ±SD	41.5±8.8	41.6±9.4	42.1±8.4	45.6±8.9	0.44

*RSV A genotype GA5 was not included in this table as this genotype was only present in one patient. In total, 112 of 134 RSV positive patients could be sequenced and a genotype could be determined.
#Hospital stay was only calculated for patients who stayed at least 24 hours in hospital.
SD = standard deviation; RTI = respiratory tract infection, RSV = Respiratory Syncytial Virus.

and the risk of RSV infection decreases with increasing age [22]. The majority of RSV-positive children presented with bronchitis/bronchiolitis followed by pneumonia and the duration of hospitalization was significantly longer compared to RSV-negative patients. However, the median duration of hospital stay of 5 days in RSV-positive patients in this study was shorter compared to previous findings of 7 days [30].

Molecular analysis of RSV-positive samples demonstrated that RSV-A was the predominant subtype which is in line with previous findings of multiple-season studies from Europe and other geographical areas [21,22]. Phylogenetic analysis revealed that the majority of RSV-A strains (n = 73, 75.3%) clustered with strains of the novel ON1 genotype with a 72-nt duplication. Phylogenetic analysis of Tsukagoshi et al. estimated that genotype ON1 evolved from genotype NA1 [35]. Recent estimates place the time of the ON1 emergence around 2008/09 [36,37].

Over the past three epidemic seasons (2010–2013) the prevalence of ON1 strains among all circulating strains varied between the different reports, but there seems to be a trend towards ON1 as the predominating RSV-A strain. In its first description in Ontario/Canada, the genotype ON1 accounted for 10% of RSV-positive samples in the season 2010-11 [14]. In the same season in Thailand, the majority of RSV isolates belonged to NA1, only few isolates belonged to ON1 [20]. One season later in 2011–12, RSV-A genotype ON1 was reported in different studies from Asia, Africa and Europe suggesting a worldwide emergence of the novel RSV-A strain. However, ON1 was only sporadically detected during that time and some countries like Pakistan did not report ON1 among circulating genotypes in 2011–12 [34]. A study from Heidelberg/Germany evaluating the genetic diversity of RSV in an outbreak in a haematology unit in 2012 also did not describe any ON1 strains [38]. In a study from Bejing, China, only one sample from February 2012 out of about 250 sequenced RSV-positive samples between 2007 and 2012 was characterized as ON1 genotype [39]. One report from Wuerzburg/Germany, assigned 10% of the identified strains to genotype ON1 in 2011–

12 [31]. In the past months an increasing number of reports about circulating genotypes in the season 2012–13 were published. In line with the findings in this study, reports from Cyprus, Italy, Kenya and South Korea described ON1 as the predominating genotype in the epidemic season 2012–13 [32,33,36,37]. Our study therefore describes a further cohort in Europe with ON1 as the predominating genotype in 2012–13 suggesting a rapid emergence of this novel strain. Further surveillance of circulating genotypes will be needed to observe the future global distribution of the ON1 strain and its trend to diversify.

The comparison of Heidelberg ON1 strains with ON1 strains from other countries revealed that Heidelberg isolates could be divided into three sub-clusters with characteristic substitutions as previously described in different countries and continents. Similar to the subdivision of RSV-B genotype BA into several sub-genotypes (BA-I – BAXII), this could be a first trend to a diversification of the ON1 genotype. However, none of the sub-clusters had bootstrap values ≥70%. Furthermore, positive selection analysis did not reveal any positively selective sites among ON1 isolates. This is also reflected by two groups of identical isolates (n = 13 and n = 18) of the ON1 genotype, suggesting the absence of selective pressure among the newly emerging strains.

Although the majority of strains was subtyped as RSV-A, 13.4% of all Heidelberg trains were subtyped as RSV-B. All RSV-B strains clustered with strains of the BA genotype with a 60-nt duplication, first described by Trento et al. in Buenos Aires, Argentina in 1999 [23], further differentiating into the genotypes BAIX (n = 10, 66.7%) and BAX (n = 5, 33.3%). Genotype BAIX separated into two sub-clusters: one including the BAIX reference sequence from Japan designated by Dapat et al. [18] who first described this genotype in 2007, and the second including the BAIX reference sequence from India described by Choudhary et al. in 2010 [40]. However, none of the two sub-clusters had bootstrap values ≥70%.

Similar to genotype BA, the nucleotide duplication of the ON1 genotype seems to result in a selection advantage compared to other RSV-A genotypes. Interestingly, despite the emergence of the ON1 virus there is conflicting data concerning the virulence in terms of disease severity [31–33]. In our cohort, retrospective analysis of basic clinical and laboratory parameters such as the duration of hospital stay, the need for intensive care as well as pCO_2 levels on admission did not reveal any association between a specific genotype and disease severity. Further surveillance of circulating RSV genotypes and corresponding clinical data is needed to understand the evolution, transmission and pathogenicity of genotype ON1 RSV infections.

Our study is subject to several limitations: We report the genetic diversity of RSV during one season in winter 2012–13 and a comparison of proportions of circulating genotypes is therefore restricted to other reports from Germany as well as worldwide. Our analysis included hospitalized children with community acquired RSV infection and therefore cannot draw conclusions for the overall population of community acquired RSV infections. However, the cohort of hospitalized children is of particular clinical relevance. Due to the retrospective study design, the evaluation of the association between pathogenicity of RSV infection and genotypes was limited to the available data. Furthermore, we did not include an analysis of further co-infections, which might also have an effect on disease severity in the evaluated study cohort. Further surveillance of the molecular epidemiology for several seasons in combination with prospectively complied clinical data is needed to directly compare the emergence of new variants and their transmissibility and virulence.

In summary, molecular characterization of RSV in Heidelberg, Germany during winter season 2012–13 confirmed the co-circulation of multiple genotypes of subtype RSV-A and RSV-B and the predominance of the novel genotype ON1. In line with the emergence of the BA genotype, it can be hypothesized that genotype ON1 could spread in a similar way and several branches might subdivide into further sub-genotypes. However, we could not find any association between disease severity and this newly emerging RSV-A genotype ON1. Continuing and long-term molecular epidemiological surveys for early detection of circulating and newly emerging genotypes in combination with clinical data are necessary to gain a better understanding of underlying genetic and antigenic mechanisms of RSV infection.

Acknowledgments

We would like to thank all nurses in the Department of Pediatrics, Heidelberg, Germany for collecting respiratory samples and all technicians in the virology diagnostic laboratory Heidelberg, Germany and Benedikt Weissbrich from the virology diagnostic laboratory at the University of Wuerzburg, Germany for excellent technical assistance. Furthermore, we cordially thank our colleague Steffen Geis from the virology diagnostic laboratory Heidelberg for the support in developing the methodology, critical reading of the manuscript as well as for his statistical advice.

Author Contributions

Conceived and designed the experiments: JT CP JGH PS. Performed the experiments: JT CP. Analyzed the data: JT CP JP. Wrote the paper: JT PS.

References

1. Glezen WP, Taber LH, Frank AL, Kasel JA (1986) Risk of primary infection and reinfection with respiratory syncytial virus. Am J Dis Child 140: 543–546.
2. Henderson FW, Collier AM, Clyde WA, Denny FW (1979) Respiratory-syncytial-virus infections, reinfections and immunity. A prospective, longitudinal study in young children. N Engl J Med 300: 530–534. doi: 10.1056/NEJM197903083001004
3. García O, Martín M, Dopazo J, Arbiza J, Frabasile S, et al. (1994) Evolutionary pattern of human respiratory syncytial virus (subgroup A): cocirculating lineages and correlation of genetic and antigenic changes in the G glycoprotein. J Virol 68: 5448–5459.
4. Hall CB, Walsh EE, Long CE, Schnabel KC (1991) Immunity to and frequency of reinfection with respiratory syncytial virus. J Infect Dis163: 693–698.
5. Storch GA, Anderson LJ, Park CS, Tsou C, Dohner DE (1991) Antigenic and genomic diversity within group A respiratory syncytial virus. 163: 858–861.
6. Pretorius MA, van Niekerk S, Tempia S, Moyes J, Cohen C, et al. (2013) Replacement and Positive Evolution of Subtype A and B Respiratory Syncytial Virus G-Protein Genotypes From 1997–2012 in South Africa. J Infect Dis 208: S227–S237. doi: 10.1093/infdis/jit477
7. Anderson LJ, Hierholzer JC, Tsou C, Hendry RM, Fernie BF, et al. (1985) Antigenic characterization of respiratory syncytial virus strains with monoclonal antibodies. J Infect Dis 151: 626–633.
8. Wertz GW, Krieger M, Ball LA (1989) Structure and cell surface maturation of the attachment glycoprotein of human respiratory syncytial virus in a cell line deficient in O glycosylation. J Virol 63: 4767–4776.
9. Johnson PR, Spriggs MK, Olmsted RA, Collins PL (1987) The G glycoprotein of human respiratory syncytial viruses of subgroups A and B: extensive sequence divergence between antigenically related proteins. Proc Natl Acad Sci USA 84: 5625–5629.
10. Peret TC, Hall CB, Schnabel KC, Golub JA, Anderson LJ (1998) Circulation patterns of genetically distinct group A and B strains of human respiratory syncytial virus in a community. J Gen Virol 79 (Pt 9): 2221–2229.
11. Peret TCT, Hall CB, Hammond GW, Piedra PA, Storch GA, et al. (2000) Circulation patterns of group A and B human respiratory syncytial virus genotypes in 5 communities in North America. J Infect Dis 181: 1891–1896. doi: 10.1086/315508
12. Venter M, Madhi SA, Tiemessen CT, Schoub BD (2001) Genetic diversity and molecular epidemiology of respiratory syncytial virus over four consecutive

seasons in South Africa: identification of new subgroup A and B genotypes. J Gen Virol 82: 2117–2124.

13. Shobugawa Y, Saito R, Sano Y, Zaraket H, Suzuki Y, et al. (2009) Emerging Genotypes of Human Respiratory Syncytial Virus Subgroup A among Patients in Japan. J Clin Microbiol 47: 2475–2482. doi: 10.1128/JCM.00115-09
14. Eshaghi A, Duvvuri VR, Lai R, Nadarajah JT, Li A, et al. (2012) Genetic variability of human respiratory syncytial virus A strains circulating in Ontario: a novel genotype with a 72 nucleotide G gene duplication. PLoS ONE 7: e32807. doi: 10.1371/journal.pone.0032807
15. Arnott A, Vong S, Mardy S, Chu S, Naughtin M, et al. (2011) A study of the genetic variability of human respiratory syncytial virus (HRSV) in Cambodia reveals the existence of a new HRSV group B genotype. J Clin Microbiol 49: 3504–3513. doi: 10.1128/JCM.01131-11
16. Blanc A, Delfraro A, Frabasile S, Arbiza J (2005) Genotypes of respiratory syncytial virus group B identified in Uruguay. Arch Virol 150: 603–609. doi: 10.1007/s00705-004-0412-x
17. Trento A, Viegas M, Galiano M, Videla C, Carballal G, et al. (2006) Natural history of human respiratory syncytial virus inferred from phylogenetic analysis of the attachment (G) glycoprotein with a 60-nucleotide duplication. J Virol 80: 975–984. doi: 10.1128/JVI.80.2.975-984.2006
18. Dapat IC, Shobugawa Y, Sano Y, Saito R, Sasaki A, et al. (2010) New Genotypes within Respiratory Syncytial Virus Group B Genotype BA in Niigata, Japan. J Clin Microbiol 48: 3423–3427. doi: 10.1128/JCM.00646-10
19. Baek YH, Choi EH, Song M-S, Pascua PNQ, Kwon H-I, et al. (2012) Prevalence and genetic characterization of respiratory syncytial virus (RSV) in hospitalized children in Korea. Arch Virol 157: 1039–1050. doi: 10.1007/s00705-012-1267-1
20. Khor C-S, Sam I-C, Hooi P-S, Chan Y-F (2013) Displacement of predominant respiratory syncytial virus genotypes in Malaysia between 1989 and 2011. Infect Genet Evol 14: 357–360. doi: 10.1016/j.meegid.2012.12.017
21. Auksornkitti V, Kamprasert N, Thongkomplew S, Suwannakarn K, Theamboonlers A, et al. (2014) Molecular characterization of human respiratory syncytial virus, 2010–2011: identification of genotype ON1 and a new subgroup B genotype in Thailand. Arch Virol 159: 499–507. doi: 10.1007/s00705-013-1773-9
22. Reiche J, Schweiger B (2009) Genetic variability of group A human respiratory syncytial virus strains circulating in Germany from 1998 to 2007. J Clin Microbiol 47: 1800–1810. doi: 10.1128/JCM.02286-08
23. Melero JA, Trento A, Videla C, Galiano M, Carballal G, et al. (2003) Major changes in the G protein of human respiratory syncytial virus isolates introduced by a duplication of 60 nucleotides. J Gen Virol 84: 3115–3120. doi: 10.1099/vir.0.19357-0
24. Trento A, Casas I, Calderón A, Garcia-Garcia ML, Calvo C, et al. (2010) Ten years of global evolution of the human respiratory syncytial virus BA genotype with a 60-nucleotide duplication in the G protein gene. J Virol 84: 7500–7512. doi: 10.1128/JVI.00345-10
25. Valley-Omar Z, Muloiwa R, Hu N-C, Eley B, Hsiao N-Y (2013) Novel respiratory syncytial virus subtype ON1 among children, Cape Town, South Africa, 2012. Emerging Infect Dis 19: 668–670. doi: 10.3201/eid1904.121465
26. Tamura K, Stecher G, Peterson D, Filipski A, Kumar S (2013) MEGA6: Molecular Evolutionary Genetics Analysis version 6.0. Mol Biol Evol 30: 2725–2729. doi: 10.1093/molbev/mst197
27. Delport W, Poon AFY, Frost SDW, Kosakovsky Pond SL (2010) Datamonkey 2010: a suite of phylogenetic analysis tools for evolutionary biology. Bioinformatics 26: 2455–2457. doi: 10.1093/bioinformatics/btq429
28. Gupta R, Jung E, Brunak S (2004) Prediction of N-glycosylation sites in human proteins. NetNGlycServer. Available: http://www.cbs.dtu.dk/services/NetNGlyc/. Accessed: 2014 Apr 6.
29. Julenius K, Mølgaard A, Gupta R, Brunak S (2005) Prediction, conservation analysis, and structural characterization of mammalian mucin-type O-glycosylation sites. Glycobiology 15: 153–164. doi: 10.1093/glycob/cwh151
30. Berner R, Schwoerer F, Schumacher RF, Meder M, Forster J (2001) Community and nosocomially acquired respiratory syncytial virus infection in a German paediatric hospital from 1988 to 1999. Eur J Pediatr 160: 541–547.
31. Prifert C, Streng A, Krempl CD, Liese J, Weissbrich B (2013) Novel respiratory syncytial virus a genotype, Germany, 2011–2012. Emerging Infect Dis 19: 1029–1030. doi: 10.3201/eid1906.121582
32. Panayiotou C, Richter J, Koliou M, Kalogirou N, Georgiou E, et al. (2014) Epidemiology of respiratory syncytial virus in children in Cyprus during three consecutive winter seasons (2010–2013): age distribution, seasonality and association between prevalent genotypes and disease severity. Epidemiol Infect: 1–6. doi: 10.1017/S0950268814000028
33. Pierangeli A, Trotta D, Scagnolari C, Ferreri ML, Nicolai A, et al. (2014) Rapid spread of the novel respiratory syncytial virus A ON1 genotype, central Italy, 2011 to 2013. Euro Surveill 19.
34. Aamir UB, Alam MM, Sadia H, Zaidi SSZ, Kazi BM (2013) Molecular Characterization of Circulating Respiratory Syncytial Virus (RSV) Genotypes in Gilgit Baltistan Province of Pakistan during 2011–2012 Winter Season. PLoS ONE 8: e74018. doi: 10.1371/journal.pone.0074018
35. Tsukagoshi H, Yokoi H, Kobayashi M, Kushibuchi I, Okamoto-Nakagawa R, et al. (2013) Genetic analysis of attachment glycoprotein (G) gene in new genotype ON1 of human respiratory syncytial virus detected in Japan. Microbiol Immunol 57: 655–659. doi: 10.1111/1348-0421.12075
36. Agoti CN, Otieno JR, Gitahi CW, Cane PA, Nokes DJ (2014) Rapid spread and diversification of respiratory syncytial virus genotype ON1, Kenya. Emerging Infect Dis 20: 950–959. doi: 10.3201/eid2006.131438
37. Kim Y-J, Kim D-W, Lee W-J, Yun M-R, Lee HY, et al. (2014) Rapid replacement of human respiratory syncytial virus A with the ON1 genotype having 72 nucleotide duplication in G gene. Infect Genet Evol 26C: 103–112. doi: 10.1016/j.meegid.2014.05.007
38. Geis S, Prifert C, Weissbrich B, Lehners N, Egerer G, et al. (2013). Molecular characterization of a respiratory syncytial virus (RSV) outbreak in a haematology unit, Heidelberg, Germany. J Clin Microbiol 51: 155–162.
39. Cui G, Qian Y, Zhu R, Deng J, Zhao L, et al. (2013) Emerging human respiratory syncytial virus genotype ON1 found in infants with pneumonia in Beijing, China. Emerg Microbes Infect 2: e22. doi: 10.1038/emi.2013.19
40. Choudhary ML, Anand SP, Wadhwa BS, Chadha MS (2013) Genetic variability of human respiratory syncytial virus in Pune, Western India. Infect Genet Evol 20C: 369–377. doi: 10.1016/j.meegid.2013.09.025

Clinical Characteristics and Immunogenetics of BCGosis/BCGitis in Chinese Children: A 6 Year Follow-Up Study

Wenjing Ying[☯], Jinqiao Sun[☯], Danru Liu[☯], Xiaoying Hui, Yeheng Yu, Jingyi Wang, Xiaochuan Wang*

Department of Clinical Immunology, Children's Hospital of Fudan University, Shanghai, China

Abstract

In this study, the clinical and immunogenetical features in a cohort of Chinese patients with BCGosis/BCGitis were investigated. For the patients with abnormal immunological functions, Sanger sequencing was used to identify the involved genes. There were 74 confirmed cases of BCGosis/BCGitis during 2007–2012. Classified by infected tissues and organs, no cases only had local infection, 39 patients had a regional infection, 21 patients had a distant infection and 14 patients had a disseminated infection. Thirty-two patients (43.2%) had definitive primary immunodeficiency diseases (PID) and chronic granulomatous disease (CGD) is the most common PID (n = 23, accounted for 71.9% of all PID patients). For CGD patients, based on the anti-tuberculosis treatment, administration of rhIFN-γ resulted in better control of BCGosis/BCGitis. The results indicate that PIDs are associated with susceptibility to BCG disease. For children with BCGosis/BCGitis, immune function evaluation is necessary, and IFN-γ treatment for BCGosis/BCGitis patients with CGD is effective.

Editor: Robert J. Wilkinson, Institute of Infectious Diseases and Molecular Medicine, South Africa

Funding: This work was supported by National Natural Science Foundation of China (81172877) and Shanghai Rising-Star Program (11QA1400700). The funders had no role in study design, data collection and analysis, decision to publish, or preparation of the manuscript.

Competing Interests: The authors have declared that no competing interests exist.

* E-mail: xchwang@shmu.edu.cn

☯ These authors contributed equally to this work.

Introduction

The Bacillus Calmette-Guerin (BCG) vaccine has existed for 80 years and is one of the most widely used of all current vaccines. The BCG vaccine has a protective effect against meningitis and disseminated tuberculosis (TB) in children [1]. The World Health Organization (WHO) recommends that all infants in highly endemic countries receive a single dose of the BCG vaccine [2]. For most children, BCG vaccination is harmless. However, infection, even disseminated infection, caused by BCG has occasionally been reported. The incidence of BCG infection is approximately 1:10,000–1:1,000,000 [3]. The BCG-induced disease phenotypes were designated as local, regional, distant, or disseminated pattern based on a revised pediatric classification proposed by Hesseling et al. [4]. The former two patterns were conventionally termed as BCGitis and the latter two as BCGosis.

Previous studies suggest that the immunological condition of children is an important factor in BCG infection. In 1995, Casanova et al. [5] reviewed 121 published cases of disseminated BCG infections. They found 61 cases of definitive immunodeficiency disease: 45 cases were severe combined immunodeficiency disease (SCID), 11 cases were chronic granulomatous disease (CGD), 4 cases were acquired immunodeficiency syndrome and 1 case had complete DiGeorge syndrome (CDGS). Norouzi et al. [6] reported that out of 158 patients with BCGosis, 120 of these patients had immunodeficiency disease. These results indicate that immunogenetic factors are critical, as these can lead to BCGosis/BCGitis. However, most of the studies on BCGosis/BCGitis are based on case reports. Until recently, there was no large sample study on the clinical characteristics and immunogenetics of BCGosis/BCGitis.

China remains one of the 22 countries that have a high TB burden that is recognized by the WHO. The prevalence of TB in China fell slightly during the past decade, but the nation still has the world's second-largest population of people with the disease [7]. The Chinese Center for Disease Control and Prevention recommends that all infants receive a single dose of the BCG vaccine immediately after birth. Some infants present with BCGosis/BCGitis after vaccination. So, we conducted this study to clarify the clinical characteristics and to describe the spectrum of primary immunodeficiency diseases (PID) in a cohort of Chinese patients with BCGosis/BCGitis.

Materials and Methods

Ethics Statement

This study was approved by the Pediatric Research Ethics Board of Clinical Pharmacology Base, Fudan University. Because all participants are children, we obtained the written informed consent from their parents, who on behalf of the children enrolled in the study.

Patients

The study began in January 2007 and was completed in December 2012. During this period, after the informed consent forms were obtained, all of the patients who were diagnosed with BCGosis/BCGitis in the Children's Hospital of Fudan University were enrolled in this study. A diagnosis of BCGosis/BCGitis was confirmed by clinical course, dermatological features, pathology, specific polymerase chain reaction (PCR) [8], and/or spoligotyping. The phenotypes of BCGosis/BCGitis were classified as local, regional, distant, and disseminated patterns, as proposed by Hesseling et al. [4].

Study design

The clinical features of all of the enrolled patients were observed and the basic immunological functions were evaluated. After evaluation of the basic immunological functions, some of the patients were diagnosed with PID. For these patients, the corresponding genes were detected according to their immune phenotype. For the patients with normal basic immunological functions, IL-12/23 and IFN-γ mediated immunity was investigated.

Routine evaluation of immunological function

The routine evaluation of immunological function involved the analysis of lymphocyte subsets; the detection of immunoglobulins G, A, M, E and complements C3, C4, and CH50; and the analysis of NADPH oxidase activity in neutrophils. Lymphocyte subsets were analyzed using a FACSCalibur flow cytometer (Becton Dickinson, Franklin Lakes, NJ, USA). Anti-CD3, CD4, CD8, CD16, CD56, CD19, and CD45 antibodies (Multitest IMK Kit, Catalog No. 340503, Becton Dickinson, Franklin Lakes, NJ, USA) were used. The immunoglobulins G, A, and M and complement C3 and C4 were detected by nephelometry. The immunoglobulin kit was purchased from Orion Diagnostica Oy (Espoo, Finland). The respiratory burst of neutrophils was determined by measuring hydrogen peroxide production, using DHR analysis [9].

Whole blood cultures and detection of IFN-γ production

According to a previous study [10], venous blood samples from patients with normal routine immunological functions were collected into heparinized tubes. These blood samples were diluted 1:2 in RPMI 1640 (Gibco) supplemented with 100 U/ml penicillin and 100 µg/ml streptomycin (Gibco). We dispensed 4.5 ml of the dilute blood sample into 3 wells (1.5 ml/well) of a 24-well plate. The plate was then incubated in an atmosphere containing 5% CO_2 and 95% air, with the following three different conditions for activation: with medium alone, with LPS (1 ng, Sigma), with LPS (1 ng, Sigma) plus IL-12 (35 ng, R&D). After 48 h, at the end of the incubation stage, the total volume of each well was recovered, centrifuged at 2500 g for 10 min, and the supernatant was stored at −80°C until the analysis. The IFN-γ concentrations were analyzed by ELISA according to the manufacturers' guidelines. The IFN-γ kits were purchased from Invitrogen (Grand Island, NY, USA).

Direct sequencing

Based on the immune phenotype of these patients, the different genes were sequenced. For patients with CGD, *CYBB*, *CYBA*, *NCF1*, *NCF2*, and *NCF4* genes were sequenced; for patients with SCID, *IL2RG*, *RAG1*, *RAG2*, *JAK3*, *IL7R*, and *LIG4* genes were sequenced; for patients with hyper IgE syndrome (HIES), *STAT3*, *TYK2*, and *DOCK8* genes were sequenced; for patients with hyper IgM syndrome (HIGM), *CD40LG*, *CD40*, *UNG*, and *AICDA* genes were sequenced; for patients with lower IFN-γ production, *IL12RB1* and *IFNGR1* genes were sequenced.

Genomic DNA was isolated from PBMCs using the RelaxGene Blood DNA System (Tiangen Biotech, Beijing, China) according to the manufacturer's instructions and amplified by PCR using synthetic oligonucleotide primers. The primer sequences were based on human genomic sequences and are available upon request. PCR products were purified by Performa DTR Gel Filtration Cartridges and directly sequenced by ABI Prism BigDye terminators. All of the entire coding regions were covered. Both strands were sequenced.

Results

Overview of the cases

There were 74 confirmed cases of BCGosis/BCGitis during the study period: 59 (79.7%) patients were boys and 15 (20.3%) patients were girls. These patients were all healthy at birth and had no contact history of TB. All patients were vaccinated with BCG within two days after birth. Among these 74 children, 32 (43.2%) had definitive PID, including 23 (31.1%) cases with CGD, 2 (2.7%) case with SCID, 2 (2.7%) cases with HIGM, 1 (1.4%) case with HIES, and 4 (5.4%) cases with Mendelian susceptibility to mycobacterial diseases (MSMD).

Clinical characteristics

Age of onset. Among the 74 patients, the median age of onset of BCGosis/BCGitis was 3.6 months old (range: 20 days to 4 years). Among the 32 patients with definitive PID, 22 (68.8%) patients presented with this condition within 1 year of vaccination, and the median age of onset is 3 months old (range: 20 days to 4 years). Among the 42 patients without definitive PID, the median age of onset is 4 months old (range: 1 month to 2 years). There is no significant difference in the age of onset of BCGosis/BCGitis between these two groups.

BCG disease classification. In the previous study [4], BCG disease was classified as local, regional, distant, and disseminated. Local or regional BCG disease was diagnosed upon confirmation of *M. bovis* BCG from fine-needle aspiration or swab samples of pus; distant or disseminated disease was diagnosed upon isolation of *M. bovis* BCG from respiratory isolates in children with respiratory symptoms or from other distant sites. Among the 74 patients, the most common tissues and organs that were affected are lymph nodes, vaccination site, and lung, regardless of whether patients had PID or not (Figure 1a). According to the above mentioned BCG disease classification, no case only had local infection, 39 (52.7%) patients had regional infection, 21 (28.4%) patients had distant infection and 14 (18.9%) patients had disseminated infection (Figure 1b). Classified by with or without definitive PID, 62.5% (20/32) patients with PID had distant or disseminated infection, and only 35.7% (15/42) patients without PID had distant or disseminated infection (Figure 1b). The results indicated that patients with PID usually had more severe BCG infection than patients without PID.

Immunological characteristics

The immunological functions of all 74 patients were evaluated. Twenty-eight patients had abnormal immunological functions. The immunological characteristics of all the 74 patients are shown in Table 1. Based on the immunological phenotype and clinical characteristic data, they were diagnosed with CGD (n = 23), SCID (n = 2), HIGM (n = 2), and HIES (n = 1), respectively. For the two SCID patients, we also detected their human immunodeficiency virus (HIV) status, because they had lower T cells counts than normal. Both are negative.

Detection of IFN-γ production

The production of IFN-γ in 46 patients with normal immune function was evaluated. We compared the production of IFN-γ in diluted whole blood after stimulation with medium alone, with LPS, and with LPS plus IL-12. We supplemented the medium

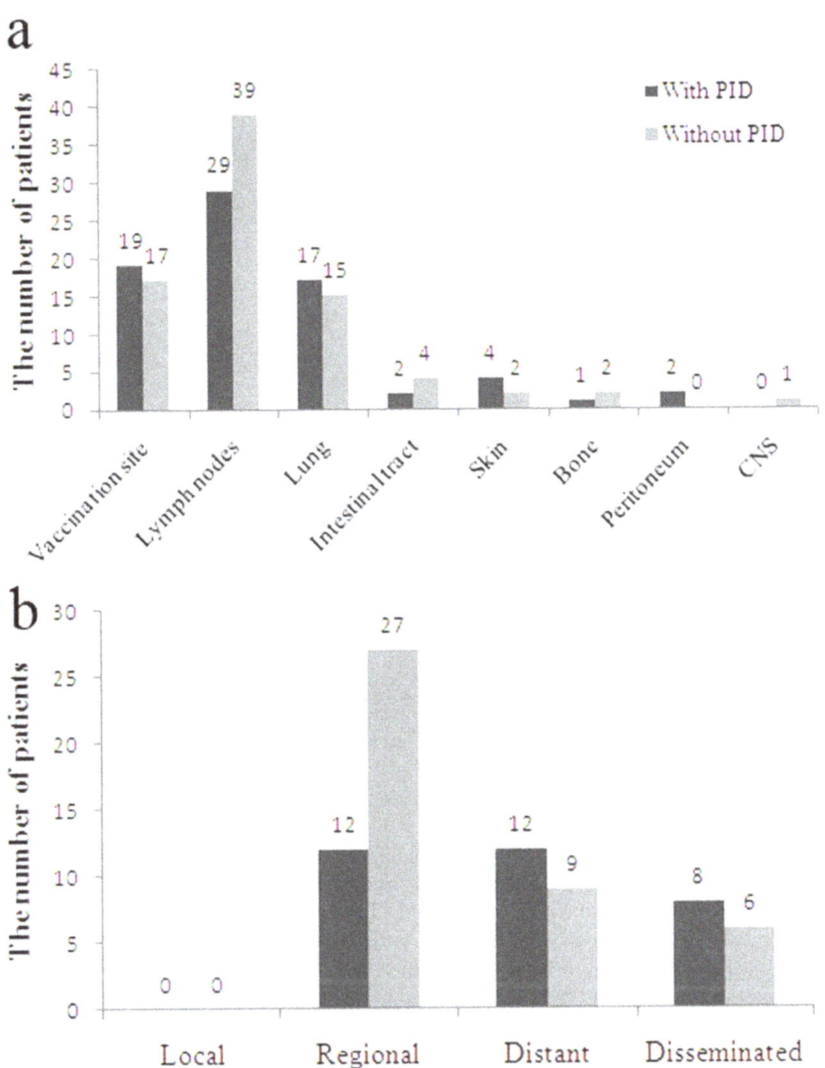

Figure 1. Clinical characteristics of 74 patients with BCGosis/BCGitis. a. infected tissues and organs; b. classification according to the infected tissues and organs. PID: primary immunodeficiency disease. CNS: central nervous system.

with IL-12, as it is a potent inducer of IFN-γ. Four patients showed significantly lower IFN-γ concentrations (37.30–37.77 pg/ml) in the supernatant after stimulation with medium alone, and IFN-γ concentrations did not significantly increase after stimulation with LPS (39.30–41.85 pg/ml) or with LPS plus IL-12 (48.10–61.59 pg/ml). Compared with these 4 patients, the remaining 42 patients showed higher IFN-γ concentrations in the supernatant after stimulation with medium alone (mean, 93.75 pg/ml) and with LPS (mean, 98.65 pg/ml), and IFN-γ concentrations had significantly increased after stimulation with LPS plus IL-12 (mean, 921.51 pg/ml).

Gene sequencing

Gene sequencing was performed for 28 patients with definitive PID and for 4 patients with lower IFN-γ production. Mutations were found in 26 patients. For 23 CGD patients, mutations in the *CYBB*, *CYBA*, *NCF1*, *NCF2* and *NCF4* genes were detected. Among the 23 CGD patients, 17 patients had a *CYBB* mutation, 1 patient had a *CYBA* mutation, 2 patients had a *NCF2* mutation, and no mutation was found in 3 cases. For 2 SCID patients, mutations in *IL2RG* were found. For 2 HIGM patients, *CD40LG*, *CD40*, *UNG*, and *AICDA* genes were sequenced. For 1 HIES patient, *STAT3*, *TYK2*, and *DOCK8* genes were sequenced. However, no mutation was found. For the 4 patients with lower IFN-γ production, we sequenced *IL12RB1* and *IFNGR1* genes. Two patients had a mutation in *IFNGR1* gene and the other 2 patients had a mutation in *IL12RB1* gene. The details of all the mutations are shown in Table 2.

Treatment and outcome

Forty-two patients without definitive PID received routine anti-TB treatment (Isoniazid, rifampicin and ethambutol). Among the 42 patients, 2 died from disseminated TB during therapy, and the remaining 40 patients were cured after 1 year of treatment.

Among the 23 CGD patients, 19 received routine anti-TB treatment, 1 was lost to follow-up, and 3 refused anti-TB treatment and died. Among the 19 patients received routine anti-TB treatment, 7 received recombinant human interferon-γ (rhIFN-γ) treatment (1 MIU/m^2, twice a week) together with anti-TB treatment. In all the 7 patients, BCGosis/BCGitis was cured after 1 year of treatment. Because the remaining 12 patients were not diagnosed with CGD when BCGosis/BCGitis was diagnosed, they

Table 1. Routine immunologic function evaluation in 74 BCGosis/BCGitis patients.

	without PID* (n = 42)	with CGD* (n = 23)	with HIGM* (n = 2)	with HIES* (n = 1)	with SCID* (n = 2)	with MSMD* (n = 4)
Lymphocyte subsets						
CD3+(%)	51–77	55–71	82; 72	94	9; 11	48–57
CD3+CD4+(%)	35–55	23–44	21; 22	52	4; 3	29–27
CD3+CD8+(%)	13–36	31–45	49; 45	27	4; 4	17–27
CD16+CD56+(%)	5–35	8–17	15; 17	2	2.5; 3.2	6–7
CD19+(%)	3–17	7–21	3; 5	4	65; 71	40–31
Immunoglobulin level						
IgG(g/L)	3.7–24.8	8.6–26	1.2; 1.75	24.6	0.98; 0.57	7.2–11.3
IgA(g/L)	0.1–2.24	0.81–3.02	1.28; 2.49	0.38	0.067; 0.03	0.23–0.98
IgM(g/L)	0.09–3.24	1.02–3.27	6.76; 55.34	3.08	0.04; 0.02	0.24–1.57
IgE(kU/L)	2.6–390	24.5–990	<2; 3.96	129000	<2	7.14–206
DHR analysis# (SI*)	>100	<10	>100	>100	>100	>100

*PID: primary immunodeficiency disease; CGD: chronic granulomatous disease; HIGM: hyper IgM syndrome; HIES: hyper IgE syndrome; MSMD: Mendelian susceptibility to mycobacterial diseases. SI: stimulation index.

#DHR analysis: The comparison was based on a stimulation index, which was defined as mean channel fluorescence intensity of PMA-stimulated neutrophils over mean channel fluorescence intensity of unstimulated neutrophils.

only received a routine anti-TB treatment. After treatment for more than 1 year, all the 12 patients were not cured and 3 died. When the remaining 9 patients were transferred to our center, they were diagnosed with CGD. They received treatment with routine anti-TB drugs and rhIFN-γ. After 1 year of treatment, BCGosis/BCGitis was cured in all the 9 patients.

Among the 4 patients with lower IFN-γ profuction, 2 cured after 2 years treatment with routine anti-TB drugs and rhIFN-γ, 1 died from disseminated TB during therapy, and 1 is still treated. Two SCID patients and 1 HIES patient also died from disseminated TB during therapy. In addition, 2 HIGM patients had received anti-TB treatment for more than 2 years, and BCGosis/BCGitis was not cured.

Discussion

The BCG vaccine has existed for 80 years and is one of the most widely used of all current vaccines, reaching >80% of neonates and infants in countries where it is part of the national childhood immunization program [1]. The BCG vaccine is widely used, and the safety of this vaccine has not been a serious issue until recently. Complications that arise from BCG vaccination are uncommon. Less than one in 1000 vaccinated individuals develop severe local reactions, and serious disseminated disease develops in less than one in a million cases [3]. There is a concern that use of the vaccine in people who are immunocompromised may result in an infection that is caused by BCG itself. The data reported by Casanova et al. [5] and Norouzi et al. [6] showed that 50% to 76% of BCG-infected patients had immunodeficiency. China is a high-TB-burden country. All full-term neonates are recommended to receive a single dose of BCG vaccine immediately after birth. With the improvement of medical technology, more children are being diagnosed with BCGosis/BCGitis in China. However, the data on the clinical characteristics and immunological conditions of these patients are lacking.

To investigate whether immunodeficiency is the main cause of BCGosis/BCGitis, we conducted the present study. The results showed that more than 40% patients with BCGosis/BCGitis had definitive PID. The proportion of patients with immunodeficiency is lower than in previous studies [5,6]. Moreover, the proportion of each type of PID is different. Casanova et al. [5] and Norouzi et al. [6] showed that SCID is the most common form of immunodeficiency in children with BCGosis/BCGitis. However, our study suggested that CGD is the most common form of immunodeficiency. This difference may be explained by the following reasons: 1. Most patients had disseminated BCG infection in the above mentioned two studies. However, only 14 patients had disseminated BCG infection in our study. Most of our patients had regional and distant infections. The difference in the types of PID between the previous study and our study may be explained by a difference in the severity of BCG infection; 2. Only a few hospitals have the ability to diagnose SCID in China. Children with SCID usually have more serious infections, and many of them die in local hospitals from complications of serious infection. These patients cannot obtain a clear diagnosis. In addition, we estimated that the incidence of SCID is lower in Chinese people. Accurate epidemiological data need further investigation.

Among the 74 patients with BCGosis/BCGitis, 23 had CGD. These results indicate that CGD patient are susceptible to BCG infection. CGD is a form of immunodeficiency that affects phagocytic leukocytes [11]. In CGD patients, leukocyte NADPH oxidase is inactive as a result of mutations in any of five genes that encode essential subunits of the enzyme, which comprise the structural components of NADPH oxidase, including gp91phox, p22phox, p47phox, p67phox and p40phox [12–14]. These molecular defects result in susceptibility to *Mycobacterium*. In our study, we found that BCGosis/BCGitis in 87% of CGD patients occurred within 1 year after BCG vaccination; 1 patient was 4 years old and the median age of onset was 3 months of age. The results suggest that the age of onset of BCGosis/BCGitis in most CGD children is earlier; however, it should be noted that in a few CGD children, the disease onset occurred later. Among the 23 CGD patients, gene mutations were found in 20 patients, including 17 CYBB mutations, 1 CYBA mutation and 2 NCF2 mutations. A correlation between gene mutations and the severity of BCG infection was not found.

Recent work showed that the IL-12/IFN-γ signaling pathway plays an important role in immunity against mycobacterial

Table 2. Details of gene mutations in 26 BCGosis/BCGitis patients with primary immunodeficiency.

Patient NO.	Gene	Mutation type	CDS level change	Protein level change
1	*CYBB*	deletion	c.1177delA	p.G393fsX404
2	*CYBB*	deletion	c.343–344delCA	p.H115fsX121
5	*CYBB*	deletion	c.76–77delTT	p.F26fsX33
6	*CYBB*	missense	c.1082G>T	p.W361L
8	*CYBB*	missense	c.1366G>A	p.D456N
9	*CYBB*	missense	c.665A>G	p.H222R
15	*CYBB*	nonsense	c.676C>T	p.R226X
23	*CYBB*	nonsense	c.1320C>A	p.Y440X
26	*CYBB*	nonsense	c.370G>T	p.E124X
28	*CYBB*	nonsense	c.676C>T	p.R226X
32	*CYBB*	nonsense	c.388C>T	p.R130X
42	*CYBB*	splice 3′	c.253-3A>G	del. Exon 4
51	*CYBB*	splice 5′	c.252+5G>A	del. Exon 3
57	*CYBB*	splice 5′	c.1150–1151+2delAAGT	del. Exon 9
59	*CYBB*	splice 5′	c.252+5G>A	del. Exon 3
63	*CYBB*	splice 5′	c.1152G>C	del. Exon 9 K384N
65	*CYBB*	splice 5′	c.252+2dupT	del. Exon 3
71	*CYBA*	nonsense	c.7C>T	p.Q3X
18	*NCF2*	deletion	c.1130–1135delACATGG	p.Asp377-Met378del
47	*NCF2*	missense	c.137T>G	p.M46R
14	*IL2RG*	missense	c.314A>G	p.Y105C
60	*IL2RG*	deletion	c.432–433delGA	p.Q144fsX22
35	*IL12RB1*	missense	c.1094T>C	p.M365T
48	*IL12RB1*	missense	c.1094T>C	p.M365T
37	*IFNGR1*	missense	c.655G>A	p.G219R
54	*IFNGR1*	missense	c.1400T>C	p.L467P

infection. The disease caused by molecular defects in the IL-12/IFN-γ signaling pathway is called MSMD. Currently, many cases of IL-12/IFN-γ signaling pathway defects have been found in a number of countries [15,16], including 2 cases with an *IL12RB1* gene mutation in China [15]. In this study, 46 patients were not found to have PID by routine immunological function evaluation. These patients had detectable IFN-γ production. Among the 46 patients, 4 had lower IFN-γ production. Two had *IL12RB1* mutation and 2 had *IFNGR1* mutation. Both *IL12RB1* mutations are homozygous. For *IFNGR1* mutation, one is homozygous mutation and the other is heterozygous mutation. The homozygous mutation site has been reported in the Human Gene Mutation Database (http://www.hgmd.org/). In the NCBI database (http://www.ncbi.nlm.nih.gov/projects/SNP/), the heterozygous mutation site has been reported as an SNP (rs1887415). However, our results showed that the patient with an *IFNGR1* heterozygous mutation had lower IFN-γ production and disseminated BCG infection. These results suggest that the site may be associated with susceptibility to mycobacterial infection. Further research into whether the site has a mutation or an SNP is needed.

A randomized, double-blind, placebo-controlled study showed that IFN-γ therapy is an effective and well-tolerated treatment for CGD patients [17]. Ahlin A., et al. found that IFN-γ treatment of patients with CGD is associated with augmented production of nitric oxide by polymorphonuclear neutrophils [18]. In our study, patients with CGD and MSMD were treated with rhIFN-γ and anti-TB drugs. The results showed that with anti-TB treatment, administration of rhIFN-γ provided better control of BCGosis/BCGitis. However, the results need to be verified by a large-sample, randomized, double-blind, placebo-controlled study.

In summary, BCGosis/BCGitis is an important indicator of immunodeficiency. CGD is the most common PID in children with BCGosis/BCGitis in China. For children with BCGosis/BCGitis, immune function evaluation is necessary, and IFN-γ treatment for BCGosis/BCGitis patients with CGD is effective.

Acknowledgments

We thank all the parents and patients who took part in this study.

Author Contributions

Conceived and designed the experiments: XW. Performed the experiments: WY JS DL XH YY JW. Analyzed the data: WY JS DL. Contributed reagents/materials/analysis tools: XW JS. Wrote the paper: XW JS.

References

1. Arbeláez MP, Nelson KE, Muñoz A. (2000) BCG vaccine effectiveness in preventing tuberculosis and its interaction with human immunodeficiency virus infection. Int J Epidemiol 29: 1085–1091.
2. Safety of BCG vaccine in HIV-infected children. World Health Organization. Available at: http://www.who.int/vaccine_safety/committee/topics/bcg/immunocompromised/Dec_2006/en/. Accessed January 18, 2013.
3. Grange JM. (1998) Complications of bacille Calmette-Guérin (BCG) vaccination and immunotherapy and their management. Commun Dis Public Health 1: 84–88.
4. Hesseling AC, Rabie H, Marais BJ, Manders M, Lips M, et al. (2006) Bacille Calmette-guerin vaccine-induced disease in HIV-infected and HIV-uninfected children. Clin Infect Dis 42: 548–558.
5. Casanova JL, Jouanguy E, Lamhamedi S, Blanche S, Fischer A. (1995) Immunological conditions of children with BCG disseminated infection. Lancet 346: 581.
6. Norouzi S, Aghamohammadi A, Mamishi S, Rosenzweig SD, Rezaei N. (2012) Bacillus Calmette-Guérin (BCG) complications associated with primary immunodeficiency diseases. J Infect 64: 543–554.
7. He GX, Zhao YL, Jiang GL, Liu YH, Xia H, et al. (2008) Prevalence of tuberculosis drug resistance in 10 provinces of China. BMC Infect Dis. 8: 166.
8. Talbot EA, Williams DL, Frothingham R. (1997) PCR identification of Mycobacterium bovis BCG. J Clin Microbiol 35: 566–569.
9. Sun J, Wang Y, Liu D, Yu Y, Wang J, et al. (2012) Prenatal diagnosis of X-linked chronic granulomatous disease by percutaneous umbilical blood sampling. Scand J Immunol 76: 512–518.
10. Feinberg J, Fieschi C, Doffinger R, Feinberg M, Leclerc T, et al. (2004) Bacillus Calmette Guerin triggers the IL-12/IFN-gamma axis by an IRAK-4- and NEMO-dependent, non-cognate interaction between monocytes, NK, and T lymphocytes. Eur J Immunol 34: 3276–3284.
11. Holland SM. (2010) Chronic granulomatous disease. Clin Rev Allergy Immunol 38: 3–10.
12. van den Berg JM, van Koppen E, Ahlin A, Belohradsky BH, Bernatowska E, et al. (2009) Chronic granulomatous disease: the European experience. PLoS One 4: e5234.
13. Matute JD, Arias AA, Wright NA, Wrobel I, Waterhouse CC, et al. (2009) A new genetic subgroup of chronic granulomatous disease with autosomal recessive mutations in p40 phox and selective defects in neutrophil NADPH oxidase activity. Blood 114: 3309–3315.
14. Chiriaco M, Di Matteo G, Sinibaldi C, Giardina E, Nardone AM, et al. (2009) Identification of deletion carriers in X-linked chronic granulomatous disease by real-time PCR. Genet Test Mol Biomarkers. 13: 785–789.
15. de Beaucoudrey L, Samarina A, Bustamante J, Cobat A, Boisson-Dupuis S, et al. (2010) Revisiting human IL-12Rβ1 deficiency: a survey of 141 patients from 30 countries. Medicine (Baltimore) 89: 381–402.
16. Sologuren I, Boisson-Dupuis S, Pestano J, Vincent QB, Fernández-Pérez L, et al. (2011) Partial recessive IFN-γR1 deficiency: genetic, immunological and clinical features of 14 patients from 11 kindreds. Hum Mol Genet 20: 1509–1523.
17. The International Chronic Granulomatous Disease Cooperative Study Group. (1991) A controlled trial of interferon gamma to prevent infection in chronic granulomatous disease. N Engl J Med 324: 509–516.
18. Ahlin A, Lärfars G, Elinder G, Palmblad J, Gyllenhammar H. (1999) Gamma interferon treatment of patients with chronic granulomatous disease is associated with augmented production of nitric oxide by polymorphonuclear neutrophils. Clin Diagn Lab Immunol 6: 420–424.

18

The Immune System in Children with Malnutrition

Maren Johanne Heilskov Rytter[1]*, Lilian Kolte[2], André Briend[1,3], Henrik Friis[1], Vibeke Brix Christensen[4]

1 Department of Nutrition, Exercise and Sports, Faculty of Science, University of Copenhagen, Frederiksberg, Denmark, **2** Department of Infectious Diseases, Copenhagen University Hospital, Hvidovre, Denmark, **3** Department for International Health, University of Tampere, School of Medicine, Tampere, Finland, **4** Department of Paediatrics, Copenhagen University Hospital Rigshospitalet, Copenhagen, Denmark

Abstract

Background: Malnourished children have increased risk of dying, with most deaths caused by infectious diseases. One mechanism behind this may be impaired immune function. However, this immune deficiency of malnutrition has not previously been systematically reviewed.

Objectives: To review the scientific literature about immune function in children with malnutrition.

Methods: A systematic literature search was done in PubMed, and additional articles identified in reference lists and by correspondence with experts in the field. The inclusion criteria were studies investigating immune parameters in children aged 1–60 months, in relation to malnutrition, defined as wasting, underweight, stunting, or oedematous malnutrition.

Results: The literature search yielded 3402 articles, of which 245 met the inclusion criteria. Most were published between 1970 and 1990, and only 33 after 2003. Malnutrition is associated with impaired gut-barrier function, reduced exocrine secretion of protective substances, and low levels of plasma complement. Lymphatic tissue, particularly the thymus, undergoes atrophy, and delayed-type hypersensitivity responses are reduced. Levels of antibodies produced after vaccination are reduced in severely malnourished children, but intact in moderate malnutrition. Cytokine patterns are skewed towards a Th2-response. Other immune parameters seem intact or elevated: leukocyte and lymphocyte counts are unaffected, and levels of immunoglobulins, particularly immunoglobulin A, are high. The acute phase response appears intact, and sometimes present in the absence of clinical infection. Limitations to the studies include their observational and often cross-sectional design and frequent confounding by infections in the children studied.

Conclusion: The immunological alterations associated with malnutrition in children may contribute to increased mortality. However, the underlying mechanisms are still inadequately understood, as well as why different types of malnutrition are associated with different immunological alterations. Better designed prospective studies are needed, based on current understanding of immunology and with state-of-the-art methods.

Editor: Taishin Akiyama, University of Tokyo, Japan

Funding: The work was supported by a PhD grant from University of Copenhagen. The funders had no role in study design, data collection and analysis, decision to publish, or preparation of the manuscript.

Competing Interests: The authors have declared that no competing interests exist.

* Email: marenrytter@hotmail.com

Introduction

Malnutrition in children is a global public health problem with wide implications. Malnourished children have increased risk of dying from infectious diseases, and it is estimated that malnutrition is the underlying cause of 45% of global deaths in children below 5 years of age [1–2]. The association between malnutrition and infections may in part be due to confounding by poverty, a determinant of both, but also possibly due to a two-way causal relationship (**Figure 1**): malnutrition increases susceptibility to infections while infections aggravate malnutrition by decreasing appetite, inducing catabolism, and increasing demand for nutrients [3]. Although it has been debated whether malnutrition increases incidence of infections, or whether it only increases severity of disease [3], solid data indicates that malnourished children are at higher risk of dying once infected [2–4]. The increased susceptibility to infections may in part be caused by impairment of immune function by malnutrition [5]. The objective of this study was to investigate the associations of different types of malnutrition with immune parameters in children, through a systematic review of the literature.

Since most infections and deaths in malnourished children occur in low-income settings, the organisms causing disease are rarely identified. Therefore, little is known about whether these differ from pathogens infecting well-nourished children, and whether malnourished children are susceptible to opportunistic

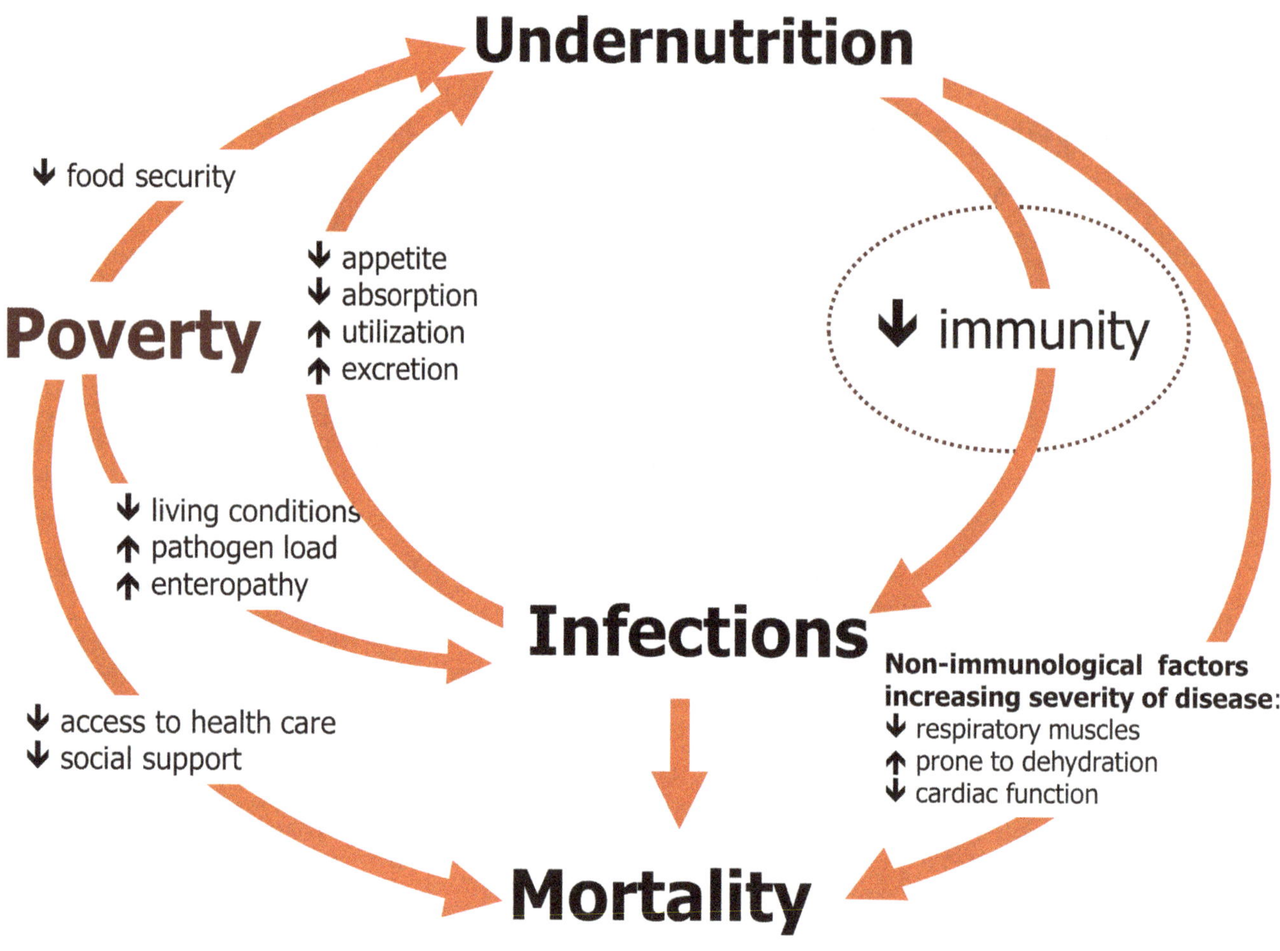

Figure 1. Conceptual framework on the relationship between malnutrition, infections and poverty.

infections. Although opportunistic infections like *Pneumocystis jirovecii* and severe varicella has been reported in malnourished children [6–7], these studies were carried out before the discovery of HIV, and may represent cases of un-diagnosed paediatric AIDS. More recent studies have found that *Pneumocystis jirovecii* pneumonia is not frequent in malnourished children not infected with HIV [8]. However, quasi-opportunistic pathogens like cryptosporidium and yeast are frequent causes of diarrhoea in malnourished children [9], and malnourished children have a higher risk of invasive bacterial infections, causing bacterial pneumonia [8], bacterial diarrhoea [10–11], and bacteraemia [12–14], with a predominance of gram negative bacteria. Due to the high prevalence of invasive bacterial infections, current guidelines recommend antibiotic treatment to all children with severe acute malnutrition, even though the evidence behind is not very strong [14].

Non-immunological factors may also contribute to increased mortality in malnourished children: reduced muscle mass may impair respiratory work with lung infections [15]; reduced electrolyte absorption from the gut [16] and impaired renal concentration capacity may increase susceptibility to dehydration from diarrhoea [5]; and diminished cardiac function may increase risk of cardiac failure [17]. Thus, immune function may only be one of several links between malnutrition, infections and increased mortality, but most likely an important one.

Definitions of malnutrition

This review considers childhood malnutrition in the sense of under-nutrition, causing growth failure or weight loss, or severe acute malnutrition, either oedematous, or non-oedematous.

Growth failure caused by malnutrition has commonly been defined by low weight-for-age (underweight), length-for-age (stunting), or weight-for-length (wasting) [5]. Generally, older studies diagnosed malnutrition using weight-for-age, while newer studies tend to use weight-for-length. Recently, mid-upper arm circumference (MUAC) has been promoted to diagnose severe acute malnutrition, because of its feasibility and because it predicts mortality risk better than other anthropometric indices [18]. Other definitions of malnutrition include specific micronutrient deficiencies, intra-uterine growth restriction, and obesity, but these conditions are outside the scope of this review.

Severe Acute Malnutrition

Two forms of severe acute malnutrition in children exist: non-oedematous malnutrition, also known as marasmus, characterized by severe wasting and currently defined by weight-for-length z-score <-3 of the WHO growth standard, or MUAC $<11{,}5$ cm; and oedematous malnutrition defined by bilateral pitting oedema (**Figure 2**) [19]. Kwashiorkor refers to a form of oedematous malnutrition, the fulminant syndrome including enlarged fatty liver, mental changes as well as skin and hair changes [20]. The term "marasmic kwashiorkor", has been used to describe children

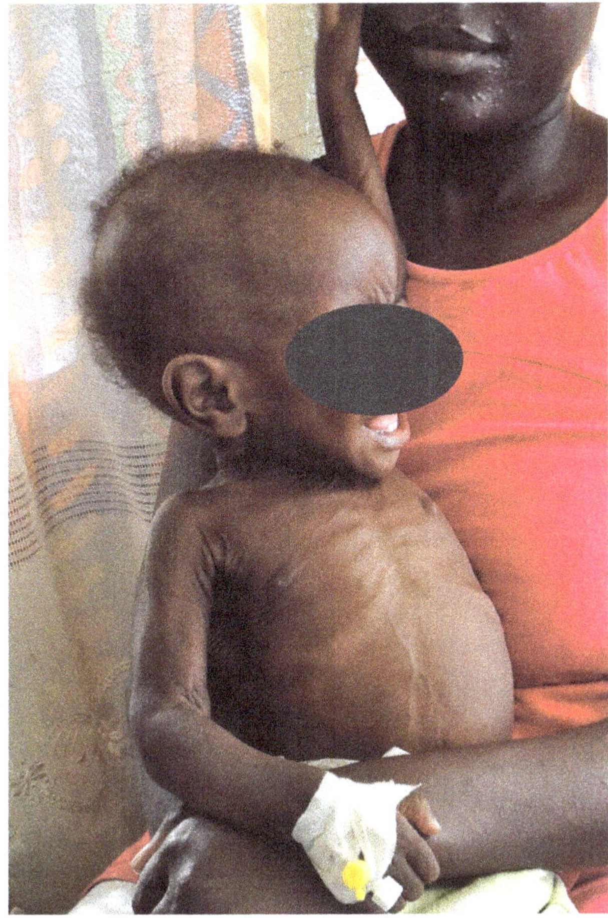
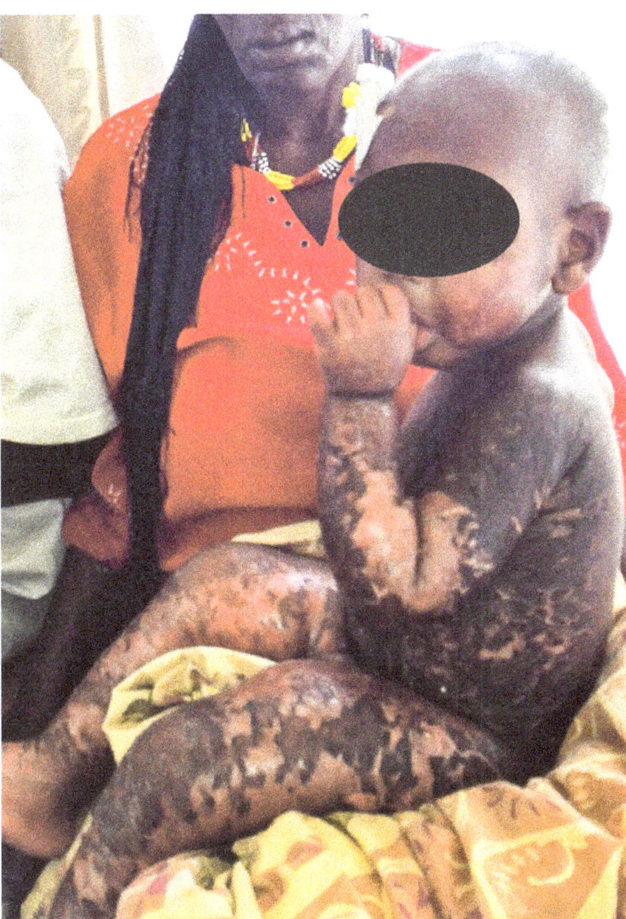

Figure 2. Clinical picture: two forms of severe acute malnutrition, oedematous and non-oedematous malnutrition.

with both wasting and oedema [21]. It is still unknown why some children develop oedematous malnutrition, and unclear whether this form of malnutrition is associated with a different degree of immune deficiency.

Materials and Methods

A systematic literature search was carried out in PubMed using combinations of the search terms related to malnutrition and immune parameters. The full search strategy and the search terms used are described in **Figure 3**.

Inclusion criteria were: studies presenting original clinical data regarding immune parameters in children, aged 1–60 months, where a comparison was made, either between malnourished and well-nourished children, or between malnourished children before and after nutritional rehabilitation. Exclusion criteria were studies of children with another primary diagnosis such as cancer, congenital heart disease or endocrine disease. Studies were accepted where children had co-morbid infections, since this is typically seen in malnourished children. Articles by RK Chandra were excluded, due to concerns about possible fraud [22]. Studies published in peer-reviewed scientific journals, as well as in books were included. Only articles in English were included.

The search was carried out in August 2013, and updated in December 2013. The search results were sorted by MJHR, based on titles, abstracts or full-text-articles. Additional literature was obtained from reference lists, text books and by personal communication with experts.

For data retrieval, studies were sorted according to whether they investigated barrier function (skin and gut), innate immunity or acquired immune system, and listed in tables based on the specific immune parameter studied. Some studies were included in more than one table. The following data was extracted from each article: year and country, number and age range of malnourished and well-nourished participants, type of malnutrition and whether included children fulfilled WHOs current diagnostic criteria for severe acute malnutrition, whether infections were present, immune parameter studied, methods used, how the parameter was associated with malnutrition, and whether children with oedematous and non-oedematous malnutrition were differentially affected.

The results of the included articles were summarized for each immune parameter. Due to the heterogeneous nature of study designs, participants and outcomes, it was not meaningful to synthesize the results in a meta-analysis. The main potential bias was presence of infection. For this reason, presence and effect of infection was considered for each study as well as for each outcome. The PRISMA (Preferred Reporting Items for Systematic Reviews and Meta-Analyses) guideline was followed, except for the items relating to meta-analysis (**Checklist S1**).

Search terms:

"malnutrition" OR "undernutrition" OR "marasmus" OR "kwashiorkor" OR "wasting" OR "stunting" OR "underweight"

AND

"immune" OR "antibodies" OR "thymus" OR "lymphatic" OR "delayed-type hypersensitivity" OR "leucocytes" OR "lymphocyte" OR "activation" OR "B-cell" OR "T-cell" OR "complement" OR "humoral" OR "cytokine" OR "chemotaxis"OR "acute phase response" OR "phagocytosis" OR "flow cytometry" OR "enteropathy" OR "barrier" OR "intestinal permeability" OR "microbiota" .

Filters: human studies, children from 0-18 years, and publications in English.

Figure 3. Full search strategy in PubMed, including search terms and filters.

Results

The search in PubMed yielded 3402 articles. By contacting experts in the field, an additional 631 papers were obtained. Reference list of all papers read were screened for relevant papers not included in the initial search. Of all the screened papers, 245 met the inclusion criteria (**Figure S1**). Another 49 articles were identified which, in addition to children 1–60 months old, also included older children. These studies were not included in the main analysis, but used in a sensitivity analysis in which all studies were included. The result of this additional analysis was essentially similar to the results obtained with studies only including children less than 60 month (results not shown). The studies were published between 1957–2014, mainly in the 1970s and 1980s. Only 33 studies were published after 2003 (**Figure 4**). The studies included 29 prospective studies that compared malnourished children to themselves after nutritional recovery, and 216 cross-sectional studies. Of the cross-sectional studies, 51 were community-based, comparing immune parameters in children according to nutritional status. The remaining 165 cross-sectional studies compared hospitalised malnourished children to well-nourished children, often recruited outside the hospital. In 53 studies, all children fulfilled WHOs diagnostic criteria for severe acute malnutrition [23]. The vast majority of these studies included children with oedematous malnutrition, while only two studies included children with non-oedematous malnutrition based on the new WHO growth standard.

The results of each immune parameter are summarized in **Table 1**, and the results of individual articles are summarized in **Tables S1–14**.

Epithelial barrier function

The barrier function of the skin and mucosal surfaces is considered the first-line defence of the immune system, upheld by the physical integrity of the epithelia, anti-microbial factors in secretions (e.g. lysozyme, secretory IgA and gastric acidity) and the commensal bacterial flora [24].

Of the articles describing barrier function in malnourished children, six described skin structure and function, 21 described structure and permeability of intestinal mucosa, 19 protective factors in secretions and 11 the microbial flora colonizing mucosal surfaces.

Skin. *Skin barrier* has mostly been studied in children with oedematous malnutrition, who may develop a characteristic dermatosis, characterized by hyper-pigmentation, cracking and scaling of the epidermis, resembling "peeling paint", providing a potential entry port for pathogens [25].

Six articles assessed barrier and immune function of the skin in malnourished children (**table S1**). Two articles describing histology reported atrophy of skin layers, but did not describe cutaneous immune cells [26–27]. Four articles described the "cutaneous inflammatory response": They made small abrasions in the skin, and placed microscopy slides over the sites. Similar or higher numbers of white blood cells migrated onto slides in malnourished children, predominantly granulocytes and a lower proportion of monocytes and macrophages [28–31]. This pattern was noted to resemble a neonatal immature immune response [30]. All four articles found this pattern in patients with oedematous malnutrition, while one study found that the response of non-oedematous children resembled that of well-nourished [30].

Structure and function of the intestinal mucosa. The intestinal mucosa of malnourished children was described in 21 articles (**table S2**). Autopsy-studies from as early as 1965 described a thin-walled intestine in malnourished children, and noted that "... the *tissue paper intestine* of kwashiorkor is well known to tropical pathologists." [32]. Small-intestinal biopsies showed thinning of the mucosa [33–36], decrease in villous height [37–43], altered villous morphology [32] [40] [44] and infiltration of lymphocytes [32] [34–38]. Electron-microscopy studies found sparse brush border with shortened microvilli and sparse endoplasmatic reticulum [42]. Others found increased intestinal permeability to lactulose [45–48]. Such an intestine may predispose to bacterial translocation, and likewise, one of the included articles described high levels of lipopolysaccharide in the blood of malnourished children, probably originating from gut bacteria translocating into the bloodstream [49]. However, the mucosal atrophy and functional changes did not only occur in malnourished children. Although sometimes found to be most severe in malnourished children [33] [35–36] [46–47], similar

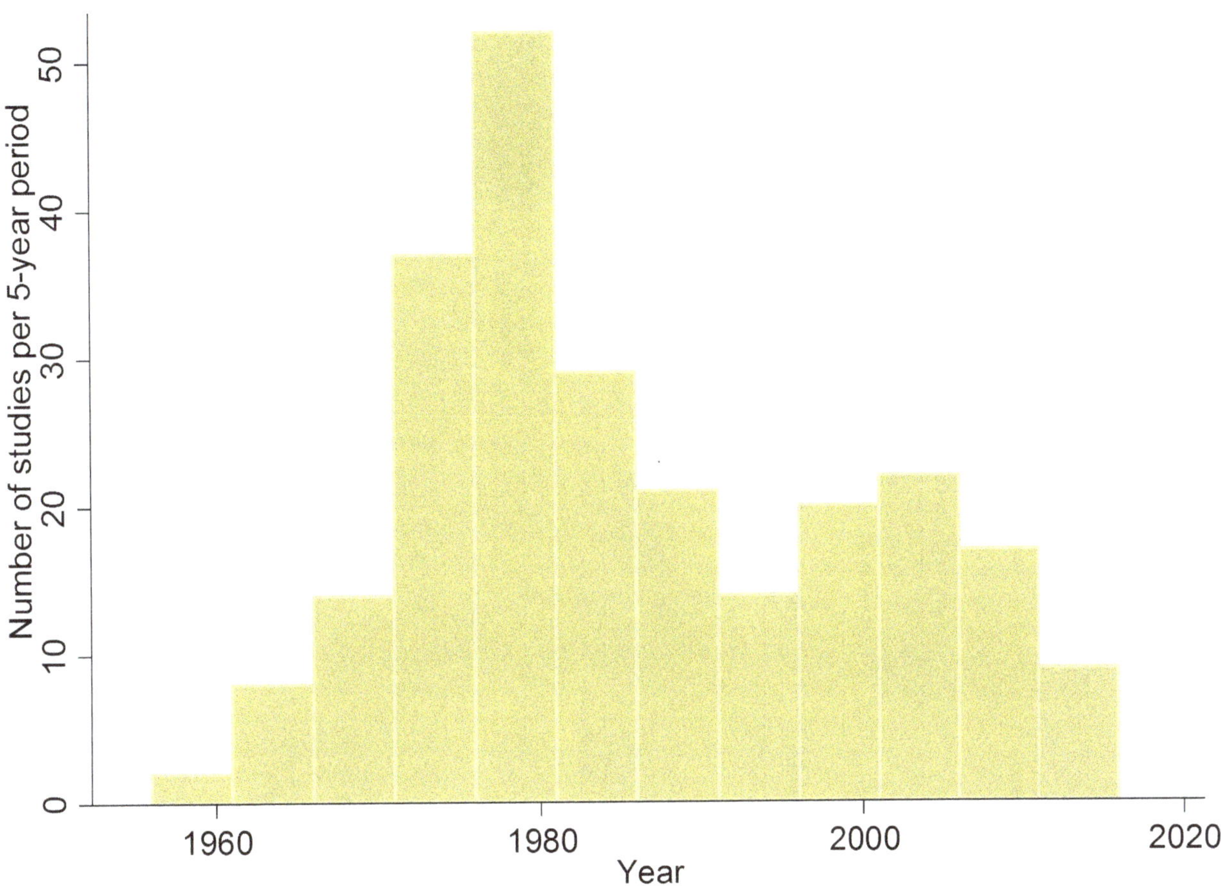

Figure 4. Number of studies published per 5-year period about immune function in malnourished children.

abnormalities were present in apparently well-nourished children from the same environment [38–40] [43] [50], and frequently persisted after nutritional recovery [34] [37] [51].

Two articles described immune cells in small intestinal biopsies from malnourished children in Gambia and Zambia: both reported increased lymphocyte infiltration, more T-cells, and cells expressing HLA-DR in malnourished children compared to English children [37–38]. However, it was similar to Gambian well-nourished children [38], and unaltered by nutritional recovery [37]. Both well-nourished and malnourished Gambian children had high levels of intestinal cytokine expression, but malnourished children had an increased ratio of cells expression pro-inflammatory to regulatory cytokines, compared to the well-nourished Gambian children [38].

The colon was only described in one article, reporting increased vascularity, atrophy of the mucosa and a tendency to rectal prolapse in children with oedematous malnutrition [52].

Four articles compared the intestine of children with oedematous and non-oedematous malnutrition: one study from South Africa found that the histological changes were most severe in those with oedema [40]. Two articles from Chile found that children with non-oedematous malnutrition had a thinner mucosa, whereas children with oedema had more villous atrophy and more cellular infiltration [35–36]. In contrast, a more recent study from Zambia found higher numbers of T-cells and cells expressing HLA-DR in the intestines of children with non-oedematous than oedematous malnutrition, while the intestines of oedematous children were deficient in sulphated glycosaminoglycan [37].

Antimicrobial factors in mucosal secretions. Nineteen articles were published on anti-microbial factors in secretions from malnourished children (**table S3**). Secretory IgA (sIgA) was investigated in 15 studies, of which 11 investigated saliva, urine, tears, nasal washings and duodenal fluid [53–63] and three investigated small intestinal biopsies [39–40] [64].

SIgA in saliva, tears and nasal washings was frequently reduced in severely malnourished children [54–55] [57–58]. One article from Egypt reported increased levels in children with oedematous malnutrition [56], but may have overestimated sIgA, since saliva flow was reduced in malnourished children, and sIgA was expressed as g/l, whereas other articles expressed it as sIgA as % of protein content. Studies of sIgA in duodenal fluid showed conflicting results [57] [59], as did studies quantifying sIgA in small intestinal biopsies [39–40] [64]. The sIgA content of urine was increased or normal in severely malnourished children [60–61]. In mild to moderately underweight children, inconsistent results were found for sIgA in tears [63] and saliva [53–54] [62–63].

Tear lysozyme content was found to be reduced in malnourished children [54] [63], while saliva lysozyme was unaffected [53–54]. Gastric acid secretion was consistently reduced in severely

Table 1. Summary of results in studies of each immune parameter.

Immune parameter	Number of studies	Period	In children with severe malnutrition?	In children with moderate malnutrition?	Different in OM compared to NOM?	Comments	Listed in table
Skin	6	1968–1989	- Atrophy - Cells in skin abrasions: ↑ GRAN, ↓ monocytes	Not assessed	Cells in abrasions only affected in OM		S1
Gut function	21	1965–2013	Thin mucosa, shorter villi, infiltration of immune cells. Increased intestinal permeability.	No linear relationship	↕	Also in well-nourished children	S2
Factors in secretions	19	1968–2012	sIgA in saliva, tears, nasal washings: ↓ in duodenal fluids: ↕, in urine: 0 Lysozyme: ↕. Gastric juice and acidity: ↓	↕	Saliva flow ↓ in OM; sIgA ↑ in OM		S3
Microbial flora	11	1972–2014	Different pattern of stool micro-biota; bacterial growth in small intestine; ↑ yeast and g. neg. bact.	↑ yeast in mouth	Not assessed		S4
White blood cells	38	1964–2009	Leukocytes in blood: 0; Microbicidal activity ↓, Chemotaxis ↓; Phagocytosis: ↕.	Leukocytes in blood: 0; NK cells: 0	Bactericidal activity ↓ in OM		S5
Acute phase	24	1970–2006	Positive APP ↑, negative APP ↓ with infection, sometimes also without clinical infection	Few studies	↕		S6
Complement	24	1973–2011	C3, C6, C1, C9, Factor B: ↓; C5, C activity: ↕; C4: 0	Not affected	All parameters ↓ in OM	Signs of in-vivo consumption in OM	S7
Lymphatic tissue	12	1956–2009	Thymic atrophy. Fewer lymphocytes in thymus cortex. Less atrophy of other lymphatic tissue.	Linear relationship of thymus size with nutritional status	↕	Also ↓ by infections and zinc deficiency	S8 and S9
DTHR	21	1965–2092	Mantoux after BCG vaccination: ↓; Reaction to other antigens: ↓	: ↕;	↕	Also ↓ by infections and zinc deficiency	S10
Lymphocytes	58	1971–2009	Total lymphocytes 0; T-cells: 0/↑; CD4 count: 0/↑; B-cells: ↓; Response to PHA: ↓	Not affected	CD4 count ↑ in OM	Conflicting result by flow cytometry older methods	S11
Antibody levels	32	1962–2008	IgG: 0; IgM: 0; IgA: ↑; IgE: ↕; IgD: ↑ in OM, ↕ in NOM	Not affected	IgA and IgD ↑ in OM		S12
Vaccination response	35	1957–2009	Antibody titre: ↓; Most acceptable sero-conversion; Possibly delay in antibody response	Antibody titre: 0; Sero-conversion: 0	Titres: ↓ in OM		S13
Cytokines	35	1975–2013	Th1-cytokines: IL1. Il2, IL12, IFN-γ: ↓; Th2 cytokines: IL10, IL14: ↑; Inflammatory cytokines (IL6, TNFα): ↕	Few studies: Same pattern as severe malnutrition	Th2-response ↑, IL6 ↑ in OM; Altered leukotrienes		S14

Legend: ↑ = higher in malnourished than well-nourished, ↓ = lower in malnourished than well-nourished, 0 = similar in malnourished and well-nourished; ↕ = inconsistent results; OM = Oedematous malnutrition, NOM = Non-oedematous malnutrition, GRAN = Granulocytes (Polymorph nuclear cells); sIgA = secretory immunoglobulin A; NK = Natural killer; APP = Acute phase protein; C = Complement component, BCG = Bacille Calmette-Guérin, PHA: phyto-hemaglutinin; Ig = immunoglobulin; IL = Interleukin; IFNγ = Interferon-gamma; TNFα = Tumour-necrosis-factor-alpha.

malnourished children [65–68], and higher pH was associated with bacterial colonization of the stomach [65].

Microbial colonization. Microbes colonizing skin and mucosa may protect against infections by competing with pathogens, by producing specific antimicrobial substances, and by stimulating host immune function [69]. Despite much recent interest in the subject, of 11 articles describing the micro-flora in malnourished children, only four were published during the last ten years (**table S4**). All found malnourished children to host a different flora from well-nourished children. Their mouths and throats contained more yeast [70–72], and their stomach and duodenum, which in healthy children is considered to be almost sterile, contained a large number of microorganisms [72–75]. Although one study found similar degree of small intestinal bacterial overgrowth in diarrhoeal patients with and without malnutrition [75], another found more small intestinal bacteria in malnourished than in well-nourished children with diarrhoea [72]. While gram positive cocci predominated in the small intestine of well-nourished children, malnourished children hosted more gram negative bacteria [65] and yeast [74].

The colonic flora, containing the vast majority of commensal bacteria, was described by sequencing bacterial DNA from stool samples in four recent articles, which consistently found that the pattern of bacteria was different in malnourished and well-nourished children [76–79]. More bacteria with pathogenic potential were found in the malnourished children [77–78], and their flora was less mature [79] and less diverse [76] [78]. A twin study from Malawi suggested that micro-flora pattern could also play a role in developing malnutrition [76]. No articles have so far reported whether the intestinal flora is different in children with oedematous and non-oedematous malnutrition.

Innate immune system

The innate immune system delivers an unspecific response relying on leukocytes (like granulocytes, monocytes and macrophages), as well as soluble factors in blood (like acute phase proteins and the complement system) [24]. Of the articles describing innate immune response, 38 described number and function of leucocytes, 25 acute phase proteins and 24 complement components and activity.

White blood cells of the innate immune system. Thirty-eight articles described number and function of leukocytes of the innate immune system (**table S5**). Most reported similar or higher numbers of total leukocytes in blood of malnourished children [49] [80–92], and three found that granulocytes were higher in malnourished children [81] [86] [93].

Two studies from Nigeria and one from Ghana found no difference in the mean percentage of natural-killer-cells among malnourished or well-nourished children [94–96], although two reported that more malnourished children had abnormally low numbers of natural-killer cells. In Zambia, levels of dendritic cells were lower in blood from malnourished children before nutritional rehabilitation than after, and elevated inflammation markers were associated with a paradoxical lower level of dendritic cell activation. This was associated with endotoxin levels in the blood, and was interpreted as a type of immune-paralysis, related to inflammation and bacterial translocation [49]. Unfortunately, it was not assessed whether this was different from well-nourished children with severe infections.

Chemotaxis of granulocytes was reduced in malnourished children in three of five studies [80] [83] [97–99], and one study found a diminished ability to adhere to foreign material [100]. Results for phagocytosis were mixed: five of 12 studies found that leukocytes of malnourished children had reduced ability to ingest particles or bacteria [81] [83] [88–89] [97–98] [101–106]. Microbicidal activity of granulocytes was reduced in malnourished children in five of seven studies [80] [83] [88] [97–98] [103] [107], while two of three studies found macrophages from malnourished children to have normal microbicidal activity [89] [108–109]. Neutrophils may kill microorganisms by producing reactive oxygen compounds; assessable by the Nitroblue Tetrazolenium (NBT) test, which, however, gave inconsistent results in malnourished children [83] [105] [110–114]. It has been hypothesized, that reactive oxygen production is involved in the pathogenesis of oedematous malnutrition [115]; however, the NBT test results did not show any clear pattern in children with oedematous compared to non-oedematous malnutrition.

One study found the levels of enzymes, like alkaline and acid phosphatase, to be increased in leukocytes from children with malnutrition [116]. More leukocytes of malnourished children were found to have markers of apoptosis (CD95) [92], and signs of DNA damage [117–118].

No articles have yet described the expression of pattern-recognition molecules, like Toll-like receptors in malnourished children, although these are fundamental to the function of the innate immune system.

Acute phase response. Acute phase responses is induced by infection or trauma, and mediated by cytokines like IL-6 and TNF-α. It involve temporal suppression of acquired, and amplification of innate immune responses, with secretion of positive acute phase proteins (APP) like C-reactive protein (CRP), serum-amyloid-A (SAA), complement factors, α-1-acid-glycoprotein or ferritin [119], while levels of other proteins are reduced, as albumin, pre-albumin, transferrin, α -2-HS-glycoprotein, and α -fetoprotein. These are sometimes called 'negative acute phase proteins', although it is not clear whether their reduced level are due to active down-regulation, or because of competition with production of positive acute phase proteins. Twenty-four articles described the levels of acute phase proteins in malnourished children with or without infection (**table S6**).

Acute phase response in children with infections. Most studies found elevated positive APP in malnourished children with infections. This included CRP [120–128], α-1 acid-glycoprotein [120–121] [129], haptoglobin [120–121] [125] [127] [129] while the results for ceruloplasmin [125] [130], and α-1-antitrysin were inconsistent [120–121] [125] [127–129]. Only one study found lower CRP levels in malnourished than well-nourished children with similar infections, despite higher levels of IL-6 [129]. So-called negative APP were uniformly low in children with malnutrition and infection, including transferrin [94] [127] [130–133], α-2-HS-glycoprotein [134–136], pre-albumin [122], fibronectin [132], and α-2-macroglobulin[127].

Acute phase response in children without infections. Three studies found elevated CRP in malnourished children without apparent infections [94] [124] [128], while two studies found similar CRP-levels in malnourished and well-nourished children [122] [137]. Results for α-1-antitrysin were inconsistent [128]. So-called negative acute phase proteins like transferrin [94] [130], α-2-HS-glycoprotein [135], fibronectin [133] [138] and pre-albumin [122] [138–139] were consistently reduced in malnourished children, even without infections.

Acute phase response to a controlled stressor. Four articles described the acute phase response induced by a vaccine. Two reported a normal [140] or increased [141] febrile response to measles vaccine in malnourished children. In another study, a similar rise in APP was seen in malnourished and well-nourished children [137], in response to a diphtheria-pertussis-tetanus-vaccination, but the increase in APP was greater when the vaccination was repeated after nutritional rehabilitation. The same was found for the febrile response to a repeated vaccine in malnourished children [142]. Since no repeated vaccine was given to well-nourished children, it is unknown whether they would also have had a stronger response to the second dose.

Complement. The complement system consists of plasma proteins secreted by the liver that, upon activation, react to recruit immune cells, opsonize and kill pathogens [24]. Three main pathways activate the complement system: the classical pathway, the alternative pathway and the lectin pathway [143], with the complement protein C3 playing a central role in all three pathways.

Twenty-four articles described levels or in-vitro activity of complement proteins (**table S7**). In 17 of 21 studies, levels of C3 were depressed in malnourished children [89] [94] [99] [106] [124–125] [127–130] [144–154]. Two studies found C3 to correlate with albumin [94] [148], and with one exception [94], C3 levels were lower in children with oedematous than non-oedematous malnutrition [89] [146] [149] [150–151] [153].

Few studies assessed C6, C9, and factor B, and most found reduced levels in malnourished children [145] [148–149] [151] [153], most so in oedematous malnutrition [148–149] [151] [153].

Levels of C1 and C4 were mostly normal in malnourished children [94] [99] [145] [148] [150–153], while two studies found reduced levels of C4 in patients with oedematous, but not non-oedematous malnutrition [89] [149]. Studies assessing C5 showed inconsistent results [145] [148–149] [151] [153].

Classical pathway activity was either unaffected [106] [145–146] [152], reduced [148] [155] [156], or reduced only in oedematous, but not in non-oedematous malnutrition [157]. Alternative pathway activity was reduced in two studies [145] [156] and unaffected in one [146]. General opsonic activity of serum was reduced in one study [156]. No articles reported the activity of the lectin pathway.

Both reduced production and increased consumption may explain the reduced levels of complement factors. Complement components are produced by the liver, and their levels correlated with albumin levels, the production of which is also impaired in malnutrition [158]. However, increased consumption is also supported by one study showing high levels of C3d, a by-product after activation of C3, in malnourished children, most pronounced in oedematous malnutrition [148].

Acquired immunity

Acquired immunity is characterized by specialized cellular and antibody-mediated immune responses, generated by T- and B-lymphocytes reacting with high specificity towards pathogens and creating long-lasting immunological memory. The acquired immune system also orchestrates tolerance to self and other non-pathogenic material like gut bacteria [24]. Of the articles describing acquired immunity, 12 described the thymo-lymphatic system, 21 delayed-type hypersensitivity responses (DTHR), 58 lymphocyte subsets in blood, 32 immunoglobulins in blood, 35 vaccination responses and 35 cytokines.

Thymus. The thymus gland is the central lymphatic organ in the acquired immune system, where maturation and proliferation of T-lymphocytes take place. The thymus is large at birth and undergoes gradual involution after childhood [159], with diminished output of T-lymphocytes [160].

Six articles reported autopsy studies of the thymo-lymphatic system in malnourished children, published between 1956 and 1988 [161–166] **table S8**). All reported thymus atrophy in malnourished children, to an extent termed "nutritional thymectomy" [164]. Histology revealed depleted thymocytes, replacement with connective tissue, and decreased cortico-medullar differentiation [163] [165–166].

Eight articles reported thymic size measured by ultrasound, in relation to nutritional status [91] [167–173] (**table S9**). Five of these studied children with severe malnutrition and found severe thymic atrophy [91] [167–170], reversible with nutritional rehabilitation, although thymic size did not reach normal levels as fast as anthropometric recovery [91] [170]. Thymic size was also measured by ultrasound in cohorts of children to determine patterns of thymic growth [159] [171], in a vaccination trial in Guinea Bissau [172] and in a pre-natal nutritional supplementation trial in Bangladesh [171]. These studies confirmed that thymus size was associated with nutritional status, even in mild malnutrition. Breastfed children often had a larger thymus than artificially fed children [174], possibly explained by IL-7 in breast milk [175], and children with a large thymus were found to have a higher chance of surviving than those with a small thymus [172] [176].

Other lymphatic tissue. Six articles reported investigations of other lymphatic tissue. Four autopsy studies found atrophy of lymph nodes, spleen, tonsils, appendix and Peyer's patches, although not as pronounced as in the thymus. Histology revealed a reduction in germinal centres and depletion of lymphocytes from para-cortical areas [161] [163–165]. Two studies in living children also found that the tonsils were smaller in malnourished than in well-nourished children [163] [177].

Delayed type hypersensitivity response (DTHR). Cellular immune function can be examined by dermal DTHR, the prototype of which is the Mantoux test. Intradermal application of substances like candida or phyto-hemaglutinin (PHA) are also used, as well as sensitizing skin with a local contact sensitizer such as 2-4-di-nitro-clorobenzene (DNCB). Twenty-one articles reported DTHR in relation to malnutrition (**table S10**).

The majority of studies found that malnourished children less frequently developed a positive Mantoux after BCG vaccination [154] [177–185]. Most also found diminished reactivity to *Candida*, PHA and other common antigens [29] [145] [179] [183] [186–190], and after sensitizing with DNCB [163] [177] [179] [183] [188] [191–192]. Conflicting results were found for DTHR in children with different types of severe malnutrition: Three studies found most impaired response in oedematous malnutrition [179] [181] [191], while one found that it was worst in non-oedematous malnutrition [184], and two studies found similar responses [186] [187].

The proportion of positive DTHR varied from study to study, both in well-nourished and malnourished children. Inconsistent results were found in moderately malnourished children [178] [180–181] [185–187] [193]. Other studies found that DTHR was improved with zinc supplementation [190] [194–195] diminished by infections [178] [181] [196], and in slightly older children, a strong interaction was seen between infections and nutritional status [197].

Lymphocytes in blood. Fifty-eight articles reported either total numbers of lymphocytes or lymphocyte subsets in blood (**table S11**). Of 16 articles, 13 reported similar or higher levels of lymphocytes in peripheral blood of malnourished children [80–83] [85–87] [90] [93] [101] [177] [179] [187] [191] [198] [199].

Three studies found that children with oedematous malnutrition had more atypical lymphocytes in blood, resembling plasma cells [81] [87] [93]. Other indicators of functional differences were higher density [200], different pattern of gene expression [201], and more markers of apoptosis in lymphocytes of malnourished children [92] [202].

T-lymphocytes in blood. Numbers of T-lymphocytes were described in 29 articles (**table S11**). Early studies identified T-lymphocytes as those forming rosettes with sheep red blood cells, while later studies used monoclonal antibodies to CD3. Using the rosette-method, 19 of 20 studies found lower levels of T-lymphocytes [28] [87] [93] [101] [128] [130] [144] [183] [186–187] [191] [199] [203–210]. Four studies using monoclonal CD3-antibodies and cell-counting by microscopy also found reduced levels of T-lymphocytes in malnourished children [144] [167–168] [207]. In contrast, only one flow cytometry study found lower levels of T-lymphocytes in malnourished children [211], while four did not [86] [94] [210] [212]. Accordingly, it seems like the rosette-based method identifies different T-lymphocytes than flow cytometry. Some studies found that the numbers of T-lymphocytes were reduced in acute infections [86] [90] [212].

Lymphocyte response to PHA stimulation. In healthy children, incubation of lymphocytes with PHA results in T-lymphocytes to proliferate. Seventeen out of 23 articles reported a reduced proliferative response to PHA in lymphocytes of malnourished children [93] [97–98] [101] [147] [154] [163] [177] [179] [186–187] [189–190] [192] [196] [203] [212–218]. Zinc supplementation improved the response in malnourished children [190].

CD4+ lymphocytes. With assessment of CD4 counts becoming widely available, it has been investigated whether the number of CD4+ lymphocytes was affected by malnutrition. In children without HIV, two of four studies using monoclonal antibodies and microscopy found reduced levels of CD4+ lymphocyte in malnourished children [144] [168] [219] [207], while all seven flow cytometry-studies except one [211] found similar or higher levels [86] [90] [91] [94] [198] [212]. Bacterial infections were noted to reduce the CD4-count [86]. For malnourished children infected with HIV, it was hoped that re-nutrition alone could increase their level of CD4+ lymphocytes. However, a study from Zambia found that CD4 counts declined during nutritional rehabilitation in HIV-infected malnourished children without anti-retroviral treatment [198]. Thus, a low level of CD4+ lymphocytes can probably not be attributed to malnutrition, regardless of whether the child has HIV or not.

Three studies noted that level of CD4+ lymphocytes were higher in children with oedematous than with non-oedematous malnutrition [91] [198] [220], and several studies have noted that children with HIV were less likely to develop oedematous malnutrition [198] [220] [221], suggesting that some level of CD4+ lymphocytes could be required to develop the syndrome.

Activation markers on T-lymphocytes. Most flow cytometry studies assessing surface markers on T-lymphocytes have been carried out in Mexico, all comparing malnourished infected children with similarly infected well-nourished children. Malnourished children were found to have fewer effector T-lymphocytes, identified as cells lacking the "naïve" markers CD62L and CD28 [90], fewer activated T-lymphocytes, with the markers CD69 and/or CD25 [212] [222] [223], and fewer memory T-lymphocytes identified by the marker CD45RO+ [86]. In contrast, a study from Ghana found similar numbers of activated T-lymphocytes, identified by HLA-DR, in malnourished and well-nourished children [94].

B-lymphocytes. Articles published before 1990 measured B-lymphocytes as those forming rosettes when incubated with sheep erythrocytes and C3, while more recent studies used monoclonal antibodies to CD20 and flow cytometry. All seven rosette-based studies found unaffected or higher B-lymphocyte counts in malnourished children [130] [186] [200] [204] [206] [213] [224], as did one study using anti-CD20 and microscopy [167]. In contrast, all four studies using flow cytometry found reduced numbers of B-lymphocytes in malnourished children [86] [94] [211] [212].

Antibody levels. Thirty-two articles described immunoglobulins in blood of malnourished children (**table S12**). Nineteen of 27 studies found no difference in IgG antibodies or total γ-globulin between malnourished and well-nourished children [94] [53] [63–64] [82] [130] [144] [147] [150] [154] [179] [186] [224–238]. Likewise, IgM levels were most frequently similar, or higher in malnourished than well-nourished children [94] [53] [63–64] [82] [130] [144] [147] [154] [179] [186] [224–225] [227–238].

IgA was elevated in malnourished children in 19 of 27 studies [94] [53] [55–56] [63–64] [82] [130] [144] [147] [150] [154] [179] [224–225] [227–238]. With a few exceptions [150] [232], all studies found elevated levels of IgA in oedematous malnutrition, while 11 of 19 studies found that IgA in non-oedematous or underweight children was normal [94] [53] [55–56] [63] [82] [130] [144] [150] [154] [179] [224] [227] [230] [233–238]. One study noted that levels of IgA correlated with the degree of dermatosis in children with Kwashiorkor [231].

IgE showed no clear pattern, but was elevated in malnourished children in three of six studies [82] [147] [211] [233] [238–239]. IgD, present in low amounts in healthy children, was elevated in children with malnutrition in two studies[130] [233], or elevated in oedematous but not non-oedematous malnutrition [179], while one study found that it was similar to well-nourished children [82].

Antibody vaccination responses. Thirty-five articles described vaccination responses to a specific antigen (**table S13**). The articles either reported *sero-conversion rates*, or *antibody titre* response. Studies assessing sero-conversion rates in children with severe malnutrition found mixed results: Six of 10 studies found reduced sero-conversion rates in children with severe malnutrition to typhoid [101] [240], diphtheria [101], tetanus[101] [206], tetanus-diphtheria-pertussis (DTP) [234], hepatitis B [241], measles [141] [149] [242] and yellow fever [243–244], and two studies found that sero-conversion was delayed in malnourished children [245] [238]. Ten of 11 studies found that severely malnourished children responded with reduced antibody titres [101] [141] [149] [206] [233–234] [238] [240–242] [246], despite some of the studies finding acceptable sero-conversion rates. No study found that children with oedematous malnutrition had a normal antibody response to vaccination. One study from 1964 found improved antibody response to DTP in children with oedematous malnutrition randomized to a high-protein diet [247]. There did not seem to be any specific vaccines whose antibody response was more affected than others by malnutrition, nor was there any pattern in terms of responses to live or dead vaccines.

In contrast, mild and moderately malnourished children were most often found to seroconvert normally when vaccinated against smallpox [248], diphtheria [101] [178] [249] [284] , DTP [178] [234], measles [139] [140] [178] [245] [250–255], polio [178] [256], meningococcus[178] [257], and hepatitis B [258], and 9 of 11 articles reported similar level of antibody titres response in moderately malnourished, as well-nourished children [101] [140] [154] [178] [234] [248–249] [252–253] [258–259].

Three of five articles reported similar adverse reactions to vaccination in malnourished as in well-nourished [140–141] [242] [245–255]. In contrast, one study found that malnourished children given measles vaccine frequently developed diarrhoea, pneumonia and fever, compared to well-nourished children, who, in turn, more often developed a rash [141].

Results were inconsistent for studies assessing levels of specific antibodies to non-vaccine antigens, like blood type antigens [260] malaria [261], H. *influenza*, E. *Coli* [235] [262], *Ascaris* [211],

Rotavirus and Lipopolysaccharide [262]. Most of these studies were done in children with moderate malnutrition.

Cytokines. Cytokines are signal molecules acting locally between immune cells, and sometimes with systemic effects. Thirty-five articles described cytokines in malnourished children (**table S14**).

Early works identified cytokines as factors in serum influencing various in-vitro functions of immune cells. Thus, three of five studies found that "Leucocyte Migration Inhibiting factor" was lower in malnourished children [84] [263–264], that serum from malnourished children contained an "E-rosette inhibiting substance" [128] [265], "lympho-cytotoxin" [266], and a substance inhibiting lymphocyte response to PHA [218] [147] [267–268], sometimes called IL-1 [269]. Similarly, Interferon (IFN) was quantified by the antiviral effect of plasma on a cell culture [95] [196]. In neither of these bioassays, the substance responsible for the effect was known. More recent studies assessed levels of cytokines by immunoassays, looking for structurally known cytokines in plasma [123] [270–272] or in cultured leucocytes [89], with flow cytometry staining for intracellular cytokines [222–223], or by identifying mRNA coding for the protein [273–274], with remarkably consistent results.

Cytokines commonly found to be low in malnourished children included IL- 1 and IL-2 [222–223] [269–270] [273–274], although one study found both cytokines to be normal in non-oedematous malnutrition and lower in oedematous malnutrition [89]. IFN-γ was low in malnourished children in six studies [49] [222–223] [273–275], unaltered in malnourished children in one [276], and elevated in one [272]. IL-12 [49] [274], IL-18 and IL-21 [274], and Granulocyte Macrophage Colony Stimulating Factor [270] were also found to be lower in malnourished children. Blunted cytokine response after in-vitro stimulation with LPS was found in malnourished children [276–278], while incubation with leptin normalized their pattern of intracellular cytokines [223].

Other cytokines were mostly found to be elevated in malnutrition: IL10 was elevated in four of five studies [49] [222–223] [272–273], so was IL-4 [211] [273] [276] and soluble receptors to Tumour Necrosis Factor-α [123]. IL-8 was elevated [277] or unaltered [272].

Tumour Necrosis Factor-α (TNFα) [49] [129] [271–273] [276] [279–280] and IL-6 [120] [122–123] [129] [271–273] [276–278] were mostly similar or higher compared to well-nourished, most often in studies of infected children.

Comparing cytokine pattern between children with oedematous and non-oedematous malnutrition, most found that the difference from well-nourished was greatest in children with oedematous malnutrition [84] [89] [123] [265] [269–270] [277], while two studies found no difference between oedematous and non-oedematous malnutrition [218] [271].

Leukotrienes (LT) are not strictly cytokines, but immune modulating molecules derived from long chain polyunsaturated fatty acids. Levels of LTC4 and LTE4 were higher, and LTB4 lower, in children with oedematous than with non-oedematous malnutrition, whose levels were similar to well-nourished [281], and prostaglandin E2 [282] was higher in children with oedematous malnutrition than in well-nourished.

Discussion

We identified and reviewed 245 articles about immune function in malnourished children. Some general problems apply to many of the studies, mostly related to their observational design. For this reason they can only describe associations, not causalities.

First, many studies were done in severely malnourished children from hospital settings, who were ill with infections, making it difficult to disentangle the immunological effect of malnutrition from the effect of infection. This problem has caused some to propose that there really is no immune impairment by malnutrition, and that all alterations seen are due to infections or underlying unknown immune deficiencies, which are also responsible for the poor growth [283]. Enteropathy could be an example of such an "invisible" condition, causing both immune deficiency and malnutrition. This hypothesis is difficult to test. However, some studies did try to account for this problem by selecting malnourished children without clinical infections, or by comparing them to well-nourished infected children. In studies from central Africa in the 1970s and 1980s, some malnourished children may have suffered from unrecognized paediatric HIV [284], giving obvious problems for interpretation.

Second, publication bias is a well-known problem, and may have occurred, particularly in older studies, where some small studies showed a dramatic effect.

Third, studies used different diagnostic criteria for malnutrition, making it difficult to determine the children's degree of malnutrition as defined by present-day criteria. While children in 52 of the studies fulfilled WHOs present criteria for severe acute malnutrition, only two diagnosed children based on the new WHO growth reference. Those defined as severely malnourished based on old growth references would most likely also be classified as severely malnourished today, since the new WHO standard tend to classify more children as severely malnourished, while some children then defined as moderately malnourished would be classified as severely malnourished today. The studies including children based on weight-for-age probably included children with stunting and wasting, without differentiating between the two.

Fourth, even using uniform criteria, malnourished children are a heterogeneous group. Anthropometric measurements are only crude markers of body composition, which - among other things - reflect nutrient deficiencies. It is unknown what specific nutrients were deficient, and to what extent infection contributed. Deficits in lean tissue and fat tissue are plausibly different physiologic conditions, and children appearing similarly malnourished may be so for entirely different reasons, with different immunological consequences. No articles have so far reported reliable measures of body composition, simultaneously with markers of immune function. Probably, the consequence of malnutrition on immune function may also depend on the pattern and load of infections. Although most studies were carried out in low-income settings with high infectious loads, a few were from middle- or high-income countries. This may also contribute to inconsistencies in the results.

In spite of these limitations, common patterns emerge from the studies, summarized below (**Figure 5**).

Immune parameters apparently not affected by malnutrition

Total white blood cell and lymphocyte counts in peripheral blood are not decreased in malnourished children, and granulocytes are frequently elevated. Likewise, T-lymphocytes and CD4 counts appear normal in malnourished children, when measured by flow cytometry, the gold standard for characterizing cell subsets. Their levels seem to be determined more by infections than by nutritional state, and do not reflect the degree of malnutrition-related immune deficiency, as high infectious mortality is seen in malnourished children, despite unaffected white blood cell counts [49].

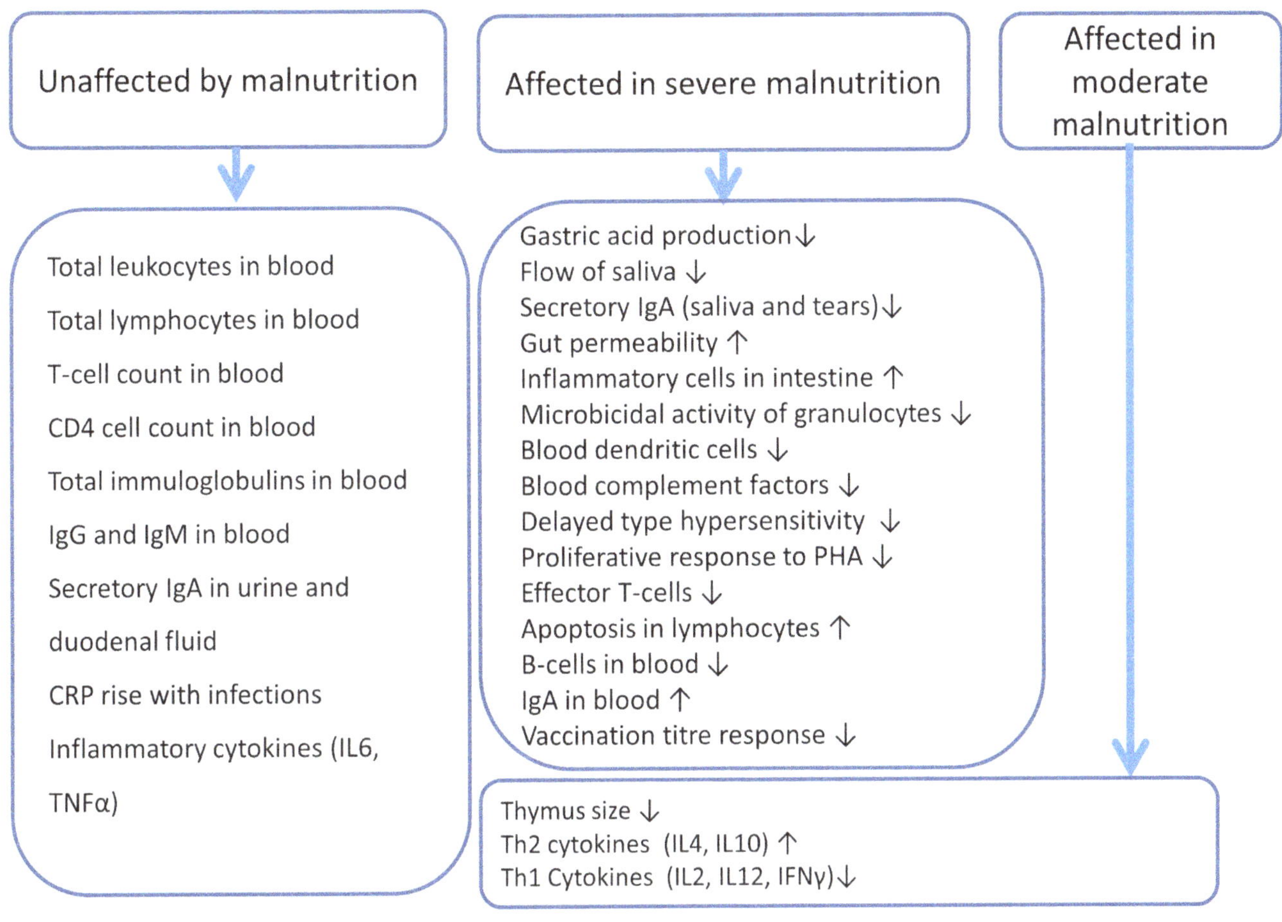

Unaffected by malnutrition
Affected in severe malnutrition
Affected in moderate malnutrition
Total leukocytes in blood
Total lymphocytes in blood
T-cell count in blood
CD4 cell count in blood
Total immuloglobulins in blood
IgG and IgM in blood
Secretory IgA in urine and duodenal fluid
CRP rise with infections
Inflammatory cytokines (IL6, TNFα)
Gastric acid production↓
Flow of saliva ↓
Secretory IgA (saliva and tears)↓
Gut permeability ↑
Inflammatory cells in intestine ↑
Microbicidal activity of granulocytes ↓
Blood dendritic cells ↓
Blood complement factors ↓
Delayed type hypersensitivity ↓
Proliferative response to PHA ↓
Effector T-cells ↓
Apoptosis in lymphocytes ↑
B-cells in blood ↓
IgA in blood ↑
Vaccination titre response ↓
Thymus size ↓
Th2 cytokines (IL4, IL10) ↑
Th1 Cytokines (IL2, IL12, IFNγ)↓

Figure 5. Summary of immune parameters affected and not affected by malnutrition.

Malnourished children can mount an acute phase response to infections, with elevated CRP and low negative acute phase reactants, and this can also be seen in absence of clinical infection. Thus, based on available evidence, the acute phase response, if anything, seems exaggerated rather than diminished. Levels of IgM and IgG are normal or elevated in malnourished children. Secretory IgA is not consistently lower in duodenal fluid, and frequently elevated in urine.

Immune parameters affected by malnutrition

The gut mucosa is atrophied and permeable in malnourished children. This enteropathy also affects well-nourished children in poor communities, but probably most severely in malnourished children. The condition appears similar to *tropical sprue* described in adults, and the term *enteropathy of malnutrition* has been replaced by the broader term *environmental enteropathy* [285]. At present, this condition is thought to result from high pathogen load rather than nutrient deficiencies, and thus primarily a cause of malnutrition, particularly of stunting [286] [287].

Production of gastric acid and flow of saliva is reduced in malnourished children. Secretory IgA is also reduced in saliva, tears and nasal washings from children with severe, but not moderate malnutrition. The small bowel of malnourished children is often colonized with abundant bacteria, and their pattern of commensal flora is altered. Granulocytes kill ingested microorganisms less effectively. Levels of complement proteins are low in blood from malnourished children, particularly in children with oedematous malnutrition, and less in children with moderate malnutrition.

Lymphatic tissue, particularly the thymus, undergoes atrophy in malnutrition in a dose-response fashion: thymic size depends on nutritional status even in milder degrees of malnutrition, and thymus size is a predictor of survival in children.

DTHR is diminished in malnourished children. Lymphocytes of malnourished children are less responsive to stimulation with PHA, fewer are activated and more cells have markers of apoptosis. Plasma IgA is mostly elevated in malnourished children, particular in those with oedema. Children with severe, but not moderate, malnutrition mount a lower specific antibody response to vaccination, although for most children sufficient to obtain protection. The lower titres seen in malnourished may be due to a delay in vaccination response.

Cytokines can be classified as those promoting a Th1 response of predominantly cellular immunity, and those promoting a Th2-response of humoral immunity [24]. Although this approach has somewhat been replaced by other classifications [288], it seems useful to describe the profile of malnourished children, whose immune system seems tuned towards a Th2 response, with high IL4 and IL10, and low levels of IL-2, IL-12 and IFN-γ. Elevated levels of IL-6 and TNFα may primarily be related to infections, and support the observation that induction of an acute phase response is intact in malnutrition. A more recent classification focuses on whether cytokines are predominantly inflammatory or anti-inflammatory [289]. Malnourished children appear to have high levels of anti-inflammatory cytokines and less clearly affected levels of pro-inflammatory cytokines in blood, in contrast to the predominantly pro-inflammatory cytokine expression in the gut of malnourished children.

Mechanisms

The mechanisms behind these immunological alterations are still not adequately understood. Some explain it by lack of energy and building blocks to synthesize the proteins required [290]. However, lack of building blocks does not explain why some immune parameters seem intact, or paradoxically elevated in malnutrition, such as plasma IgA, acute-phase proteins, leucocytes in blood, and production of Th2 cytokines. If it was simply a matter of lack of building blocks, all parameters of the immune system should be equally affected. The fact that the pattern of cytokines in malnourished children is tuned towards at Th2-response fits with their high levels of immunoglobulins, reduction in thymus size and diminished DTHR. Still, the pathophysiology behind this Th2 skewedness remains unexplained.

Infections could obviously contribute to the changes seen, and interactions have been noted between infection and malnutrition in their respective effects on immune parameters [197]. However, although many of the immunological changes appear to be synergistically affected by malnutrition and infections, malnutrition also seems to be independently associated with altered immune function.

Animal studies suggest hormonal factors to be involved in the immune profile of malnutrition. Leptin [291], prolactin [292] and growth hormone [293] all stimulate thymic growth and function, and their levels are low in malnourished children. In support of this, a recent study found that a low leptin level was associated with a higher risk of death in malnourished children [272]. Growth hormone therapy increased thymic size and output in adult HIV patients [294]. In contrast, cortisol and adrenalin induce thymic atrophy in mice [295–296], and cortisol is high in children with malnutrition and other forms of stress. It is plausible that this hormonal interplay is implicated in the immune deficiency in malnourished children.

This hormonal profile is similar to that of an acute phase response, where thymus atrophy also occurs, acquired immunity is temporarily suppressed and innate immunity takes over [296]. This could explain why some malnourished children have elevated positive APP and most have depressed negative APP in absence of clinical infections. Zinc deficiency causes thymic atrophy [297–298], and acute phase responses lower plasma zinc, so zinc status may contribute to the immune deficiency of both malnutrition and acute phase responses.

In HIV infection, persisting subclinical inflammation and immune activation is frequently present, and may be partly responsible for immune deficiency and disease manifestations [299]. Given the frequent finding of elevated acute phase proteins in malnourished children, it seems plausible that a similar state of subclinical inflammation could be involved in both the impairment of immune function, and in the vicious circle of catabolism and deterioration of the nutritional status. However, in spite of elevated acute phase proteins, most studies have reported unaffected or even paradoxically lowered levels of activated T-cell and dendritic cells in malnourished children.

The intracellular receptor, *mammalian target of Raptomycin* (mTOR), is present in most cells. It responds to concentrations of nutrients in the cell's surroundings, and to other signs of stress, such as hypoxia, enabling the cell to adapt its metabolism to locally available nutrients. Immune cells also use mTOR to regulate their state of activation. Nutrient availability may thereby determine whether an immune cell is activated [300], and whether T-cells differentiate towards a pro-inflammatory or a tolerance-inducing phenotype [301]. Some immune cells may even deplete the micro-environment of certain nutrients, to manipulate the activation of mTOR. Accordingly, the significance of nutrients in the micro-environment expands from simple building blocks to signal molecules. Obviously, this mechanism could be involved in the immunological profile in malnutrition. However, no articles have yet described the activity of mTOR in malnourished children.

A research group working with animal models of malnutrition has proposed a theory called the "tolerance hypothesis" [302]. This suggests that the depression of cellular immunity in malnutrition is an adaptive response to prevent autoimmune reactions, which would otherwise occur as a result of catabolism and release of self-antigens. Although adaptive in this sense, it happens at the price of increased susceptibility to infections [303]. However, if this tolerance hypothesis holds true, one would expect to see occasional break-through of auto-immune reactions in malnourished children. Such phenomena have apparently not been studied.

The pathogenesis of oedematous malnutrition is still unknown. Many immune parameters seem affected to a different degree in children with oedematous malnutrition, with higher levels of IgA, higher levels of abnormal antibodies like IgD, poorer vaccination responses and cytokines more skewed towards a Th2-response; their complement levels are lower, which may partly be caused by increased consumption of complement in-vivo. The pattern of leukotrienes is different in children with oedematous compared to non-oedematous malnutrition. This immunological profile resembles that seen in autoimmune diseases such as lupus erythematosus [304–305]. Moreover, elevated immunoglobulins in children with oedematous malnutrition seem to correlate with its unexplainable manifestations, like dermatosis and oedema [231] [233]. It could be speculated whether this syndrome could indeed represent some kind of autoimmune reaction to malnutrition, perhaps resulting from a failure to induce efficient tolerance.

Conclusion

In spite of the prevalence of malnutrition, and its fatal consequences, scientific interest in the immune deficiency of malnutrition seems dwindling, and little research has been carried out on the topic during the last ten years. For this reason, most evidence on the subject relies on immunological methods used 30 to 40 years ago, many of which are no longer in use, and little research has been done with modern methods, and with the present understanding of immunology. Moreover, most studies have looked at isolated aspects of immune function, despite the fact that the parameters are interdependent, and the division into innate and adaptive immune function seems to be a simplification. Thus, our understanding of immune function in malnutrition is still very limited.

This review illuminates the little that we know about the immunological alterations associated with malnutrition, and also points to significant gaps in our knowledge. Future well designed prospective cohort studies should examine how immune parameters are related to morbidity and mortality in malnourished children, with detailed characteristic of nutritional status, preferably body composition, of infections, enteropathy and of low-grade inflammation. When testing nutritional and medical interventions for malnutrition, immune parameters should be included as outcomes. Studies should investigate newer immunological parameters in malnutrition, like expression of innate pattern recognition receptors (as the Toll-like receptor), the lectin pathway of the complement system and mTOR expression and activity. It should be investigated whether a small thymus is associated with lower output of recent thymic-derived T-cells, and how it correlates with hormones like leptin, cortisol, insulin and Insulin Growth Factor-1. Innate and adaptive immune parameters should be assessed simultaneously, taking into account their dynamic interdependency. To understand whether malnutrition is indeed associated with active down-regulation of immune reactivity (as formulated in the "tolerance hypothesis"), the balance between regulatory T-lymphocytes and their counterparts, Th17 lymphocytes should be measured. Finally, prospective studies among children at risk should assess whether immune profiles differ in those who subsequently develop oedematous and non-oedematous malnutrition, and it should be investigated whether children with oedematous malnutrition have markers suggestive of auto-immune or inflammatory diseases. Such studies would reduce our current ignorance on the interplay between malnutrition and infectious diseases.

Supporting Information

Figure S1 PRISMA Flow diagram showing study retrieval and selection.

Table S1 Articles describing barrier and immune function of skin in malnourished children.

Table S2 Articles describing intestinal function and mucosal structure in children with malnutrition.

Table S3 Articles describing anti-microbial factors in mucosal secretions of malnourished children.

Table S4 Articles describing commensal flora in children with malnutrition.

Table S5 Articles describing function of innate immune cells: polymorph-nuclear cells and monocytes/macrophages in children with malnutrition.

Table S6 Articles describing acute phase response in malnourished children.

Table S7 Articles describing complement in malnourished children.

Table S8 Articles describing thymus and other lymphatic tissue in autopsies of malnourished children.

Table S9 Articles describing ultrasound scans of thymus in malnourished children.

Table S10 Articles describing delayed type hypersensitivity response in children with malnutrition.

Table S11 Articles describing lymphocyte subsets in children with malnutrition.

Table S12 Articles describing antibody levels in children with malnutrition.

Table S13 Articles describing humoral vaccination responses in children with malnutrition.

Table S14 Articles describing cytokines in malnourished children.

Checklist S1 PRISMA Checklist.

Acknowledgments

We are grateful to Dr Michael Golden for providing an extensive list of literature on the subject, and to Professor Kim Fleischer Michaelsen and Charlotte Gylling Mortensen for critically reviewing the manuscript.

Author Contributions

Conceived and designed the experiments: MJHR VBC. Performed the experiments: MJHR. Analyzed the data: MJHR. Contributed to the writing of the manuscript: MJHR LK AB HF VBC.

References

1. Black RE, Victora CG, Walker SP, Bhutta ZA, Christian P, et al. (2013) Maternal and child undernutrition and overweight in low-income and middle-income countries. Lancet 382: 427–451. doi:10.1016/S0140-6736(13)60937-X.
2. Pelletier DL, Frongillo EA Jr, Schroeder DG, Habicht JP (1995) The effects of malnutrition on child mortality in developing countries. Bull World Health Organ 73: 443–448.
3. Tomkins A, Watson F (1989) Malnutrition and Infection - A Review - Nutrition Policy Discussion Paper No. 5. United Nations - Administrative Commitee on Coordination - Subcommitee on Nutrition.
4. Chisti MJ, Tebruegge M, La Vincente S, Graham SM, Duke T (2009) Pneumonia in severely malnourished children in developing countries - mortality risk, aetiology and validity of WHO clinical signs: a systematic review. Trop Med Int Health TM IH 14: 1173–1189. doi:10.1111/j.1365-3156.2009.02364.x.
5. Waterlow JC (1992) Protein Energy malnutrition, 2nd ed. London: Hodder&Stouton.
6. Dutz W, Jennings-Khodadad E, Post C, Kohout E, Nazarian I, et al. (1974) Marasmus and Pneumocystis carinii pneumonia in institutionalised infants. Observations during an endemic. Z Für Kinderheilkd 117: 241–258.
7. Purtilo DT, Connor DH (1975) Fatal infections in protein-calorie malnourished children with thymolymphatic atrophy. Arch Dis Child 50: 149–152.
8. Ikeogu MO, Wolf B, Mathe S (1997) Pulmonary manifestations in HIV seropositivity and malnutrition in Zimbabwe. Arch Dis Child 76: 124–128.
9. Amadi B, Kelly P, Mwiya M, Mulwazi E, Sianongo S, et al. (2001) Intestinal and systemic infection, HIV, and mortality in Zambian children with persistent diarrhea and malnutrition. J Pediatr Gastroenterol Nutr 32: 550–554.
10. Mondal D, Haque R, Sack RB, Kirkpatrick BD, Petri WA Jr (2009) Attribution of malnutrition to cause-specific diarrheal illness: evidence from a prospective study of preschool children in Mirpur, Dhaka, Bangladesh. Am J Trop Med Hyg 80: 824–826.
11. Khatun F, Faruque ASG, Koeck JL, Olliaro P, Millet P, et al. (2011) Changing species distribution and antimicrobial susceptibility pattern of Shigella over a 29-year period (1980–2008). Epidemiol Infect 139: 446–452. doi:10.1017/S0950268810001093.
12. Berkley JA, Lowe BS, Mwangi I, Williams T, Bauni E, et al. (2005) Bacteremia among children admitted to a rural hospital in Kenya. N Engl J Med 352: 39–47. doi:10.1056/NEJMoa040275.
13. Aiken AM, Mturi N, Njuguna P, Mohammed S, Berkley JA, et al. (2011) Risk and causes of paediatric hospital-acquired bacteraemia in Kilifi District Hospital, Kenya: a prospective cohort study. Lancet 378: 2021–2027. doi:10.1016/S0140-6736(11)61622-X.
14. Alcoba G, Kerac M, Breysse S, Salpeteur C, Galetto-Lacour A, et al. (2013) Do children with uncomplicated severe acute malnutrition need antibiotics? A systematic review and meta-analysis. PloS One 8: e53184. doi:10.1371/journal.pone.0053184.

15. Soler-Cataluña JJ, Sánchez-Sánchez L, Martínez-García MA, Sánchez PR, Salcedo E, et al. (2005) Mid-arm muscle area is a better predictor of mortality than body mass index in COPD. Chest 128: 2108–2115. doi:10.1378/chest.128.4.2108.
16. Roediger WE (1990) The starved colon–diminished mucosal nutrition, diminished absorption, and colitis. Dis Colon Rectum 33: 858–862.
17. Faddan NHA, Sayh KIE, Shams H, Badrawy H (2010) Myocardial dysfunction in malnourished children. Ann Pediatr Cardiol 3: 113–118. doi:10.4103/0974-2069.74036.
18. Myatt M, Khara T, Collins S (2006) A review of methods to detect cases of severely malnourished children in the community for their admission into community-based therapeutic care programs. Food Nutr Bull 27: S7–23.
19. World Health Organization, United Nations Children's Fund (2009) WHO child growth standards and the identification of severe acute malnutrition in infants and children A Joint Statement. Available: http://www.who.int/maternal_child_adolescent/documents/9789241598163/en/. Accessed 2014 Aug 5.
20. Williams C (1935) Kwashiorkor - a nutritional disease in children associated with a maize diet. The Lancet nov 16, 1935: 1151–1152.
21. Wellcome Trust Working Party (1970) Classification of infantile malnutrition. The Lancet aug 8: 302–303.
22. Smith R (2005) Investigating the previous studies of a fraudulent author. BMJ 331: 288–291. doi:10.1136/bmj.331.7511.288.
23. WHO (2009) WHO child growth standards and the identification of severe acute malnutrition in infants and children. Geneva: WHO. Available: http://www.who.int/nutrition/publications/severemalnutrition/9789241598163_eng.pdf. Accessed 7 July 2013.
24. Murphy K (2012) Janeways's Immunobiology. 2012th ed. Garland Science, Taylor & Francis Group.
25. Heilskov S, Rytter MJH, Vestergaard C, Briend A, Babirekere E, et al. (2014) Dermatosis in children with oedematous malnutrition (Kwashiorkor): a review of the literature. J Eur Acad Dermatol Venereol JEADV. doi:10.1111/jdv.12452.
26. Sims RT (1968) The ultrastructure of depigmented skin in kwashiorkor. Br J Dermatol 80: 822–832.
27. Thavaraj V, Sesikeran B (1989) Histopathological changes in skin of children with clinical protein energy malnutrition before and after recovery. J Trop Pediatr 35: 105–108.
28. Kulapongs P, Edelman R, Suskind R, Olson RE (1977) Defective local leukocyte mobilization in children with kwashiorkor. Am J Clin Nutr 30: 367–370.
29. Bhaskaram P, Reddy V (1982) Cutaneous inflammatory response in kwashiorkor. Indian J Med Res 76: 849 853.
30. Freyre EA, Chabes A, Poémape O, Chabes A (1973) Abnormal Rebuck skin window response in kwashiorkor. J Pediatr 82: 523–526.
31. Edelman R, Suskind R, Olson RE, Sirisinha S (1973) Mechanisms of defective delayed cutaneous hypersensitivity in children with protein-calorie malnutrition. Lancet 1: 506–508.
32. Burman D (1965) The jejunal mucosa in kwashiorkor. Arch Dis Child 40: 526–531.
33. Brunser O, Castillo C, Araya M (1976) Fine structure of the small intestinal mucosa in infantile marasmic malnutrition. Gastroenterology 70: 495–507.
34. Schneider RE, Viteri FE (1972) Morphological aspects of the duodenojejunal mucosa in protein-calorie malnourished children and during recovery. Am J Clin Nutr 25: 1092–1102.
35. Brunser O, Reid A, Monckeberg F, Maccioni A, Contreras I (1968) Jejunal mucosa in infant malnutrition. Am J Clin Nutr 21: 976–983.
36. Brunser O, Reid A, Mönckeberg F, Maccioni A, Contreras I (1966) Jejunal biopsies in infant malnutrition: with special reference to mitotic index. Pediatrics 38: 605–612.
37. Amadi B, Fagbemi AO, Kelly P, Mwiya M, Torrente F, et al. (2009) Reduced production of sulfated glycosaminoglycans occurs in Zambian children with kwashiorkor but not marasmus. Am J Clin Nutr 89: 592–600. doi:10.3945/ajcn.2008.27092.
38. Campbell DI, Murch SH, Elia M, Sullivan PB, Sanyang MS, et al. (2003) Chronic T cell-mediated enteropathy in rural west African children: relationship with nutritional status and small bowel function. Pediatr Res 54: 306–311. doi:10.1203/01.PDR.0000076666.16021.5E.
39. Green F, Heyworth B (1980) Immunoglobulin-containing cells in jejunal mucosa of children with protein-energy malnutrition and gastroenteritis. Arch Dis Child 55: 380–383.
40. Kaschula RO, Gajjar PD, Mann M, Hill I, Purvis J, et al. (1979) Infantile jejunal mucosa in infection and malnutrition. Isr J Med Sci 15: 356–361.
41. Theron JJ, Wittmann W, Prinsloo JG (1971) The fine structure of the jejunum in kwashiorkor. Exp Mol Pathol 14: 184–199.
42. Shiner M, Redmond AO, Hansen JD (1973) The jejunal mucosa in protein-energy malnutrition. A clinical, histological, and ultrastructural study. Exp Mol Pathol 19: 61–78.
43. Römer H, Urbach R, Gomez MA, Lopez A, Perozo-Ruggeri G, et al. (1983) Moderate and severe protein energy malnutrition in childhood: effects on jejunal mucosal morphology and disaccharidase activities. J Pediatr Gastroenterol Nutr 2: 459–464.
44. Stanfield JP, Hutt MS, Tunnicliffe R (1965) Intestinal biopsy in kwashiorkor. Lancet 2: 519–523.
45. Behrens RH, Lunn PG, Northrop CA, Hanlon PW, Neale G (1987) Factors affecting the integrity of the intestinal mucosa of Gambian children. Am J Clin Nutr 45: 1433–1441.
46. Brewster DR, Manary MJ, Menzies IS, O'Loughlin EV, Henry RL (1997) Intestinal permeability in kwashiorkor. Arch Dis Child 76: 236–241.
47. Hossain MI, Nahar B, Hamadani JD, Ahmed T, Roy AK, et al. (2010) Intestinal mucosal permeability of severely underweight and nonmalnourished Bangladeshi children and effects of nutritional rehabilitation. J Pediatr Gastroenterol Nutr 51: 638–644. doi:10.1097/MPG.0b013e3181eb3128.
48. Boaz RT, Joseph AJ, Kang G, Bose A (2013) Intestinal permeability in normally nourished and malnourished children with and without diarrhea. Indian Pediatr 50: 152–153.
49. Hughes SM, Amadi B, Mwiya M, Nkamba H, Tomkins A, et al. (2009) Dendritic cell anergy results from endotoxemia in severe malnutrition. J Immunol Baltim Md 1950 183: 2818–2826. doi:10.4049/jimmunol.0803518.
50. Mishra OP, Dhawan T, Singla PN, Dixit VK, Arya NC, et al. (2001) Endoscopic and histopathological evaluation of preschool children with chronic diarrhoea. J Trop Pediatr 47: 77–80.
51. Sullivan PB, Lunn PG, Northrop-Clewes C, Crowe PT, Marsh MN, et al. (1992) Persistent diarrhea and malnutrition–the impact of treatment on small bowel structure and permeability. J Pediatr Gastroenterol Nutr 14: 208–215.
52. Redmond AO, Kaschula RO, Freeseman C, Hansen JD (1971) The colon in kwashiorkor. Arch Dis Child 46: 470–473.
53. McMurray DN, Rey H, Casazza LJ, Watson RR (1977) Effect of moderate malnutrition on concentrations of immunoglobulins and enzymes in tears and saliva of young Colombian children. Am J Clin Nutr 30: 1944–1948.
54. Watson RR, McMurray DN, Martin P, Reyes MA (1985) Effect of age, malnutrition and renutrition on free secretory component and IgA in secretions. Am J Clin Nutr 42: 281–288.
55. Sirisinha S, Suskind R, Edelman R, Asvapaka C, Olson RE (1975) Secretory and serum IgA in children with protein-calorie malnutrition. Pediatrics 55: 166–170.
56. Ibrahim AM, el-Hawary MF, Sakr R (1978) Protein-calorie malnutrition (PCM) in Egypt immunological changes of salivary protein in PCM. Z Für Ernährungswissenschaft 17: 145–152.
57. Reddy V, Raghuramulu N, Bhaskaram C (1976) Secretory IgA in protein-calorie malnutrition. Arch Dis Child 51: 871–874.
58. Yakubu AM (1982) Secretory IgA in nasal secretions of children with acute gastroenteritis and kwashiorkor. Ann Trop Paediatr 2: 139–142.
59. Bell RG, Turner KJ, Gracey M, Suharjono Sunoto (1976) Serum and small intestinal immunoglobulin levels in undernourished children. Am J Clin Nutr 29: 392–397.
60. Buchanan N, Fairburn JA, Schmaman A (1973) Urinary tract infection and secretory urinary IgA in malnutrition. South Afr Med J Suid-Afr Tydskr Vir Geneeskd 47: 1179–1181.
61. Marei MA, al-Hamshary AM, Abdalla KF, Abdel-Maaboud AI (1998) A study on secretory IgA in malnourished children with chronic diarrhoea associated with parasitic infections. J Egypt Soc Parasitol 28: 907–913.
62. Miller EM, McConnell DS (2012) Brief communication: chronic undernutrition is associated with higher mucosal antibody levels among Ariaal infants of northern Kenya. Am J Phys Anthropol 149: 136–141. doi:10.1002/ajpa.22108.
63. Watson RR, Reyes MA, McMurray DN (1978) Influence of malnutrition on the concentration of IgA, lysozyme, amylase and aminopeptidase in children's tears. Proc Soc Exp Biol Med Soc Exp Biol Med N Y N 157: 215–219.
64. Beatty DW, Napier B, Sinclair-Smith CC, McCabe K, Hughes EJ (1983) Secretory IgA synthesis in Kwashiorkor. J Clin Lab Immunol 12: 31–36.
65. Gilman RH, Partanen R, Brown KH, Spira WM, Khanam S, et al. (1988) Decreased gastric acid secretion and bacterial colonization of the stomach in severely malnourished Bangladeshi children. Gastroenterology 94: 1308–1314.
66. Shashidhar S, Shah SB, Acharya PT (1976) Gastric acid, pH and pepsin in healthy and protein calorie malnourished children. Indian J Pediatr 43: 145–151.
67. Gracey M, Cullity GJ, Suharjono S (1977) The stomach in malnutrition. Arch Dis Child 52: 325–327.
68. Adesola AO (1968) The influence of severe protein deficiency (kwashiorkor) on gastric acid secretion in Nigerian children. Br J Surg 55: 866.
69. Vael C, Desager K (2009) The importance of the development of the intestinal microbiota in infancy. Curr Opin Pediatr 21: 794–800. doi:10.1097/MOP.0b013e328332351b.
70. Scheutz F, Matee MI, Simon E, Mwinula JH, Lyamuya EF, et al. (1997) Association between carriage of oral yeasts, malnutrition and HIV-1 infection among Tanzanian children aged 18 months to 5 years. Community Dent Oral Epidemiol 25: 193–198.
71. Matee MI, Simon E, Christensen MF, Kirk K, Andersen L, et al. (1995) Association between carriage of oral yeasts and malnutrition among Tanzanian infants aged 6–24 months. Oral Dis 1: 37–42.
72. Omoike IU, Abiodun PO (1989) Upper small intestinal microflora in diarrhea and malnutrition in Nigerian children. J Pediatr Gastroenterol Nutr 9: 314–321.
73. Mata LJ, Jiménez F, Cordón M, Rosales R, Prera E, et al. (1972) Gastrointestinal flora of children with protein–calorie malnutrition. Am J Clin Nutr 25: 118–126.

74. Gracey M, Stone DE, Suharjono Sunoto (1974) Isolation of Candida species from the gastrointestinal tract in malnourished children. Am J Clin Nutr 27: 345–349.
75. Neto UF, Toccalino H, Dujovney F (1976) Stool bacterial aerobic overgrowth in the small intestine of children with acute diarrhoea. Acta Paediatr Scand 65: 609–615.
76. Smith MI, Yatsunenko T, Manary MJ, Trehan I, Mkakosya R, et al. (2013) Gut microbiomes of Malawian twin pairs discordant for kwashiorkor. Science 339: 548–554. doi:10.1126/science.1229000.
77. Monira S, Nakamura S, Gotoh K, Izutsu K, Watanabe H, et al. (2011) Gut microbiota of healthy and malnourished children in bangladesh. Front Microbiol 2: 228. doi:10.3389/fmicb.2011.00228.
78. Gupta SS, Mohammed MH, Ghosh TS, Kanungo S, Nair GB, et al. (2011) Metagenome of the gut of a malnourished child. Gut Pathog 3: 7. doi:10.1186/1757-4749-3-7.
79. Subramanian S, Huq S, Yatsunenko T, Haque R, Mahfuz M, et al. (2014) Persistent gut microbiota immaturity in malnourished Bangladeshi children. Nature. doi:10.1038/nature13421.
80. Rosen EU, Geefhuysen J, Anderson R, Joffe M, Rabson AR (1975) Leucocyte function in children with kwashiorkor. Arch Dis Child 50: 220–224.
81. Schopfer K, Douglas SD (1976) Fine structural studies of peripheral blood leucocytes from children with kwashiorkor: morphological and functional properties. Br J Haematol 32: 573–577.
82. Purtilo DT, Riggs RS, Evans R, Neafie RC (1976) Humoral immunity of parasitized, malnourished children. Am J Trop Med Hyg 25: 229–232.
83. Schopfer K, Douglas SD (1976) Neutrophil function in children with kwashiorkor. J Lab Clin Med 88: 450–461.
84. Fongwo NP, Arinola OG, Salimonu LS (1999) Leucocyte migration inhibition factor (L-MIF) in malnourished Nigerian children. Afr J Med Med Sci 28: 17–20.
85. Nájera O, González C, Toledo G, López L, Cortés E, et al. (2001) CD45RA and CD45RO isoforms in infected malnourished and infected well-nourished children. Clin Exp Immunol 126: 461–465.
86. Nájera O, González C, Toledo G, López L, Ortiz R (2004) Flow cytometry study of lymphocyte subsets in malnourished and well-nourished children with bacterial infections. Clin Diagn Lab Immunol 11: 577–580. doi:10.1128/CDLI.11.3.577-580.2004.
87. Keusch G, Urritia J, Guerrero O, Castenada G, Douglas S (1977) Rosette-Forming Lymphocytes in Guatemalan Children with Protein-Calorie Malnutrition. Malnutrition and the Immune Response, Edited by Robert M Suskind. New York: Raven Press, Vol. 1977.pp. 117–124.
88. Keusch G, Urrutia JJ, Fernandez R, Guerrero O, Casteneda G (1977) Humoral and Cellular Aspects of Intracellular Bactericidal killing in Guatemalan Children with Protein-Energy Malnutrition. Malnutrition and the Immune Response, Edited by Robert M Suskind. New York: Raven Press.pp. 245–251.
89. Lotfy OA, Saleh WA, el-Barbari M (1998) A study of some changes of cell-mediated immunity in protein energy malnutrition. J Egypt Soc Parasitol 28: 413–428.
90. Nájera O, González C, Cortés E, Toledo G, Ortiz R (2007) Effector T lymphocytes in well-nourished and malnourished infected children. Clin Exp Immunol 148: 501–506. doi:10.1111/j.1365-2249.2007.03369.x.
91. Nassar MF, Younis NT, Tohamy AG, Dalam DM, El Badawy MA (2007) T-lymphocyte subsets and thymic size in malnourished infants in Egypt: a hospital-based study. East Mediterr Health J Rev Santé Méditerranée Orient Al-Majallah Al-Ṣiḥḥīyah Li-Sharq Al-Mutawassiṭ 13: 1031–1042.
92. Nassar MF, El-Batrawy SR, Nagy NM (2009) CD95 expression in white blood cells of malnourished infants during hospitalization and catch-up growth. East Mediterr Health J Rev Santé Méditerranée Orient Al-Majallah Al-Ṣiḥḥīyah Li-Sharq Al-Mutawassiṭ 15: 574–583.
93. Schopfer K, Douglas SD (1976) In vitro studies of lymphocytes from children with kwashiorkor. Clin Immunol Immunopathol 5: 21–30.
94. Rikimaru T, Taniquchi K, Yartey J, Kennedy D, Nkrumah F (1998) Humoral and cell-mediated immunity in malnourished children in Ghana. Eur J Clin Nutr 1998 May; 52: 344–350.
95. Salimonu LS, Ojo-Amaize E, Williams AI, Johnson AO, Cooke AR, et al. (1982) Depressed natural killer cell activity in children with protein-calorie malnutrition. Clin Immunol Immunopathol 24: 1–7.
96. Salimonu LS, Ojo-Amaize E, Johnson AO, Laditan AA, Akinwolere OA, et al. (1983) Depressed natural killer cell activity in children with protein–calorie malnutrition. II. Correction of the impaired activity after nutritional recovery. Cell Immunol 82: 210–215.
97. Vásquez-Garibay E, Campollo-Rivas O, Romero-Velarde E, Méndez-Estrada C, García-Iglesias T, et al. (2002) Effect of renutrition on natural and cell-mediated immune response in infants with severe malnutrition. J Pediatr Gastroenterol Nutr 34: 296–301.
98. Vásquez-Garibay E, Méndez-Estrada C, Romero-Velarde E, García-Iglesias MT, Campollo-Rivas O (2004) Nutritional support with nucleotide addition favors immune response in severely malnourished infants. Arch Med Res 35: 284–288. doi:10.1016/j.arcmed.2004.03.002.
99. Rich K, Neumann C, Stiehm R (1977) Neutrophil Chemotaxis in Malnourished Ghaninan Children. In: Suskind RM, editor.Malnutrition and the Immune Response.New York: Raven Press. pp. 271–275.
100. Goyal HK, Kaushik SK, Dhamieja JP, Suman RK, Kumar KK (1981) A study of granulocyte adherence in protein calorie malnutrition. Indian Pediatr 18: 287–292.
101. Reddy V, Jagadeesan V, Ragharamulu N, Bhaskaram C, Srikantia SG (1976) Functional significance of growth retardation in malnutrition. Am J Clin Nutr 29: 3–7.
102. Tejada C, Argueta V, Sanchez M, Albertazzi C (1964) Phagocytic and alkaline phosphatase activity of leucocytes in kwashiorkor. J Pediatr 64: 753–761.
103. Douglas SD, Schopfer K (1974) Phagocyte function in protein-calorie malnutrition. Clin Exp Immunol 17: 121–128.
104. Leitzmann C, Vithayasai V, Windecker P, Suskind R, Olson R (1977) Phagocytosis and Killing Function of Polymorphnuclear Leukocytes in Thai Children with Protein-Energy Malnutrition. In: Suskind RM, editor.Malnutri-Malnutrition and the Immune Response.New York: Raven Press. pp. 253–257.
105. Shousha S, Kamel K (1972) Nitro blue tetrazolium test in children with kwashiorkor with a comment on the use of latex particles in the test. J Clin Pathol 25: 494–497.
106. Forte WCN, Martins Campos JV, Leao RC (1984) Non specific immunological response in moderate malnutrition. Allergol Immunopathol (Madr) 12: 489–496.
107. Chhangani L, Sharma ML, Sharma UB, Joshi N (1985) In vitro study of phagocytic and bactericidal activity of neutrophils in cases of protein energy malnutrition. Indian J Pathol Microbiol 28: 199–203.
108. Bhaskaram P (1980) Macrophage function in severe protein energy malnutrition. Indian J Med Res 71: 247–250.
109. Bhaskaram P, Reddy V (1982) Macrophage function in kwashiorkor. Indian J Pediatr 49: 497–499.
110. Shilotri PG (1976) Hydrogen peroxide production by leukocytes in protein-calorie malnutrition. Clin Chim Acta Int J Clin Chem 71: 511–514.
111. Raman TS (1992) Nitroblue tetrazolium test in protein energy malnutrition. Indian Pediatr 29: 355–356.
112. Altay C, Dogramaci N, Bingol A, Say B (1972) Nitroblue tetrazolium test in children with malnutrition. J Pediatr 81: 392–393.
113. Machado RM, da Costa JC, de Lima Filho EC, Brasil MR, da Rocha GM (1985) Longitudinal study of the nitroblue tetrazolium test in children with protein-calorie malnutrition. J Trop Pediatr 31: 74–77.
114. Wolfsdorf J, Nolan R (1974) Leucocyte function in protein deficiency states. South Afr Med J Suid-Afr Tydskr Vir Geneeskd 48: 528–530.
115. Golden MH, Ramdath D (1987) Free radicals in the pathogenesis of kwashiorkor. Proc Nutr Soc 46: 53–68.
116. Shousha S, Kamel K, Ahmad KK (1974) Cytochemistry of polymorphonuclear neutrophil leukocytes in kwashiorkor. J Egypt Med Assoc 57: 298–308.
117. González C, Nájera O, Cortés E, Toledo G, López L, et al. (2002) Hydrogen peroxide-induced DNA damage and DNA repair in lymphocytes from malnourished children. Environ Mol Mutagen 39: 33–42.
118. González C, Nájera O, Cortés E, Toledo G, López L, et al. (2002) Susceptibility to DNA damage induced by antibiotics in lymphocytes from malnourished children. Teratog Carcinog Mutagen 22: 147–158.
119. Berczi I, Quintanar-Stephano A, Kovacs K (2009) Neuroimmune regulation in immunocompetence, acute illness, and healing. Ann N Y Acad Sci 1153: 220–239. doi:10.1111/j.1749-6632.2008.03975.x.
120. Reid M, Badaloo A, Forrester T, Morlese JF, Heird WC, et al. (2002) The acute-phase protein response to infection in edematous and nonedematous protein-energy malnutrition. Am J Clin Nutr 76: 1409–1415.
121. Morlese JF, Forrester T, Jahoor F (1998) Acute-phase protein response to infection in severe malnutrition. Am J Physiol 275: E112–117.
122. Malavé I, Vethencourt MA, Pirela M, Cordero R (1998) Serum levels of thyroxine-binding prealbumin, C-reactive protein and interleukin-6 in protein-energy undernourished children and normal controls without or with associated clinical infections. J Trop Pediatr 44: 256–262.
123. Sauerwein RW, Mulder JA, Mulder L, Lowe B, Peshu N, et al. (1997) Inflammatory mediators in children with protein-energy malnutrition. Am J Clin Nutr 65: 1534–1539.
124. Ekanem E, Umotong A, Raykundalia C, Catty D (1997) Serum C-reactive protein and C3 complement protein levels in severely malnourished Nigerian children with and without bacterial infections. Acta Pædiatrica 86: 1317–1320. doi:10.1111/j.1651-2227.1997.tb14905.x.
125. Razban SZ, Olusi SO, Ade-Serrano MA, Osunkoya BO, Adeshina HA, et al. (1975) Acute phase proteins in children with protein-calorie malnutrition. J Trop Med Hyg 78: 264–266.
126. El-Sayed HL, Nassar MF, Habib NM, Elmasry OA, Gomaa SM (2006) Structural and functional affection of the heart in protein energy malnutrition patients on admission and after nutritional recovery. Eur J Clin Nutr 60: 502–510. doi:10.1038/sj.ejcn.1602344.
127. McFarlane H (1977) Acute-Phase Proteins in Malnutrition. In: Suskind RM, editor.Malnutrition and the Immune Response.New York: Raven Press. pp. 403–405.
128. Salimonu LS (1985) Soluble immune complexes, acute phase proteins and E-rosette inhibitory substance in sera of malnourished children. Ann Trop Paediatr 5: 137–141.
129. Manary MJ, Yarasheski KE, Berger R, Abrams ET, Hart CA, et al. (2004) Whole-body leucine kinetics and the acute phase response during acute infection in marasmic Malawian children. Pediatr Res 55: 940–946. doi:10.1203/01.pdr.0000127017.44938.6d.

130. Nahani J, Nik-Aeen A, Rafii M, Mohagheghpour N (1976) Effect of malnutrition on several parameters of the immune system of children. Nutr Metab 20: 302–306.
131. Parent MA, Loening WE, Coovadia HM, Smythe PM (1974) Pattern of biochemical and immune recovery in protein calorie malnutrition. South Afr Med J Suid-Afr Tydskr Vir Geneeskd 48: 1375–1378.
132. Akenami FO, Koskiniemi M, Siimes MA, Ekanem EE, Bolarin DM, et al. (1997) Assessment of plasma fibronectin in malnourished Nigerian children. J Pediatr Gastroenterol Nutr 24: 183–188.
133. Hassanein el-S A, Assem HM, Rezk MM, el-Maghraby RM (1998) Study of plasma albumin, transferrin, and fibronectin in children with mild to moderate protein-energy malnutrition. J Trop Pediatr 44: 362–365.
134. Schelp FP, Thanangkul O, Supawan V, Pongpaew P (1980) α2HS-glycoprotein serum levels in protein–energy malnutrition. Br J Nutr 43: 381–383. doi:10.1079/BJN19800101.
135. Abiodun PO, Ihongbe JC, Dati F (1985) Decreased levels of alpha 2 HS-glycoprotein in children with protein-energy-malnutrition. Eur J Pediatr 144: 368–369.
136. Abiodun PO, Olomu IN (1987) Alpha 2 HS-glycoprotein levels in children with protein-energy malnutrition and infections. J Pediatr Gastroenterol Nutr 6: 271–275.
137. Doherty JF, Golden MH, Raynes JG, Griffin GE, McAdam KP (1993) Acute-phase protein response is impaired in severely malnourished children. Clin Sci Lond Engl 1979 84: 169–175.
138. Yoder MC, Anderson DC, Gopalakrishna GS, Douglas SD, Polin RA (1987) Comparison of serum fibronectin, prealbumin, and albumin concentrations during nutritional repletion in protein-calorie malnourished infants. J Pediatr Gastroenterol Nutr 6: 84–88.
139. Dao H, Delisle H, Fournier P (1992) Anthropometric status, serum prealbumin level and immune response to measles vaccination in Mali children. J Trop Pediatr 38: 179–184.
140. McMurray DN, Loomis SA, Casazza LJ, Rey H (1979) Influence of moderate malnutrition on morbidity and antibody response following vaccination with live, attenuated measles virus vaccine. Bull Pan Am Health Organ 13: 52–57.
141. Idris S, El Seed AM (1983) Measles vaccination in severely malnourished Sudanese children. Ann Trop Paediatr 3: 63–67.
142. Doherty JF, Golden MH, Griffin GE, McAdam KP (1989) Febrile response in malnutrition. West Indian Med J 38: 209–212.
143. Degn SE, Thiel S, Jensenius JC (2007) New perspectives on mannan-binding lectin-mediated complement activation. Immunobiology 212: 301–311. doi:10.1016/j.imbio.2006.12.004.
144. Ozkan H, Olgun N, Saşmaz E, Abacioğlu H, Okuyan M, et al. (1993) Nutrition, immunity and infections: T lymphocyte subpopulations in protein–energy malnutrition. J Trop Pediatr 39: 257–260.
145. Sakamoto M, Nishioka K (1992) Complement system in nutritional deficiency. World Rev Nutr Diet 67: 114–139.
146. Kumar R, Kumar A, Sethi RS, Gupta RK, Kaushik AK, et al. (1984) A study of complement activity in malnutrition. Indian Pediatr 21: 541–547.
147. Beatty DW, Dowdle EB (1978) The effects of kwashiorkor serum on lymphocyte transformation in vitro. Clin Exp Immunol 32: 134–143.
148. Haller L, Zubler RH, Lambert PH (1978) Plasma levels of complement components and complement haemolytic activity in protein-energy malnutrition. Clin Exp Immunol 34: 248–252.
149. Hafez M, Aref GH, Mehareb SW, Kassem AS, El-Tahhan H, et al. (1977) Antibody production and complement system in protein energy malnutrition. J Trop Med Hyg 80: 36–39.
150. Olusi SO, McFarlane H, Osunkoya BO, Adesina H (1975) Specific protein assays in protein-calorie malnutrition. Clin Chim Acta Int J Clin Chem 62: 107–116.
151. Olusi SO, McFarlane H, Ade-Serrano M, Osunkoya BO, Adesina H (1976) Complement components in children with protein-calorie malnutrition. Trop Geogr Med 28: 323–328.
152. Forte WC, Forte AC, Leão RC (1992) Complement system in malnutrition. Allergol Immunopathol (Madr) 20: 157–160.
153. Sirisinha S, Edelman R, Suskind R, Charupatana C, Olson RE (1973) Complement and C3-proactivator levels in children with protein-calorie malnutrition and effect of dietary treatment. Lancet 1: 1016–1020.
154. Kielman A (1977) Nutritional and Immune Responses of Subclinically Malnourished Indian Children. In: Suskind RM, editor.Malnutrition and the Immune Response.New York: Raven Press. pp. 429–440.
155. Abdulrhman MA, Nassar MF, Mostafa HW, El-Khayat ZA, Abu El Naga MW (2011) Effect of honey on 50% complement hemolytic activity in infants with protein energy malnutrition: a randomized controlled pilot study. J Med Food 14: 551–555. doi:10.1089/jmf.2010.0082.
156. Keusch GT, Torun B, Johnston RB Jr, Urrutia JJ (1984) Impairment of hemolytic complement activation by both classical and alternative pathways in serum from patients with kwashiorkor. J Pediatr 105: 434–436.
157. Suskind R, Edelman R, Kulapongs P, Pariyanonda A, Sirisinha S (1976) Complement activity in children with protein-calorie malnutrition. Am J Clin Nutr 29: 1089–1092.
158. Jahoor F, Badaloo A, Reid M, Forrester T (2008) Protein metabolism in severe childhood malnutrition. Ann Trop Paediatr 28: 87–101. doi:10.1179/146532808X302107.
159. Hasselbalch H, Ersbøll AK, Jeppesen DL, Nielsen MB (1999) Thymus size in infants from birth until 24 months of age evaluated by ultrasound. A longitudinal prediction model for the thymic index. Acta Radiol Stockh Swed 1987 40: 41–44.
160. Gui J, Mustachio LM, Su D-M, Craig RW (2012) Thymus Size and Age-related Thymic Involution: Early Programming, Sexual Dimorphism, Progenitors and Stroma. Aging Dis 3: 280–290.
161. Naeye RL (1965) Organ and cellular development in congenital heart disease and in alimentary malnutrition. J Pediatr 67: 447–458.
162. Watts T (1969) Thymus weights in malnourished children. J Trop Pediatr 15: 155–158.
163. Smythe PM, Brereton-Stiles GG, Grace HJ, Mafoyane A, Schonland M, et al. (1971) Thymolymphatic deficiency and depression of cell-mediated immunity in protein-calorie malnutrition. Lancet 2: 939–943.
164. Schonland M (1972) Depression of immunity in protein-calorie malnutrition: a post-mortem study. J Trop Pediatr Environ Child Health 18: 217–224.
165. Aref GH, Abdel-Aziz A, Elaraby II, Abdel-Moneim MA, Hebeishy NA, et al. (1982) A post-mortem study of the thymolymphatic system in protein energy malnutrition. J Trop Med Hyg 85: 109–114.
166. Jambon B, Ziegler O, Maire B, Hutin MF, Parent G, et al. (1988) Thymulin (facteur thymique serique) and zinc contents of the thymus glands of malnourished children. Am J Clin Nutr 48: 335–342.
167. Parent G, Chevalier P, Zalles L, Sevilla R, Bustos M, et al. (1994) In vitro lymphocyte-differentiating effects of thymulin (Zn-FTS) on lymphocyte subpopulations of severely malnourished children. Am J Clin Nutr 60: 274–278.
168. Chevalier P, Sevilla R, Zalles L, Sejas E, Belmonte G, et al. (1994) Study of thymus and thymocytes in Bolivian preschool children during recovery from severe acute malnutrition. J Nutr Immunol Vol 3, 1994: 27–39.
169. Chevalier P (1997) Thymic ultrasonography in children, a non-invasive assessment of nutritional immune deficiency. Nutr Res 17: 1271–1276. doi:10.1016/S0271-5317(97)00110-3.
170. Chevalier P, Sevilla R, Sejas E, Zalles L, Belmonte G, et al. (1998) Immune recovery of malnourished children takes longer than nutritional recovery: implications for treatment and discharge. J Trop Pediatr 44: 304–307.
171. Collinson AC, Moore SE, Cole TJ, Prentice AM (2003) Birth season and environmental influences on patterns of thymic growth in rural Gambian infants. Acta Paediatr Oslo Nor 1992 92: 1014–1020.
172. Garly M-L, Trautner SL, Marx C, Danebod K, Nielsen J, et al. (2008) Thymus size at 6 months of age and subsequent child mortality. J Pediatr 153: 683–688, 688.e1–3. doi:10.1016/j.jpeds.2008.04.069.
173. Moore SE, Prentice AM, Wagatsuma Y, Fulford AJC, Collinson AC, et al. (2009) Early-life nutritional and environmental determinants of thymic size in infants born in rural Bangladesh. Acta Paediatr Oslo Nor 1992 98: 1168–1175. doi:10.1111/j.1651-2227.2009.01292.x.
174. Hasselbalch H, Jeppesen DL, Engelmann MD, Michaelsen KF, Nielsen MB (1996) Decreased thymus size in formula-fed infants compared with breastfed infants. Acta Paediatr Oslo Nor 1992 85: 1029–1032.
175. Ngom PT, Collinson AC, Pido-Lopez J, Henson SM, Prentice AM, et al. (2004) Improved thymic function in exclusively breastfed infants is associated with higher interleukin 7 concentrations in their mothers' breast milk. Am J Clin Nutr 80: 722–728.
176. Moore SE, Fulford AJ, Wagatsuma Y, Persson LÅ, Arifeen SE, et al. (2013) Thymus development and infant and child mortality in rural Bangladesh. Int J Epidemiol. doi:10.1093/ije/dyt232.
177. McMurray DN, Loomis SA, Casazza LJ, Rey H, Miranda R (1981) Development of impaired cell-mediated immunity in mild and moderate malnutrition. Am J Clin Nutr 34: 68–77.
178. Greenwood BM, Bradley-Moore AM, Bradley AK, Kirkwood BR, Gilles HM (1986) The immune response to vaccination in undernourished and well-nourished Nigerian children. Ann Trop Med Parasitol 80: 537–544.
179. McMurray DN, Watson RR, Reyes MA (1981) Effect of renutrition on humoral and cell-mediated immunity in severely malnourished children. Am J Clin Nutr 34: 2117–2126.
180. Seth V, Kukreja N, Sundaram KR, Malaviya AN (1981) Delayed hypersensitivity after BCG in preschool children in relation to their nutritional status. Indian J Med Res 74: 392–398.
181. Satyanarayana K, Bhaskaram P, Seshu VC, Reddy V (1980) Influence of nutrition on postvaccinial tuberculin sensitivity. Am J Clin Nutr 33: 2334–2337.
182. Heyworth B (1977) Delayed hypersensitivity to PPD-S following BCG vaccination in African children–an 18-month field study. Trans R Soc Trop Med Hyg 71: 251–253.
183. Smith N, Khadroui S, Lopez V, Hamza B (1977) Cellular Immune Response in Tunisian Children with Severe Infantile Malnutrition. Malnutrition and the Immune Response, Edited by Robert Suskind. New York: Raven Press, Vol. 1977.
184. Abbassy AS, el-Din MK, Hassan AI, Aref GH, Hammad SA, et al. (1974) Studies of cell-mediated immunity and allergy in protein energy malnutrition. I. Cell-mediated delayed hypersensitivity. J Trop Med Hyg 77: 13–17.
185. Harland PS (1965) Tuberculin reactions in malnourished children. Lancet 2: 719–721.
186. Puri V, Misra PK, Saxena KC, Saxsena PN, Saxena RP, et al. (1980) Immune status in malnutrition. Indian Pediatr 17: 127–133.

187. Bhaskaram C, Reddy V (1974) Cell mediated immunity in protein-calorie malnutrition. J Trop Pediatr Environ Child Health 20: 284–286.
188. Edelman R (1973) Cutaneous hypersensitivity in protein-calorie malnutrition. Lancet 1: 1244–1245.
189. Geefhuysen J, Rosen EU, Katz J, Ipp T, Metz J (1971) Impaired cellular immunity in kwashiorkor with improvement after therapy. Br Med J 4: 527–529.
190. Castillo-Duran C, Heresi G, Fisberg M, Uauy R (1987) Controlled trial of zinc supplementation during recovery from malnutrition: effects on growth and immune function. Am J Clin Nutr 45: 602–608.
191. Fakhir S, Ahmad P, Faridi MA, Rattan A (1989) Cell-mediated immune responses in malnourished host. J Trop Pediatr 35: 175–178.
192. Schlesinger L, Stekel A (1974) Impaired cellular Immunity in marasmic infants. Am J Clin Nutr 27: 615–620.
193. Ziegler HD, Ziegler PB (1975) Depression of tuberculin reaction in mild and moderate protein-calorie malnourished children following BCG vaccination. Johns Hopkins Med J 137: 59–64.
194. Golden MH, Harland PS, Golden BE, Jackson AA (1978) Zinc and immunocompetence in protein-energy malnutrition. Lancet 1: 1226–1228.
195. Schlesinger L, Arevalo M, Arredondo S, Diaz M, Lönnerdal B, et al. (1992) Effect of a zinc-fortified formula on immunocompetence and growth of malnourished infants. Am J Clin Nutr 56: 491–498.
196. Schlesinger L, Ohlbaum A, Grez L, Stekel A (1977) Cell-mediated Immune studies in Marasmic Children from Chile: Delayed Hypersensitivity, Lymphocyte transformation, and Interferon Production. Suskind RM, editor. Malnutrition and the Immune Response. New York: Raven Press, Vol. 1977.
197. Wander K, Shell-Duncan B, Brindle E, O'Connor K (2013) Predictors of delayed-type hypersensitivity to Candida albicans and anti-Epstein-Barr virus antibody among children in Kilimanjaro, Tanzania. Am J Phys Anthropol 151: 183–190. doi:10.1002/ajpa.22250.
198. Hughes SM, Amadi B, Mwiya M, Nkamba H, Mulundu G, et al. (2009) CD4 counts decline despite nutritional recovery in HIV-infected Zambian children with severe malnutrition. Pediatrics 123: e347–351. doi:10.1542/peds.2008-1316.
199. Olusi SO, Thurman GB, Goldstein AL (1980) Effect of thymosin on T-lymphocyte rosette formation in children with kwashiorkor. Clin Immunol Immunopathol 15: 687–691.
200. Mahalanabis D, Jalan KN, Chatterjee A, Maitra TK, Agarwal SK, et al. (1979) Evidence for altered density characteristics of the peripheral blood lymphocytes in kwashiorkor. Am J Clin Nutr 32: 992–996.
201. González C, González H, Rodríguez L, Cortés L, Nájera O, et al. (2006) Differential gene expression in lymphocytes from malnourished children. Cell Biol Int 30: 610–614. doi:10.1016/j.cellbi.2006.02.011.
202. El-Hodhod MAA, Nassar MF, Zaki MM, Moustafa A (2005) Apoptotic changes in lymphocytes of protein energy malnutrition patients. Nutr Res 25: 21–29. doi:10.1016/j.nutres.2004.10.005.
203. Ferguson AC, Lawlor GJ Jr, Neumann CG, Oh W, Stiehm ER (1974) Decreased rosette-forming lymphocytes in malnutrition and intrauterine growth retardation. J Pediatr 85: 717–723.
204. Bang BG, Mahalanabis D, Mukherjee KL, Bang FB (1975) T and B lymphocyte rosetting in undernourished children. Proc Soc Exp Biol Med Soc Exp Biol Med N Y N 149: 199–202.
205. Rabson AR, Geefhuyzen J, Rosen EU, Joffe M (1975) Letter: Rosette-forming T-lymphocytes in malnutrition. Br Med J 1: 40.
206. Salimonu LS, Johnson AO, Williams AI, Adeleye GI, Osunkoya BO (1982) Lymphocyte subpopulations and antibody levels in immunized malnourished children. Br J Nutr 48: 7–14.
207. Joffe MI, Kew M, Rabson AR (1983) Lymphocyte subtypes in patients with atopic eczema, protein calorie malnutrition, SLE and liver disease. J Clin Lab Immunol 10: 97–101.
208. Cruz JR, Chew F, Fernandez RA, Torun B, Goldstein AL, et al. (1987) Effects of nutritional recuperation on E-rosetting lymphocytes and in vitro response to thymosin in malnourished children. J Pediatr Gastroenterol Nutr 6: 387–391.
209. Keusch GT, Cruz JR, Torun B, Urrutia JJ, Smith H Jr, et al. (1987) Immature circulating lymphocytes in severely malnourished Guatemalan children. J Pediatr Gastroenterol Nutr 6: 265–270.
210. Fakhir S, Ahmed P, Faridi MM, Rattan A (1988) Early rosette forming T cell–a marker of cellular immunodeficiency in PEM. Indian Pediatr 25: 1017–1018.
211. Hagel I, Lynch NR, Puccio F, Rodriguez O, Luzondo R, et al. (2003) Defective regulation of the protective IgE response against intestinal helminth Ascaris lumbricoides in malnourished children. J Trop Pediatr 49: 136–142.
212. Nájera O, González C, Cortés E, Betancourt M, Ortiz R, et al. (2002) Early Activation of T, B and NK Lymphocytes in Infected Malnourished and Infected Well-Nourished Children. J Nutr Immunol 5: 85–97. doi:10.1300/J053v05n03_07.
213. Kulapongs P, Suskind R, Vithayasai V, Olson R (1977) In Vitro Cell-Mediated Immune Response in Thai Children with Protein-Calorie Malnutrition. Malnutrition and the Immune Response, Edited by Robert M Suskind. New York: Raven Press, Vol. 1977.
214. Grace HJ, Armstrong D, Smythe PM (1972) Reduced lymphocyte transformation in protein calorie malnutrition. South Afr Med J Suid-Afr Tydskr Vir Geneeskd 46: 402–403.
215. Murthy PB, Rahiman MA, Tulpule PG (1982) Lymphocyte proliferation kinetics in malnourished children measured by differential chromatid staining. Br J Nutr 47: 445–450.
216. Ortiz R, Campos C, Gómez JL, Espinoza M, Ramos-Motilla M, et al. (1995) Effect of renutrition on the proliferation kinetics of PHA stimulated lymphocytes from malnourished children. Mutat Res 334: 235–241.
217. Moore DL, Heyworth B, Brown J (1974) PHA-induced lymphocyte transformations in leucocyte cultures from malarious, malnourished and control Gambian children. Clin Exp Immunol 17: 647–656.
218. Moore DL, Heyworth B, Brown J (1977) Effects of autologous plasma on lymphocyte transformation in malaria and in acute protein-energy malnutrition. Comparison of purified lymphocyte and whole blood cultures. Immunology 33: 777–785.
219. Noureldin MS, Shaltout AA, El Hamshary EM, Ali ME (1999) Opportunistic intestinal protozoal infections in immunocompromised children. J Egypt Soc Parasitol 29: 951–961.
220. Bachou H, Tylleskär T, Downing R, Tumwine JK (2006) Severe malnutrition with and without HIV-1 infection in hospitalised children in Kampala, Uganda: differences in clinical features, haematological findings and CD4+ cell counts. Nutr J 5: 27–27. doi:10.1186/1475-2891-5-27.
221. Ndagije F, Baribwira C, Coulter JBS (2007) Micronutrients and T-cell subsets: a comparison between HIV-infected and uninfected, severely malnourished Rwandan children. Ann Trop Paediatr 27: 269–275. doi:10.1179/146532807X245652.
222. Rodríguez L, González C, Flores L, Jiménez-Zamudio L, Graniel J, et al. (2005) Assessment by flow cytometry of cytokine production in malnourished children. Clin Diagn Lab Immunol 12: 502–507. doi:10.1128/CDLI.12.4.502-507.2005.
223. Rodríguez L, Graniel J, Ortiz R (2007) Effect of leptin on activation and cytokine synthesis in peripheral blood lymphocytes of malnourished infected children. Clin Exp Immunol 148: 478–485. doi:10.1111/j.1365-2249.2007.03361.x.
224. Fakhir S, Ahmad P, Faridi MM, Rattan A (1988) Serum immunoglobulins and B cell count in protein energy malnutrition. Indian Pediatr 25: 960–965.
225. Rosen EU, Geefhuysen J, Ipp T (1971) Immunoglobulin levels in protein calorie malnutrition. South Afr Med J Suid-Afr Tydskr Vir Geneeskd 45: 980–982.
226. Cohen S, Hansen JD (1962) Metabolism of albumin and gamma-globulin in kwashiorkor. Clin Sci 23: 351–359.
227. Najjar SS, Stephan M, Asfour RY (1969) Serum levels of immunoglobulins in marasmic infants. Arch Dis Child 44: 120–123.
228. Keet MP, Thom H (1969) Serum immunoglobulins in kwashiorkor. Arch Dis Child 44: 600–603.
229. Watson CE, Freesemann C (1970) Immunoglobulins in protein-calorie malnutrition. Arch Dis Child 45: 282–284.
230. el-Gholmy A, Helmy O, Hashish S, Ragan HA, el-Gamal Y (1970) Immunoglobulins in marasmus. J Trop Med Hyg 73: 196–199.
231. el-Gholmy A, Hashish S, Helmy O, Aly RH, el-Gamal Y (1970) A study of immunoglobulins in kwashiorkor. J Trop Med Hyg 73: 192–195.
232. Aref GH, el-Din MK, Hassan AI, Araby II (1970) Immunoglobulins in kwashiorkor. J Trop Med Hyg 73: 186–191.
233. Suskind R, Sirishinha S, Vithayasai V, Edelman R, Damrongsak D, et al. (1976) Immunoglobulins and antibody response in children with protein-calorie malnutrition. Am J Clin Nutr 29: 836–841.
234. Awdeh ZL, Kanawati AK, Alami SY (1977) Antibody response in marasmic children during recovery. Acta Paediatr Scand 66: 689–692.
235. Cripps AW, Otczyk DC, Barker J, Lehmann D, Alpers MP (2008) The relationship between undernutrition and humoral immune status in children with pneumonia in Papua New Guinea. P N G Med J 51: 120–130.
236. Casazza LJ, Sunoto S, Sugiono M (1972) Immunoglobulin levels in malnourished children. Paediatr Indones 12: 263–270.
237. Taddesse WW (1988) Immunoglobulins in kwashiorkor. East Afr Med J 65: 393–396.
238. Suskind R, Sirisinha S, Edelman R, Vithayasai V, Damrongsak D, et al. (1977) Immunoglobulins and Antibody Response in Thai Children with Protein-Calirie Malnutrition. Suskind RM, editor. Malnutrition and the Immune Response. New York: Raven Press, Vol. 1977.
239. Forte WCN, Santos de Menezes MC, Horta C, Carneiro Leão Bach R (2003) Serum IgE level in malnutrition. Allergol Immunopathol (Madr) 31: 83–86.
240. Pretorius PJ, De Villiers LS (1962) Antibody response in children with protein malnutrition. Am J Clin Nutr 10: 379–383.
241. el-Gamal Y, Aly RH, Hossny E, Afify E, el-Taliawy D (1996) Response of Egyptian infants with protein calorie malnutrition to hepatitis B vaccination. J Trop Pediatr 42: 144–145.
242. Powell GM (1982) Response to live attenuated measles vaccine in children with severe kwashiorkor. Ann Trop Paediatr 2: 143–145.
243. Brown RE, Katz M (1966) Failure of antibody production to yellow fever vaccine in children with kwashiorkor. Trop Geogr Med 18: 125–128.
244. Brown RE, Katz M (1965) Antigenic Stimulation in Undernourished Children. East Afr Med J 42: 221–232.
245. Wesley A, Coovadia HM, Watson AR (1979) Immunization against measles in children at risk for severe disease. Trans R Soc Trop Med Hyg 73: 710–715.

246. el-Molla A, el-Ghoroury A, Hussein M, Badr-el-Din MK, Hassen AH, et al. (1973) Antibody production in protein calorie malnutrition. J Trop Med Hyg 76: 248–250.
247. Reddy V, Srikantia SG (1964) Antibody Response in Kwashiorkor. Indian J Med Res 52: 1154–1158.
248. Brown RE, Katz M (1966) Smallpox vaccination in malnourished children. Trop Geogr Med 18: 129–132.
249. Paul S, Saini L, Grover S, Ray K, Ray SN, et al. (1979) Immune response in malnutrition–study following routine DPT immunization! Indian Pediatr 16: 3–10.
250. Ekunwe EO (1985) Malnutrition and seroconversion following measles immunization. J Trop Pediatr 31: 290–291.
251. Halsey NA, Boulos R, Mode F, Andre J, Bowman L, et al. (1985) Response to measles vaccine in Haitian infants 6 to 12 months old. Influence of maternal antibodies, malnutrition, and concurrent illnesses. N Engl J Med 313: 544–549. doi:10.1056/NEJM198508293130904.
252. Baer CL, Bratt DE, Edwards R, McFarlane H, Utermohlen V (1986) Response of mildly to moderately malnourished children to measles vaccination. West Indian Med J 35: 106–111.
253. Smedman L, Silva MC, Gunnlaugsson G, Norrby E, Zetterstrom R (1986) Augmented antibody response to live attenuated measles vaccine in children with Plasmodium falciparum parasitaemia. Ann Trop Paediatr 6: 149–153.
254. Smedman L, Gunnlaugsson G, Norrby E, Silva MC, Zetterström R (1988) Follow-up of the antibody response to measles vaccine in a rural area of Guinea-Bissau. Acta Paediatr Scand 77: 885–889.
255. Bhaskaram P, Madhusudan J, Radhrakrishna KV, Raj S (1986) Immunological response to measles vaccination in poor communities. Hum Nutr Clin Nutr 40: 295–299.
256. Chopra K, Kundu S, Chowdhury DS (1989) Antibody response of infants in tropics to five doses of oral polio vaccine. J Trop Pediatr 35: 19–23.
257. Greenwood BM, Bradley AK, Blakebrough IS, Whittle HC, Marshall TF, et al. (1980) The immune response to a meningococcal polysaccharide vaccine in an African village. Trans R Soc Trop Med Hyg 74: 340–346.
258. Asturias EJ, Mayorga C, Caffaro C, Ramirez P, Ram M, et al. (2009) Differences in the immune response to hepatitis B and Haemophilus influenzae type b vaccines in Guatemalan infants by ethnic group and nutritional status. Vaccine 27: 3650–3654. doi:10.1016/j.vaccine.2009.03.035.
259. Waibale P, Bowlin SJ, Mortimer EA Jr, Whalen C (1999) The effect of human immunodeficiency virus-1 infection and stunting on measles immunoglobulin-G levels in children vaccinated against measles in Uganda. Int J Epidemiol 28: 341–346.
260. Kahn E, Stein H, Zoutendyk A (1957) Isohemagglutinins and immunity in malnutrition. Am J Clin Nutr 5: 70–71.
261. Fillol F, Sarr JB, Boulanger D, Cisse B, Sokhna C, et al. (2009) Impact of child malnutrition on the specific anti-Plasmodium falciparum antibody response. Malar J 8: 116. doi:10.1186/1475-2875-8-116.
262. Brüssow H, Sidoti J, Dirren H, Freire WB (1995) Effect of malnutrition in Ecuadorian children on titers of serum antibodies to various microbial antigens. Clin Diagn Lab Immunol 2: 62–68.
263. Lomnitzer R, Rosen EU, Geefhuysen J, Rabson AR (1976) Defective leucocyte inhibitory factor (LIF) production by lymphocytes in children with kwashiorkor. South Afr Med J Suid-Afr Tydskr Vir Geneeskd 50: 1820–1822.
264. Heresi GP, Saitúa MT, Schlesinger L (1981) Leukocyte migration inhibition factor production in marasmic infants. Am J Clin Nutr 34: 909–913.
265. Salimonu LS, Johnson AO, Williams AI, Adeleye GI, Osunkoya BO (1982) The occurrence and properties of E rosette inhibitory substance in the sera of malnourished children. Clin Exp Immunol 47: 626–634.
266. Kobielowa Z, Turowski G, Szumera B, Lankosz-Lauterbach J (1979) Direct lymphocytotoxic test in protein-calorie malnutrition in infants. Acta Med Pol 20: 265–272.
267. Beatty DW, Dowdle EB (1979) Deficiency in kwashiorkor serum of factors required for optimal lymphocyte transformation in vitro. Clin Exp Immunol 35: 433–442.
268. Heyworth B, Moore DL, Brown J (1975) Depression of lymphocyte response to phytohaemagglutinin in the presence of plasma from children with acute protein energy malnutrition. Clin Exp Immunol 22: 72–77.
269. Bhaskaram P, Sivakumar B (1986) Interleukin-1 in malnutrition. Arch Dis Child 61: 182–185.
270. Aslan Y, Erduran E, Gedik Y, Mocan H, Okten A, et al. (1996) Serum interleukin-1 and granulocyte-macrophage colony-stimulating factor levels in protein malnourished patients during acute infection. Cent Afr J Med 42: 179–184.
271. Dülger H, Arik M, Sekeroğlu MR, Tarakçioğlu M, Noyan T, et al. (2002) Pro-inflammatory cytokines in Turkish children with protein-energy malnutrition. Mediators Inflamm 11: 363–365. doi:10.1080/09629350210000051566.
272. Bartz S, Mody A, Hornik C, Bain J, Muehlbauer M, et al. (2014) Severe acute malnutrition in childhood: hormonal and metabolic status at presentation, response to treatment, and predictors of mortality. J Clin Endocrinol Metab 99: 2128–2137. doi:10.1210/jc.2013-4018.
273. González-Martínez H, Rodríguez L, Nájera O, Cruz D, Miliar A, et al. (2008) Expression of cytokine mRNA in lymphocytes of malnourished children. J Clin Immunol 28: 593–599. doi:10.1007/s10875-008-9204-5.
274. González-Torres C, González-Martínez H, Miliar A, Nájera O, Graniel J, et al. (2013) Effect of malnutrition on the expression of cytokines involved in Th1 cell differentiation. Nutrients 5: 579–593. doi:10.3390/nu5020579.
275. Solis B, Samartín S, Gómez S, Nova E, de la Rosa B, et al. (2002) Probiotics as a help in children suffering from malnutrition and diarrhoea. Eur J Clin Nutr 56 Suppl 3: S57–59. doi:10.1038/sj.ejcn.1601488.
276. Palacio A, Lopez M, Perez-Bravo F, Monkeberg F, Schlesinger L (2002) Leptin levels are associated with immune response in malnourished infants. J Clin Endocrinol Metab 87: 3040–3046.
277. Abo-Shousha SA, Hussein MZ, Rashwan IA, Salama M (2005) Production of proinflammatory cytokines: granulocyte-macrophage colony stimulating factor, interleukin-8 and interleukin-6 by peripheral blood mononuclear cells of protein energy malnourished children. Egypt J Immunol Egypt Assoc Immunol 12: 125–131.
278. Doherty JF, Golden MH, Remick DG, Griffin GE (1994) Production of interleukin-6 and tumour necrosis factor-alpha in vitro is reduced in whole blood of severely malnourished children. Clin Sci Lond Engl 1979 86: 347–351.
279. Giovambattista A, Spinedi E, Sanjurjo A, Chisari A, Rodrigo M, et al. (2000) Circulating and mitogen-induced tumor necrosis factor (TNF) in malnourished children. Medicina (Mex) 60: 339–342.
280. Hemalatha R, Bhaskaram P, Balakrishna N, Saraswathi I (2002) Association of tumour necrosis factor alpha & malnutrition with outcome in children with acute bacterial meningitis. Indian J Med Res 115: 55–58.
281. Mayatepek E, Becker K, Hoffmann G, Leichsenring M, Gana L (1993) Leukotrienes in the pathophysiology of kwashiorkor. The Lancet 342: 958–960. doi:10.1016/0140-6736(93)92003-C.
282. Iputo JE, Sammon AM, Tindimwebwa G (2002) Prostaglandin E2 is raised in kwashiorkor. South Afr Med J Suid-Afr Tydskr Vir Geneeskd 92: 310–312.
283. Morgan G (1997) What, if any, is the effect of malnutrition on immunological competence? Lancet 349: 1693–1695. doi:10.1016/S0140-6736(96)12038-9.
284. Saxinger WC, Levine PH, Dean AG, de Thé G, Lange-Wantzin G, et al. (1985) Evidence for exposure to HTLV-III in Uganda before 1973. Science 227: 1036–1038.
285. Prendergast A, Kelly P (2012) Enteropathies in the developing world: neglected effects on global health. Am J Trop Med Hyg 86: 756–763. doi:10.4269/ajtmh.2012.11-0743.
286. Keusch GT, Rosenberg IH, Denno DM, Duggan C, Guerrant RL, et al. (2013) Implications of acquired environmental enteric dysfunction for growth and stunting in infants and children living in low- and middle-income countries. Food Nutr Bull 34: 357–364.
287. Campbell DI, Elia M, Lunn PG (2003) Growth faltering in rural Gambian infants is associated with impaired small intestinal barrier function, leading to endotoxemia and systemic inflammation. J Nutr 133: 1332–1338.
288. Basso AS, Cheroutre H, Mucida D (2009) More stories on Th17 cells. Cell Res 19: 399–411. doi:10.1038/cr.2009.26.
289. Opal SM, DePalo VA (2000) Anti-inflammatory cytokines. Chest 117: 1162–1172.
290. Manary MJ, Yarasheski KE, Smith S, Abrams ET, Hart CA (2004) Protein quantity, not protein quality, accelerates whole-body leucine kinetics and the acute-phase response during acute infection in marasmic Malawian children. Br J Nutr 92: 589–595.
291. Howard JK, Lord GM, Matarese G, Vendetti S, Ghatei MA, et al. (1999) Leptin protects mice from starvation-induced lymphoid atrophy and increases thymic cellularity in ob/ob mice. J Clin Invest 104: 1051–1059. doi:10.1172/JCI6762.
292. De Mello-Coelho V, Savino W, Postel-Vinay MC, Dardenne M (1998) Role of prolactin and growth hormone on thymus physiology. Dev Immunol 6: 317–323.
293. Savino W, Postel-Vinay MC, Smaniotto S, Dardenne M (2002) The thymus gland: a target organ for growth hormone. Scand J Immunol 55: 442–452.
294. Hansen BR, Kolte L, Haugaard SB, Dirksen C, Jensen FK, et al. (2009) Improved thymic index, density and output in HIV-infected patients following low-dose growth hormone therapy: a placebo controlled study. AIDS Lond Engl 23: 2123–2131. doi:10.1097/QAD.0b013e3283303307.
295. Barone KS, O'Brien PC, Stevenson JR (1993) Characterization and mechanisms of thymic atrophy in protein-malnourished mice: role of corticosterone. Cell Immunol 148: 226–233. doi:10.1006/cimm.1993.1105.
296. Haeryfar SM, Berczi I (2001) The thymus and the acute phase response. Cell Mol Biol Noisy-Gd Fr 47: 145–156.
297. Golden MH, Jackson AA, Golden BE (1977) Effect of zinc on thymus of recently malnourished children. Lancet 2: 1057–1059.
298. Chevalier P (1995) Zinc and duration of treatment of severe malnutrition. Lancet 345: 1046–1047.
299. Miedema F, Hazenberg MD, Tesselaar K, van Baarle D, de Boer RJ, et al. (2013) Immune Activation and Collateral Damage in AIDS Pathogenesis. Front Immunol 4: 298. doi:10.3389/fimmu.2013.00298.
300. Cobbold SP (2013) The mTOR pathway and integrating immune regulation. Immunology. doi:10.1111/imm.12162.
301. Peter C, Waldmann H, Cobbold SP (2010) mTOR signalling and metabolic regulation of T cell differentiation. Curr Opin Immunol 22: 655–661. doi:10.1016/j.coi.2010.08.010.
302. Monk JM, Steevels TAM, Hillyer LM, Woodward B (2011) Constitutive, but not challenge-induced, interleukin-10 production is robust in acute pre-

pubescent protein and energy deficits: new support for the tolerance hypothesis of malnutrition-associated immune depression based on cytokine production in vivo. Int J Environ Res Public Health 8: 117–135. doi:10.3390/ijerph8010117.
303. Monk JM, Richard CL, Woodward B (2011) A non-inflammatory form of immune competence prevails in acute pre-pubescent malnutrition: new evidence based on critical mRNA transcripts in the mouse. Br J Nutr: 1–5. doi:10.1017/S0007114511004399.
304. Lo MS, Zurakowski D, Son MB, Sundel RP (2013) Hypergammaglobulinemia in the pediatric population as a marker for underlying autoimmune disease: a retrospective cohort study. Pediatr Rheumatol Online J 11: 42. doi:10.1186/1546-0096-11-42.
305. Chen M, Daha MR, Kallenberg CGM (2010) The complement system in systemic autoimmune disease. J Autoimmun 34: J276–J286. doi:10.1016/j.jaut.2009.11.014.

19

A Robust Parameter Estimation Method for Estimating Disease Burden of Respiratory Viruses

King Pan Chan[1], Chit Ming Wong[1]*, Susan S. S. Chiu[2]*, Kwok Hung Chan[3], Xi Ling Wang[1], Eunice L. Y. Chan[2], J. S. Malik Peiris[1,4], Lin Yang[1,5]

1 School of Publish Health, The University of Hong Kong, Hong Kong Special Administrative Region, China, **2** Department of Paediatrics and Adolescent Medicine, The University of Hong Kong, Hong Kong Special Administrative Region, China, **3** Department of Microbiology, The University of Hong Kong, Hong Kong Special Administrative Region, China, **4** HKU - Pasteur Research Centre, Hong Kong Special Administrative Region, China, **5** Squina International Centre for Infection Control, School of Nursing, The Hong Kong Polytechnic University, Hong Kong Special Administrative Region, China

Abstract

Background: Poisson model has been widely applied to estimate the disease burden of influenza, but there has been little success in providing reliable estimates for other respiratory viruses.

Methods: We compared the estimates of excess hospitalization rates derived from the Poisson models with different combinations of inference methods and virus proxies respectively, with the aim to determine the optimal modeling approach. These models were validated by comparing the estimates of excess hospitalization attributable to respiratory viruses with the observed rates of laboratory confirmed paediatric hospitalization for acute respiratory infections obtained from a population based study.

Results: The Bayesian inference method generally outperformed the classical likelihood estimation, particularly for RSV and parainfluenza, in terms of providing estimates closer to the observed hospitalization rates. Compared to the other proxy variables, age-specific positive counts provided better estimates for influenza, RSV and parainfluenza, regardless of inference methods. The Bayesian inference combined with age-specific positive counts also provided valid and reliable estimates for excess hospitalization associated with multiple respiratory viruses in both the 2009 H1N1 pandemic and interpandemic period.

Conclusions: Poisson models using the Bayesian inference method and virus proxies of age-specific positive counts should be considered in disease burden studies on multiple respiratory viruses.

Editor: Edward Goldstein, Harvard School of Public Health, United States of America

Funding: This work was supported by the Research Fund for the Control of Infectious Diseases [RFCID 11100582] and the Area of Excellence Scheme of the University Grants Committee [AoE/M-12/06] of the Hong Kong Special Administrative Region Government. The funders had no role in study design, data collection and analysis, decision to publish, or preparation of the manuscript.

Competing Interests: The authors have declared that no competing interests exist.

* E-mail: hrmrwcm@hku.hk (CMW); ssschiu@hkucc.hku.hk (SSSC)

Introduction

Acute respiratory infections accounted for 11–22% of global deaths of children under five, with a significant proportion caused by respiratory viruses [1]. However, obtaining reliable population based estimates for disease burden of respiratory viruses remains a challenge. These viruses usually cause overlapping clinical syndromes, making it difficult to assign viral aetiology based on the clinical presentations of patients [2]. Moreover, laboratory tests necessary for case confirmation are not always conducted in clinical settings owing to limited laboratory capacity [3]. Previous studies have used several statistical methods to quantify the morbidity and mortality burden associated with influenza and respiratory syncytial viruses (RSV) [4]. These methods first established a baseline level with the assumption of no virus circulation, and then defined the excess hospitalization or mortality as the difference between the observed and baseline. However, few of these methods were able to separately determine the burden attributable to different respiratory viruses and even fewer studies have assessed the burden of respiratory viruses other than influenza and RSV. One commonly used method, Poisson regression modeling, allows simultaneous assessment of co-circulating viruses and has become increasingly popular recently. But our previous study showed that the point estimates derived by the classical maximum likelihood method for respiratory viruses other than influenza were unrealistically small and even negative [5]. The challenge lies in resolving the overlapping peaks of these co-circulating viruses, and also in adjusting for the confounding effects of other seasonal factors such as temperature or humidity [6]. An alternative estimation method, Bayesian inference, could be used as it has the advantage of incorporating the prior knowledge on parameter distributions [7]. Another unsolved problem in disease burden studies is the choice of virus proxy variables. The numbers or proportions of specimens positive for different viruses in all specimens tested have been widely used in previous studies [8,9]. Other less frequently used proxies include influenza-like illness rates multiplied by laboratory-test positive proportions (ILI×LAB) [10]. Although virus attack rates could be different across age groups due to the heterogeneity in prior immunity and exposure risks [11–13], no studies have hitherto integrated age-specific virus data into the models, largely due to the lack of such data in most regions. In this study we evaluated the performance of various combinations of model assumption, virus proxy variables and inference methods, in estimating excess hospitalization attributable to several co-circulating respiratory viruses. The estimates have been validated by comparison with observed rates of laboratory confirmed paediatric hospitalization rates for acute respiratory infections obtained from a population based study.

Methods

Data source

Hospital admission records of the two major public hospitals on the Hong Kong Island (Queen Mary Hospital (QMH) and Pamela Youde Nethersole Eastern Hospital (PYNEH) were obtained from the Hong Kong Hospital Authority during the study period of October 2003–September 2010. We compiled weekly numbers of hospital admissions with any listed discharge diagnosis of acute respiratory diseases (ARD) for the age groups of <1, 1–5 and 6–17 years, according to the International Classification of Diseases (9th Revision, ICD9) codes 460–466 or 480–487. Age specific virology data were obtained from the Microbiology Laboratory of QMH, which provides virology diagnostic services for both QMH and PYNEH, for influenza A (seasonal subtypes H3N2, sH1N1 and pandemic strain pH1N1), influenza B, respiratory syncytial virus (RSV), adenovirus and parainfluenza virus types 1–3. This laboratory tested a total of 80 611 specimens collected from both QMH and PYNEH during the study period, by using direct immunofluorescence tests (IF) and viral culture. Reverse transcription polymerase chain reaction (RT-PCR) was only routinely carried out during the 2009 pandemic [14]. Meteorological data were obtained from the Hong Kong Observatory.

Poisson model

Poisson models were first fitted to the age-stratified weekly admission numbers of acute respiratory diseases. A typical form of this model is

$$E[\log Y_t] =$$
$$\beta_0 + \beta_1 fluA_t + \beta_2 fluB_t + \beta_3 RSV_t + \beta_5 adeno_t + \beta_4 paraflu_t + s(t) + s(Temp_t)$$
$$+ s(Humd_t)$$

$$\beta_1, \beta_2, \beta_3, \beta_4, \beta_5 \sim Uniform[0,\theta] \qquad \text{(Model 1)}$$

where Y_t denotes the numbers of age-specific hospital admissions at week t $(t = 1,2,\ldots,366)$, and follows a Poisson distribution with mean μ_t and variance $\varphi\mu_t$. Here φ is an over-dispersion factor to adjust for the unequal mean and variance [15]. $fluA_t$, $fluB_t$, RSV_t, $adeno_t$ and $paraflu_t$ denote the age-specific weekly counts of specimens positive for influenza A and B, RSV, adenovirus or parainfluenza viruses, respectively. $s(t)$, $s(Temp_t)$ and $s(Humd_t)$ are the natural spline functions of time, weekly average temperature and relative humidity, respectively. Five degrees of freedom per year were used for the seasonal trend and two degrees of freedom for temperature and relative humidity. We used a Bayesian inference process based on Gibbs sampling (BUGS) [16] to estimate the parameters. A variety of Bayesian approaches have been widely applied to calculate the genetic distance in phylogenetic analysis [17] and to describe the transmission dynamics of influenza viruses [18]. By incorporating prior knowledge on the distribution of parameter with available data, the Bayesian inference method could provide a posterior distribution closer to the true underlying distribution [19]. Due to the known adverse effects of the viruses on hospital admissions, we assumed that the parameter of virus proxy variable followed a non-negative distribution. Therefore the coefficients of these variables β_1, β_2, β_3, β_4 and β_5 were estimated by a Bayesian process, under the distribution assumption of $Uniform[0,\theta]$. The posterior distribution of each covariate parameter was estimated by repeating a Monte Carlo Markov Chain simulation for 50,000 iterations with 25,000 burn-in iterations. Based on our previous findings [20], the starting point of θ was set to 10, to cover the range of excess risk from 0–20% associated with 10% increase in virus proxies.

In addition to age-specific positive counts, we tried different combinations of virus proxies with the Bayesian inference method on virus coefficients: age-specific proportions of positive specimens (Model 2), all-ages proportions (Model 3) or all-ages influenza-like illness rates multiplied by all-ages proportions (ILI×LAB, model 4). Besides the commonly adopted log linear Poisson regression models that assumed multiplicative effects of viruses, we also tried linear Gaussian models that assumed additive effects of influenza (Model 5) [10,21]. To compare the Bayesian approach with our previous models based on classical likelihood estimation, we fitted the classical log linear Poisson models with the proxies of age-specific counts (Model 6), age-specific proportions (Model 7) and all-ages proportions (Model 8).

Model validation

Baseline hospitalization for influenza A subtype H3N2 was first calculated from the model as the expected weekly numbers of admissions when the H3N2 proxy variable was set to zero and all the other variables were kept as the observed values. Excess hospitalization attributable to H3N2 was defined as the sum of difference between the observed and baseline hospitalization [22]. Similar calculation was repeated for other subtypes of influenza A, influenza B, RSV, adenovirus and parainfluenza, respectively. Annual excess rate of hospitalization was separately calculated for each year, by dividing the annual total number of excess hospitalization by the mid-year age-specific population in the Hong Kong Island obtained from the year 2006 census.

Annual excess rates estimated by these statistical methods were then compared with the directly observed admission rates for a population based systematic sample of laboratory confirmed cases of respiratory virus infections, who were admitted into the QMH and PYNEH with any listed diagnosis of ARD during the same period. The details of data collection for the directly observed virologically confirmed hospitalization rates have been described elsewhere [23]. Briefly, nasopharyngeal aspirates from patients who were younger than 18 years and admitted with symptoms of acute respiratory infection on one chosen day (Wednesday or Thursday) of each week, were all tested for five respiratory viruses by IF. Since these two hospitals provide acute paediatric hospital services for approximately 70% of the population in Hong Kong Island, we could estimate the population based age-specific hospitalization rates from this cohort. We calculated the mean of absolute percentage difference between the annual age-specific estimates and corresponding virologically confirmed observed hospitalization rates, and chose the most optimal model as that with the smallest mean difference. We also assessed the lag effects of these viruses by replacing the virus proxy variables with the proxies at the weeks up to three weeks before the current (lag1, 2

Table 1. Mean absolute percentage difference between annual age-specific excess hospitalization rates and annual hospitalization rates of laboratory confirmed infections in a pediatric cohort.

	Model 1	Model 2	Model 3	Model 4	Model 5	Model 6	Model 7	Model 8
Link function	**Log**	**Log**	**Log**	**Log**	**Linear**	**Log**	**Log**	**Log**
Inference	**Bayesian**	**Bayesian**	**Bayesian**	**Bayesian**	**Bayesian**	**Classical**	**Classical**	**Classical**
Prior	**Uniform**	**Uniform**	**Uniform**	**Uniform**	**Uniform**	**NA**	**NA**	**NA**
Virus proxies	**Age-specific count**	**Age-specific proportion**	**All-ages proportion**	**ILI×LAB**	**Age-specific count**	**Age-specific count**	**Age-specific proportion**	**All-ages proportion**
Influenza A								
sH1N1	38.4	43.3	40.6	33.9	46.6	41.0	77.4	44.0
H3N2	38.8	28.4	71.4	33.9	48.0	38.7	27.7	93.8
pH1N1	37.8	74.5	47.1	43.6	41.5	37.0	48.7	49.7
Influenza B	54.3	43.2	57.3	58.7	64.9	57.0	53.9	74.3
RSV	39.1	46.1	45.3	55.7	43.6	39.4	78.3	279.4
Parainfluenza	53.8	61.6	71.1	81.4	49.2	53.6	88.1	215.3
Adenovirus	63.4	79.1	68.8	65.3	68.3	68.2	108.9	145.0

Abbreviations: RSV, respiratory syncytial virus; NA, not available.

Table 2. Mean absolute percentage difference of excess hospitalization rates from annual hospitalization rates of laboratory confirmed infections in a pediatric cohort.

Lag weeks	Lag 1	Lag 2	Lag 3
Influenza A			
sH1N1	52.5	70.9	81.5
H3N2	44.5	62.5	70.0
pH1N1	57.8	68.5	78.5
Influenza B	41.7	62.7	72.5
RSV	62.2	102.6	77.6
Parainfluenza	65.2	94.9	86.4
Adenovirus	65.4	71.6	62.8

Excess rates were estimated from the log-linear Poisson model using a Bayesian approach with the virus proxies of age-specific positive counts at the different lag weeks.

and 3), to take into account of the potential delay between the virus infection and hospital admissions. For simplicity, the same lag was used for all the virus proxies in the model. In order to assess whether our method could differentiate the impacts of viruses during the interpandemic and pandemic periods, we calculated the excess rates separately for the 2009 H1N1 influenza pandemic period of May 2009 to August 2010, and for the preceding interpandemic period of October 2003 to April 2009. All the analysis was performed by the statistical packages R (version 2.5.1) and WinBUGS (version 1.4.3).

Ethical approval was obtained from the Institutional Review Board of the University of Hong Kong/Hospital Authority Hong Kong West Cluster (UW 11-264). Informed consent was not obtained because patient records were anonymized and de-identified prior to analysis.

Results

The mean absolute percentage difference between the annual age-specific rates of excess hospitalization derived from different models and the corresponding observed rates is shown in Table 1. In the models using the same virus proxies, the estimates from the models using the Bayesian inference showed smaller deviations from the observed rates than the classical likelihood estimates, particularly for RSV, parainfluenza and adenovirus. In the models using the Bayesian inference, compared to the other virus proxies, age-specific counts provided the estimates with smaller deviation from the true observed rates for most viruses (Table 1). The log-link models (Model 1) offered the estimates closer to the observed rates than the identity-link models (Model 5), with the exception of parainfluenza. Overall, the log-link Poisson models using the Bayesian inference and the proxies of age-specific counts (Model 1) provided the most reliable estimates for the excess hospitalization associated with influenza A and B, RSV, parainfluenza and adenoviruses. Therefore we chose this model as the final one and presented the estimates from this model in the rest part of this paper. The lag effects up to three weeks were separately assessed by replacing the age-specific positive counts virus at the current week (lag 0) with those at one to three weeks before (lag 1–3). These models with different lag week consistently provided the estimates more deviant from the observed rates, compared to the proxy variables at the current week (Table 2).

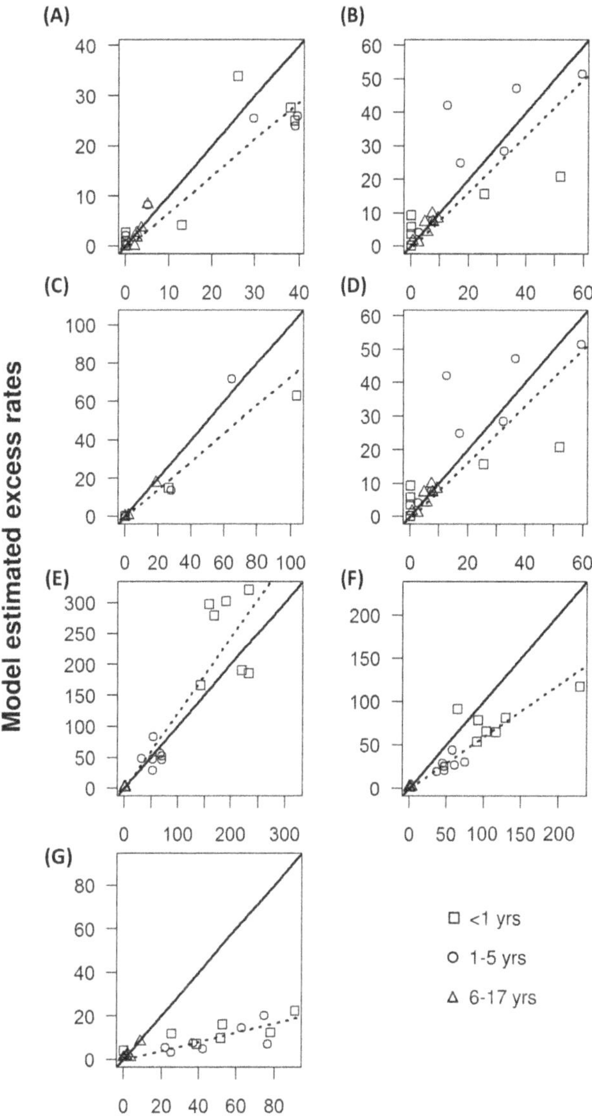

Figure 1. Comparison of annual excess hospitalization rates per 10,000 population and directly observed rates during each of the seven seasons, for (A) sH1N1, (B) H3N2, (C) pH1N1, (D) influenza B, (E) respiratory syncytial virus (RSV), (F) parainfluenza and (G) adenovirus. Excess hospitalization rates were derived from the WinBUGS models with age-specific counts as virus proxy.

Annual excess rates of hospitalization were slightly lower than the directly observed rates for influenza A subtypes sH1N1, H3N2, pH1N1 and influenza B in all the age groups, without any pattern of consistent under- or over-estimation observed in any of these age groups (Figure 1). For RSV, excess rates tended to be higher than the observed hospitalization rates, particularly for the <1 age groups. Most of the estimates for parainfluenza were smaller than the observed rates. The greatest deviation from the observed rates was found in adenovirus.

Compared to the interpandemic period, the 2009 H1N1 pandemic was associated with an obvious increase in the observed rates of laboratory confirmed cases for RSV, but a decrease in other viruses (Table 3). Overall the model provided the estimates similar to the directly observed rates of all the viruses under study

Table 3. Comparison of weekly directly observed rates (per 100,000 population) and excess rates of hospitalization associated with influenza estimated by the Bayesian approach, during the interpandemic period (4 January 2004–25 April 2009) and pandemic period (26 April 2009–14 August 2010).

Virus/Age group	Interpandmic		Pandemic	
	Directly observed rates	Excess rates (95% CI)	Directly observed rates	Excess rates (95% CI)
sH1N1				
<1	4.2	3.2 (0.3, 6.6)	0.0	0.4 (0.0, 1.0)
1–5	3.9	2.9 (1.0, 4.6)	0.7	0.8 (0.3, 1.3)
6–17	0.6	0.6 (0.3, 0.9)	0.1	0.1 (0.0, 0.1)
H3N2				
<1	8.9	12.0 (6.9, 17.3)	5.7	8.1 (4.6, 11.6)
1–5	6.2	9.0 (7.0, 11.0)	5.1	6.4 (4.9, 8.0)
6–17	0.7	0.9 (0.6, 1.2)	0.3	0.9 (0.6, 1.3)
pH1N1				
<1	na	na	17.2	11.3 (1.2, 21.9)
1–5	na	na	12.4	12.2 (8.2, 16.3)
6–17	na	na	2.9	2.6 (2.0, 3.2)
Influenza B				
<1	2.8	1.9 (0.1, 5.1)	0.0	0.8 (0.0, 2.2)
1–5	5.6	5.9 (4.0, 8.0)	0.7	5.2 (3.4, 7.0)
6–17	1.0	1.1 (0.8, 1.4)	1.0	1.1 (0.8, 1.6)
RSV				
<1	36.5	48.1 (38.7, 57.0)	45.8	48.3 (39.3, 57.9)
1–5	10.6	9.0 (5.1, 12.6)	12.7	12.4 (7.0, 17.2)
6–17	0.1	0.3 (0.0, 0.7)	0.2	0.4 (0.0, 1.1)
Parainfluenza				
<1	24.8	15.9 (8.0, 23.7)	13.3	11.6 (5.7, 17.6)
1–5	9.9	5.0 (1.8, 8.0)	10.9	6.3 (2.2, 10.3)
6–17	0.1	0.2 (0.1, 0.4)	0.3	0.4 (0.1, 0.8)
Adenovirus				
<1	10.3	2.4 (0.1, 5.4)	5.7	2.2 (0.1, 5.1)
1–5	9.6	1.7 (0.1, 4.3)	5.5	1.0 (0.0, 2.6)
6–17	0.6	0.5 (0.2, 0.9)	0.1	0.2 (0.1, 0.3)

Abbreviations: RSV, respiratory syncytial virus; NA, not available.

during the pandemic period, except slight overestimation in H3N2 and influenza B, and underestimation in adenovirus. The model performance was comparable between the interpandemic and pandemic periods for all the viruses.

Discussion

Time series models have widely adopted by recent studies to estimate the disease burden of influenza and RSV [24,25]. In this study we compared the Bayesian inference method with the classical likelihood estimation, in terms of obtaining more reliable estimates for the disease burden of co-circulating viruses including influenza, RSV, parainfluenza and adenovirus. Under the assumption of positive association between respiratory virus activity and hospitalization, the Bayesian inference method successfully separated the individual effects of multiple respiratory viruses, which the previous models have not or only partially achieved [5,26]. With the exception of adenovirus, the model estimates closely matched the true hospitalization rates across different age groups that were observed in a pediatric cohort under a systematic surveillance for respiratory virus infections. We speculated that underestimation in adenovirus was probably due to its less clear seasonal pattern and relatively lower positive isolation rate compared to the other viruses (Figure 2). Nevertheless, the models overall offered the satisfactory estimates which were within the close range of true hospitalization rates without exaggeration.

Taking the advantage of long standing virology data with linked age information in Hong Kong, this study for the first time added the age-specific virology data as proxy in the time series models for disease burden studies. We found that age-specific counts showed the best performance among all the proxies when combined with either the Bayesian or classical likelihood inference methods. In previous studies, we used all-ages proportion as proxy because it took into account the temporal variations in total numbers of specimens collected. However, this might not be the case for age-specific virology data, as relatively small numbers of total

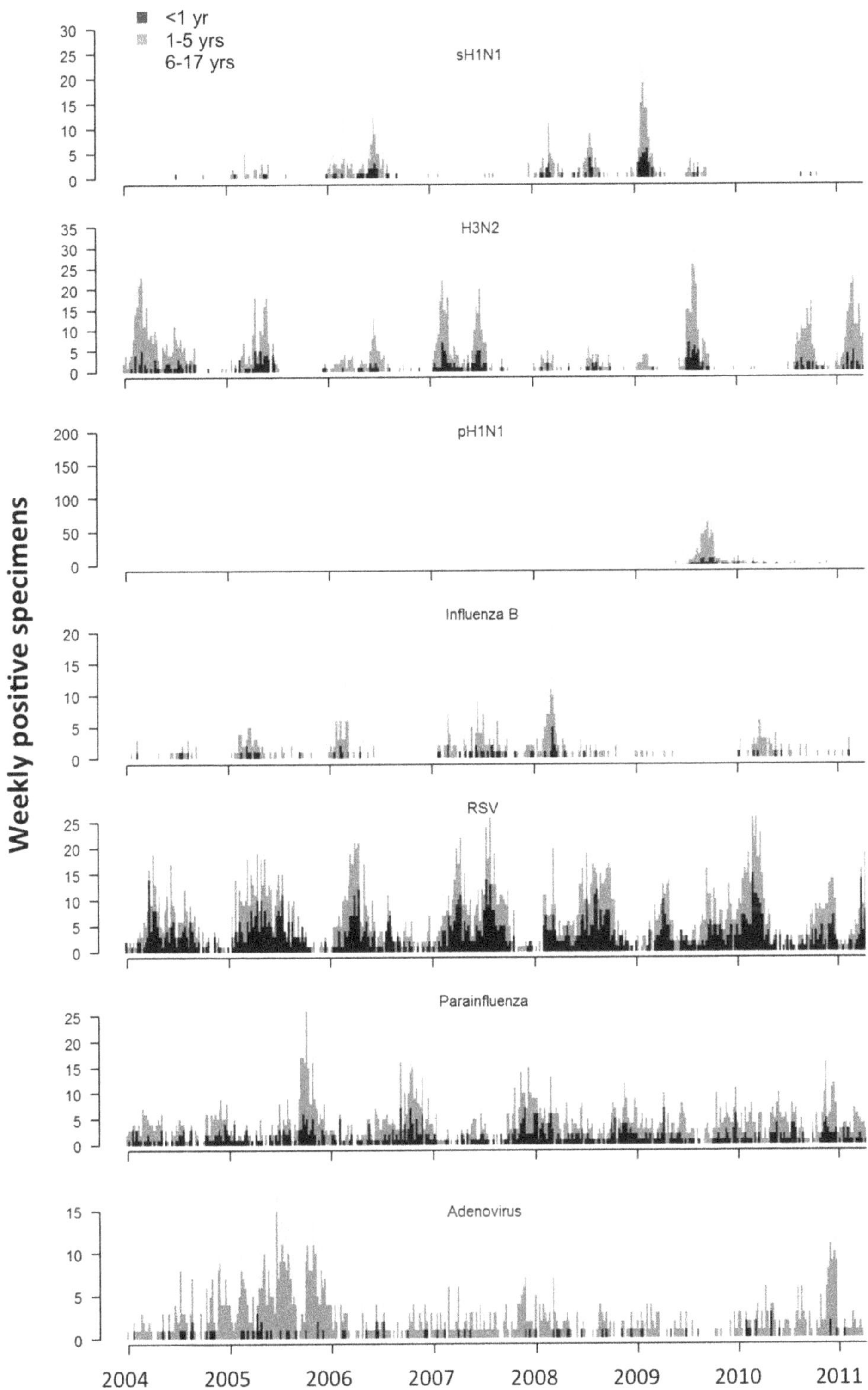

Figure 2. Weekly numbers of specimens positive for influenza A or B, RSV, parainfluenza and adenovirus in the age groups of <1, 1–5 and 6–17 years.

specimens tested in some age groups could have introduced spurious peaks in age-specific proportions. We also evaluated the performance of ILI×LAB proxy, which was found more closely correlated with the true incidence of influenza during the interpandemic or pandemic period [21,27]. We found this proxy provides the estimates closer to the observed rates than age-specific and all-ages proportions, but slightly worse than the proxy of age-specific counts in most viruses (Table 1 and Figure 3). Taken

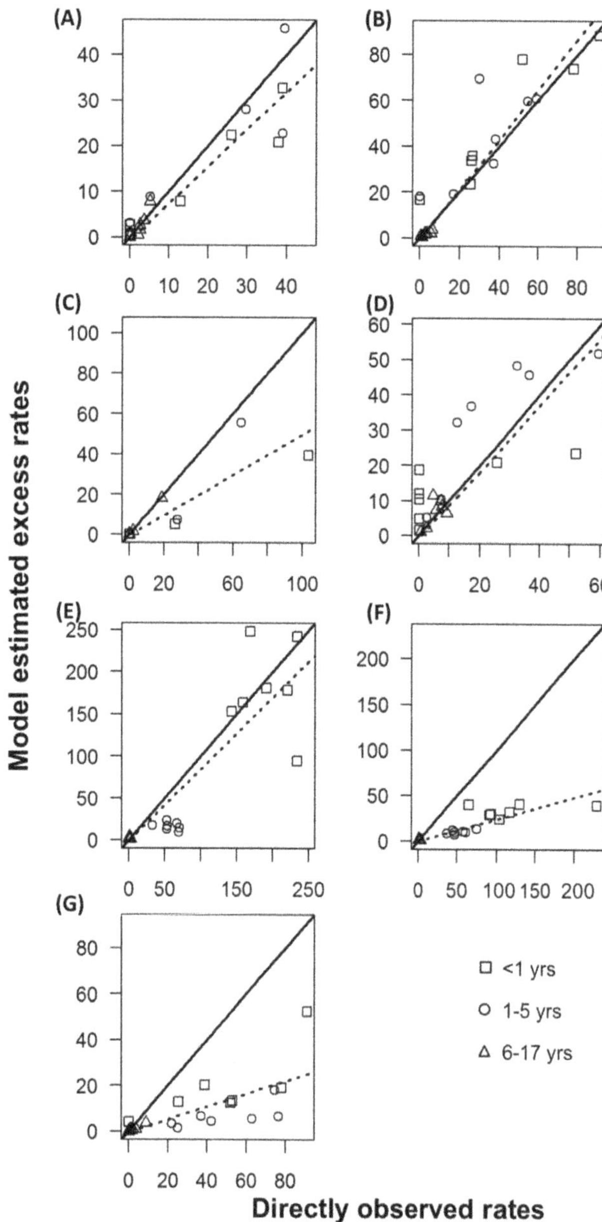

Figure 3. Comparison of annual excess hospitalization rates per 10,000 population and directly observed rates during each of the seven seasons, for (A) sH1N1, (B) H3N2, (C) pH1N1, (D) influenza B, (E) respiratory syncytial virus (RSV), (F) parainfluenza and (G) adenovirus. Excess hospitalization rates were derived from the Poisson models with the virus proxies of influenza-like illness rates multiplied by virus proportions (ILI×LAB).

together, age-specific counts shall be recommended as proxy variables if such data are available. If age information is unavailable, ILI×LAB is probably the proxy that shall be considered.

The 2009 H1N1 pandemic was characterized with dramatically increased attack rates among children and young adults, but the severity of pandemic infections was comparable to the seasonal virus strains [28,29]. ARD admission rates in our pediatric cohort increased by a proportion ranging from 7% to 170% during the pandemic (Table 1), and many other studies also reported a similar magnitude of increase [30–33]. However, the admissions due to non-influenza infections decreased in the pandemic, except RSV. Our model estimates were able to capture this trend, showing the same change directions as the observed rates. However, large deviations were also observed in some age-virus categories, such as influenza B in the <1 and 1–5 age groups. Further studies are warranted to fine tune our modeling approach in order to derive reliable estimates for different periods.

It has been widely accepted that Poisson distribution is appropriate to fit the low-frequency count data, but the log-link function commonly adopted in Poisson models has been criticized for its assumption of exponential increase in health outcomes along with one unit increase in virus proxies [8,34]. Some of recent studies switched to a more "reasonable" assumption of linear relation by adopting an identity-link function in Poisson models [35,36]. In this study we found that the log-link function yielded the estimates slightly closer to the true incidence of influenza hospitalizations than the identity-link. However, the key assumption on the association of virus proxies and health outcomes in Poisson models still remain to be proved. Further evidence on the mechanism of influenza transmission and pathogenicity in human community could probably help resolve this problem.

Our study has potential limitations. First, the Bayesian estimates are sensitive to the prior distributions and the prior assumption of nonnegative coefficient for virus proxy variables needs to be carefully justified. Since our virology data were obtained from the laboratory surveillance based on hospitalized inpatients, it is reasonable to assume that these virology data were positively associated with the increase of hospital admissions with viral respiratory infections. However, overestimation might exist if the assumption of prior distribution is not well justified, and caution needs to be taken when extending this approach to estimate the excess mortality of other respiratory viruses, as most viruses other than influenza cause only mild symptoms that might not necessarily lead to death [37]. Second, age-specific virus data requires long standing and intensive virology surveillance for multiple respiratory viruses, but such surveillance networks may not be available for influenza in many countries. Nevertheless, the importance of simultaneous assessment on other respiratory viruses, particularly RSV, has started to be recognized [26,38]. So we can expect these data will become available in more and more countries in the near future. Third, we only estimated the excess hospitalization of five respiratory viruses due to limited virology data. There are many other respiratory viruses (e.g. rhinovirus) and bacteria (e.g. *Streptococcus pneumonia*) also contribute greatly to ARD hospitalization in children, although the clinical significance of detection of some of these (e.g. rhinovirus) remains unclear. Further studies are needed to assess whether addition of more virology data could alter the performance of models.

In conclusion, age-specific counts of positive specimens are probably the best proxies for virus activity and should be used in the disease burden models if such data are available. In the absence of age-specific data, the Bayesian inference proposed in this study is superior to the classical likelihood inference method, as the former provides more reliable estimates on excess hospitalization respectively associated with multiple respiratory viruses.

Acknowledgments

We thank Dr Ben Cowling and Dr Eric HY Lau for helpful discussions. We also thank the Research Fund for the Control of Infectious Diseases

[RFCID 11100582] and the Area of Excellence Scheme of the University Grants Committee [AoE/M-12/06] of the Hong Kong Special Administrative Region Government.

Author Contributions

Conceived and designed the experiments: LY CMW SSSC JSMP. Performed the experiments: KHC. Analyzed the data: KPC XLW ELYC. Wrote the paper: LY KPC CMW.

References

1. Williams BG, Gouws E, Boschi-Pinto C, Bryce J, Dye C (2002) Estimates of world-wide distribution of child deaths from acute respiratory infections. Lancet Infect Dis 2: 25–32.
2. Monto AS, Gravenstein S, Elliott M, Colopy M, Schweinle J (2000) Clinical signs and symptoms predicting influenza infection. ArchInternMed 160: 3243–3247.
3. Fleming DM, Elliot AJ, Cross KW (2007) Morbidity profiles of patients consulting during influenza and respiratory syncytial virus active periods. EpidemiolInfect 135: 1099–1108.
4. Thompson WW, Weintraub E, Dhankhar P, Cheng PY, Brammer L, et al. (2009) Estimates of US influenza-associated deaths made using four different methods. InfluenzaOther RespiViruses 3: 37–49.
5. Yang L, Chiu SS, Chan KP, Chan KH, Wong WH, et al. (2011) Validation of statistical models for estimating hospitalization associated with influenza and other respiratory viruses. PLoS One 6: e17882.
6. Dowell SF (2001) Seasonal variation in host susceptibility and cycles of certain infectious diseases. EmergInfect Dis 7: 369–374.
7. Dellaportas P, Smith AFM (1993) Bayesian Inference for Generalized Linear and Proportional Hazards Models via Gibbs Sampling. Journal of the Royal Statistical Society Series C (Applied Statistics) 42: 443–459.
8. Thompson WW, Shay DK, Weintraub E, Brammer L, Cox N, et al. (2003) Mortality associated with influenza and respiratory syncytial virus in the United States. JAMA 289: 179–186.
9. Wong CM, Chan KP, Hedley AJ, Peiris JSM (2004) Influenza-associated mortality in Hong Kong. Clin Infect Dis 39: 1611–1617.
10. Wu P, Goldstein E, Ho LM, Yang L, Nishiura H, et al. (2012) Excess mortality associated with influenza A and B virus in Hong Kong, 1998–2009. Journal of Infectious Diseases 206: 1862–1871.
11. Hui SL, Chu LW, Peiris JSM, Chan KH, Chu D, et al. (2006) Immune response to influenza vaccination in community-dwelling Chinese elderly persons. Vaccine 24: 5371–5380.
12. Munoz FM (2003) Influenza virus infection in infancy and early childhood. Paediatric Respiratory Reviews 4: 99–104.
13. Olson DR, Heffernan RT, Paladini M, Konty K, Weiss D, et al. (2007) Monitoring the impact of influenza by age: emergency department fever and respiratory complaint surveillance in New York City. PLoS Med 4: e247.
14. Chan KH, Peiris JS, Lim W, Nicholls JM, Chiu SS (2008) Comparison of nasopharyngeal flocked swabs and aspirates for rapid diagnosis of respiratory viruses in children. J Clin Virol 42: 65–69.
15. Hastie TJ, Tibshirani RJ (1990) Generalized additive models. London: Chapman and Hall.
16. Lunn DJ, Thomas A, Best N, Spiegelhalter D (2000) WinBUGS - A Bayesian modelling framework: Concepts, structure, and extensibility. Statistics and Computing 10: 325–337.
17. Bahl J, Nelson MI, Chan KH, Chen R, Vijaykrishna D, et al. (2011) Temporally structured metapopulation dynamics and persistence of influenza A H3N2 virus in humans. Proc Natl Acad Sci U S A 108: 19359–19364.
18. Birrell PJ, Ketsetzis G, Gay NJ, Cooper BS, Presanis AM, et al. (2011) Bayesian modeling to unmask and predict influenza A/H1N1pdm dynamics in London. Proceedings of the National Academy of Sciences 108: 18238–18243.
19. Christensen R, Johnson W, Branscum A, Hanson TE (2011) Bayesian ideas and data analysis. US: CRC Press.
20. Yang L, Chen PY, He JF, Chan KP, Ou CQ, et al. (2011) Effect modification of environmental factors on influenza-associated mortality: a time-series study in two Chinese cities. BMC Infect Dis 11: 342.
21. Goldstein E, Viboud C, Charu V, Lipsitch M (2012) Improving the Estimation of Influenza-Related Mortality Over a Seasonal Baseline. Epidemiology 23: 829–838.
22. Wong CM, Yang L, Chan KP, Leung GM, Chan KH, et al. (2006) Influenza-associated hospitalization in a subtropical city. PLoS Med 3: e121.
23. Chiu SS, Chan KH, Chen H, Young BW, Lim W, et al. (2009) Virologically confirmed population-based burden of hospitalization caused by influenza A and B among children in Hong Kong. Clin Infect Dis 49: 1016–1021.
24. Charu V, Simonsen L, Lustig R, Steiner C, Viboud C (2013) Mortality burden of the 2009–10 influenza pandemic in the United States: improving the timeliness of influenza severity estimates using inpatient mortality records. Influenza Other Respi Viruses.
25. Redlberger-Fritz M, Aberle JH, Popow-Kraupp T, Kundi M (2012) Attributable deaths due to influenza: a comparative study of seasonal and pandemic influenza. Eur J Epidemiol 27: 567–575.
26. van Asten L, van den Wijngaard C, van Pelt W, van de Kassteele J, Meijer A, et al. (2012) Mortality Attributable to 9 Common Infections: Significant effect of influenza A, RSV, influenza B, norovirus and parainfluenza in the elderly. J Infect Dis 206: 628–639.
27. Wong JY, Wu P, Nishiura H, Goldstein E, Lau EH, et al. (2013) Infection Fatality Risk of the Pandemic A(H1N1)2009 Virus in Hong Kong. Am J Epidemiol 177: 834–840.
28. Wu JT, Ho A, Ma ES, Lee CK, Chu DK, et al. (2011) Estimating Infection Attack Rates and Severity in Real Time during an Influenza Pandemic: Analysis of Serial Cross-Sectional Serologic Surveillance Data. PLoSMed 8: e1001103.
29. Belongia EA, Irving SA, Waring SC, Coleman LA, Meece JK, et al. (2010) Clinical characteristics and 30-day outcomes for influenza A 2009 (H1N1), 2008–2009 (H1N1), and 2007–2008 (H3N2) infections. JAMA 304: 1091–1098.
30. Hernandez JE, Grainger J, Simonsen L, Collis P, Edelman L, et al. (2012) Impact of the 2009/2010 influenza A (H1N1) pandemic on trends in influenza hospitalization, diagnostic testing, and treatment. Influenza Other Respi Viruses 6: 305–308.
31. Engelhard D, Bromberg M, Averbuch D, Tenenbaum A, Goldmann D, et al. (2011) Increased extent of and risk factors for pandemic (H1N1) 2009 and seasonal influenza among children, Israel. Emerg Infect Dis 17: 1740–1743.
32. Karageorgopoulos DE, Vouloumanou EK, Korbila IP, Kapaskelis A, Falagas ME (2011) Age distribution of cases of 2009 (H1N1) pandemic influenza in comparison with seasonal influenza. PLoS ONE 6: e21690.
33. Song X, DeBiasi RL, Campos JM, Fagbuyi DB, Jacobs BR, et al. (2012) Comparison of pandemic and seasonal influenza A infections in pediatric patients: were they different? Influenza Other Respi Viruses 6: 25–27.
34. Thompson WW, Ridenhour BL, Barile JP, Shay DK (2012) Time-series analyses of count data to estimate the burden of seasonal infectious diseases. Epidemiology 23: 839–842.
35. Newall AT, Viboud C, Wood JG (2010) Influenza-attributable mortality in Australians aged more than 50 years: a comparison of different modelling approaches. Epidemiol Infect 138: 836–842.
36. Lemaitre M, Carrat F, Rey G, Miller M, Simonsen L, et al. (2012) Mortality burden of the 2009 A/H1N1 influenza pandemic in France: comparison to seasonal influenza and the A/H3N2 pandemic. PLoS One 7: e45051.
37. Foppa IM, Hossain MM (2008) Revised estimates of influenza-associated excess mortality, United States, 1995 through 2005. Emerg Themes Epidemiol 5: 26.
38. Zhou H, Thompson WW, Viboud CG, Ringholz CM, Cheng PY, et al. (2012) Hospitalizations Associated With Influenza and Respiratory Syncytial Virus in the United States, 1993–2008. Clin Infect Dis 54: 1427–1436.

20

Poor Clinical Outcomes for HIV Infected Children on Antiretroviral Therapy in Rural Mozambique: Need for Program Quality Improvement and Community Engagement

Sten H. Vermund[1,2,6]*, Meridith Blevins[1,3], Troy D. Moon[1,2,6], Eurico José[6], Linda Moiane[6], José A. Tique[1,6], Mohsin Sidat[7], Philip J. Ciampa[1,5], Bryan E. Shepherd[1,3], Lara M. E. Vaz[1,4,6¤]

1 Vanderbilt Institute for Global Health, Vanderbilt University School of Medicine, Nashville, Tennessee, United States of America, **2** Department of Pediatrics, Vanderbilt University School of Medicine, Nashville, Tennessee, United States of America, **3** Department of Biostatistics, Vanderbilt University School of Medicine, Nashville, Tennessee, United States of America, **4** Department of Preventive Medicine, Vanderbilt University School of Medicine, Nashville, Tennessee, United States of America, **5** Department of Medicine, Vanderbilt University School of Medicine, Nashville, Tennessee, United States of America, **6** Friends in Global Health, Quelimane and Maputo, Mozambique, **7** School of Medicine, Universidade Eduardo Mondlane, Maputo, Mozambique

Abstract

Introduction: Residents of Zambézia Province, Mozambique live from rural subsistence farming and fishing. The 2009 provincial HIV prevalence for adults 15–49 years was 12.6%, higher among women (15.3%) than men (8.9%). We reviewed clinical data to assess outcomes for HIV-infected children on combination antiretroviral therapy (cART) in a highly resource-limited setting.

Methods: We studied rates of 2-year mortality and loss to follow-up (LTFU) for children $<$15 years of age initiating cART between June 2006–July 2011 in 10 rural districts. National guidelines define LTFU as $>$60 days following last-scheduled medication pickup. Kaplan-Meier estimates to compute mortality assumed non-informative censoring. Cumulative LTFU incidence calculations treated death as a competing risk.

Results: Of 753 children, 29.0% (95% CI: 24.5, 33.2) were confirmed dead by 2 years and 39.0% (95% CI: 34.8, 42.9) were LTFU with unknown clinical outcomes. The cohort mortality rate was 8.4% (95% CI: 6.3, 10.4) after 90 days on cART and 19.2% (95% CI: 16.0, 22.3) after 365 days. Higher hemoglobin at cART initiation was associated with being alive and on cART at 2 years (alive: 9.3 g/dL vs. dead or LTFU: 8.3–8.4 g/dL, $p<0.01$). Cotrimoxazole use within 90 days of ART initiation was associated with improved 2-year outcomes Treatment was initiated late (WHO stage III/IV) among 48% of the children with WHO stage recorded in their records. Marked heterogeneity in outcomes by district was noted ($p<0.001$).

Conclusions: We found poor clinical and programmatic outcomes among children taking cART in rural Mozambique. Expanded testing, early infant diagnosis, counseling/support services, case finding, and outreach are insufficiently implemented. Our quality improvement efforts seek to better link pregnancy and HIV services, expand coverage and timeliness of infant diagnosis and treatment, and increase follow-up and adherence.

Editor: David W. Dowdy, Johns Hopkins Bloomberg School of Public Health, United States of America

Funding: This research was supported by the President's Emergency Plan for AIDS Relief (PEPFAR) through the Centers for Disease Control and Prevention (grant #U2GPS000631). The findings and conclusions in this report are those of the authors and do not necessarily represent the official position of the CDC. Dr. Tique was supported by the Fogarty AIDS International Training and Research Program, National Institutes of Health #D43TW001035. The funders had no role in study design, data collection and analysis, decision to publish, or preparation of the manuscript.

Competing Interests: Dr. Vermund is a member of the PLOS ONE editorial board. This does not alter the authors' adherence to PLOS ONE editorial policies and criteria.

* Email: sten.vermund@vanderbilt.edu

¤ Current address: Save the Children, Washington DC, United States of America

Introduction

Mozambique is one of the most HIV-affected countries with an estimated national HIV prevalence in 2009 of 11.5%, translating into approximately 1.4 million adults living with HIV. [1,2] Because of its heavy HIV burden, Mozambique is a priority nation for support from the U.S. President's Emergency Plan for AIDS Relief (PEPFAR). [3] National combination antiretroviral therapy (cART) coverage is low; only an estimated 52% of adults and 20% of children in need of cART were believed to be receiving it as of the end of 2011. [4] In 2010, an estimated 70.8% of pregnant women in their first antenatal care appointment received HIV counseling and testing and 40.2% of HIV-infected pregnant women received ARV prophylaxis for the prevention of mother-to-child transmission (PMTCT), typically single-dose nevirapine [5].

Under 5 (U5) mortality rates have been falling rapidly in Mozambique with 2011 national U5 mortality estimated at 135/1000 live births compared to 219/1000 live births in 1990, in large part because of improvements in vaccination coverage and efforts to manage childhood diarrheal and acute respiratory illnesses. [6] The most recent national estimate is 97/1000 live births, from the latest Demographic Health Survey [7], still shy of the 2015 Millennium Development Goal of 73 deaths per 1000 live births. HIV/AIDS contributes 10% to the U5 mortality nationally [6].

Zambézia Province is a very low-income region of 4.2 million persons in north-central Mozambique whose majority of residents are rural subsistence farmers and fishermen. Zambézia has the nation's second largest provincial population, representing ≈20% of Mozambique's total. [1,8] Provincial HIV prevalence among adults 15–49 years in 2009 was estimated at 12.6% overall, 15.3% among women and 8.9% among men, all higher than national averages, e.g., 13.1% for women 15–49 nationally. [1] Current U5 mortality estimates show Zambézia as having the worst U5 mortality of all provinces, with deaths estimated at 142/1000 live births. [9] Leading causes of U5 deaths in Zambézia in 2009 include neonatal deaths (26.1%), malaria (27.7%) and acute lower respiratory infection (13.7%). HIV/AIDS-related deaths account for 11.5% of U5 deaths in the province [9,10].

Children with HIV are not in care at as high a proportion as adults with HIV in Africa, and their outcomes are not as good in most programs. [11–71] To assess mortality for HIV-infected children on cART, we reviewed data from PEPFAR-supported clinics run by the Zambézia Provincial Health Directorate (Direcção Provincial de Saúde, DPS) in 10 districts where a Vanderbilt University non-governmental organization (NGO) provides technical assistance.

Methods

Both the Mozambican National Bioethics Committee for Health (*Comité Nacional de Bioética em Saúde* [CNBS]) and the Institutional Review Board of Vanderbilt University approved this analysis. Analysis was performed on routinely collected, de-identified, aggregate patient level data and no individual informed consent was obtained. The CNBS and the Vanderbilt Institutional Review Board explicitly waived the need for written informed consent from the participants.

We analyzed data from a cohort of HIV-infected children <15 years of age initiating cART between June 2006–July 2011 in 10 of 17 rural districts in Zambézia Province. Details of our Friends in Global Health NGO clinical program with the DPS and the Ministry of Health (Ministério de Saúde [MISAU]) have been reported previously. [72] Two districts for which we were responsible did not have electronic medical records at the time of analysis and so were excluded;[73] five additional districts were supported by another NGO in this time period. [74] Patients who transferred from another facility after starting cART were not included in this analysis as data on their care history was incomplete (N = 156).

Patient characteristics at treatment initiation of those alive, lost, and dead at the end of 2 years' follow-up were compared using rank sum and chi-square tests. Deaths were ascertained from both clinical records and from parental testimonials. Mozambican national guidelines define loss to follow-up (LTFU) as no effective clinical contact within 60 days after the last scheduled medication pickup. [75] Two additional definitions of LTFU from the literature were also applied for the purpose of cross-cohort comparisons. The 'universal' definition classifies patients as LTFU if there is no effective clinical contact within 180 days of database closure. [76] The 'reference' definition assigns 1 day of follow-up to any individual who does not return following treatment initiation, includes only individuals initiating ART 6 months prior to the database closure, and classifies patients as LTFU if there is no effective clinical contact within 180 days of database closure. [77] All three LTFU definitions deem the patient lost at the date of last contact as opposed to the date of missed visit. Kaplan-Meier estimates were used to compute mortality and the combined endpoint of mortality and LTFU. Cumulative incidence of LTFU was calculated by treating death as a competing risk. Mortality estimates assumed non-informative censoring, i.e., patients LTFU were assumed to have rates of death similar to patients not LTFU. This likely implies that our mortality calculations are underestimates of true mortality.

Our study did not include children enrolled in HIV care who never initiated treatment. [78] Cotrimoxazole (CTX) data were treated as a tick box for "yes", collected each visit for the corresponding visit date. If a patient was on CTX anywhere from 0 to 365 days before ART initiation, we considered the patient as "CTX use prior to cART". If a patient was on CTX anywhere from 90 days before to 90 days after ART initiation, we considered the patient as "current CTX use".

Results

During five years of PEPFAR support, 753 HIV-infected children <15 years of age initiated cART. Of these children, 678 (90.0%) were <8 years of age at cART initiation, 397 (52.7%) were <2 years, and 191 (25.4%) were <1 years. Girls represented 57% of the pediatric cART patients. Median CD4+ T-lymphocyte cell count (CD4 counts) and percentage (CD4 percentage) at cART initiation were 497 and 15, respectively, although these quantities were missing for 62% and 70% of patients. Nearly half (48%) of children initiated cART very late in their disease progression (WHO stage III or IV), although WHO stage was missing for 58% of patients.

Two years after cART initiation, 152 patients had died and 240 were LTFU. At two years, the estimated probability of death was 29.0% (95% confidence interval [CI] 24.5–33.2), the cumulative incidence of LTFU was 38.7 (95% CI 34.8–42.9), and the probability of either death or LTFU was 62.0% (95% CI 57.6–65.9). We observed substantial heterogeneity between districts in two-year outcomes (Figure 1). Two year LTFU ranged from a district low of 25% to a high of 70% (Fig. 1A; $p<0.001$), mortality ranged from 16–34% (Fig. 1B; $p = 0.19$), and death or LTFU ranged from 51.1–88.1% (Fig. 1C; $p<0.001$). The association between treatment duration and mortality rate did not suggest a marked decline in mortality over time. At 90 days on cART, the mortality rate was 8.4% (95% CI: 6.3, 10.4). At 365 days on cART, the mortality rate was 19.2% (95% CI: 16.0, 22.3) and at 730 days (two years) on cART, the mortality rate was 29.0% (95% CI: 24.5%, 33.2%). Cumulative incidence of LTFU was lower when applying two definitions from the literature. [75] The cumulative incidence of LTFU using the 'universal' definition was 26.0% (95% CI 22.6–29.9) at 2 years. [76] The cumulative incidence of LTFU using the 'reference' definition was 26.4% (95% CI 22.9–30.2) at 2 years [77].

Table 1 compares patient characteristics at cART initiation between those who were alive, dead, and lost after two years. We did not detect any difference in CD4 counts or percentage at cART initiation in children who were alive and on treatment at 2 years compared to those who were either not alive or not in care at

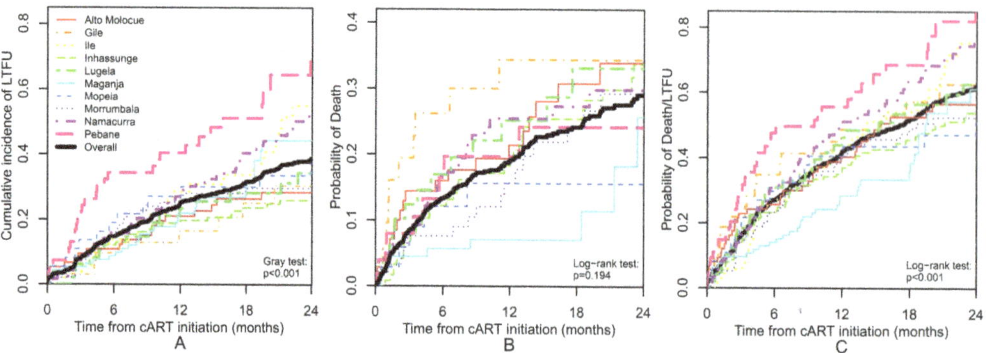

Figure 1. Variation by district in pediatric loss to follow up (LTFU), death, and death or LTFU for 2 years following combination antiretroviral therapy initiation, 10 districts of Zambézia Province, Mozambique, 2006–2011.

that time (p = 0.6), though we had high rates of missing data. We observed higher hemoglobin at the time of cART initiation among those children alive and on treatment at 2 years (alive: median 9.3 g/dL; 8.3 for dead; 8.4 g/dL for LTFU, p<0.01 for alive vs. dead or LTFU). Any cotrimoxazole use in the year prior to ART initiation was associated with improved 2-year outcomes (alive: 76%, dead: 49%, lost: 55%). Cotrimoxazole use within 90 days of ART initiation was associated with improved 2-year outcomes (alive: 69%, dead: 58%, lost: 59%).

Discussion

The experience from our PEPFAR cART program found that 29% of children initiating cART were dead within two years. It is likely that many of the 39% LTFU are at high risk of death or have already died. HIV care for children is not yet optimized in this impoverished setting with a backdrop of health workforce shortages, poor health care infrastructures, challenging transportation, poor maternal and child health outcomes, high rates of tuberculosis and malaria infections, high levels of malnutrition, low adult and pediatric cART and maternal ARV prophylaxis coverage rates, and limited formal counseling/social support programs. Similar challenges are reported elsewhere, particularly where cART is initiated late and co-infections are already extant. [20,79,80] Considerably better outcomes are reported from LMIC outside of Africa. [81–92] While a number of pediatric cART programs have reported much better success, we do not know the extent to which there is a reporting bias in the literature, i.e., overrepresentation in the literature of more favorable program outcomes. [11,44,60,64,65,68,69,85,93–110] Challenges we face have been reported from many low and middle-income nations, though we think our results are especially worrisome [25,111–117].

We observed a wide range of LTFU in different districts, suggesting possible inconsistent fidelity across sites to the active case-finding (*busca activa*) program that is in place, as well as variations in the quality of care, system infrastructure and/or community engagement. [118] In PMTCT work in Zambia and subsequently in the multinational PEARL study, similar clinic-by-clinic diversity has been seen, documenting that the specific component of the continuum of care that is "broken" in lower functioning clinics may differ by clinic [119–123].

In a poorly functioning clinic in Mozambique, we may find health providers who are able to speak only Portuguese with clients, rather than the local language. We have learned from pediatric and obstetric quality improvement work that mothers frequently do not understand complex instructions in Portuguese from health providers who often come from other provinces and may not speak one of the local languages spoken in this ethnically diverse province. [8,118,124] On aggregate, Zambézia residents have low health literacy and numeracy rates, likely contributing to patient/caregiver-provider miscommunication and, possibly to LTFU and suboptimal adherence [125].

Another common occurrence in a poorly functioning clinic generally is the failure of pyschosocial services to effectively engage caregivers fully in chronic pediatric care services, as well as HIV services for themselves. Prior to HIV services, long-term follow-up of chronic diseases was not something with which residents of Zambézia Province were familiar. It is common, especially in rural Africa, that asymptomatic or improving children, parents or guardians do not recognize the need for ongoing services. [126–132] The same applies to parents themselves; they may be LTFU once they feel better. [72,78] We have also had anecdotal reports of parents in our program avoiding care for their children (or themselves) due to stigma and fear of persons learning of the HIV infections in their children. These are daunting challenges that call for more effective counseling and trust-building between providers and clients, and potentially for earlier engagement of children in their health care. The active case-finding approach (*busca active*) of the DPS/MISAU needs serious review and improvement in the face of high mortality and LTFU data in children. It is also possible that traditional active case-finding efforts need to be tailored for special populations, such as children. Improved counseling and family-centered treatment approaches need further exploration. Any innovation in engaging HIV-infected women in their own care can be expected to improve follow-up for their children as well. [133–135] A recent review found that although there is evidence of effectiveness of interventions to improve access and adherence to cART, there is less known about major barriers and ways to address them among vulnerable groups such as women, children and adolescents [136].

There is little tradition of long-term pediatric care in rural Zambézia Province. Mothers take children for vaccines and acute illnesses, but only a tuberculosis diagnosis results in chronic care involving long-term drug administration that can reasonably be expected to be available (such medications as insulin and oncology drugs are not available in the rural clinics). In fact, loss to follow-up rates for children with HIV are high throughout southern Africa. [137] Mothers have told us that they and/or their fathers do not want the stigma of having them take the child for HIV care, that they live too far away and cannot afford the time or money for care, they do not know the health workers due to high turnover rates, and that health workers often mistreat them and violate their confidentiality and their privacy [124,138,139].

Table 1. Characteristics of children at initiation of combination antiretroviral therapy by 2 year outcome in 10 districts of Zambézia Province, Mozambique, 2006–2011 (PITC = Provider-initiated testing and counseling; PMTCT = Prevention of mother-to-child HIV transmission; BMI = Body Mass Index or weight in kg divided by height squared).

	Alive	Dead	Lost	Combined	P-value
	(n = 361)	(n = 152)	(n = 240)	(n = 753)	
Female, n(%)	204 (57%)	73 (48%)	118 (49%)	395 (52%)	0.1
Age (years), median (IQR)	2 (1, 4)	1 (0, 2)	1 (1, 3)	1 (0, 4)	<0.001
District, n(%)					0.002
Alto Molócuè	38 (11%)	19 (12%)	19 (8%)	76 (10%)	
Gilé	15 (4%)	10 (7%)	8 (3%)	33 (4%)	
Ile	23 (6%)	10 (7%)	22 (9%)	55 (7%)	
Inhassunge	69 (19%)	31 (20%)	30 (12%)	130 (17%)	
Lugela	22 (6%)	13 (9%)	15 (6%)	50 (7%)	
Maganja	58 (16%)	9 (6%)	28 (12%)	95 (13%)	
Mopeia	19 (5%)	5 (3%)	13 (5%)	37 (5%)	
Morrumbala	52 (14%)	18 (12%)	26 (11%)	96 (13%)	
Namacurra	47 (13%)	28 (18%)	50 (21%)	125 (17%)	
Pebane	18 (5%)	9 (6%)	29 (12%)	56 (7%)	
Referral site[4], n(%)					0.7
Missing	297 (83%)	134 (88%)	193 (80%)	624 (83%)	
External consultation (PITC)	10 (16%)	4 (22%)	6 (13%)	20 (16%)	
Medical inpatient (PITC)	2 (3%)	0 (0%)	4 (9%)	6 (5%)	
Tuberculosis care (PITC)	1 (2%)	0 (0%)	0 (0%)	1 (<1%)	
PMTCT site	7 (11%)	3 (17%)	8 (17%)	18 (14%)	
Voluntary counseling and testing site	44 (69%)	11 (61%)	29 (62%)	84 (65%)	
Height (cm), median (IQR)[1]	85 (67, 109)	70 (63, 84.2)	72 (66, 81.8)	75 (66, 103.5)	0.04
Missing	206 (57%)	118 (78%)	174 (72%)	498 (66%)	
Weight (kg), median (IQR)[1]	8.5 (6.3, 14)	6.7 (5, 9.5)	7 (5.8, 10)	7.5 (6, 12.4)	<0.001
Missing	4 (1%)	10 (7%)	24 (10%)	38 (5%)	
BMI (kg/m^2), median (IQR)[1]	15.2 (14.1, 16.6)	14.4 (13.8, 17.4)	14.9 (14.2, 16.6)	15.1 (14.1, 16.8)	1
Missing	274 (76%)	132 (87%)	197 (82%)	603 (80%)	
CD4+ cell count/μL, median (IQR)[2]	458 (248, 760)	595 (164, 734)	513 (314, 841)	497 (237, 774)	0.7
Missing	222 (61%)	90 (59%)	149 (62%)	461 (61%)	
CD4 percentage, median (IQR)[2]	15 (10, 21)	15 (12, 22)	15 (8, 21)	15 (10, 21)	0.6
Missing	251 (70%)	107 (70%)	171 (71%)	529 (70%)	
Hemoglobin (g/dL), median (IQR)[2]	9.3 (8, 10.4)	8.3 (7, 9.3)	8.4 (7.4, 9.4)	8.9 (7.6, 9.9)	<0.001
Missing	237 (66%)	100 (66%)	163 (68%)	500 (66%)	
WHO stage, n(%)[2]					0.1
Missing	224 (62%)	75 (49%)	130 (54%)	429 (57%)	
I	47 (34%)	18 (23%)	32 (29%)	97 (30%)	
II	30 (22%)	11 (14%)	29 (26%)	70 (22%)	
III	43 (31%)	39 (51%)	37 (34%)	119 (37%)	
IV	17 (12%)	9 (12%)	12 (11%)	38 (12%)	
Cotrimoxazole use (prior to ART), n(%)[3]	273 (76%)	75 (49%)	132 (55%)	480 (64%)	<0.001
Cotrimoxazole use (current), n(%)[3]	249 (69%)	88 (58%)	142 (59%)	479 (64%)	0.01

Percentages are computed using the number of patients with a non-missing value.
[1]Weight, height, and BMI are collected at enrollment. [2]Collected within 90 days before and 14 days after ART initiation. [3]Prior to ART means any cotrimoxazole (CTX) use recorded in 365 days prior to ART initiation. Current means any CTX use in 90 days before or 90 days after ART initiation. CTX use is recorded along with the visit date; data is not collected on non-users so we are unable to assess missing data. [4]When PITC referral sites are grouped: p = 0.9.

There is evidence from this study and elsewhere that early infant diagnosis, provider initiated testing and counseling, case finding of older children, and family support and outreach are not sufficiently developed in rural Mozambique.

[8,73,78,118,124,125,134,135,140–152] As of 2011, all HIV-infected children <2 years of age should be started on cART as per Mozambican national guidelines, based on results of the South African CHER trial. [79] As of May 2013, Mozambican guidelines changed further to mandate cART for all infected children <5 years of age, independent of clinical status or CD4+ cell count. Yet our study suggests that poor adherence by health workers to standards of screening and HIV staging and subsequent CD4 monitoring impairs pediatric outcomes by delaying recognition of children in need of cART and prophylaxis for opportunistic infections (OI). OI prophylaxis with cotrimoxazole was a protective factor for adverse outcomes in our study. We do not believe that co-trimoxazole benefits are explained by urban-rural differences, as all our sites were rural, nor by family income or assets. All HIV-related services provided by the Ministry, which includes all of the services in this study, are available free of cost, including provision of cotrimoxazole. Family income is not recorded on the clinical record, only patient (or parent) profession; we are thus unable to distinguish subsistence farmers from those who sell their crops, small merchants from larger ones. Over 80 percent of the overall population in the province subsists on less than USD 2 per day as we have documented in a baseline USAID report (Vergara, AE, Blevins M, Vaz LME, et al (2011). Baseline survey report: Improving livelihoods and health of children, women and families in the Province of Zambézia, Republic of Mozambique (available at [http://globalhealth.vanderbilt.edu/programs/scip/]).

Since many children are not diagnosed early or begun on cART early and/or fail to stay in (or adhere to) cART-based care, adverse events are high. [118] We believe that poor interpretation of the guidelines by providers and an overall reluctance to place young children on cART is playing a major role. Quality improvement efforts are essential [148] and are underway to improve infant diagnosis and treatment initiation. [124,135] Linkages across MCH services are being forged to improve treatment outcomes.

Health worker shortages contribute to poor quality of pediatric care. Given severe health care worker shortages and structural impediments to effective long-term care services, we believe that international support, such as that available from PEPFAR and the Global Fund to Fight AIDS, Tuberculosis and Malaria, will be needed for many years to come. [153–157] Whether traditional healers, far more numerous than allopathic practitioners, can be engaged in a productive way for early referral and for assistance in adherence and follow up is unknown. [158,159] More effective community engagement is essential and some success has been had with church-based outreach. [159,160] It is also unknown the extent to which efforts such as the Medical Education Partnership Initiative,[161] the Royal Society-DFID Africa Capacity Building Initiative,[162] or the Consortium of New Southern African Medical Schools [163] will make a major difference over the next 5–10 years in addressing chronic health worker shortages in rural Africa. [164–167] Task-shifting would be a reasonable approach, but nursing and medical assistants (*técnicos de medicina* in Mozambique) are also in very short supply. [8] Creative approaches to patient-to-patient adherence and retention show promise [168–170].

Our data have limitations that affect the completeness of our study. Missing data were frequent, particularly CD4 counts, CD4%, and WHO stage, limiting our ability to examine delays in initiation of treatment. Multivariable analyses were not performed to estimate independent associations with clinical outcomes due to large amounts of missing data and potential for misclassification among those LTFU. We only ask age (in years) of the child such that age subgroups are less reliable, particularly for younger ages, than if we had reliable birthdate; however, rural populations often do not know specific birthdates. Information on cotrimoxazole use was recorded; however, the nature of the documentation is to record use and thus we are unable to differentiate between non-users and missing data. If data are not missing completely at random, there would be bias in the summary statistics of non-missing data. Generalizability of findings to the whole province was limited because data were available for 10 of the total 17 districts. Our database does not collect information on risk factors for poor clinical outcomes external to the patient visit; prospective data collection on such factors (e.g., health facility staffing, drug stock-outs, family support) would permit more robust risk assessment. Nonetheless, we believe that our data clearly indicate a seriously underperforming pediatric care program in need of aggressive quality improvement; despite limitations, we have found these real-world data to be adequate to guide programmatic improvement and community engagement. These efforts are beginning to bear fruit [124,135,148].

There are many challenges not likely to be resolved soon: health care worker shortages and high turnover rates, particularly in remote rural settings, drug and supply stockouts, language barriers, gender-power distortions, literacy and numeracy challenges, poor attitudes of health care workers towards patients, lack of appreciation of the germ theory of disease, crushing rural poverty, poor transportation infrastructures, and structural barriers within the clinical care setting. [73,78,146,148,153,171–173] Co-infections prevalent in the tropics and food shortages are recurring challenges that are far less prevalent in higher income nations. [174–177] Drug resistance has not been studied widely in Mozambique [178].

Even in the face of these obstacles, we and others are having some success in pediatric care HIV quality improvement. [124,135,179–181] That our real-world findings of co-trimoxazole benefit to children in HIV care reinforces clinical trial results suggesting that HIV-infected children benefit from continued co-trimoxazole (protecting against both malaria and non-malarial disease), even when they are on cART. [182] To better retain children on cART and co-trimoxazole, more comprehensive quality improvement efforts are needed to identify staff, structural, cultural, social and policy challenges and to craft solutions for support to pediatric patients, their caregivers, and health care providers.

Acknowledgments

The authors thank Megan Pask, Wilson Silva, Tito Jequicene, Jairzinho Tereso, Carlos Castel-Branco, Ferreira Ferreira, Kulssum Faque, and Deidra Parrish for their help with this work.

Disclosures: This research was supported by the President's Emergency Plan for AIDS Relief (PEPFAR) through the Centers for Disease Control and Prevention (grant #U2GPS000631). The findings and conclusions in this report are those of the authors and do not necessarily represent the official position of the CDC. Dr. Tique was supported by the Fogarty AIDS International Training and Research Program, National Institutes of Health #D43TW001035).

Author Contributions

Conceived and designed the experiments: SHV MB TDM EJ BES LMEV. Performed the experiments: MB TDM EJ LM JAT MS LMEV. Analyzed the data: SHV MB BES LMEV. Contributed reagents/materials/analysis tools: SHV MB TDM EJ LM LMEV. Wrote the paper: SHV MB TDM BES LMEV. Edited and improved the paper: SHV MB TDM EJ LM JAT MS PJC BES LMEV.

References

1. Ministério da Saúde Instituto Nacional de Saúde (INS), Instituto Nacional de Estatística (INE), ICF Macro (2010) Inquérito Nacional de Prevalência, Riscos Comportamentais e Informação sobre o HIV e SIDA (INSIDA) em Moçambique 2009. Calverton, Maryland, EUA: INS, INE, e ICF Macro.
2. Auld AF, Mbofana F, Shiraishi RW, Sanchez M, Alfredo C, et al. (2011) Four-year treatment outcomes of adult patients enrolled in Mozambique's rapidly expanding antiretroviral therapy program. PLoS One 6: e18453.
3. U.S. State Department (2011) The United States President's Emergency Plan for AIDS Relief.
4. Republic of Mozambique, National AIDS Council, CNCS (2012) 2012 Global AIDS Response Progress Report for the Period 2010–2011. Mozambique: Ministério da Saúde Instituto Nacional de Saúde (INS).
5. National Public Health Directorate MoH, Republic of Mozambique (2011) Preliminary Report of the National Evaluation of the Prevention of Mother-to-Child Transmission Program.
6. WHO (2012) Partnership for Maternal, Newborn & Child Health, World Health Organization. Countdown to 2015: Building a Future for Women and Children, Mozambique Country Reports.
7. Instituto Nacional de Estatistica, Ministerio da Saude, US AID (2013) Moçambique Inquérito Demográfico e de Saúde 2011. Calverton, Maryland, USA.
8. Audet CM, Burlison J, Moon TD, Sidat M, Vergara AE, et al. (2010) Sociocultural and epidemiological aspects of HIV/AIDS in Mozambique. BMC Int Health Hum Rights 10: 15.
9. Institute NS (2009) Preliminary Report on the Multiple Indicator Cluster Survey, 2008. Maputo, Mozambique.
10. Republic of Mozambique, Ministry of Health, National Institute of Health (2009) Mozambique National Child Mortality Study 2009 Summary.
11. Bolton-Moore C, Mubiana-Mbewe M, Cantrell RA, Chintu N, Stringer EM, et al. (2007) Clinical outcomes and CD4 cell response in children receiving antiretroviral therapy at primary health care facilities in Zambia. JAMA 298: 1888–1899.
12. Bland RM, Ndirangu J, Newell ML (2013) Maximising opportunities for increased antiretroviral treatment in children in an existing HIV programme in rural South Africa. BMJ 346: f550.
13. Patel SD, Larson E, Mbengashe T, O'Bra H, Brown JW, et al. (2012) Increases in pediatric antiretroviral treatment, South Africa 2005–2010. PLoS One 7: e44914.
14. Munyagwa M, Baisley K, Levin J, Brian M, Grosskurth H, et al. (2012) Mortality of HIV-infected and uninfected children in a longitudinal cohort in rural south-west Uganda during 8 years of follow-up. Trop Med Int Health 17: 836–843.
15. Meyers T, Dramowski A, Schneider H, Gardiner N, Kuhn L, et al. (2012) Changes in pediatric HIV-related hospital admissions and mortality in Soweto, South Africa, 1996–2011: light at the end of the tunnel? J Acquir Immune Defic Syndr 60: 503–510.
16. Johnson LF, Davies MA, Moultrie H, Sherman GG, Bland RM, et al. (2012) The effect of early initiation of antiretroviral treatment in infants on pediatric AIDS mortality in South Africa: a model-based analysis. Pediatr Infect Dis J 31: 474–480.
17. Bland RM (2011) Management of HIV-infected children in Africa: progress and challenges. Arch Dis Child 96: 911–915.
18. Eley B (2006) Addressing the paediatric HIV epidemic: a perspective from the Western Cape Region of South Africa. Trans R Soc Trop Med Hyg 100: 19–23.
19. De Baets AJ, Bulterys M, Abrams EJ, Kankassa C, Pazvakavambwa IE (2007) Care and treatment of HIV-infected children in Africa: issues and challenges at the district hospital level. Pediatr Infect Dis J 26: 163–173.
20. Braitstein P, Nyandiko W, Vreeman R, Wools-Kaloustian K, Sang E, et al. (2009) The clinical burden of tuberculosis among human immunodeficiency virus-infected children in Western Kenya and the impact of combination antiretroviral treatment. Pediatr Infect Dis J 28: 626–632.
21. Nicoll A, Timaeus I, Kigadye RM, Walraven G, Killewo J (1994) The impact of HIV-1 infection on mortality in children under 5 years of age in sub-Saharan Africa: a demographic and epidemiologic analysis. AIDS 8: 995–1005.
22. Martinson NA, Moultrie H, van Niekerk R, Barry G, Coovadia A, et al. (2009) HAART and risk of tuberculosis in HIV-infected South African children: a multi-site retrospective cohort. Int J Tuberc Lung Dis 13: 862–867.
23. Sutcliffe CG, van Dijk JH, Bolton-Moore C, Cotham M, Tambatamba B, et al. (2010) Differences in presentation, treatment initiation, and response among children infected with human immunodeficiency virus in urban and rural Zambia. Pediatr Infect Dis J 29: 849–854.
24. Sutcliffe CG, van Dijk JH, Bolton C, Persaud D, Moss WJ (2008) Effectiveness of antiretroviral therapy among HIV-infected children in sub-Saharan Africa. Lancet Infect Dis 8: 477–489.
25. van Dijk JH, Sutcliffe CG, Munsanje B, Hamangaba F, Thuma PE, et al. (2009) Barriers to the care of HIV-infected children in rural Zambia: a cross-sectional analysis. BMC Infect Dis 9: 169.
26. Feucht UD, Kinzer M, Kruger M (2007) Reasons for delay in initiation of antiretroviral therapy in a population of HIV-infected South African children. J Trop Pediatr 53: 398–402.
27. Thomas TA, Shenoi SV, Heysell SK, Eksteen FJ, Sunkari VB, et al. (2010) Extensively drug-resistant tuberculosis in children with human immunodeficiency virus in rural South Africa. Int J Tuberc Lung Dis 14: 1244–1251.
28. Adjorlolo-Johnson G, Wahl Uheling A, Ramachandran S, Strasser S, Kouakou J, et al. (2013) Scaling up pediatric HIV care and treatment in Africa: clinical site characteristics associated with favorable service utilization. J Acquir Immune Defic Syndr 62: e7–e13.
29. Kabue MM, Buck WC, Wanless SR, Cox CM, McCollum ED, et al. (2012) Mortality and clinical outcomes in HIV-infected children on antiretroviral therapy in Malawi, Lesotho, and Swaziland. Pediatrics 130: e591–599.
30. Okomo U, Togun T, Oko F, Peterson K, Townend J, et al. (2012) Treatment outcomes among HIV-1 and HIV-2 infected children initiating antiretroviral therapy in a concentrated low prevalence setting in West Africa. BMC Pediatr 12: 95.
31. Grimwood A, Fatti G, Mothibi E, Malahlela M, Shea J, et al. (2012) Community adherence support improves programme retention in children on antiretroviral treatment: a multicentre cohort study in South Africa. J Int AIDS Soc 15: 17381.
32. Chhagan MK, Kauchali S, Van den Broeck J (2012) Clinical and contextual determinants of anthropometric failure at baseline and longitudinal improvements after starting antiretroviral treatment among South African children. Trop Med Int Health 17: 1092–1099.
33. Satti H, McLaughlin MM, Omotayo DB, Keshavjee S, Becerra MC, et al. (2012) Outcomes of comprehensive care for children empirically treated for multidrug-resistant tuberculosis in a setting of high HIV prevalence. PLoS One 7: e37114.
34. Laughton B, Cornell M, Grove D, Kidd M, Springer PE, et al. (2012) Early antiretroviral therapy improves neurodevelopmental outcomes in infants. AIDS 26: 1685–1690.
35. Haberer JE, Kiwanuka J, Nansera D, Ragland K, Mellins C, et al. (2012) Multiple measures reveal antiretroviral adherence successes and challenges in HIV-infected Ugandan children. PLoS One 7: e36737.
36. Kekitiinwa A, Asiimwe AR, Kasirye P, Korutaro V, Kitaka S, et al. (2012) Prospective long-term outcomes of a cohort of Ugandan children with laboratory monitoring during antiretroviral therapy. Pediatr Infect Dis J 31: e117–125.
37. Musiime V, Kayiwa J, Kiconco M, Tamale W, Alima H, et al. (2012) Response to antiretroviral therapy of HIV type 1-infected children in urban and rural settings of Uganda. AIDS Res Hum Retroviruses 28: 1647–1657.
38. Workneh G, Scherzer L, Kirk B, Draper HR, Anabwani G, et al. (2013) Evaluation of the effectiveness of an outreach clinical mentoring programme in support of paediatric HIV care scale-up in Botswana. AIDS Care 25: 11–19.
39. Heidari S, Mofenson LM, Hobbs CV, Cotton MF, Marlink R, et al. (2012) Unresolved antiretroviral treatment management issues in HIV-infected children. J Acquir Immune Defic Syndr 59: 161–169.
40. Kim MH, Cox C, Dave A, Draper HR, Kabue M, et al. (2012) Prompt initiation of ART With therapeutic food is associated with improved outcomes in HIV-infected Malawian children with malnutrition. J Acquir Immune Defic Syndr 59: 173–176.
41. Zyl GU, Rabie H, Nuttall JJ, Cotton MF (2011) It is time to consider third-line options in antiretroviral-experienced paediatric patients? J Int AIDS Soc 14: 55.
42. Reubenson G (2011) Pediatric drug-resistant tuberculosis: a global perspective: a global perspective. Paediatr Drugs 13: 349–355.
43. Geddes R, Giddy J, Butler LM, Van Wyk E, Crankshaw T, et al. (2011) Dual and triple therapy to prevent mother-to-child transmission of HIV in a resource-limited setting - lessons from a South African programme. S Afr Med J 101: 651–654.
44. Fatti G, Bock P, Eley B, Mothibi E, Grimwood A (2011) Temporal trends in baseline characteristics and treatment outcomes of children starting antiretroviral treatment: an analysis in four provinces in South Africa, 2004–2009. J Acquir Immune Defic Syndr 58: e60–67.
45. Ahoua L, Guenther G, Rouzioux C, Pinoges L, Anguzu P, et al. (2011) Immunovirological response to combined antiretroviral therapy and drug resistance patterns in children: 1- and 2-year outcomes in rural Uganda. BMC Pediatr 11: 67.
46. Desmonde S, Coffie P, Aka E, Amani-Bosse C, Messou E, et al. (2011) Severe morbidity and mortality in untreated HIV-infected children in a paediatric care programme in Abidjan, Cote d'Ivoire, 2004–2009. BMC Infect Dis 11: 182.
47. Ciaranello AL, Perez F, Maruva M, Chu J, Engelsmann B, et al. (2011) WHO 2010 guidelines for prevention of mother-to-child HIV transmission in Zimbabwe: modeling clinical outcomes in infants and mothers. PLoS One 6: e20224.
48. Bakanda C, Birungi J, Mwesigwa R, Nachega JB, Chan K, et al. (2011) Survival of HIV-infected adolescents on antiretroviral therapy in Uganda: findings from a nationally representative cohort in Uganda. PLoS One 6: e19261.
49. Schneider K, Puthanakit T, Kerr S, Law MG, Cooper DA, et al. (2011) Economic evaluation of monitoring virologic responses to antiretroviral therapy in HIV-infected children in resource-limited settings. AIDS 25: 1143–1151.

50. Frohoff C, Moodley M, Fairlie L, Coovadia A, Moultrie H, et al. (2011) Antiretroviral therapy outcomes in HIV-infected children after adjusting protease inhibitor dosing during tuberculosis treatment. PLoS One 6: e17273.
51. De Maayer T, Saloojee H (2011) Clinical outcomes of severe malnutrition in a high tuberculosis and HIV setting. Arch Dis Child 96: 560–564.
52. McCollum ED, Preidis GA, Golitko CL, Siwande LD, Mwansambo C, et al. (2011) Routine inpatient human immunodeficiency virus testing system increases access to pediatric human immunodeficiency virus care in sub-Saharan Africa. Pediatr Infect Dis J 30: e75–81.
53. Ndondoki C, Dabis F, Namale L, Becquet R, Ekouevi D, et al. (2011) [Survival, clinical and biological outcomes of HIV-infected children treated by antiretroviral therapy in Africa: systematic review, 2004–2009]. Presse Med 40: e338–357.
54. Peacock-Villada E, Richardson BA, John-Stewart GC (2011) Post-HAART outcomes in pediatric populations: comparison of resource-limited and developed countries. Pediatrics 127: e423–441.
55. Fatti G, Bock P, Grimwood A, Eley B (2010) Increased vulnerability of rural children on antiretroviral therapy attending public health facilities in South Africa: a retrospective cohort study. J Int AIDS Soc 13: 46.
56. Buck WC, Kabue MM, Kazembe PN, Kline MW (2010) Discontinuation of standard first-line antiretroviral therapy in a cohort of 1434 Malawian children. J Int AIDS Soc 13: 31.
57. Musoke PM, Mudiope P, Barlow-Mosha LN, Ajuna P, Bagenda D, et al. (2010) Growth, immune and viral responses in HIV infected African children receiving highly active antiretroviral therapy: a prospective cohort study. BMC Pediatr 10: 56.
58. Sutcliffe CG, Bolton-Moore C, van Dijk JH, Cotham M, Tambatamba B, et al. (2010) Secular trends in pediatric antiretroviral treatment programs in rural and urban Zambia: a retrospective cohort study. BMC Pediatr 10: 54.
59. Nyandiko WM, Mwangi A, Ayaya SO, Nabakwe EC, Tenge CN, et al. (2009) Characteristics of HIV-infected children seen in Western Kenya. East Afr Med J 86: 364–373.
60. Sauvageot D, Schaefer M, Olson D, Pujades-Rodriguez M, O'Brien DP (2010) Antiretroviral therapy outcomes in resource-limited settings for HIV-infected children <5 years of age. Pediatrics 125: e1039–1047.
61. Davies MA, Keiser O, Technau K, Eley B, Rabie H, et al. (2009) Outcomes of the South African National Antiretroviral Treatment Programme for children: the IeDEA Southern Africa collaboration. S Afr Med J 99: 730–737.
62. Leyenaar JK, Novosad PM, Ferrer KT, Thahane LK, Mohapi EQ, et al. (2010) Early clinical outcomes in children enrolled in human immunodeficiency virus infection care and treatment in lesotho. Pediatr Infect Dis J 29: 340–345.
63. Ciaranello AL, Chang Y, Margulis AV, Bernstein A, Bassett IV, et al. (2009) Effectiveness of pediatric antiretroviral therapy in resource-limited settings: a systematic review and meta-analysis. Clin Infect Dis 49: 1915–1927.
64. Janssen N, Ndirangu J, Newell ML, Bland RM (2010) Successful paediatric HIV treatment in rural primary care in Africa. Arch Dis Child 95: 414–421.
65. Memirie ST (2009) Clinical outcome of children on HAART at police referral hospital, Addis Ababa, Ethiopia. Ethiop Med J 47: 159–164.
66. Ntanda H, Olupot-Olupot P, Mugyenyi P, Kityo C, Lowes R, et al. (2009) Orphanhood predicts delayed access to care in Ugandan children. Pediatr Infect Dis J 28: 153–155.
67. Van Winghem J, Telfer B, Reid T, Ouko J, Mutunga A, et al. (2008) Implementation of a comprehensive program including psycho-social and treatment literacy activities to improve adherence to HIV care and treatment for a pediatric population in Kenya. BMC Pediatr 8: 52.
68. Kiboneka A, Wangisi J, Nabiryo C, Tembe J, Kusemererwa S, et al. (2008) Clinical and immunological outcomes of a national paediatric cohort receiving combination antiretroviral therapy in Uganda. AIDS 22: 2493–2499.
69. Jaspan HB, Berrisford AE, Boulle AM (2008) Two-year outcomes of children on non-nucleoside reverse transcriptase inhibitor and protease inhibitor regimens in a South African pediatric antiretroviral program. Pediatr Infect Dis J 27: 993–998.
70. Bock P, Boulle A, White C, Osler M, Eley B (2008) Provision of antiretroviral therapy to children within the public sector of South Africa. Trans R Soc Trop Med Hyg 102: 905–911.
71. Walker AS, Ford D, Mulenga V, Thomason MJ, Nunn A, et al. (2009) Adherence to both cotrimoxazole and placebo is associated with improved survival among HIV-infected Zambian children. AIDS Behav 13: 33–41.
72. Moon TD, Burlison JR, Sidat M, Pires P, Silva W, et al. (2010) Lessons Learned while Implementing an HIV/AIDs Care and Treatment Program in Rural Mozambique. Retrovirology: Research and Treatment 3: 1.
73. Manders EJ, Jose E, Solis M, Burlison J, Nhampossa JL, et al. (2010) Implementing OpenMRS for patient monitoring in an HIV/AIDS care and treatment program in rural Mozambique. Stud Health Technol Inform 160: 411–415.
74. Lahuerta M, Lima J, Elul B, Okamura M, Alvim MF, et al. (2011) Patients enrolled in HIV care in Mozambique: baseline characteristics and follow-up outcomes. J Acquir Immune Defic Syndr 58: e75–86.
75. Shepherd BE, Blevins M, Vaz LM, Moon TD, Kipp AM, et al. (2013) Impact of Definitions of Loss to Follow-up on Estimates of Retention, Disease Progression, and Mortality: Application to an HIV Program in Mozambique. Am J Epidemiol.
76. Chi BH, Yiannoutsos CT, Westfall AO, Newman JE, Zhou J, et al. (2011) Universal definition of loss to follow-up in HIV treatment programs: a statistical analysis of 111 facilities in Africa, Asia, and Latin America. PLoS Med 8: e1001111.
77. Grimsrud AT, Cornell M, Egger M, Boulle A, Myer L (2013) Impact of definitions of loss to follow-up (LTFU) in antiretroviral therapy program evaluation: variation in the definition can have an appreciable impact on estimated proportions of LTFU. J Clin Epidemiol.
78. Moon TD, Burlison JR, Blevins M, Shepherd BE, Baptista A, et al. (2011) Enrolment and programmatic trends and predictors of antiretroviral therapy initiation from president's emergency plan for AIDS Relief (PEPFAR)-supported public HIV care and treatment sites in rural Mozambique. Int J STD AIDS 22: 621–627.
79. Violari A, Cotton MF, Gibb DM, Babiker AG, Steyn J, et al. (2008) Early antiretroviral therapy and mortality among HIV-infected infants. N Engl J Med 359: 2233–2244.
80. Ylitalo N, Brogly S, Hughes MD, Nachman S, Dankner W, et al. (2006) Risk factors for opportunistic illnesses in children with human immunodeficiency virus in the era of highly active antiretroviral therapy. Arch Pediatr Adolesc Med 160: 778–787.
81. Rath BA, von Kleist M, Castillo ME, Kolevic L, Caballero P, et al. (2013) Antiviral resistance and correlates of virologic failure in the first cohort of HIV-infected children gaining access to structured antiretroviral therapy in Lima, Peru: a cross-sectional analysis. BMC Infect Dis 13: 1.
82. Christie CD, Pierre RB (2012) Eliminating vertically-transmitted HIV/AIDS while improving access to treatment and care for women, children and adolescents in Jamaica. West Indian Med J 61: 396–404.
83. Hansudewechakul R, Naiwatanakul T, Katana A, Faikratok W, Lolekha R, et al. (2012) Successful clinical outcomes following decentralization of tertiary paediatric HIV care to a community-based paediatric antiretroviral treatment network, Chiangrai, Thailand, 2002 to 2008. J Int AIDS Soc 15: 17358.
84. Diniz LM, Maia MM, Camargos LS, Amaral LC, Goulart EM, et al. (2011) Impact of HAART on growth and hospitalization rates among HIV-infected children. J Pediatr (Rio J) 87: 131–137.
85. Lumbiganon P, Kariminia A, Aurpibul L, Hansudewechakul R, Puthanakit T, et al. (2011) Survival of HIV-infected children: a cohort study from the Asia-Pacific region. J Acquir Immune Defic Syndr 56: 365–371.
86. Oliveira R, Krauss M, Essama-Bibi S, Hofer C, Robert Harris D, et al. (2010) Viral load predicts new world health organization stage 3 and 4 events in HIV-infected children receiving highly active antiretroviral therapy, independent of CD4 T lymphocyte value. Clin Infect Dis 51: 1325–1333.
87. Rodriguez de Schiavi MS, Scrigni A, Garcia Arrigoni P, Bologna R, Barboni G, et al. (2009) [Highly active antiretroviral therapy in HIV sero-positive children. Disease progression by baseline clinical, immunological and virological status]. Arch Argent Pediatr 107: 212–220.
88. Prasitsuebsai W, Bowen AC, Pang J, Hesp C, Kariminia A, et al. (2010) Pediatric HIV clinical care resources and management practices in Asia: a regional survey of the TREAT Asia pediatric network. AIDS Patient Care STDS 24: 127–131.
89. McConnell MS, Chasombat S, Siangphoe U, Yuktanont P, Lolekha R, et al. (2010) National program scale-up and patient outcomes in a pediatric antiretroviral treatment program, Thailand, 2000–2007. J Acquir Immune Defic Syndr 54: 423–429.
90. Souza E, Santos N, Valentini S, Silva G, Falbo A (2010) Long-term follow-up outcomes of perinatally HIV-infected adolescents: infection control but school failure. J Trop Pediatr 56: 421–426.
91. Kumarasamy N, Venkatesh KK, Devaleenol B, Poongulali S, Mothi SN, et al. (2009) Safety, tolerability and effectiveness of generic HAART in HIV-infected children in South India. J Trop Pediatr 55: 155–159.
92. Noel F, Mehta S, Zhu Y, Rouzier Pde M, Marcelin A, et al. (2008) Improving outcomes in infants of HIV-infected women in a developing country setting. PLoS One 3: e3723.
93. Reddi A, Leeper SC, Grobler AC, Geddes R, France KH, et al. (2007) Preliminary outcomes of a paediatric highly active antiretroviral therapy cohort from KwaZulu-Natal, South Africa. BMC Pediatr 7: 13.
94. Puthanakit T, Aurpibul L, Oberdorfer P, Akarathum N, Kanjananit S, et al. (2007) Hospitalization and mortality among HIV-infected children after receiving highly active antiretroviral therapy. Clin Infect Dis 44: 599–604.
95. Puthanakit T, Oberdorfer A, Akarathum N, Kanjanavanit S, Wannarit P, et al. (2005) Efficacy of highly active antiretroviral therapy in HIV-infected children participating in Thailand's National Access to Antiretroviral Program. Clin Infect Dis 41: 100–107.
96. Janssens B, Raleigh B, Soeung S, Akao K, Te V, et al. (2007) Effectiveness of highly active antiretroviral therapy in HIV-positive children: evaluation at 12 months in a routine program in Cambodia. Pediatrics 120: e1134–1140.
97. Nyandiko WM, Ayaya S, Nabakwe E, Tenge C, Sidle JE, et al. (2006) Outcomes of HIV-infected orphaned and non-orphaned children on antiretroviral therapy in western Kenya. J Acquir Immune Defic Syndr 43: 418–425.
98. Wamalwa DC, Obimbo EM, Farquhar C, Richardson BA, Mbori-Ngacha DA, et al. (2010) Predictors of mortality in HIV-1 infected children on antiretroviral therapy in Kenya: a prospective cohort. BMC Pediatr 10: 33.
99. O'Brien DP, Sauvageot D, Zachariah R, Humblet P, Medecins Sans F (2006) In resource-limited settings good early outcomes can be achieved in children

using adult fixed-dose combination antiretroviral therapy. AIDS 20: 1955–1960.

100. Adje-Toure C, Hanson DL, Talla-Nzussouo N, Borget MY, Kouadio LY, et al. (2008) Virologic and immunologic response to antiretroviral therapy and predictors of HIV type 1 drug resistance in children receiving treatment in Abidjan, Cote d'Ivoire. AIDS Res Hum Retroviruses 24: 911–917.
101. Song R, Jelagat J, Dzombo D, Mwalimu M, Mandaliya K, et al. (2007) Efficacy of highly active antiretroviral therapy in HIV-1 infected children in Kenya. Pediatrics 120: e856–861.
102. Kline MW, Matusa RF, Copaciu L, Calles NR, Kline NE, et al. (2004) Comprehensive pediatric human immunodeficiency virus care and treatment in Constanta, Romania: implementation of a program of highly active antiretroviral therapy in a resource-poor setting. Pediatr Infect Dis J 23: 695–700.
103. Kabue MM, Kekitiinwa A, Maganda A, Risser JM, Chan W, et al. (2008) Growth in HIV-infected children receiving antiretroviral therapy at a pediatric infectious diseases clinic in Uganda. AIDS Patient Care STDS 22: 245–251.
104. Kline MW, Rugina S, Ilie M, Matusa RF, Schweitzer AM, et al. (2007) Long-term follow-up of 414 HIV-infected Romanian children and adolescents receiving lopinavir/ritonavir-containing highly active antiretroviral therapy. Pediatrics 119: e1116–1120.
105. Evans-Gilbert T, Pierre R, Steel-Duncan JC, Rodriguez B, Whorms S, et al. (2004) Antiretroviral drug therapy in HIV-infected Jamaican children. West Indian Med J 53: 322–326.
106. Pierre RB, Steel-Duncan JC, Evans-Gilbert T, Rodriguez B, Moore J, et al. (2008) Effectiveness of antiretroviral therapy in treating paediatric HIV/AIDS in Jamaica. West Indian Med J 57: 223–230.
107. Eley B, Davies MA, Apolles P, Cowburn C, Buys H, et al. (2006) Antiretroviral treatment for children. S Afr Med J 96: 988–993.
108. Collins IJ, Jourdain G, Hansudewechakul R, Kanjanavanit S, Hongsiriwon S, et al. (2010) Long-term survival of HIV-infected children receiving antiretroviral therapy in Thailand: a 5-year observational cohort study. Clin Infect Dis 51: 1449–1457.
109. Meyers TM, Yotebieng M, Kuhn L, Moultrie H (2011) Antiretroviral therapy responses among children attending a large public clinic in Soweto, South Africa. Pediatr Infect Dis J 30: 974–979.
110. van Kooten Niekerk NK, Knies MM, Howard J, Rabie H, Zeier M, et al. (2006) The first 5 years of the family clinic for HIV at Tygerberg Hospital: family demographics, survival of children and early impact of antiretroviral therapy. J Trop Pediatr 52: 3–11.
111. Kamya MR, Mayanja-Kizza H, Kambugu A, Bakeera-Kitaka S, Semitala F, et al. (2007) Predictors of long-term viral failure among ugandan children and adults treated with antiretroviral therapy. J Acquir Immune Defic Syndr 46: 187–193.
112. Zanoni BC, Phungula T, Zanoni HM, France H, Feeney ME (2011) Risk factors associated with increased mortality among HIV infected children initiating antiretroviral therapy (ART) in South Africa. PLoS One 6: e22706.
113. Bong CN, Yu JK, Chiang HC, Huang WL, Hsieh TC, et al. (2007) Risk factors for early mortality in children on adult fixed-dose combination antiretroviral treatment in a central hospital in Malawi. AIDS 21: 1805–1810.
114. Callens SF, Shabani N, Lusiama J, Lelo P, Kitetele F, et al. (2009) Mortality and associated factors after initiation of pediatric antiretroviral treatment in the Democratic Republic of the Congo. Pediatr Infect Dis J 28: 35–40.
115. Raguenaud ME, Isaakidis P, Zachariah R, Te V, Soeung S, et al. (2009) Excellent outcomes among HIV+ children on ART, but unacceptably high pre-ART mortality and losses to follow-up: a cohort study from Cambodia. BMC Pediatr 9: 54.
116. Taye B, Shiferaw S, Enquselassie F (2010) The impact of malnutrition in survival of HIV infected children after initiation of antiretroviral treatment (ART). Ethiop Med J 48: 1–10.
117. Anaky MF, Duvignac J, Wemin L, Kouakoussui A, Karcher S, et al. (2010) Scaling up antiretroviral therapy for HIV-infected children in Cote d'Ivoire: determinants of survival and loss to programme. Bull World Health Organ 88: 490–499.
118. Groh K, Audet CM, Baptista A, Sidat M, Vergara A, et al. (2011) Barriers to antiretroviral therapy adherence in rural Mozambique. BMC Public Health 11: 650.
119. Stringer EM, Sinkala M, Stringer JS, Mzyece E, Makuka I, et al. (2003) Prevention of mother-to-child transmission of HIV in Africa: successes and challenges in scaling-up a nevirapine-based program in Lusaka, Zambia. AIDS 17: 1377–1382.
120. Stringer JS, Sinkala M, Maclean CC, Levy J, Kankasa C, et al. (2005) Effectiveness of a city-wide program to prevent mother-to-child HIV transmission in Lusaka, Zambia. AIDS 19: 1309–1315.
121. Reithinger R, Megazzini K, Durako SJ, Harris DR, Vermund SH (2007) Monitoring and evaluation of programmes to prevent mother to child transmission of HIV in Africa. BMJ 334: 1143–1146.
122. Stringer EM, Ekouevi DK, Coetzee D, Tih PM, Creek TL, et al. (2010) Coverage of nevirapine-based services to prevent mother-to-child HIV transmission in 4 African countries. JAMA 304: 293–302.
123. Stringer EM, Chintu NT, Levy JW, Sinkala M, Chi BH, et al. (2008) Declining HIV prevalence among young pregnant women in Lusaka, Zambia. Bull World Health Organ 86: 697–702.
124. Ciampa PJ, Burlison JR, Blevins M, Sidat M, Moon TD, et al. (2011) Improving retention in the early infant diagnosis of HIV program in rural Mozambique by better service integration. J Acquir Immune Defic Syndr 58: 115–119.
125. Ciampa PJ, Vaz LM, Blevins M, Sidat M, Rothman RL, et al. (2012) The association among literacy, numeracy, HIV knowledge and health-seeking behavior: a population-based survey of women in rural Mozambique. PLoS One 7: e39391.
126. Nyandiko W, Vreeman R, Liu H, Shangani S, Sang E, et al. (2013) Nonadherence to clinic appointments among HIV-infected children in an ambulatory care program in western Kenya. J Acquir Immune Defic Syndr 63: e49–55.
127. Sengayi M, Dwane N, Marinda E, Sipambo N, Fairlie L, et al. (2013) Predictors of loss to follow-up among children in the first and second years of antiretroviral treatment in Johannesburg, South Africa. Glob Health Action 6: 19248.
128. Wachira J, Middlestadt SE, Vreeman R, Braitstein P (2012) Factors underlying taking a child to HIV care: implications for reducing loss to follow-up among HIV-infected and -exposed children. SAHARA J 9: 20–29.
129. Langat NT, Odero W, Gatongi P (2012) Antiretroviral drug adherence by HIV infected children attending Kericho District Hospital, Kenya. East Afr J Public Health 9: 101–104.
130. McNairy ML, Lamb MR, Carter RJ, Fayorsey R, Tene G, et al. (2012) Retention of HIV-infected children on antiretroviral treatment in HIV care and treatment programs in Kenya, Mozambique, Rwanda and Tanzania. J Acquir Immune Defic Syndr.
131. Okomo U, Togun T, Oko F, Peterson K, Jaye A (2012) Mortality and loss to programme before antiretroviral therapy among HIV-infected children eligible for treatment in The Gambia, West Africa. AIDS Res Ther 9: 28.
132. Chetty T, Knight S, Giddy J, Crankshaw TL, Butler LM, et al. (2012) A retrospective study of Human Immunodeficiency Virus transmission, mortality and loss to follow-up among infants in the first 18 months of life in a prevention of mother-to-child transmission programme in an urban hospital in KwaZulu-Natal, South Africa. BMC Pediatr 12: 146.
133. Audet CM, Silva Matos C, Blevins M, Cardoso A, Moon TD, et al. (2012) Acceptability of cervical cancer screening in rural Mozambique. Health Educ Res 27: 544–551.
134. Moon TD, Silva-Matos C, Cordoso A, Baptista AJ, Sidat M, et al. (2012) Implementation of cervical cancer screening using visual inspection with acetic acid in rural Mozambique: successes and challenges using HIV care and treatment programme investments in Zambezia Province. J Int AIDS Soc 15: 17406.
135. Ciampa PJ, Tique JA, Juma N, Sidat M, Moon TD, et al. (2012) Addressing poor retention of infants exposed to HIV: a quality improvement study in rural Mozambique. J Acquir Immune Defic Syndr 60: e46–52.
136. Scanlon ML, Vreeman RC (2013) Current strategies for improving access and adherence to antiretroviral therapies in resource-limited settings. HIV AIDS (Auckl) 5: 1–17.
137. Fenner L, Brinkhof MW, Keiser O, Weigel R, Cornell M, et al. (2010) Early mortality and loss to follow-up in HIV-infected children starting antiretroviral therapy in Southern Africa. Journal of acquired immune deficiency syndromes (1999) 54: 524.
138. Groh K, Audet C, Baptista A, Sidat M, Vergara A, et al. (2011) Barriers to antiretroviral therapy adherence in rural Mozambique. BMC public health 11: 650.
139. Audet CM, Groh K, Moon TD, Vermund SH, Sidat M (2012) Poor-quality health services and lack of programme support leads to low uptake of HIV testing in rural Mozambique. African Journal of AIDS Research 11: 327–335.
140. Geelhoed D, Lafort Y, Chissale E, Candrinho B, Degomme O (2013) Integrated maternal and child health services in Mozambique: structural health system limitations overshadow its effect on follow-up of HIV-exposed infants. BMC Health Serv Res 13: 207.
141. Lambdin BH, Micek MA, Sherr K, Gimbel S, Karagianis M, et al. (2013) Integration of HIV care and treatment in primary health care centers and patient retention in central Mozambique: a retrospective cohort study. J Acquir Immune Defic Syndr 62: e146–152.
142. Audet CM, Sidat M, Blevins M, Moon TD, Vergara A, et al. (2012) HIV knowledge and health-seeking behavior in Zambezia Province, Mozambique. SAHARA J 9: 41–46.
143. Ciampa PJ, Skinner SL, Patricio SR, Rothman RL, Vermund SH, et al. (2012) Comprehensive knowledge of HIV among women in rural Mozambique: development and validation of the HIV knowledge 27 scale. PLoS One 7: e48676.
144. Lehe JD, Sitoe NE, Tobaiwa O, Loquiha O, Quevedo JI, et al. (2012) Evaluating operational specifications of point-of-care diagnostic tests: a standardized scorecard. PLoS One 7: e47459.
145. Bandali S (2013) HIV Risk Assessment and Risk Reduction Strategies in the Context of Prevailing Gender Norms in Rural Areas of Cabo Delgado, Mozambique. J Int Assoc Provid AIDS Care 12: 50–54.
146. Yao J, Murray AT, Agadjanian V, Hayford SR (2012) Geographic influences on sexual and reproductive health service utilization in rural Mozambique. Appl Geogr 32: 601–607.

147. Wandeler G, Keiser O, Pfeiffer K, Pestilli S, Fritz C, et al. (2012) Outcomes of antiretroviral treatment programs in rural Southern Africa. J Acquir Immune Defic Syndr 59: e9–16.
148. Cook RE, Ciampa PJ, Sidat M, Blevins M, Burlison J, et al. (2011) Predictors of successful early infant diagnosis of HIV in a rural district hospital in Zambezia, Mozambique. J Acquir Immune Defic Syndr 56: e104–109.
149. Noden BH, Gomes A, Ferreira A (2010) Influence of religious affiliation and education on HIV knowledge and HIV-related sexual behaviors among unmarried youth in rural central Mozambique. AIDS Care 22: 1285–1294.
150. Posse M, Baltussen R (2009) Barriers to access to antiretroviral treatment in Mozambique, as perceived by patients and health workers in urban and rural settings. AIDS Patient Care STDS 23: 867–875.
151. Agadjanian V, Sen S (2007) Promises and challenges of faith-based AIDS care and support in Mozambique. Am J Public Health 97: 362–366.
152. Vuylsteke B, Bastos R, Barreto J, Crucitti T, Folgosa E, et al. (1993) High prevalence of sexually transmitted diseases in a rural area in Mozambique. Genitourin Med 69: 427–430.
153. Vermund SH, Sidat M, Weil LF, Tique JA, Moon TD, et al. (2012) Transitioning HIV care and treatment programs in southern Africa to full local management. AIDS 26: 1303–1310.
154. Gormley W, McCaffery J, Quain EE (2011) Moving forward on human resources for health: next steps for scaling up toward universal access to HIV/AIDS prevention, treatment, and care. J Acquir Immune Defic Syndr 57 Suppl 2: S113–115.
155. Lambdin BH, Micek MA, Koepsell TD, Hughes JP, Sherr K, et al. (2011) Patient volume, human resource levels, and attrition from HIV treatment programs in central Mozambique. J Acquir Immune Defic Syndr 57: e33–39.
156. Fulton BD, Scheffler RM, Sparkes SP, Auh EY, Vujicic M, et al. (2011) Health workforce skill mix and task shifting in low income countries: a review of recent evidence. Hum Resour Health 9: 1.
157. Adjorlolo-Johnson G, Wahl A, Ramachandran S, Strasser S, Kouakou J, et al. (2012) Scaling up Pediatric HIV Care and Treatment in Africa: Clinical Site Characteristics Associated with Favorable Service Utilization. J Acquir Immune Defic Syndr.
158. Audet CM, Blevins M, Moon TD, Shepherd BE, Vergara A, et al. (2012) Knowledge and Treatment of HIV/AIDS by traditional healers in central Mozambique. J Altern Comlement Med [In Press].
159. Audet CM, Blevins M, Moon TD, Sidat M, Shepherd BE, et al. (2012) Traditional healers in rural Mozambique: Qualitative survey of HIV/AIDS-related attitudes and practices. Journal of Social Aspects of HIV/AIDS [In Press].
160. Agadjanian V, Menjivar C (2011) Fighting down the scourge, building up the church: organisational constraints in religious involvement with HIV/AIDS in Mozambique. Glob Public Health 6 Suppl 2: S148–162.
161. MEPI (Medical Education Partnership Initiative) (2010)Medical Education Partnership Initiative.
162. The Africa Capacity Building Initiative (1991) The Africa Capacity Building Initiative.
163. CONSAMS (Consortium of New Southern African Medical Schools) (2011) Consortium of New Southern African Medical Schools.
164. Eichbaum Q, Nyarango P, Bowa K, Odonkor P, Ferrao J, et al. (2012) "Global networks, alliances and consortia" in global health education - The case for south-to-south partnerships. J Acquir Immune Defic Syndr.
165. Chen C, Buch E, Wassermann T, Frehywot S, Mullan F, et al. (2012) A survey of Sub-Saharan African medical schools. Hum Resour Health 10: 4.
166. Mullan F, Frehywot S, Omaswa F, Sewankambo N, Talib Z, et al. (2012) The Medical Education Partnership Initiative: PEPFAR's effort to boost health worker education to strengthen health systems. Health Aff (Millwood) 31: 1561–1572.
167. Mullan F, Frehywot S, Omaswa F, Buch E, Chen C, et al. (2011) Medical schools in sub-Saharan Africa. Lancet 377: 1113–1121.
168. Decroo T, Telfer B, Biot M, Maikere J, Dezembro S, et al. (2011) Distribution of antiretroviral treatment through self-forming groups of patients in Tete Province, Mozambique. J Acquir Immune Defic Syndr 56: e39–44.
169. Decroo T, Panunzi I, das Dores C, Maldonado F, Biot M, et al. (2009) Lessons learned during down referral of antiretroviral treatment in Tete, Mozambique. J Int AIDS Soc 12: 6.
170. Decroo T, Van Damme W, Kegels G, Remartinez D, Rasschaert F (2012) Are Expert Patients an Untapped Resource for ART Provision in Sub-Saharan Africa? AIDS Res Treat 2012: 749718.
171. Bandali S (2012) HIV Risk Assessment and Risk Reduction Strategies in the Context of Prevailing Gender Norms in Rural Areas of Cabo Delgado, Mozambique. J Int Assoc Physicians AIDS Care (Chic).
172. Bandali S (2011) Norms and practices within marriage which shape gender roles, HIV/AIDS risk and risk reduction strategies in Cabo Delgado, Mozambique. AIDS Care 23: 1171–1176.
173. Lahuerta M, Lima J, Nuwagaba-Biribonwoha H, Okamura M, Alvim MF, et al. (2012) Factors associated with late antiretroviral therapy initiation among adults in Mozambique. PLoS One 7: e37125.
174. Hendriksen IC, Ferro J, Montoya P, Chhaganlal KD, Seni A, et al. (2012) Diagnosis, Clinical Presentation, and In-Hospital Mortality of Severe Malaria in HIV-Coinfected Children and Adults in Mozambique. Clin Infect Dis 55: 1144–1153.
175. Naniche D, Letang E, Nhampossa T, David C, Menendez C, et al. (2011) Alterations in T cell subsets in human immunodeficiency virus-infected adults with co-infections in southern Mozambique. Am J Trop Med Hyg 85: 776–781.
176. Modjarrad K, Vermund SH (2010) Effect of treating co-infections on HIV-1 viral load: a systematic review. Lancet Infect Dis 10: 455–463.
177. Modjarrad K, Vermund SH (2011) An addition to the effect of treating co-infections on HIV-1 viral load. Lancet Infect Dis 11: 81.
178. Vaz P, Augusto O, Bila D, Macassa E, Vubil A, et al. (2012) Surveillance of HIV drug resistance in children receiving antiretroviral therapy: a pilot study of the World Health Organization's generic protocol in Maputo, Mozambique. Clin Infect Dis 54 Suppl 4: S369–374.
179. Holmes CB, Blandford JM, Sangrujee N, Stewart SR, DuBois A, et al. (2012) PEPFAR's past and future efforts to cut costs, improve efficiency, and increase the impact of global HIV programs. Health Aff (Millwood) 31: 1553–1560.
180. Jani IV, Sabatier J, Vubil A, Subbarao S, Bila D, et al. (2012) Evaluation of a high-throughput diagnostic system for detection of HIV-1 in dried blood spot samples from infants in Mozambique. J Clin Microbiol 50: 1458–1460.
181. Jani IV, Sitoe NE, Alfai ER, Chongo PL, Quevedo JI, et al. (2011) Effect of point-of-care CD4 cell count tests on retention of patients and rates of antiretroviral therapy initiation in primary health clinics: an observational cohort study. Lancet 378: 1572–1579.
182. Bwakura-Dangarembizi M, Kendall L, Bakeera-Kitaka S, Nahirya-Ntege P, Keishanyu R, et al. (2014) A Randomized Trial of Prolonged Co-trimoxazole in HIV-Infected Children in Africa. New England Journal of Medicine 370: 41–53.

Diagnostic Testing of Pediatric Fevers: Meta-Analysis of 13 National Surveys Assessing Influences of Malaria Endemicity and Source of Care on Test Uptake for Febrile Children under Five Years

Emily White Johansson[1]*, Peter W. Gething[2], Helena Hildenwall[3], Bonnie Mappin[2], Max Petzold[4], Stefan Swartling Peterson[1,3,5], Katarina Ekholm Selling[1]

1 International Maternal and Child Health, Department of Women's and Children's Health, Uppsala University, Uppsala, Sweden, 2 Spatial Ecology and Epidemiology Group, Department of Zoology, University of Oxford, Oxford, United Kingdom, 3 Global Health, Department of Public Health Sciences, Karolinska Institutet, Stockholm, Sweden, 4 Center for Applied Biostatistics, University of Gothenburg, Gothenburg, Sweden, 5 School of Public Health, College of Health Sciences, Makerere University, Kampala, Uganda

Abstract

Background: In 2010, the World Health Organization revised guidelines to recommend diagnosis of all suspected malaria cases prior to treatment. There has been no systematic assessment of malaria test uptake for pediatric fevers at the population level as countries start implementing guidelines. We examined test use for pediatric fevers in relation to malaria endemicity and treatment-seeking behavior in multiple sub-Saharan African countries in initial years of implementation.

Methods and Findings: We compiled data from national population-based surveys reporting fever prevalence, care-seeking and diagnostic use for children under five years in 13 sub-Saharan African countries in 2009–2011/12 (n = 105,791). Mixed-effects logistic regression models quantified the influence of source of care and malaria endemicity on test use after adjusting for socioeconomic covariates. Results were stratified by malaria endemicity categories: low ($PfPR_{2-10}<5\%$), moderate ($PfPR_{2-10}$ 5–40%), high ($PfPR_{2-10}>40\%$). Among febrile under-fives surveyed, 16.9% (95% CI: 11.8%–21.9%) were tested. Compared to hospitals, febrile children attending non-hospital sources (OR: 0.62, 95% CI: 0.56–0.69) and community health workers (OR: 0.31, 95% CI: 0.23–0.43) were less often tested. Febrile children in high-risk areas had reduced odds of testing compared to low-risk settings (OR: 0.51, 95% CI: 0.42–0.62). Febrile children in least poor households were more often tested than in poorest (OR: 1.63, 95% CI: 1.39–1.91), as were children with better-educated mothers compared to least educated (OR: 1.33, 95% CI: 1.16–1.54).

Conclusions: Diagnostic testing of pediatric fevers was low and inequitable at the outset of new guidelines. Greater testing is needed at lower or less formal sources where pediatric fevers are commonly managed, particularly to reach the poorest. Lower test uptake in high-risk settings merits further investigation given potential implications for diagnostic scale-up in these areas. Findings could inform continued implementation of new guidelines to improve access to and equity in point-of-care diagnostics use for pediatric fevers.

Editor: Joshua Yukich, Tulane University School of Public Health and Tropical Medicine, United States of America

Funding: Uppsala University provides salary support for SSP, KES and also funds EWJ. Karolinska Institutet provides salary support for SSP. HH receives funding from the Swedish Research Council for Health, Working Life and Welfare/the European Commission under a COFAS Marie Curie Post-Doctoral Fellowship. Salary support for MP is from University of Gothenburg. PWG is a Medical Research Council Career Development Fellow and receives funding from the Bill and Melinda Gates Foundation that also funds BM. The funders had no role in study design, data collection and analysis, decision to publish, or preparation of the manuscript.

Competing Interests: The authors have declared that no competing interests exist.

* E-mail: emily.johansson@kbh.uu.se

Introduction

For many years presumptive anti-malarial treatment for febrile children was promoted in malaria-endemic African countries due to lack of diagnostic tools, resulting in widespread malaria over-diagnosis [1], non-rational use of anti-malarial drugs [2], and poor quality treatment of other fever causes [3]. In 2010, however, the World Health Organization (WHO) revised guidelines to recommend diagnosis of all suspected malaria cases before starting treatment based on expert recommendations and increasing availability of malaria rapid diagnostic tests (mRDTs) [4]. Higher anti-malarial drug costs also drive the need for better precision in treatment [5].

The shift from presumptive treatment of febrile children to test-based case management has great potential to improve malaria surveillance, rational drug use and appropriate management of febrile illnesses [6]. By 2010, 37 African countries had a malaria

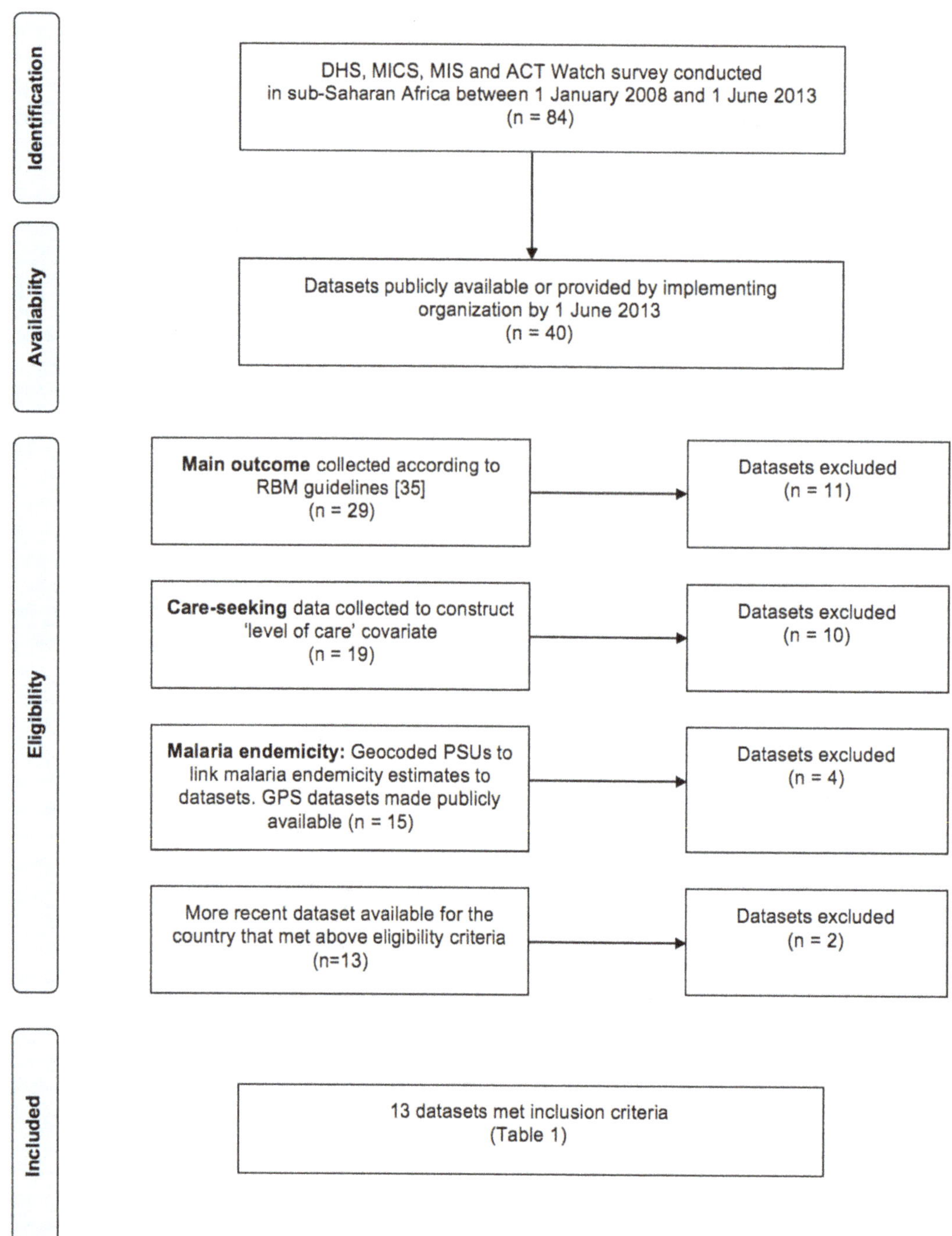

Figure 1. Flow chart of inclusion criteria for study.

diagnosis policy for all age groups and programs are now investing in wide-scale mRDT provision [7].

Despite this investment, evidence to date regarding malaria diagnostic test practices in sub-Saharan Africa is largely derived from adherence studies in limited health facility settings [8–22], or from qualitative interviews of health workers with limited external validity [23–27]. There has been no large-scale, systematic assessment of malaria test use at the population level as countries start scaling up diagnostics in line with revised international guidelines. There is also a limited understanding of factors associated with diagnostic test uptake for pediatric fevers, particularly in relation to patterns of malaria endemicity and treatment seeking behavior that may vary substantially within countries.

Malaria transmission intensity has long been known to influence the management of acute febrile illnesses in children, resulting in common malaria over-diagnosis in malaria-endemic settings [28]. Malaria endemicity has also been hypothesized to specifically affect malaria diagnostic testing practices [29] similar to how local disease epidemiology influences diagnostic use for pediatric infections in high-income countries [30]. Yet, there is currently limited understanding of this key relationship between local malaria epidemiology and the use of diagnostic tests to confirm malaria infection.

Similarly, it is likely that treatment-seeking behavior greatly influences whether a febrile child gets tested for malaria. Microscopy has historically been concentrated at hospitals and higher-level health facilities [31], and initial mRDT implementation has also targeted formal health system sources [6]. Yet, most pediatric febrile illnesses are managed at home or in community settings where diagnostic tests are near absent [32]. Recent research indicates that the largest contributor to reduced systems effectiveness of malaria case management in Zambia is where care was sought for the sick child [33]. Individual characteristics, notably maternal education, may also affect test use given their well-known role in the uptake of other child survival interventions [34]. Yet, there is no evidence about such factors, nor if these individual influences are conditioned by the child's residence or malaria risk.

In 2009, Roll Back Malaria (RBM) recommended asking a question on malaria diagnostic test use in national population-based surveys [35]. Since this time, comparable data have been collected in Demographic and Health Surveys (DHS) [36], Multiple Indicator Cluster Surveys (MICS) [37], Malaria Indicator Surveys (MIS) [38] and ACT Watch Household Surveys [39]. We analyzed these new data to assess extent and determinants of malaria diagnostic test use for pediatric fevers in multiple sub-Saharan African countries during initial years of implementing new guidelines. This paper represents an early assessment against which future progress in diagnostic scale-up may be measured.

Methods

Data Sources

National population-based cross-sectional surveys from DHS, MICS, MIS and ACT Watch conducted in sub-Saharan Africa since 2008 were systematically reviewed for inclusion in this study (Figure 1). 84 surveys were conducted in sub-Saharan African countries between 1 January 2008 and 1 June 2013; 40 datasets were publicly available by 1 June 2013 or were made available by the implementing organization. All datasets were included if they measured the outcome according to RBM guidelines [35], and main covariates as described below. 11 surveys did not collect the outcome measure, or data were collected using non-standard methods. 14 surveys did not collect information to measure main covariates (source of care or malaria endemicity). Two datasets were excluded because a more recent survey was available for the country.

13 DHS and MIS met inclusion criteria, which spanned the period 2009–2011/12 (Table 1). Survey methods are described elsewhere [36]. All surveys with one exception were conducted after national policies were changed to recommend parasitological diagnosis for all age groups prior to treatment, although countries were at different stages of operationalizing these policies at the time of survey fieldwork [40]. For this reason, country-level results are included as a supplement to this paper (Table S1).

Outcome and Explanatory Covariates

Malaria diagnostic test use is measured by asking caregivers of children under five with reported fever in the past two weeks if "At any time during the illness did (name) have blood taken from his/her finger or heel for testing?" This question does not differentiate between diagnostic tests, and is assumed to refer to either microscopy or mRDT.

There were two main covariates: source of care and malaria endemicity. Source of care is measured by asking caregivers of febrile children if they sought advice or treatment for the illness, and if so, from where care was sought. Multiple responses are allowed, and response categories are standardized across countries with some modifications to account for different health system structures. This covariate was categorized as: (1) hospital (2) non-hospital formal medical (3) community health worker (CHW) (4) pharmacy (5) other (6) no care sought. Hospital, CHW, and pharmacy include any such listed response. Non-hospital includes any formal health system source that is not a hospital or CHW, including health centers or posts, outreach or mobile clinics, and private doctors. Some countries include additional sources for this category, such as maternities or municipal clinics. Other includes shops, traditional practitioners, relatives, and non-specified sources. 'Hospital' and 'non-hospital' categories were further dichotomized into public or private sources to analyze test uptake across different managing authorities.

The questionnaire does not explicitly record where testing occurred, but plausibly happened where care was sought. If the child visited multiple sources (e.g. hospital and pharmacy), it was assumed testing occurred at the highest level attended and the covariate was coded using a hierarchical stepwise approach. We conducted a sensitivity analysis by comparing adjusted odds ratios with a covariate constructed by excluding febrile children visiting both hospital and non-hospital sources. In this approach, 732 febrile children visited multiple sources in 13 countries; 367 were excluded that visited both hospital and non-hospital sources. No significant difference was found between approaches (data not shown).

Malaria Atlas Project estimates of malaria endemicity were included in the model, which are described elsewhere [41]. Briefly, the geographical limits of malaria transmission were estimated using routine reporting data and biological models of transmission-limiting aridity and temperature conditions. Within these limits, parasite prevalence survey data were assembled, geolocated, and used within a Bayesian geostatistical model to interpolate a continuous space-time posterior prediction of age-standardized *Plasmodium falciparum* parasite rate in 2–10 year olds ($PfPR_{2-10}$) for every 5×5-km pixel for the year 2010. Malaria endemicity estimates were linked to survey datasets through geocoded PSUs. All individual observations were assigned their PSU-level malaria risk value, which was then categorized into one of five malaria endemicity classes: malaria free; unstable transmission; and low ($PfPR_{2-10}<5\%$), medium ($PfPR_{2-10}$ 5%–40%), and high ($PfPR_{2-10}>40\%$) stable endemic transmission.

Socioeconomic covariates associated with child survival intervention uptake were incorporated in the model. These included child's age and sex, maternal age and education, household wealth and density, and residence [42,43]. Child's age was categorized as 0–5, 6–11, 12–23, 24–35, 36–47, 48–59 months. Maternal age was categorized as 15–24, 25–29, 30–34, 35–39, 40–49 years. Maternal education was categorized as no education, primary and at least secondary education attendance. A household wealth index is pre-specified in datasets and described elsewhere [44]. Household density was categorized as 1–4, 5–8, 9–12 and 13 or more household members [45]. Residence was dichotomized as urban or rural.

Among 29,245 febrile children under five surveyed in 13 countries, 300 had missing values for the outcome, 312 for source of care, 752 for malaria endemicity, and one for maternal education. 36 had missing values for two or more variables. Listwise deletion was used to exclude observations with any missing value from the analysis.

Table 1. Survey information for 13 countries.

Country	Survey	Year	Fieldwork months	*n* PSUs	*n* Under-fives	Percent under-fives with fever (95% CI)[a]		*n* Febrile under-fives	Percent febrile under-fives tested (95% CI)[b]		Year of national policy change[c]
Angola	MIS	2011	January-May	240	7,782	34.1	(31.9–36.2)	2,652	25.9	(23.0–28.9)	2010
Burkina Faso	DHS	2010–2011	May-January	574	14,001	20.6	(19.5–21.7)	2,886	5.3	(4.3–6.3)	2009
Burundi	DHS	2010–2011	August-January	376	7,418	30.1	(28.6–31.7)	2,236	27.0	(24.4–29.6)	2007
Lesotho	DHS	2009–2010	October-January	400	3,348	17.2	(15.7–18.8)	577	10.0	(6.7–13.2)	–
Liberia	MIS	2011	September-December	150	2,876	49.2	(46.4–52.1)	1,416	33.3	(28.9–37.7)	2005
Madagascar	MIS	2011	April-May	268	6,377	14.7	(13.0–16.4)	938	6.2	(4.0–8.5)	2006
Malawi	DHS	2010	June-November	849	18,013	34.5	(33.0–36.0)	6,214	17.4	(15.8–19.1)	2011
Nigeria	MIS	2010	October-December	239	5,519	35.4	(32.3–38.6)	1,956	5.4	(4.1–6.8)	2006
Rwanda	DHS	2010–2011	September-March	492	8,605	15.8	(14.8–16.7)	1,355	21.0	(18.5–23.5)	2009
Senegal	DHS	2010–2011	October-April	391	10,893	22.6	(20.8–24.4)	2,463	9.7	(7.8–11.6)	2007
Tanzania	AIS/MIS	2011–2012	December-May	583	8,216	20.4	(18.8–22.0)	1,675	24.9	(21.2–28.7)	2009 (mainland); 2006 (Zanzibar)
Uganda	DHS	2011	June-December	404	7,535	40.4	(38.1–42.7)	3,042	25.9	(23.2–28.6)	1997
Zimbabwe	DHS	2010–2011	September-March	406	5,208	9.7	(8.8–10.7)	506	7.4	(4.9–9.8)	2008
Total					**105,791**	**26.5**	**(21.0–32.0)**	**27,916**	**16.9**	**(11.8–21.9)**	

DHS refers to Demographic and Health Survey. MIS refers to Malaria Indicator Survey. AIS refers to AIDS Indicator Survey. PSU refers to primary sampling unit.
[a]Children less than five years old reportedly having fever in the 2 weeks prior to the interview.
[b]Febrile children less than five years old reportedly receiving a finger or heel stick for testing.
[c][40] Refers to year national policy changed to recommend parasitological diagnosis in patients of all ages prior to treatment.

Data Analysis

Mixed-effects logistic regression models were used to quantify the influence of covariates on malaria test use in pooled and individual country datasets. PSUs were nested within country identifiers and normal distribution of the random effects was assumed. Covariates were included as categorical fixed effects nested within PSUs. Crude odds ratios of main covariates (malaria endemicity and source of care) were initially estimated for their effect on the outcome. Main covariates were then included simultaneously in one model and, subsequently, odds ratios were adjusted for the effect of all covariates, as listed above. We tested for an interaction between maternal education and malaria endemicity in the final model, and separately for an equivalent interaction between maternal education and residence. Results were stratified by malaria endemicity categories and separately by residence to examine effect differences across contexts. The level of statistical significance was set to 0.05. National point estimates were tabulated using sample weights pre-specified in datasets, and proportions for the pooled dataset were estimated using meta-analytical methods. Standard error estimation accounted for data clustering in survey designs. Stata 12 (STATA Corp, College Station, TX) was used for all analyses.

We also crudely estimated total pediatric fevers attending and tested at different sources of care in 2010 across studied countries to further contextualize findings in our discussion. This was done by applying proportions tested from our analysis to published estimates of total pediatric fevers updated to 2010 [46]. This crude analysis helps visualize the rough magnitude of tested and untested pediatric fevers at different sources of care in order to further inform discussion of results.

Results

105,791 children under five years old were surveyed in 13 countries (Table 1). 27,916 (26.5%, 95% CI: 21.0%–32.0%) had reported fever in the two weeks prior to the survey interview, and 4,990 (16.9%, 95% CI: 11.8%–21.9%) were tested.

Table 2 indicates that 35.3% (95% CI: 26.1%–44.6%) of febrile children attending hospitals were tested compared to 26.0% (95% CI: 18.2%–33.9%) visiting non-hospital formal medical sources, and 16.5% (95% CI: 10.6%–22.3%) visiting CHWs. 22.8% (95% CI: 14.5%–31.1%) of febrile children in low-risk areas were tested compared to 20.0% (95% CI: 13.6%–26.4%) in moderate stable transmission areas, and 16.3% (95% CI: 10.8%–21.7%) in high transmission settings. 11.1% (95% CI: 9.2%–13.1%) of febrile children in malaria-free areas were reportedly tested.

Main Covariates

Febrile children in high-risk areas were less often tested than those in low-risk areas (Table 3). Compared to low-risk areas, the odds of testing declined by 49% for febrile children in high-risk areas (OR: 0.51, 95% CI: 0.42–0.62), and by 54% (OR: 0.46, 95% CI: 0.34–0.63) in malaria-free areas. There was a non-significant difference in the odds of testing febrile children in moderate stable transmission areas when compared to low-risk areas (OR: 1.04, 95% CI: 0.86–1.25). Comparisons with unstable transmission areas are limited given few observations in these areas in our analysis.

Source of care was consistently and significantly associated with malaria test uptake after controlling for other covariates (Table 3). Compared to hospitals, the odds of testing febrile children decreased by 38% if attending non-hospital sources (OR: 0.62, 95% CI: 0.56–0.69), and by 69% (OR: 0.31, 95% CI: 0.23–0.43) if visiting CHWs. Nine countries had similar results (Figure 2 and Table S1). In Uganda, however, the odds of testing febrile children visiting non-hospital formal medical sources was 2.10 (95% CI: 1.67–2.64) times higher than if visiting hospitals. Figure 3 further illustrates the rough magnitude of tested and untested pediatric fevers at different sources of care in studied countries in 2010 to provide context to regression model results.

Crude analyses indicate a non-significant difference in test uptake among febrile children attending public (34.8%, 95% CI: 25.0%–44.5%) versus private (36.5%, 95% CI: 26.3%–46.8%) hospitals across studied countries ($p = 0.315$), and lower uptake at public (25.0%, 95% CI: 17.5%–32.5%) compared to private (30.8%, 95% CI: 16.5%–45.1%) non-hospital sources ($p = 0.022$).

Other Covariates

Residence was significantly associated with test use in the adjusted analysis (Table 3). Compared to urban areas, the odds of testing febrile children decreased by 29% in rural settings (OR: 0.71, 95% CI: 0.62–0.82). For febrile children in least poor households, the odds of testing was 1.63 (95% CI: 1.39–1.91) times higher than for those in poorest households after adjusting for other covariates. Febrile children of mothers that attended primary or at least secondary education had 1.32 (95% CI: 1.19–1.46) and 1.33 (95% CI: 1.16–1.54) times higher odds of getting tested, respectively, than those having mothers with no education. Febrile children over 12 months were more often tested than infants aged 0–11 months. Compared to older infants (6–11 months), the odds of younger infants (0–5 months) getting tested declined by 28% in the adjusted analysis (OR: 0.72, 95% CI: 0.59–0.87). Maternal age and child's sex were non-significant covariates.

Stratification by Malaria Endemicity

There was evidence of an interaction between categorical variables maternal education and malaria endemicity (p-values ranged from 0.009 to 0.467 for stable transmission categories) when incorporated into the final model. To further explore this result, the final model was stratified by low ($PfPR_{2-10}$<5%), medium ($PfPR_{2-10}$ 5%–40%), and high ($PfPR_{2-10}$>40%) stable malaria transmission categories. In high-risk settings, the odds of testing febrile children with mothers who attended primary or at least secondary education was 1.71 (95% CI: 1.44–2.02) and 2.23 (95% CI: 1.76–2.82) times higher, respectively, than if the mother had no education after controlling for other covariates (Figure 4). This effect was negligible in moderate- and low-risk areas. The stratified model by urban and rural residence indicated no significant difference in maternal education's effect on test use between contexts (data not shown).

Discussion

Overall, diagnostic testing of pediatric fevers was low and inequitable in studied countries at the outset of new guidelines. Test uptake was lowest at locations where pediatric fevers are more often managed, particularly for poorest children, and in areas with the highest risk of malaria infection. Our findings also demonstrate an important socioeconomic dimension to malaria testing.

We found seeking care from lower levels or less formal sources greatly reduced the likelihood of testing, as occurs with other facility-based interventions [47]. This is most plausibly explained by lower test availability at these locations, including their near absence among CHWs and pharmacies [48]. It is also possible that patients attending hospitals are systematically different from those

Table 2. Characteristics of febrile children less than five years old reportedly tested in 13 countries.

		n febrile under-fives[a]	Percent febrile under-fives tested (95% CI)[b]	
Total		*27,916*	*16.9*	*(11.8–21.9)*
Source of care[c]	Hospital	5,279	35.3	(26.1–44.6)
	Non-hospital formal medical	9,938	26.0	(18.2–33.9)
	Community health worker	381	16.5	(10.6–22.3)
	Pharmacy	1,742	6.2	(3.4–9.0)
	Other	1,769	6.9	(4.3–9.4)
	No care sought	8,618	3.3	(2.3–4.3)
Malaria endemicity[d]	No transmission	1,023	11.1	(9.2–13.1)
	Unstable transmission	7	42.9	(15.8–75.0)
	Low stable transmission	2,797	22.8	(14.5–31.1)
	Moderate stable transmission	12,211	20.0	(13.6–26.4)
	High stable transmission	11,287	16.3	(10.8–21.7)
Child's age (in months)	0–5	2,174	12.7	(8.3–17.0)
	6–11	4,094	17.1	(11.6–22.7)
	12–23	7,191	18.1	(12.5–23.8)
	24–35	6,006	17.8	(12.3–23.2)
	36–47	4,782	16.0	(11.3–20.7)
	48–59	4,021	15.9	(10.7–21.1)
Child's sex	Male	14,297	17.0	(12.0–22.0)
	Female	13,620	16.7	(11.7–21.8)
Maternal age (in years)	15–24	8,798	17.7	(12.7–22.8)
	25–29	7,725	16.8	(11.1–22.5)
	30–34	5,237	16.4	(11.2–21.5)
	35–39	3,829	16.3	(11.3–21.3)
	40–49	2,331	16.3	(11.5–21.2)
Maternal education	No education	9,989	14.0	(9.8–18.2)
	Primary attendance	13,883	17.4	(13.1–21.7)
	Secondary or higher attendance	4,047	27.0	(18.6–35.5)
Household wealth index	Poorest	6,107	12.4	(8.6–16.3)
	Second	5,797	12.8	(9.1–16.5)
	Middle	5,838	14.6	(10.1–19.1)
	Fourth	5,609	18.5	(12.6–24.5)
	Least poor	4,574	27.6	(18.0–37.3)
Number of household members	0–4	7,239	18.1	(12.8–23.4)
	5–8	14,156	17.0	(12.1–21.9)
	9–12	4,241	16.3	(10.9–21.6)
	13 or more	2,280	14.6	(10.1–19.1)
Residence	Urban	5,651	27.4	(17.8–37.1)
	Rural	22,264	14.6	(10.4–18.7)

[a]Children less than five years old reportedly having fever in the 2 weeks prior to the interview.
[b]Febrile children less than five years old reportedly receiving a finger or heel stick for testing.
[c]Non-hospital formal medical refers to any formal medical source that is not a hospital or CHW. Other refers to traditional practitioners, shops, relatives/friends, or other non-specified locations.
[d]No transmission refer to non-endemic areas. Unstable transmission refers to areas of very low but non-zero malaria transmission. Stable transmission categories refer to low ($PfPR_{2-10}<5\%$), moderate ($PfPR_{2-10}$ 5%–40%) and high ($PfPR_{2-10}>40\%$).

attending other sources in ways that influence testing (e.g. more severe illness).

Crude estimates of total pediatric fevers attending and tested at different sources of care further illustrates that diagnostic testing is not reaching sources of care bearing the disproportionate burden of fever cases. This is a particular challenge to improve equitable access to diagnostic testing in the future since these are the same sources where poor and marginalized families often seek care [32]. There is an urgent need to improve quantification of diagnostic

Table 3. Effect of source of care, malaria endemicity and socioeconomic covariates on test uptake.

		AOR[a]	95% CI	p-value
Source of care[b]	Hospital	1.00		
	Non-hospital formal medical	0.62	0.56–0.69	<0.001
	Community health worker	0.31	0.23–0.43	<0.001
	Pharmacy	0.06	0.05–0.09	<0.001
	Other	0.10	0.08–0.13	<0.001
	No care sought	0.05	0.04–0.06	<0.001
Malaria endemicity[c]	No transmission	0.46	0.34–0.63	<0.001
	Unstable transmission	1.32	0.11–15.50	0.823
	Low stable transmission	1.00		
	Moderate stable transmission	1.04	0.86–1.25	0.697
	High stable transmission	0.51	0.42–0.62	<0.001
Child's age (in months)	0–5	0.72	0.59–0.87	0.001
	6–11	1.00		
	12–23	1.24	1.09–1.41	0.001
	24–35	1.27	1.11–1.45	<0.001
	36–47	1.10	0.95–1.26	0.203
	48–59	1.18	1.02–1.37	0.030
Child's sex	Male	1.00		
	Female	0.98	0.91–1.06	0.676
Maternal age (in years)	15–24	1.00		
	25–29	1.01	0.91–1.12	0.891
	30–34	1.06	0.94–1.20	0.336
	35–39	1.06	0.92–1.21	0.425
	40–49	0.99	0.83–1.17	0.890
Maternal education	No education attendance	1.00		
	Primary attendance	1.32	1.19–1.46	<0.001
	Secondary or higher attendance	1.33	1.16–1.54	<0.001
Household wealth index	Poorest	1.00		
	Second	0.99	0.87–1.13	0.850
	Middle	1.03	0.90–1.18	0.670
	Fourth	1.21	1.06–1.40	0.006
	Least poor	1.63	1.39–1.91	<0.001
Number of household members	0–4	1.00		
	5–8	0.95	0.86–1.05	0.307
	9–12	0.87	0.76–0.99	0.036
	13 or more	0.66	0.54–0.80	<0.001
Residence	Urban	1.00		
	Rural	0.71	0.62–0.82	<0.001

CI refers to confidence interval. AOR refers to adjusted odds ratio. COR refers to crude odds ratio.
[a]Mixed-effects logistic regression model in pooled dataset of 13 surveys, adjusted for data clustering and above covariates.
[b]COR (source of care): non-hospital = 0.56 (95% CI: 0.51–0.62); community health worker = 0.30 (95% CI: 0.21–0.41); pharmacy = 0.06 (95% CI: 0.05–0.08); other = 0.09 (95% CI: 0.07–0.12); no care sought = 0.04 (95% CI: 0.04–0.05). Non-hospital formal medical refers to any formal medical source that is not a hospital or CHW. Other refers to traditional practitioners, shops, relatives/friends, or other non-specified locations.
[c]COR (malaria endemicity): no transmission = 0.51 (95% CI: 0.38–0.70); unstable transmission = 5.67 (95% CI: 0.44–73.6); moderate stable transmission = 1.35 (95% CI: 1.12–1.63); high stable transmission = 0.67 (95% CI: 0.55–0.81). No risk areas refer to non-endemic areas. Unstable malaria transmission refers to areas of very low but non-zero transmission. Stable transmission categories refer to low ($PfPR_{2-10}<5\%$), moderate ($PfPR_{2-10}$ 5%–40%) and high ($PfPR_{2-10}>40\%$).

need along these lines in order to inform mRDT forecasting and procurement as countries work toward universal test coverage.

Our results also indicate febrile children at the highest malaria risk are less often tested than those at lower risk. Some countries have prioritized mRDT to low-risk areas to increase diagnostic availability in these settings [49]. Reduced uptake in high-risk areas could also be due to entrenched presumptive treatment practices [50]. In locations where diagnostic tests commonly indicate malaria infection – or as malaria 'suspicion' rises – there may be less perceived value of testing over habitual presumptive

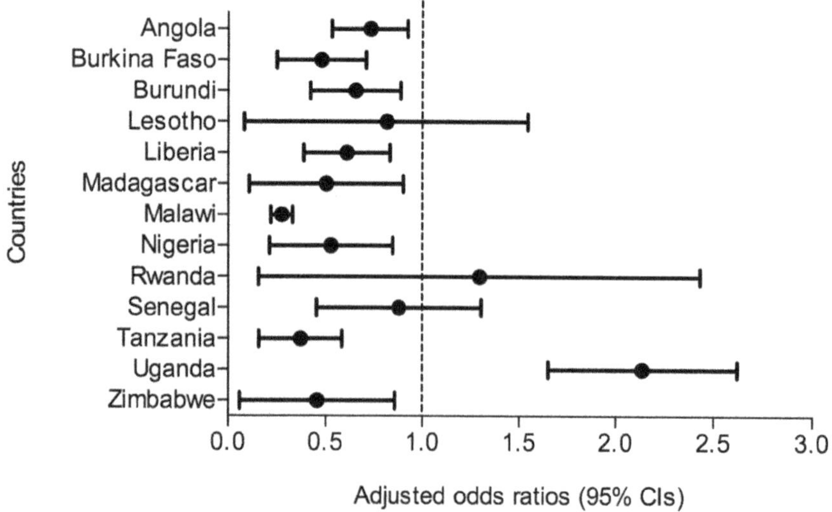

Figure 2. Forest plot of test uptake at non-hospital sources versus hospitals in each country. Figure legend: CI refers to confidence interval. Mixed-effects logistic regression models adjusted for data clustering and Table 3 covariates. AOR <1.0 indicates reduced odds of testing at non-hospital sources compared to hospitals.

treatment practices by caregivers and/or health workers. Similarly, less testing in malaria-free areas is likely due to lower malaria 'suspicion' in these settings. This finding merits further investigation given potential implications for mRDT scale-up in high-risk areas.

Different influences of maternal education on test use in low- and high-risk settings could further support this theory. Independent of other factors, our findings show febrile children of educated mothers in high-risk areas have twice the odds of getting tested than those with non-educated mothers, while this effect was negligible in low- and moderate-risk settings. Again, a perceived lesser value of testing in high-risk areas could exacerbate an 'early adopter' effect among better-educated mothers [51]. Poorly educated mothers, or those less open to new technologies or medical procedures, could be less inclined to change treatment habits in areas where testing commonly provides the same result as presumptive practices, particularly if time or cost is associated with testing. Health workers, too, could less often test children in high-risk settings without caregiver demand, which favors educated mothers. In low-risk areas where a malaria diagnosis is less clear, a wider range of caregivers and/or health workers may be more inclined toward testing, potentially coupled with higher test availability depending on country implementation strategies.

Results show infants are less often tested than older children, and younger infants (0–5 months) are less often tested than older ones (six to 11 months). This finding has not been previously reported to our knowledge. Mean age of malaria onset is about six months [52]. Health workers may therefore not suspect malaria in young infants and test less often. Alternatively, fever in infants is often a clinical 'red flag' given higher mortality rates in this age group. This could cause backsliding to habitual presumptive treatment practices. This result merits further investigation since malaria infection is still possible in young infants. In fact, testing could arguably be more informative for this group since diagnosis is less clear, and differential diagnosis of childhood illnesses with overlapping symptoms (e.g. malaria and pneumonia) is important [53].

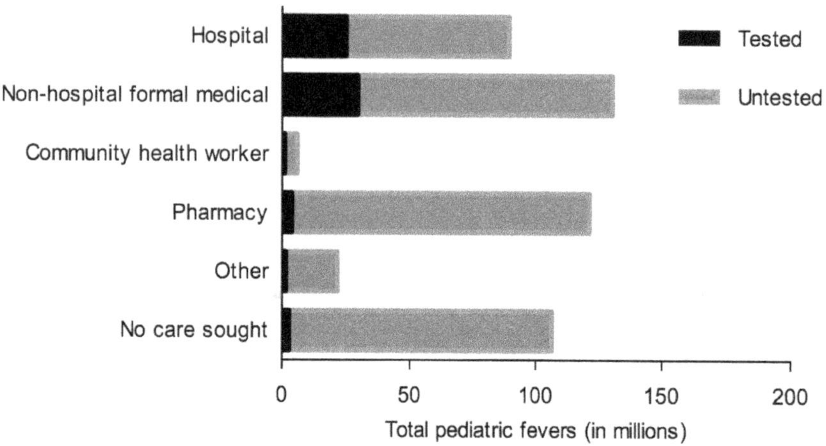

Figure 3. Estimated pediatric fevers attending and tested by source of care in 13 countries in 2010. Figure legend: All totals are given in '000 s.

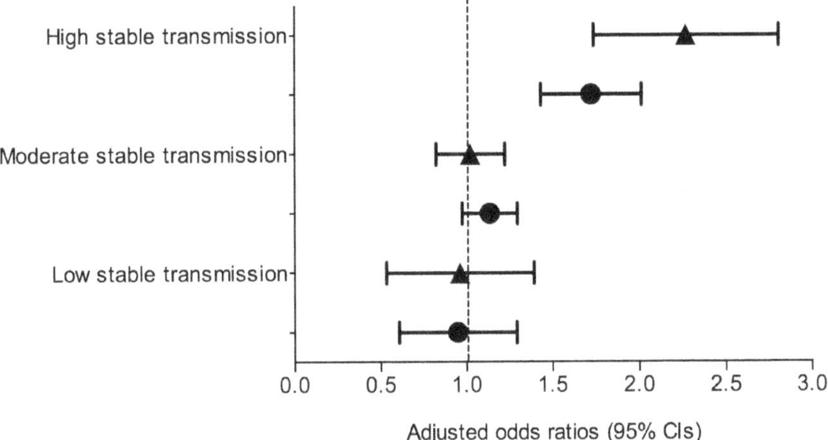

Figure 4. Effect of maternal education on test uptake in different malaria endemicities. Figure legend: ▲, Secondary or higher schooling versus no schooling; ●, Primary schooling versus no schooling. Mixed-effects logistic regression model in pooled dataset of 13 surveys, adjusted for data clustering and Table 3 covariates. Stable transmission categories refer to low ($PfPR_{2-10}$<5%), moderate ($PfPR_{2-10}$ 5%–40%) and high ($PfPR_{2-10}$> 40%).

Our study further demonstrates a socioeconomic dimension to malaria testing. Independent of other factors, febrile children in poorest households are less often tested, as are those with poorly educated mothers. Rural settings are associated with less testing, as are large households in the adjusted analysis. This is likely due to lower test availability where marginalized families often seek care. Integrated community case management is a promising approach to improve equitable access to testing and care [54]. Studies show that CHWs can appropriately use rapid diagnostic tests to manage pediatric fevers [55].

These results should be viewed in light of some data limitations. First, findings indicate differences in test uptake across population groups but do not explain reasons for observed practices. Second, surveys only measure whether blood was taken for testing, and as such, do not differentiate between microscopy and mRDT. Higher coverage at certain locations, such as hospitals, may be due to long-standing microscopy availability rather than targeted mRDT roll out. Moreover, testing practices could differ for microscopy and mRDT, particularly since mRDT requires less training and time to use effectively [56–58]. Data in this analysis may largely reflect testing by microscopy given our early assessment with countries at different stages of mRDT implementation. Future analyses based on more recent data, once available, could potentially provide a different result if a greater proportion of testing is conducted using mRDT rather than microscopy. Third, data indicate test use but not appropriate treatment based on test results. Fourth, surveys do not measure facility or clinician factors that may greatly influence uptake.

Finally, a recent validation study found caregiver recall of testing was not highly sensitive (61.9%) but had reasonable specificity (90.0%) when compared to direct facility observation of malaria diagnostic test receipt [59]. The authors found no significant differences in recall across examined caregiver characteristics. Other studies have shown poor caregiver recall of child morbidities or previous health events, particularly among poor, rural or less educated mothers [60,61]. Findings could overestimate differences in test uptake between these groups.

Conclusion

Based on 105,791 children under age five years surveyed in 13 countries in 2009–2011/12, our findings demonstrate low and inequitable testing of pediatric fevers as countries start to implement new guidelines. Malaria diagnostic testing has become increasingly important in the context of malaria control and elimination to improve surveillance, rational drug use and appropriate fever management [62]. Countries are now working toward universal test coverage of all suspected malaria cases in line with revised international guidelines. This paper represents an early assessment against which to measure future progress in diagnostic scale-up, and highlights inequities in testing that need to be addressed going forward. Research is urgently needed to better understand reasons for reduced testing among the youngest children and in high-risk settings, which could plausibly be due to a perceived lesser value of testing for these populations. This analysis should be repeated in the near-term as mRDT implementation matures, and additional data become available for the years 2012–2014. Similar analyses are also needed to examine testing practices for older children and adults. Current findings could inform continued mRDT implementation in order to improve access to and equity in point-of-care diagnostics use for pediatric fevers.

Author Contributions

Conceived and designed the experiments: EWJ KES SSP HH MP PWG. Performed the experiments: EWJ. Analyzed the data: EWJ MP KES SSP PWG BM HH. Contributed reagents/materials/analysis tools: EWJ KES

MP SSP. Wrote the paper: EWJ. Analyzed and modeled populations at malaria risk: PWG BM. Estimated total pediatric fevers tested in 2010: PWG BM EWJ. Contributed to interpretation of findings: EWJ PWG SSP HH KES. Reviewed, revised and contributed writing to paper: EWJ PWG HH BM SSP MP KES.

References

1. Gwer C, Newton CJRC, Berkley JA (2007) Over-diagnosis and co-morbidity of severe malaria in African children: a guide for clinicians. Am J Trop Med Hyg 77: 6–13.
2. World Health Organization (2000) The use of anti-malarial drugs: report of a WHO informal consultation. Geneva: World Health Organization.
3. Källander K, Nsungwa-Sabiiti J, Peterson S (2004) Symptom overlap for malaria and pneumonia – policy implications for home management strategies. Acta Trop 90: 211–4.
4. World Health Organization (2010) Guidelines for the treatment of malaria. Geneva: World Health Organization.
5. Mosha JF, Conteh L, Tediosi F, Gesase S, Bruce J (2010) Cost implications of improving malaria diagnosis: findings from north-eastern Tanzania. PLoS One 5(1): e8707.
6. World Health Organization (2012) T3: Test. Treat. Track. Scaling up diagnostic testing, treatment and surveillance for malaria. Geneva: World Health Organization.
7. World Health Organization (2011) World malaria report 2011. Geneva: World Health Organization.
8. Bruxvoort K, Kalolella A, Nchimba H, Festo C, Taylor M, et al. (2013) Getting antimalarials on target: impact of national roll-out of malaria rapid diagnostic tests on health facility treatment in three regions of Tanzania. Trop Med Int Health 18: 1269–82.
9. Shakeley D, Elfving K, Aydin-Schmidt B, Msellem MI, Morris U, et al. (2013) The usefulness of rapid diagnostic tests in the new context of low malaria transmission in Zanzibar. PLoS One 8: e72912.
10. Mubi M, Kakoko D, Ngasala B, Premji Z, Peterson S, et al. (2013) Malaria diagnosis and treatment practices following introduction of rapid diagnostic tests in Kibaha District, Coast Region, Tanzania. Malar J 12: 293.
11. Bottieau E, Gillet P, De Weggheleire A, Scheirlinck A, Stokx J, et al. (2013) Treatment practices in patients with suspected malaria in Provincial Hospital of Tete, Mozambique. Trans R Soc Trop Med Hyg 107(3): 176–82.
12. Yukich JO, Bennett A, Albertini A, Incardona S, Moonga H, et al. (2012) Reductions in artemisinin-based combination therapy consumption after the nationwide scale up of routine malaria rapid diagnostic testing in Zambia. Am J Trop Med Hyg 87(3): 437–46.
13. Masanja IM, Selemani M, Amuri B, Kajungu D, Khatib R, et al. (2012) Increased use of malaria rapid diagnostic tests improves targeting of anti-malarial treatment in rural Tanzania: implications for nationwide rollout of malaria rapid diagnostic tests. Malar J 11: 221.
14. D'Acremont V, Kahama-Maro J, Swai N, Mtasiwa D, Genton B, et al. (2011) Reduction of anti-malarial consumption after rapid diagnostic tests implementation in Dar Es Salaam: a before-after and cluster randomized controlled study. Malar J 10: 107.
15. Bastiaens GJ, Schaftenaar E, Ndaro A, Keuter M, Bousema T, et al. (2011) Malaria diagnostic testing and treatment practices in three different Plasmodium falciparum transmission settings in Tanzania: before and after a government policy change. Malar J 10: 76.
16. Juma E, Zurovac D (2011) Changes in health workers' malaria diagnosis and treatment practices in Kenya. Malar J 10: 1.
17. Masanja MI, McMorrow M, Kahigwa E, Kachur SP, McElroy PD (2010) Health workers' use of malaria rapid diagnostic tests (RDTs) to guide clinical decision making in rural dispensaries, Tanzania. Am J Trop Med Hyg 83(6): 1238–41.
18. Kyabayinze DJ, Asiime C, Nakanjako D, Nabakooza J, Counihan H, et al. (2010) Use of RDTs to improve malaria diagnosis and fever case management at primary health care facilities in Uganda. Malar J 9: 200.
19. Skarbinski J, Ouma PO, Causer LM, Kariuki SK, Barnwell JW, et al. (2009) Effect of malaria rapid diagnostic tests on the management of uncomplicated malaria with artemethur-lumefantrine in Kenya: a cluster randomized trial. Am J Trop Med Hyg 80(6): 919–26.
20. Msellem MI, Mårtensson A, Rotllant G, Bhattarai A, Strömberg J, et al. (2009) Influence of rapid malaria diagnostic tests on treatment and health outcome in fever patients, Zanzibar: a crossover validation study. PLoS Med 6(4): e100070.
21. Zurovac D, Njogu J, Akhwale W, Hamer DH, Larson BA, et al. (2008) Effects of revised diagnostic recommendations on malaria treatment practices across age groups in Kenya. Trop Med Int Health 13(6): 784–7.
22. Hamer DH, Ndhlovu M, Zurovac D, Fox M, Yeboah-Antwi K, et al. (2007) Improved diagnostic testing and malaria treatment practices in Zambia. JAMA 297(20): 2227–31.
23. Ushasoro MD, Okoli CC, Uzochukwu BS (2013) Qualitative study of presumptive treatment of childhood malaria in third-tier tertiary hospitals in southeast Nigeria: a focus group and in-depth study. Malar J 12: 436.
24. Baltzell K, Elfving K, Shakely D, Ali AS, Msellem MI, et al. (2013) Febrile illness management in children under five years of age: a pilot study on primary health care workers' practices in Zanzibar. Malar J 12: 37.
25. Ezeoke OP, Ezumah NN, Chandler CC, Mangham-Jeffries LJ, Onwujekwe OE, et al. (2012) Exploring health providers' and community perceptions and experiences with malaria tests in South-East Nigeria: a critical step towards appropriate treatment. Malar J 11: 368.
26. Uzochukwu BS, Onwujekwe E, Ezuma NN, Exeoke OP, Ajuba MO, et al. (2011) Improving rational treatment of malaria: perceptions and influence of RDTs on prescribing behavior of health workers in southeast Nigeria. PloS One 6: e14627.
27. Chandler C, Jones C, Boniface G, Juma K, Reyburn H, et al. (2008) Guidelines and mindlines: why do clinical staff over-diagnose malaria in Tanzania? A qualitative study. Malar J 7: 53.
28. Reyburn H, Mbatia R, Drakeley C, Carneiro I, Mwakasungula E, et al. (2004) Overdiagnosis of malaria in patients with severe febrile illness in Tanzania: a prospective study. BMJ 329: 1212.
29. Graz B, Willcox M, Szeless T, Rougemont A (2011) "Test and treat" or presumptive treatment for malaria in high transmission situations? A reflection on the latest WHO guidelines. Malar J 10: 136.
30. Bisno AL, Gerber MA, Gwaltney JM, Kaplan EL, Schwartz RH (2002) Practice guidelines for the diagnosis and management of Group A Streptococcal Pharyngitis. Clin Inf D 35: 113–125.
31. Petti CA, Polage CR, Quinn TC, Ronald AR, Sande MA (2006) Laboratory medicine in Africa: a barrier to effective health care. Clin Infect Dis 42: 377–382.
32. Orem JM, Mugisha F, Okui AP, Musango L, Kirigia JM (2013) Health care seeking patterns and determinants of out-of-pocket expenditure for malaria for the children under-five in Uganda. Malar J 12: 175.
33. Littrell M, Miller JM, Ndhlovu M, Hamainza B, Hawela M, et al. (2013) Documenting malaria case management coverage in Zambia: a systems effectiveness approach. Malar J 12: 371.
34. Mosley WH, Chen L (1984) An analytic framework for the study of child survival in developing countries. Population and Development Review 10: 25–45.
35. Roll Back Malaria (2009) Guidelines for core population-based indicators. Calverton, Maryland: ICF Macro.
36. MEASURE DHS (2013) Demographic and health surveys. Available: http://www.measuredhs.com. Accessed 5 June 2013.
37. United Nations Children's Fund (2013) Childinfo: multiple indicator cluster surveys. Available: http://www.childinfo.org/mics.html. Accessed: 5 June 2013.
38. Roll Back Malaria (2013) Malaria indicator surveys. Available: http://www.malariasurveys.org. Accessed: 5 June 2013.
39. ACT Watch (2013) ACT Watch: Evidence for malaria medicine policy. Available: http://www.actwatch.info. Accessed 5 June 2013.
40. World Health Organization (2012) World malaria report 2012. Geneva: World Health Organization.
41. Hay SI, Smith DL, Snow RW (2008) Measuring malaria endemicity from intense to interrupted transmission. Lancet Infect Dis 8: 369–378.
42. Hwang J, Graves PM, Jima D, Reithinger R, Kachur SP, et al. (2010) Knowledge of malaria and its association with malaria-related behaviors – results from the malaria indicator survey, Ethiopia, 2007. PLoS ONE 5(7): e11692.
43. Watsierah CA, Jura WG, Raballah E, Kaseje D, Abong'o B, et al. (2011) Knowledge and behavior as determinants of anti-malarial drug use in a peri-urban population from malaria holoendemic region of western Kenya. Malar J 10: 99.
44. MEASURE DHS (2004) The DHS wealth index - DHS comparative reports. Calverton, Maryland: ICF Macro.
45. MEASURE DHS (1997) Demographic and socioeconomic characteristics of households - DHS comparative studies. Calverton, Maryland: ICF Macro.
46. Gething PW, Kirui VC, Alegana VA, Okiro EA, Noor AM, et al. (2010) Estimating the number of paediatric fevers associated with malaria infection presenting to Africa's public health sector in 2007. PLoS Med 7(7): e1000301.
47. Gabrysch S, Cousens S, Cox J, Campbell OMR (2011) The influence of distance and level of care on delivery place in rural Zambia: a study linked national data in a geographic information system. PLoS Med 8(1): e1000394.
48. Hamer DH, Marsh DR, Peterson S, Pagnoni F (2012) Integrated community case management: next steps in addressing the implementation research agenda. Am J Trop Med Hyg 87: 151–153.
49. Republic of Uganda (2009) Uganda national malaria strategic plan, 2011–2015. Kampala: Ministry of Health.
50. Mwanziva C, Shekalaghe S, Ndaro A, Mengerink B, Megiroo S, et al. (2008) Overuse of artemisinin-combination therapy in Mto wa Mbu (rivier of mosquitoes), an area misinterpreted as high endemic for malaria. Malar J 7: 232.
51. Pai NP, Vadnais C, Denkinger C, Engel N, Pai M (2012) Point-of-care testing for infectious diseases: diversity, complexity and barriers in low- and middle-income countries. PLoS Med 9(9): e1001306.
52. Achidi EW, Salimonu LS, Perlmann H, Perlmann P, Berzins K, et al. (1996) Lack of association between levels of transplacentally acquired Plasmodium falciparum-specific antibodies and age of onset of clinical malaria in infants in a malaria endemic area of Nigeria. Acta Trop 61: 315–326.

53. World Health Organization (1991) The overlap in the clinical presentation and treatment of malaria and pneumonia in children: report of a meeting. Geneva: World Health Organization.
54. Marsh DR, Hamer DH, Pagnoni F, Peterson S (2012) Evidence for the implementation, effects and impact of the integrated community case management strategy to treat childhood infection. Am J Trop Med Hyg 87: 2–5.
55. Mukanga DA, Tiono AB, Anyorigiya T, Källander K, Konate AT, et al. (2012) Integrated community case management of fevers in children under five using rapid diagnostic tests and respiratory rate counting: a multi-country cluster randomized trial. Am J Trop Med Hyg 87: 21–29.
56. Strom GE, Haanshuus CG, Fataki M, Langeland N, Blomberg B (2013) Challenges in diagnosing pediatric malaria in Dar Es Salaam, Tanzania. Malar J 12: 228.
57. Kahama-Maro J, D'Acremont V, Mtasiwa D, Genton B, Lengeler C (2011) Low quality of routine microscopy for malaria at different levels of the health system in Dar Es Salaam. Malar J 10: 332.
58. Harchut K, Standley C, Dobson A, Klaassen B, Rambaud-Althaus C, et al. (2013) Over-diagnosis of malaria by microscopy in the Kilombero Valley, Southern Tanzania: an evaluation of the utility and cost-effectiveness of rapid diagnostic tests. Malar J 12: 159.
59. Eisele TP, Silumbe K, Yukich J, Hamainza B, Keating J, et al. (2013) Accuracy of measuring diagnosis and treatment of childhood malaria from household surveys in Zambia. PLoS Med 10(5): e1001417.
60. Feiken DR, Audi A, Olack B, Bigogo GM, Polyak C, et al. (2010) Evaluation of the optimal recall period for disease symptoms in home-based morbidity surveillance in rural and urban Kenya. Int J Epidemiol 39(2): 450–8.
61. Hildenwall H, Lindkvist J, Tumwine JK, Bergqvist Y, Pariyo G, et al. (2008) Low validity of caretakers' reports on use of selected antimalarials and antibiotics in children with severe pneumonia at an urban hospital in Uganda. Trans Roy Soc Trop Med Hyg 103: 95–101.
62. Cotter C, Sturrock HJW, Hsiang MS, Liu J, Phillips AA, et al. (2013) The changing epidemiology of malaria elimination: new strategies for new challenges. Lancet 382: 900–911.

Prolonged Seasonality of Respiratory Syncytial Virus Infection among Preterm Infants in a Subtropical Climate

Chyong-Hsin Hsu[1]*, Chia-Ying Lin[1], Hsin Chi[2], Jui-Hsing Chang[1], Han-Yang Hung[1], Hsin-An Kao[1], Chun-Chih Peng[1], Wai-Tim Jim[1]

1 Department of Pediatrics, Division of Neonatology, Mackay Memorial Hospital, Taipei, Taiwan, **2** Department of Pediatrics, Division of Infectious Disease, Mackay Memorial Hospital, Taipei, Taiwan

Abstract

Objective: There is limited epidemiological data on the seasonality of respiratory syncytial virus (RSV) infection in subtropical climates, such as in Taiwan. This study aimed to assess RSV seasonality among children ≤24 months of age in Taiwan. We also assessed factors (gestational age [GA], chronologic age [CA], and bronchopulmonary dysplasia [BPD]) associated with RSV-associated hospitalization in preterm infants to confirm the appropriateness of the novel Taiwanese RSV prophylactic policy.

Study Design: From January 2000 to August 2010, 3572 children aged ≤24-months were admitted to Taipei Mackay Memorial Hospital due to RSV infection. The monthly RSV-associated hospitalization rate among children aged ≤24 months was retrospectively reviewed. Among these children, 378 were born preterm. The associations between GA, CA, and BPD and the incidence of RSV-associated hospitalization in the preterm infants were assessed.

Results: In children aged ≤24 months, the monthly distribution of RSV-associated hospitalization rates revealed a prolonged RSV season with a duration of 10 months. Infants with GAs ≤32 weeks and those who had BPD had the highest rates of RSV hospitalization ($P<0.001$). Preterm infants were most vulnerable to RSV infection within CA 9 months.

Conclusions: Given that Taiwan has a prolonged (10-month) RSV season, the American Academy of Pediatrics' recommendations for RSV prophylaxis are not directly applicable. The current Taiwanese guidelines for RSV prophylaxis, which specify palivizumab injection (a total six doses until CA 8–9 months) for preterm infants (those born before $28^{6/7}$ weeks GA or before $35^{6/7}$ weeks GA with BPD), are appropriate. This prophylaxis strategy may be applicable to other countries/regions with subtropical climates.

Editor: Oliver Schildgen, Kliniken der Stadt Köln gGmbH, Germany

Funding: The authors received no specific funding for this work.

Competing Interests: The authors have declared that no competing interests exist.

* Email: t200441@mmh.org.tw

Introduction

Respiratory syncytial virus (RSV) is the major pathogen of acute lower respiratory tract infection (ALRTI) in infancy and childhood [1,2]. Of note, premature infants are ten-fold more likely than term infants to develop complicated RSV [3] and experience higher rates of hospitalization and mortality [4]. As there is no effective etiopathogenetic treatment once an infant is infected by RSV, effective RSV prophylaxis is extremely important [5].

Since 1998, the American Academy of Pediatrics (AAP) has recommended the use of palivizumab for passive immunization against RSV [6]. The AAP recommendations account for seasonality of RSV infection ie, in temperate climates, RSV infection rates typically peak during the cold season, whereas in tropical climates RSV infection rates typically peak during the rainy season [7]. To date, however, there is limited information regarding RSV seasonality in subtropical climates [6,8]. As RSV surveillance is a globally important issue, a thorough understanding of RSV epidemiology in subtropical climates, such as that in Taiwan, is important for the optimization of global RSV prevention strategies. The current Taiwanese recommendations (published in 2010 December) for RSV prophylaxis specify six doses of palivizumab, targeting preterm infants born before $28^{6/7}$ weeks gestational age (GA) or those born before $35^{6/7}$ weeks GA with bronchopulmonary dysplasia (BPD), until a chronologic age (CA) of 8–9 months.

The purpose of this study was to determine the seasonality of RSV infection among children aged ≤24 months in Taiwan, a subtropical area. We also examined the effects of gestational age (GA), CA, and BPD on the incidence of RSV infection in preterm infants to confirm the appropriateness of the novel RSV prophylactic policy for premature infants in Taiwan.

Methods

Study Design and Data Collection

This retrospective single-center cohort study was conducted at Taipei Mackay Memorial Hospital, a tertiary medical center serving the greater Taipei metropolitan area in Northern Taiwan. Eligible participants were children aged ≤24 months who had a discharge diagnosis of RSV-associated bronchiolitis and/or pneumonia (ICD-9 CM Codes 466.11, 480.1, or 079.6) from January 2000 to August 2010. Preterm infants were included in the study if they were born in Taipei Mackay Memorial Hospital, had a GA <37 weeks, and were discharged alive from the neonatal intensive care unit (NICU) from 1 January 2000 to 31 August 2010. Prematurity was defined as birth before 37 weeks of GA (ie, GA ≤36 weeks and 6 days) in accordance with ICD-9 codes 765.10~765.19 and 765.01–765.09. Infants were excluded from the study if they had congenital heart disease, other than patent ductus arteriosus or a septal defect that was hemodynamically insignificant, or any congenital anomaly. Repeat admission infants were also excluded because repeated admission may be related to other potentially confounding factors (aside from GA, CA, and BPD) eg, the level of neutralizing antibodies in the serum, etc.

A case manager from the Premature Baby Foundation of Taiwan assisted with the contact of preterm babies with very low birth weight (≤1500 g), almost all of whom had regular outpatient department follow-up visits after their discharge from Taipei Mackay Memorial Hospital. Note: for reasons of convenience, most preterm infants return to Taipei Mackay Memorial Hospital for any additional care requirements after discharge.

The diagnosis of RSV infection was confirmed by examination of nasopharyngeal specimens using either RSV antigen-specific direct immunofluorescence assay or virus culture. We defined a respiratory illness as being attributable to RSV if the patient had RSV infection necessitating hospitalization and was for positive the RSV-specific antigen or had a positive virus culture between 7 days before and 3 days after admission [8]. As the incubation period for RSV is typically 3 to 5 days, patients who had symptoms that appeared ≥5 days after admission were considered to have nosocomial RSV infection [7–9]. In addition to RSV testing, patients underwent throat virus cultures after admission (no comorbid viruses were detected).

We obtained the following information from neonatal chart records: GA, birth weight, gender, dates of nursery admission and discharge, and time on oxygen in the NICU. The presence of BPD was also recorded. BPD was defined as persistent oxygen dependency 28 days after birth [10], the need for oxygen at 36 weeks postmenstrual age [11], and the presence of a characteristic chest roentgenographic finding in accordance with ICD-9 code 770.7. De-identified patient data were collated by a single neonatologist. All links between the final data analyzed and the original data were removed. The study was approved by the local Study Review Board and Ethics Committee of Taipei Mackay Memorial Hospital. Written informed consent was given by next of kin of the participants.

Outcome Measures

The monthly incidence of RSV-associated hospitalization for children aged ≤24 months was calculated for the study period to determine the seasonal activity of RSV infection at Taipei Mackay Memorial Hospital. We used the surveillance model for seasonality proposed by the Taiwan Centers for Disease Control (CDC) (Taiwan-CDC) [12,13] as well as the seasonality model of the US CDC [14] to determine RSV seasonality in Taiwan. The RSV season was defined as a period of two or more consecutive months in which the RSV-associated hospitalization rate was above the baseline rate. The baseline RSV-associated hospitalization rate was calculated by firstly determining the monthly RSV-associated hospitalization rate for children aged ≤24 months old as follows:

$$X_i = \frac{\text{Number of RSV hospitalizations}}{\text{Total number of hospitalizations}},$$

$$i = 1, 2, \ldots, 12 \text{ (from January to December).}$$

The average monthly RSV-associated hospitalization rate was then calculated as follows: $\frac{1}{12}\sum_{i=1}^{12} X_i = 29.67$ (‰)

The months with RSV-associated hospitalization rates <29.67 ‰ were defined as "non-epidemic months". The average monthly RSV-associated hospitalization rate of "non-epidemic months" was defined as the "baseline rate".

Infants who were born preterm were categorized into three GA-based groups for comparison of RSV-related hospitalization: ≤28, 29–32, and 33–36 weeks.

Children who were born preterm with RSV infection were further stratified into three subgroups according to their CA of onset for comparison: ≤9, 10–15, and 16–24 months.

RSV-infected premature infants with underlying BPD were identified for subgroup data analyses.

Statistical Analyses

Categorical variables are presented as counts and percentages, and were compared by chi-square test. Birth weight data are presented as median and full range. Statistical analyses were two-sided and carried out using SPSS software, version 20 (SPSS Inc., Chicago, IL). Statistical significance was indicated by $P<0.05$.

Results

Study Population

From January 2000 to August 2010, a total of 123,975 children aged ≤24 months were admitted to Taipei Mackay Memorial Hospital, 3,572 for RSV infection (Figure 1). Of these 5,572 children who were born premature (boys: n = 3048; girls: n = 2524; median birth weight: 1848 g [range: 522–3386 g]), 413 were admitted for RSV infection. After the exclusion of repeated admissions and infants who had nosocomial infections (Figure 1), 378 preterm infants were included in the study (boys: n = 230; girls: n = 148; median birth weight: 1859 g [range: 522–2864 g]). Of these infants, 67 had underlying BPD and 311 did not. Hence, 10.6% (378/3572) of the admissions due to RSV infection were preterm infants. The attributable mortality rate for RSV infection among the preterm infants was 7.9 ‰ (n = 3) in our study population.

Monthly Incidence of RSV-Associated Hospitalization and Assessment of Seasonality

The monthly incidence of RSV-associated hospitalization among children aged ≤24 months in the study period is shown in Figure 2. Figure 2A summarizes the monthly RSV-associated hospitalization rate for the entire observation period. Figure 2B summarizes the average monthly RSV-associated hospitalization rate from January to December for the observation period. The baseline monthly RSV-related hospitalization rate was 18.52 ‰. The RSV season was defined as a period of two or more

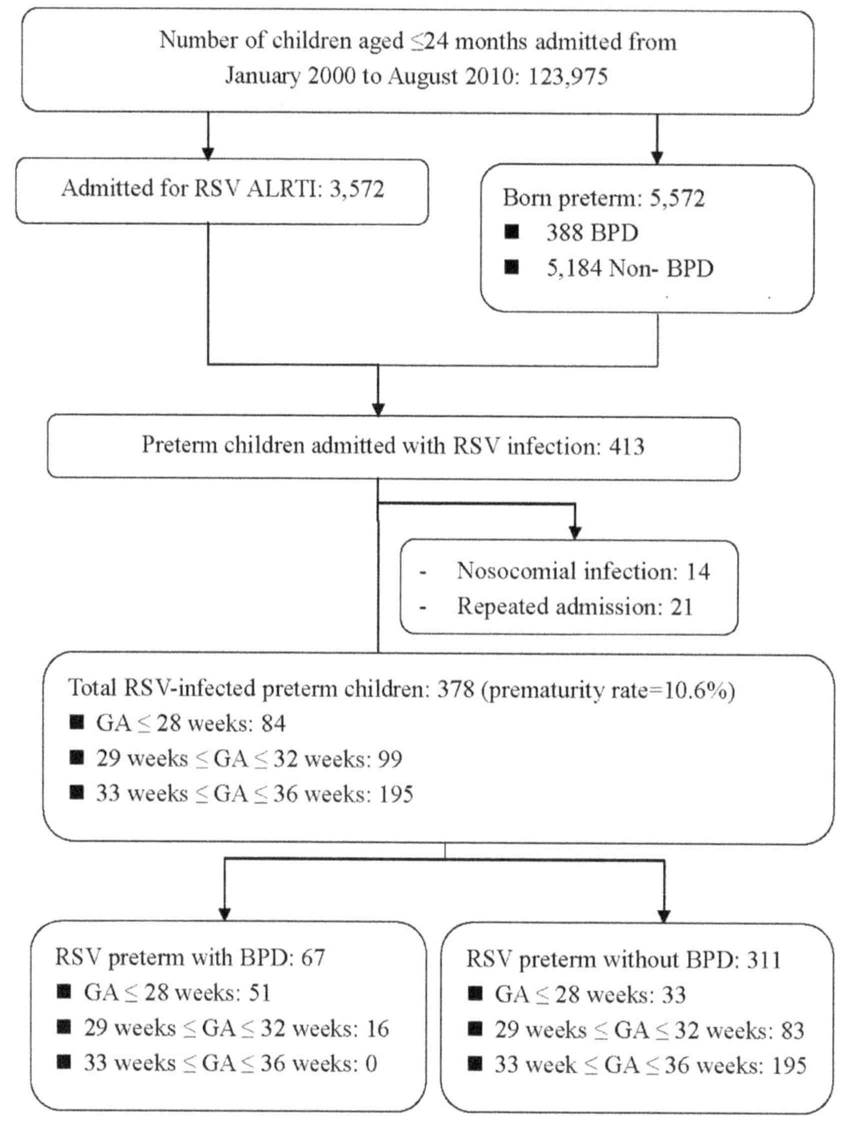

Figure 1. Flow chart of infants aged ≤24 months included in the study. ALRTI, acute lower respiratory tract infection; BPD, bronchopulmonary dysplasia; GA, gestational age; RSV, respiratory syncytial virus.

consecutive months, in which the RSV-associated hospitalization rate was above the basal rate. In our study, there was a prolonged, continuous RSV season lasting 10 months.

The Impact of Gestational Age (GA) on RSV-Associated Hospitalization

The proportion of infants with RSV infection by GA (among the 5,572 infants who were born preterm) is summarized overall and by BPD status in Table 1. There were no differences in the rate of RSV infection by GA among infants who had underlying BPD. Of the non-BPD infants, those with GAs ≤28 weeks and 29–32 weeks had a significantly higher rate of RSV-associated hospitalization compared with those with a GA 33–36 weeks ($P<$ 0.001).

Effect of BPD on RSV Infection

Of the 5,572 premature infants, 388 had BPD and 5184 did not. A significantly higher proportion of infants who had BPD experienced RSV infection compared infants who did not have BPD (67/388; 17.3% vs 311/5184; 6.0%, $P<0.001$).

Trends in RSV-Related Hospitalization by CA and Prematurity

The proportion of infants hospitalized due to RSV infection by CA of onset (categorized by GA and BPD status) is presented in Figure 3. As most extremely low birth weight preterm infants (birth weight ≤1000 g) and very low birth weight infants (birth weight ≤1500 g) usually remained in hospital for 2–3 months after birth, we used a CA of 9 months (ie, almost 6 months after discharge) as the first cut-off point, and thereafter stratified the cut-off points by 6-month blocks to assess the timing of when preterm neonates were most vulnerable to RSV infection after discharge. Therefore, RSV-associated hospitalization rates were analyzed for infants grouped into three age cohorts: (≤9 months, 10 to 15 months, and 16 to 24 months). Moreover, the preterm infants with RSV with and without BPD were divided into 3 GA categories to

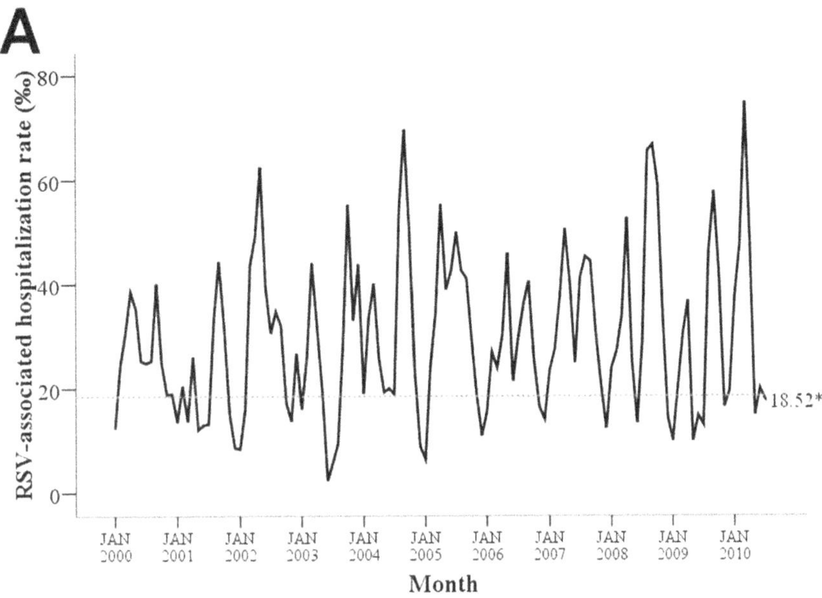

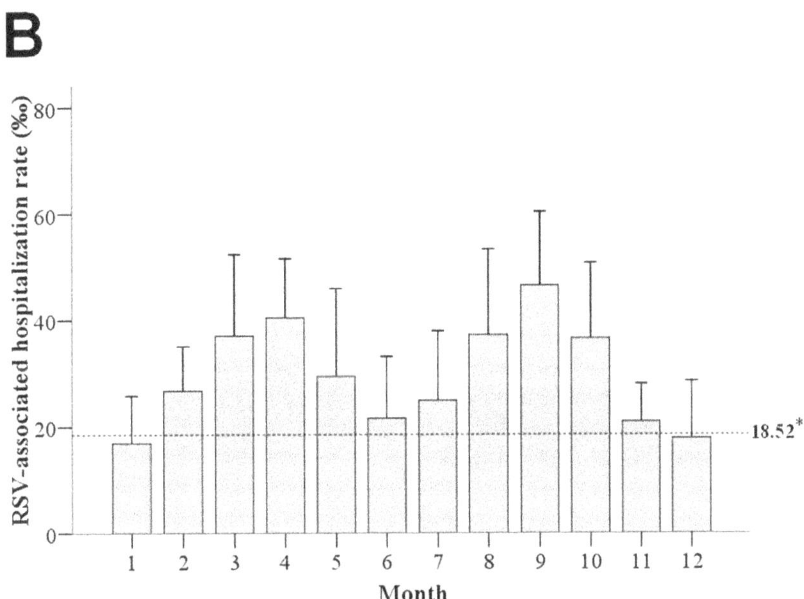

Figure 2. Monthly distribution of the RSV-associated hospitalization rate among all infants aged ≤24 months in the study (from January 2000 to August 2010). *The baseline rate of RSV infection was 18.52 ‰. RSV, respiratory syncytial virus. (A) Monthly RSV-associated hospitalization rates for the entire observation period. (B) Average monthly RSV-associated hospitalization rates from January to December for the observation period.

Table 1. Respiratory syncytial virus infection by gestational age for infants aged ≤24 months who were born premature (overall and by bronchopulmonary dysplasia status).

Infants	Gestational Age			*P* Value
	≤28 weeks	29–32 weeks	33–36 weeks	
Overall (378/5572), n/N (%)	84/584 (14.4)*	99/935 (10.6)*	195/4053 (4.8)	<0.001
With underlying BPD (67/388), n/N (%)	51/301 (16.9)	16/83 (19.3)	0/4 (0)	0.825
Without underlying BPD (311/5184), n/N (%)	33/283 (11.6)*	83/852 (9.7)*	195/4049 (4.8)	<0.001

BPD, bronchopulmonary dysplasia.
N = total premature babies (by gestational age); n = RSV-infected premature babies (by gestational age).
*Indicates a significant difference compared with gestational age 33–36 weeks.

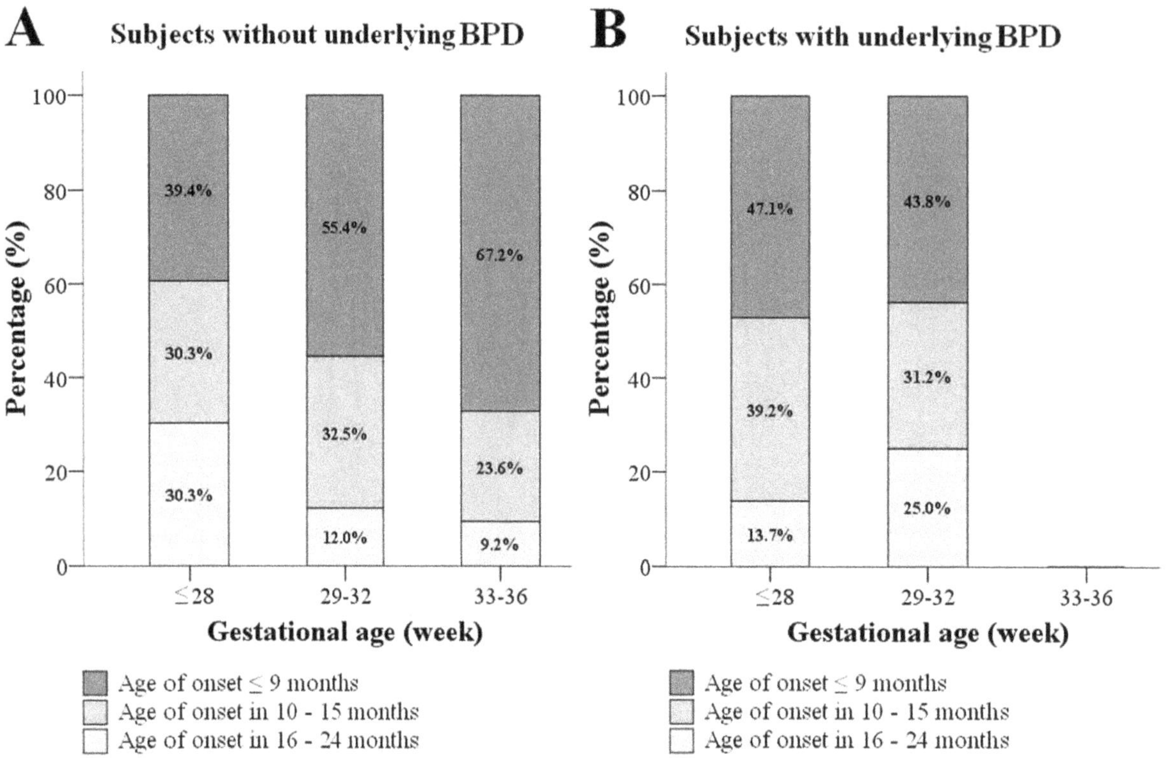

Figure 3. Percentage of infants (born premature) aged ≤24 months-with respiratory syncytial virus infection by age of onset (chronologic age), by gestational age, and BPD status (A: without BPD, n = 311; B: with BPD, n = 67). Note: there were no infants with underlying BPD at gestational age 33–36 months. BPD, bronchopulmonary dysplasia.

facilitate GA comparisons: ≤28 weeks, 29–32 weeks, and 33–36 weeks.

Overall. Overall, 58.5% (221/378) of infants admitted due to RSV infections experienced onset within 9 months, 28.5% (108/378) experienced onset within 10–15 months, and 12.9% (49/378) experienced onset within 16–24 months. Regardless of BPD status and GA, RSV infection most frequently occurred within 9 months, followed by 10–15 months, and 16–24 months.

Without underlying BPD. The results for infants without underlying BPD are summarized in Figure 3A. Regardless of GA, RSV infection was most common within 9 months, followed by 10–15 months, and then 16–24 months.

With underlying BPD. The results for infants with underlying BPD are summarized in Figure 3B. There were no infants born at GA 33–36 weeks with BPD. Regardless of GA, RSV infection was most common within 9 months, followed by 10–15 months, and then 16–24 months.

Discussion

RSV-prophylaxis strategies are globally important given that RSV circulates throughout the world. To the best of our knowledge, this is the first population-based, retrospective cohort study demonstrating prolonged seasonality of RSV infection (duration = 10 months) among children aged ≤24 months in a subtropical climate. This is different from RSV epidemiology data obtained in the United States, Canada, and European countries. The prolonged RSV seasonality makes the establishment of an RSV prevention policy challenging because one of the most important elements of the current RSV prophylactic guideline recommended by AAP is the existence of a distinct RSV season for 5 months from November to March (or from December to April) in temperate climate zones [15]. Other countries located in subtropical climate regions, such as Hong Kong, Northern Vietnam, and southern China [16,17] are also faced with the potential problem of RSV being present throughout the year, which complicates the development of effective prophylactic programs.

Taiwan is located at 23°0′N~25°5′N latitude and 120° 39' E~121° 33' E longitude; hence, the entire country is located in a subtropical climate region. Our result confirmed that there is a prolonged RSV season in Taiwan. In a previous report, Huang et al [6]reported that there was RSV infection year-round in Taiwan. Two previous retrospective studies [3,18] also reported an apparent biannual pattern of RSV infection in Taiwan. The explanation for the disparate study findings may relate to differences in study design, unequal-aged based populations, population characteristics, and sample size. The prolonged seasonality in our study may be explained by the lack of marked seasonal changes in temperature and the lack of any profound effect of rainfall in Taiwan [19].

Given our finding of prolonged RSV seasonality, the AAP guideline on RSV prophylaxis with palivizumab are not directly applicable in Taiwan. The AAP guidelines specify a total of 5 doses (as the maximum) of monthly palivizumab to prevent RSV infection because the average duration of RSV season in temperate climates is 5 months [15]. The AAP guidelines also specify that palivizumab should be given during the RSV season to protect high-risk groups such as premature infants (GA $\leq 28^{6/7}$ weeks) or infants with BPD. Such an approach is not practical in a subtropical area with an RSV season lasting 10 months. Indeed, high-risk preterm infants would require 10 doses of palivizumab during the RSV season in Taiwan according to the AAP guidelines; this is not economically feasible. Hence, factors aside from seasonality must be considered in developing a reasonable and practical prophylaxis strategy in Taiwan (and presumably other countries in subtropical climate regions). Our findings suggest that GA, CA, and BPD are three important factors that should be considered in the establishment of cost–effective palivizumab prophylaxis strategies.

Our finding that preterm infants who have BPD have an increased risk for RSV infection are consistent with those determined in the IMpact RSV and other studies [5,18,20–22]. Our findings are also in keeping with those of the IRIS study group [21] who reported that preterm infants with either a GA ≤ 32 weeks or those with BPD have a very high risk of RSV-associated hospitalization. Of note, we found that CA ≤9 months was the most susceptible period for RSV infection among preterm infants in a subtropical climate with prolonged RSV seasonality. Only one previous report has examined this relationship and found that RSV-related hospitalization was most commonly observed among (predominantly term-born) infants aged 3–6 months [23]. Different to the findings from the IRIS and FLIP studies, which indicate that the risk of RSV infection is highest among infants with a CA <3 or 6 months at the start of the RSV season, our findings suggest that once preterm infants are discharged, monthly palivizumab should be administered for a total 6 doses until CA 8–9 months. There are several potential explanations for our finding regarding CA and the risk of RSV infection. First, preterm infants typically remain in the intensive care unit during the first 2–3 months after birth, so the risk of infection is highest within the first 6 months after discharge ie, 8–9 months of CA. Second, before CA 9 months, parents may become less vigilant about the potential risks of infection due to the relatively improved physiological conditions of their premature infants. Third, infants with underlying BPD (or other co-morbidities) often require frequent outpatient follow-up visits or interventions before CA 9 months, which may increase their likelihood of exposure to RSV. Finally, in Taiwan, infants' mothers return to work around this time and infants are typically cared for by babysitters thereafter. These babysitters usually look after more than one infant, thus increasing the risk of cross-infection. Our findings indicate that CA ≤9 months is a critical period for re-admission of preterm infants; hence, the first dose of palivizumab should be given 3–4 days before discharge and monthly thereafter until CA 8–9 months.

Although we employed a number of measures to minimize potential bias, our study does have several limitations. First, palivizumab was not widely available until 2010 December in Taiwan; hence, we could not conduct a prospective study to assess seasonality before 2010. Widespread prophylaxis with palivizumab from 2010 will make it difficult to collect the necessary epidemiologic data to analyze the risk factors for RSV-induced ALRTI in the future. For the same reason, there was no control group in our study. Despite being retrospective in nature, our study did encompass a significant (10-year) period of time and thus, we believe, contributes important epidemiological information. Second, although the RSV screening method used had very high sensitivity (93%) and specificity (98%), it is possible that some relevant cases of RSV infection were missed. Third, not all infants with ALRTI underwent RSV rapid test or throat virus culture. Hence, the RSV infection rate may have been underestimated. Fourth, as this study was carried out at a single institution, an additional population-based study acquiring data from multiple centers is warranted to confirm our findings and provide valuable information that could be used to optimize RSV prophylaxis. Despite the aforementioned limitations, we suggest that the data presented herein are extremely important, and provide a reasonable representation of RSV infection among children aged ≤24 months in a subtropical climate.

In our study, both GA≤28 weeks and GA 29–32 weeks were high-risk groups for RSV infection. Since December 2010, the Taiwan Society of Neonatology advised the Bureau of National Health Insurance in Taiwan to provide a total six monthly doses of palivizumab injections to premature infants with a GA $\leq 28^{6/7}$ weeks or prematurity with BPD and born before GA $35^{6/7}$ weeks, including the first dose before discharge and continuing until five months after discharge. Therefore, eligible infants will be protected by CA of 8–9 months, the most critical period of susceptibility to RSV infection. The current policy in Taiwan, subtropical climate country with prolonged RSV seasonality, is appropriate and may serve as a reference for other countries in subtropical climates in which the AAP guideline may not be applicable for RSV prophylaxis.

Acknowledgments

The authors acknowledge the kind assistance and wonderful team work provided by the staff at Taipei Mackay Memorial Hospital.

Author Contributions

Conceived and designed the experiments: CHH. Performed the experiments: CYL. Analyzed the data: CYL. Contributed reagents/materials/analysis tools: CHH CYL HC JHC HYH HAK CCP WTJ. Wrote the paper: CHH CYL HC JHC HYH HAK CCP WTJ.

References

1. Hall CB, Weinberg GA, Iwane MK, Blumkin AK, Edwards KM, et al. (2009) The burden of respiratory syncytial virus infection in young children. N Engl J Med. 360: 588–598.
2. Nair H, Nokes DJ, Gessner BD, Dherani M, Madhi SA, et al. (2010) Global burden of acute lower respiratory infections due to respiratory syncytial virus in young children: a systematic review and meta-analysis. Lancet. 375: 1545–1555.
3. Chi H, Chang IS, Tsai FY, Huang LM, Shao PL, et al. (2011) Epidemiological study of hospitalization associated with respiratory syncytial virus infection in Taiwanese children between 2004 and 2007. J Formos Med Assoc. 110: 388–396.
4. Tatochenko V, Uchaikin V, Gorelov A, Gudkov K, Campbell A, et al. (2010) Epidemiology of respiratory syncytial virus in children </=2 years of age hospitalized with lower respiratory tract infections in the Russian Federation: a prospective, multicenter study. Clin Epidemiol. 2: 221–227.
5. (1998) Palivizumab, a humanized respiratory syncytial virus monoclonal antibody, reduces hospitalization from respiratory syncytial virus infection in high-risk infants. The IMpact-RSV Study Group. Pediatrics. 102: 531–537.
6. Huang YC, Lin TY, Chang LY, Wong KS, Ning SC (2001) Epidemiology of respiratory syncytial virus infection among paediatric inpatients in northern Taiwan. Eur J Pediatr. 160: 581–582.
7. Carbonell-Estrany X, Quero J, Group IS (2001) Hospitalization rates for respiratory syncytial virus infection in premature infants born during two consecutive seasons. Pediatr Infect Dis J. 20: 874–879.
8. Joffe S, Escobar GJ, Black SB, Armstrong MA, Lieu TA (1999) Rehospitalization for respiratory syncytial virus among premature infants. Pediatrics. 104: 894–899.
9. Figueras-Aloy J, Carbonell-Estrany X, Quero-Jimenez J, Fernandez-Colomer B, Guzman-Cabanas J, et al. (2008) FLIP-2 Study: risk factors linked to respiratory syncytial virus infection requiring hospitalization in premature infants born in Spain at a gestational age of 32 to 35 weeks. Pediatr Infect Dis J. 27: 788–793.
10. Northway WH Jr., Rosan RC, Porter DY (1967) Pulmonary disease following respirator therapy of hyaline-membrane disease. Bronchopulmonary dysplasia. N Engl J Med. 276: 357–368.
11. Christine AG, Sherin UD (2012) Avery's disease of the newborn (9th ed). Philadelphia, PA: Elsevier.

12. Chu SC, Wang ET, Liu DP (2013) A review of prevention and control for enterovirus infections in Asia. Taiwan CDC Taiwan Epidemiology Bulletin. 29.
13. Wu TN, Tsai SF, Li SF, Lee TF, Huang TM, et al. (1999) Sentinel surveillance for enterovirus 71, Taiwan, 1998. Emerg Infect Dis. 5: 458–460.
14. US CDC (2013) Overview of influenza surveillance in the US. 17 October 2013.
15. Committee on Infectious Diseases (2009) From the American Academy of Pediatrics: Policy statements–Modified recommendations for use of palivizumab for prevention of respiratory syncytial virus infections. Pediatrics. 124: 1694–1701.
16. Chan PK, Sung RY, Fung KS, Hui M, Chik KW, et al. (1999) Epidemiology of respiratory syncytial virus infection among paediatric patients in Hong Kong: seasonality and disease impact. Epidemiol Infect. 123: 257–262.
17. Stensballe LG, Devasundaram JK, Simoes EA (2003) Respiratory syncytial virus epidemics: the ups and downs of a seasonal virus. Pediatr Infect Dis J. 22: S21–32.
18. Lee JT, Chang LY, Wang LC, Kao CL, Shao PL, et al. (2007) Epidemiology of respiratory syncytial virus infection in northern Taiwan, 2001–2005 – seasonality, clinical characteristics, and disease burden. J Microbiol Immunol Infect. 40: 293–301.
19. Tsai HP, Kuo PH, Liu CC, Wang JR (2001) Respiratory viral infections among pediatric inpatients and outpatients in Taiwan from 1997 to 1999. J Clin Microbiol. 39: 111–118.
20. Kusuda S, Takahashi N, Saitoh T, Terai M, Kaneda H, et al. (2011) Survey of pediatric ward hospitalization due to respiratory syncytial virus infection after the introduction of palivizumab to high-risk infants in Japan. Pediatr Int. 53: 368–373.
21. Carbonell-Estrany X, Quero J, Bustos G, Cotero A, Domenech E, et al. (2000) Rehospitalization because of respiratory syncytial virus infection in premature infants younger than 33 weeks of gestation: a prospective study. IRIS Study Group. Pediatr Infect Dis J. 19: 592–597.
22. Boyce TG, Mellen BG, Mitchel EF Jr., Wright PF, Griffin MR (2000) Rates of hospitalization for respiratory syncytial virus infection among children in medicaid. J Pediatr. 137: 865–870.
23. Fryzek JP, Martone WJ, Groothuis JR (2011) Trends in chronologic age and infant respiratory syncytial virus hospitalization: an 8-year cohort study. Adv Ther. 28: 195–201.

23

Caregiver Perceptions and Motivation for Disclosing or Concealing the Diagnosis of HIV Infection to Children Receiving HIV Care in Mbarara, Uganda: A Qualitative Study

Julius Kiwanuka[1]*, Edgar Mulogo[2], Jessica E. Haberer[3,4]

1 Department of Paediatrics and Child Health, Mbarara University of Science and Technology, Mbarara, Uganda, 2 Department of Community Health, Mbarara University of Science and Technology, Mbarara, Uganda, 3 Massachusetts General Hospital, Center for Global Health, Boston, Massachusetts, United States of America, 4 Harvard Medical School, Boston, Massachusetts, United States of America

Abstract

Background: Disclosure of the diagnosis of HIV to HIV-infected children is challenging for caregivers. Despite current recommendations, data suggest that levels of disclosure of HIV status to HIV-infected children receiving care in resource-limited settings are very low. Few studies describe the disclosure process for children in these settings, particularly the motivators, antecedent goals, and immediate outcomes of disclosure to HIV-infected children. This study examined caregivers' perception of the disclosure concept prior to disclosure, their motivation towards or away from disclosure, and their short- and long-term intentions for disclosure to their HIV-infected children.

Methods: In-depth interviews were conducted with primary caregivers of 40 HIV-infected children (ages 5–15 years) who were receiving HIV care but did not know their HIV status.

Results: Caregivers of HIV-infected children mainly perceived disclosure as a single event rather than a process of gradual delivery of information about the child's illness. They viewed disclosure as potentially beneficial both to children and themselves, as well as an opportunity to explain the parents' role in the transmission of HIV to the children. Caregivers desired to personally conduct the disclosure; however, most reported being over-whelmed with fear of negative outcomes and revealed a lack of self-efficacy towards managing the disclosure process. Consequently, most cope by deception to avoid or delay disclosure until they perceive their own readiness to disclose.

Conclusions: Interventions for HIV disclosure should consider that caregivers may desire to be directly responsible for disclosure to children under their care. They, however, need to be empowered with practical skills to recognize opportunities to initiate the disclosure process early, as well as supported to manage it in a phased, developmentally appropriate manner. The potential role for peer counselors in the disclosure process deserves further study.

Editor: Grace C. John-Stewart, University of Washingto, United States of America

Funding: The study was funded by a mentorship grant from the Canada-Africa Prevention Trials (CAPT) Network (captnetwork.org). Dr. Haberer was supported by the US National Institutes of Health (K23MH087228). The funders had no role in study design, data collection and analysis, decision to publish, or preparation of the manuscript.

Competing Interests: The authors have declared that no competing interests exist.

* E-mail: jpkiwanuka@gmail.com

Introduction

Globally, paediatric HIV infection continues to be a major problem. Approximately 3.3 million children younger than 15 years are living with HIV, with 2.9 million of them in sub-Saharan Africa [1]. In Uganda, just over 7% of the adult population and about 1% of children less than 5 years are HIV-infected [2]. There has been considerable progress in recent years towards making comprehensive HIV treatment accessible to children in Uganda; paediatric antiretroviral therapy (ART) services have been scaled up to over 300 health facilities throughout the country. With increasing availability of accessible, effective combination ART, paediatric HIV has been transformed from a rapidly fatal infection to a chronic disease requiring complex lifelong treatment and support [3].

The increasing survival of perinatally HIV-infected children into adolescence and adulthood has brought to the fore new and important challenges relating to adherence to long-term treatment, as well as development issues including, among many, peer relationships, puberty, and sexuality [4,5]. The issue of HIV status disclosure - whether, when, and how to inform HIV-infected children about their HIV status - has gained increased attention in recent years [6,7].

Disclosure of HIV status is one of the most complex challenges facing individuals who live with HIV/AIDS. It entails communication about a highly stigmatized, life-threatening, transmissible and, currently, still incurable infection. It is usually approached with much anxiety and fear of negative consequences, notably stigmatization and discrimination, and is often avoided altogether [8]. Although unintended disclosure may occur, HIV-infected adults typically make a choice to disclose their status to others. The motivation to disclose and the immediate consequences of disclosure are viewed from the affected individual's viewpoint [9].

The disclosure process in paediatric HIV is more complex and less well understood. In children, the process involves consideration, by the caregiver, of the child's developmental and emotional readiness to receive the information about his/her HIV status, as well as attitudes and motivations/goals of the caregiver and/or health worker towards disclosure [9,10]. Caregivers and health-care workers are presented with many challenges around disclosure, including deciding what is in the child's best interest and when, why, and how much information about his/her HIV status should be shared with him/her [11].

The World Health Organization and national paediatric HIV guidelines [6,12] recommend developmentally appropriate HIV status disclosure to adolescents and school-age children. The WHO made the strong recommendation that children of school age should be told their HIV positive status; younger children should be told their status incrementally to accommodate their cognitive skills and emotional maturity, in preparation for full disclosure [13]. Expected benefits of disclosure include enhanced access to support services, better treatment adherence, improved family communication, and better long-term health and emotional well-being for the child [14,15]. Reports generally indicate positive outcomes associated with disclosure in children, although stigma and depression have been reported, especially in the short-term [16-19].

However, current data from resource-limited settings show typically low rates of disclosure to children, ranging between 10–38% [7,18,20–22]. In a recent study conducted in the Mbarara Regional Referral Hospital in Uganda, caregivers reported that only 31% of children between 5 and 17 years had received full disclosure of their HIV status [23]. A much smaller proportion (about 7%) of children was classified as receiving partial disclosure, despite being within the age range for which initiation of the disclosure process is recommended. Additionally, because disclosure of perinatal HIV is generally delayed until late childhood or adolescence, children usually receive ART for long durations of time before the reasons for this prolonged therapy are fully discussed with them.

Reasons for these low rates of disclosure are not fully understood. In studies mainly from the developed world, caregivers cite a belief that the child is either not old enough or not ready [24,25] or is not sufficiently mature to understand and/or cope with the diagnosis [26]; concern that if they disclosed, their child would not keep the diagnosis private; or worry that children would be exposed to ostracism and negative reactions from community and family [24–26]. Some HIV-infected mothers have reported the concern that their child will be angry with them for transmitting the virus [25]. Further research is needed to understand the disclosure process in low resource settings.

Moreover, few interventions to support disclosure are available and are limited to developed settings. Further data is needed to develop effective, locally appropriate HIV disclosure interventions that can be used to facilitate and support effective and beneficial disclosure in developing settings. Such interventions require an understanding of the disclosure process, including factors that affect the likelihood and the outcomes of disclosure, as well as the drivers of caregivers' decision-making towards disclosure (or concealment) of HIV status to children under their care [9]. This study examines caregivers' perception of the disclosure concept prior to disclosure, their motivation towards or away from disclosure, and their short- and long-term intentions for disclosure to their HIV-infected children in a rural Ugandan population.

Methods

Ethical statement

This study was approved by the Mbarara University Institutional Research Ethics Committee (MUST-IREC) and the Uganda National Council for Science and Technology. Written, informed consent was obtained from all caregivers

Overview

In-depth interviews were conducted with the primary caregivers of HIV-infected children (ages 5–15 years) who were receiving HIV care but did not know their HIV status.

Study setting

The study was conducted in the Paediatric HIV Clinic of the Mbarara Regional Referral Hospital, Mbarara, Uganda, located about 250 km southwest of Kampala. The hospital is a tertiary centre serving the predominantly rural population of southwestern Uganda and also serves as a primary health care facility for the population of Mbarara Municipality (approximately 100,000 people). The Paediatric HIV Clinic began providing ART in 2002 and has treated over 1,000 children cumulatively. Approximately 700 children are currently registered for comprehensive HIV care in the clinic. The children have access to free care and treatment, including ART, and the quality of medical care is considerably higher than that available elsewhere in the region. Counseling for ART adherence is offered routinely to caregivers; however, no specific training is given to caregivers to assist them with disclosure.

Participants

The study enrolled adults who identified themselves as the current primary caregivers of children receiving HIV care in the hospital. A primary caregiver was defined as an adult, living in the same household as the child in question, who was ordinarily responsible for supervising the care of the child in the home and for bringing the child to hospital for his/her regular clinic visits. Caregivers were eligible for the study if they were above 18 years of age, had a child between 5 and 15 years in the clinic, and, to the caregiver's knowledge, disclosure of the child's HIV status had not taken place. Participants were enrolled consecutively during clinic visits. Interviews were reviewed continually until theme saturation was achieved [27]. No selection was made based on age or gender. Institutionalized children and those in boarding school were excluded, as the circumstances for disclosure likely differ greatly from those of children living in households.

Interviews

Individual in-depth interviews were conducted, by a research assistant trained in qualitative interview methods, in a closed room away from other clinic patients and the children, to ensure privacy and avoid unplanned disclosure to the children. According to the individual subject's choice, interviews were conducted in English or Runyankore (the main local dialect in the region). With permission, all interviews were digitally recorded and later transcribed. Runyankore transcripts were translated into English post-hoc. Each caregiver was interviewed one time for 50–60 minutes on average.

Interviews began with structured questions on individual characteristics (e.g., demographics, time since diagnosis, educational levels of both caregiver and child), family characteristics (e.g., relationship of caregiver to child, marital status, child's orphan status) and the health and HIV status of the caregiver. An interview guide was developed using a *priori* themes that were anticipated based on a review of the literature and consideration of what the study team considered would emerge based on their experience interacting with HIV-infected children and their caregivers. The interviewer started the interview with open-ended questions in four main areas. First, they were asked for their personal experiences caring for HIV-infected children. Second, caregivers were asked questions to explore their perception of disclosure to children both in terms of the content and scope of the disclosure conversation. They were asked whether and when children should be told their HIV status, how much they should be told, how they should be told, and by whom. The interviewer then defined four main components as essential elements of full disclosure: 1) naming the disease (using the label HIV/AIDS or its equivalent in local dialect), 2) discussing the consequences and implications of having HIV infection, 3) discussing the origin/source of the child's HIV infection and 4) discussing the fact that the child's HIV infection can be transmitted to others. Caregivers were then asked to discuss if they would find aspects of disclosure easy or difficult. They were also asked their thoughts on potential mediating factors that may facilitate or hinder successful disclosure. Third, the interviewer asked caregivers to discuss both benefits and perceived potential harms from disclosing to the children. Finally, information was also collected on the caregivers' specific intentions regarding disclosure to children in their care, including whether and when they intended to disclose, and their personal goals for any disclosure.

Data analysis

Data were analysed using directed content analysis [28]. Recorded interviews were transcribed and, if needed, translated directly into English by the primary interviewer. The lead investigator (JK) reviewed the transcripts for accuracy by playing back the recordings while reading through the transcripts. Thematic category construction methods were used to inductively analyze and represent the data [29]. The content analysis proceeded in three phases. In the first phase, two analysts (JK, EM) reviewed the transcripts and created codes based on topics that arose frequently and/or had relevance to perceptions, motivations, or intentions around disclosure. A preliminary codebook was developed based on 20% of the interviews and refined on review of another 20% of interviews. Key definitions of the codes were then generated and further modifications were conducted iteratively after applying the codes to the remainder of the interviews. Once the codebook was complete, the analysts conducted open coding, in which they applied a code from the codebook to a block of text to indicate the primary theme or idea being expressed. During the second phase the two analysts grouped similar codes and identified relationships between codes to identify emerging patterns of experience expressed in the data. In the third phase, summary coding, the investigative team (JK, EM, and JH) identified the central themes that emerged from analysis and separated them from outliers, to summarize the key findings across all interviews.

Results

Description of participants

A summary of the main characteristics of the participants is presented in Table 1. Overall, 44 eligible caregivers were approached to participate. Four caregivers declined because of time constraints. Forty caregivers were interviewed, 33 of whom were the HIV-infected biological parents (32 mothers and one father) of the children for whom they cared. The rest were HIV-uninfected or untested. All except one were females, and 31 of them were receiving ART. Most HIV-infected caregivers reported having disclosed their own status to someone in their family or community. The majority of children were between 5 and 10 years, and more than 75% were receiving ART at the time of the study.

Key themes

Five major themes were identified (Table 2): 1) Caregiver understanding of the concept of HIV disclosure, 2) Caregiver attitudes, motivations, and goals for disclosure, 3) Avoiding disclosure, 4) Coping before disclosure through deception, and 5) Intentions for disclosure.

Caregiver understanding of the concept of HIV disclosure

Before hearing the interviewer's definition of the components of full disclosure, caregivers emphasized two points about their understanding of the concept: 1) openness in telling the truth about the disease and 2) the importance of complete disclosure, meaning the source of the child's infection, the health implications of HIV, and potential to transmit the infection to others.

Telling the truth. Most of the caregivers discussed disclosure as a "truth-telling" event, primarily focused on naming the disease. It involved being honest and open, for the first time, to the child about his/her HIV status and specifically using the terms HIV or AIDS.

> *"...it means telling the truth about the disease... It means you to be open and telling her that you are HIV-infected" (37-year-old mother of 10-year-old girl)*

Many caregivers discussed this truth telling as a single event that could not be drawn out into more than a single disclosure conversation. Thus, one caregiver stated:

> *"Once you have prepared yourself to disclose to the child you have to say each and everything. You tell the child that she has HIV, and she got it from me. Because if you do not mention that then what will you say she is suffering from?" (35-year-old aunt of 10-year-old girl)*

Importance of complete disclosure. Caregivers discussed what they felt were critical components of complete disclosure. Three elements emerged, namely discussing the source of the child's infection, health implications of having HIV, and potential to transmit the infection to others.

A significant proportion of caregivers emphasized the importance of telling the child where and how he/she was infected with HIV. They recognised that this would mean inevitable disclosure of their own status. They felt, however, that they needed to dispel confusion in the child's mind since the child may only know HIV to be sexually transmitted. For some caregivers this discussion also needed to include a clarification that the transmission of HIV from the mother was unintentional.

Table 1. Characteristics of caregivers and children (n = 40).

Characteristic	Frequency	Percent
Caregiver's age (years)		
21–30	10	25.0%
31–40	20	50.0%
41–50	6	15.0%
51–60	3	7.5%
61–70	1	2.5%
Caregiver's sex		
Male	1	2.50%
Female	39	97.5%
Caregiver's relationship to the child		
Mother	32	80.0%
Father	1	2.5%
Grandmother	3	7.5%
Aunt	4	10.0%
Highest education level attained		
No school	3	7.5%
Primary school	28	70.0%
Secondary school	7	17.5%
Tertiary education	2	5.0%
Caregiver's HIV status		
Infected	33	82.5%
Uninfected or untested	7	17.5%
Caregiver on HAART		
Yes	31	77.5%
No	9	22.5%
Child's age (years)		
5–7	16	40.0%
8–10	17	42.5%
11–15	7	17.5%
Child's sex		
Male	20	50.0%
Female	20	50.0%
Child's age at diagnosis (years)		
0–0.9	3	7.5%
1–4.9	24	60.0%
5–9.9	12	30.0%
10–14.9	1	2.5%
Child on HAART		
Yes	31	77.5%
No	9	22.5%

HAART = highly active antiretroviral therapy.

"I understand that you should tell the child the truth.... and you explain to him in detail how she got the disease. Tell her that you got it from me. Tell her that me as a parent I did not intend this to happen." (32-year-old mother of 8-year-old girl)

Many caregivers included a discussion of the long-term consequences of HIV to the child as a necessary component of disclosure.

Table 2. Summary of categories/themes.

Caregiver understanding of the concept of HIV disclosure
Telling the truth
Complete disclosure; important components of full disclosure
Caregiver motivations for disclosure
The child should know
Benefits of disclosing
The caregiver has a responsibility to disclose
Avoiding disclosure
Fear of negative outcomes
Feeling unable to disclose
Coping before disclosure through deception
Intentions for disclosure

"You have to tell her that the disease you have is not curable, it will not go away. You will have to take medicine constantly. You will have to continue taking it, and never interrupt it. If you do that you will die." (33-year-old mother of 9-year-old boy)

The majority of caregivers discussed the importance of emphasizing to the child that they could transmit HIV to others through some forms of contact in the course of regular activities, like play for young children or through sexual activity in older children. As such, including this component in the disclosure package was justified as necessary to protect the child's contacts from accidental exposure to HIV. In some cases, this emphasis was used as a means for controlling the child's behaviour around sexuality.

"Tell him that once you are of age, be careful and don't engage yourself in acts of sexual immorality. The most important thing the child should understand is not to have sexual intercourse. Other things will be told to him along the way." (38-year-old father of 13-year-old boy)

Caregiver motivations for disclosure

Caregivers were unequivocal in their affirmation that children should be told that they have HIV. The three main sub-themes around their motivations for such disclosure included 1) the child should know, 2) benefits for the care of the child, and 3) the caregiver's responsibility to disclose.

The child should know. Caregivers generally felt that HIV-infected children needed to know their HIV status to make sense of whatever was going on in their lives, especially in terms of their health. They felt that the child has a right to this explanation.

"Yes, it is right to tell them. When the child is with other children, and they keep on teasing him because they know his mother had HIV, and they know that he has HIV and for him he doesn't know... Once you tell him and he knows, even if he gets annoyed he still knows what he is suffering from." (26-year-old aunt of 11-year-old boy)

Benefits of disclosing. Caregivers perceived a range of potential benefits in the HIV-infected child knowing his/her status. As the caregivers had not yet disclosed, these represented their beliefs rather than experiences of the benefits of disclosure.

The main benefits of disclosing to an HIV-infected child that caregivers discussed included health benefits and protection of others.

Most caregivers hoped that disclosure would motivate the child to take his/her ART consistently and take more personal responsibility for his/her own care generally. Responses emphasized caregivers' faith in ART, and their acceptance that consistent adherence would be central to the child's survival and quality of life. As such, many caregivers focused on the incurable, and ultimately fatal, nature of untreated HIV/AIDS. They anticipated that this would motivate the child to be adherent to medication.

> *"The child should understand that if he stops taking his medicine he will die. You should tell the child that HIV has no cure. He has to continue taking his medicine and if he ever stops, he will die." (33-year-old mother of 9-year-old girl)*

Getting children to understand this point was especially important for most caregivers and in some cases could lead to mutual support for adherence in both the child and caregiver.

> *"Once you have told the child, he will know that he needs to take his drugs. And let's say he is at school and he doesn't want his fellow children to see him swallowing the medicine, he may decide not to take it. But once you have disclosed to him, he will try by all means and make sure he swallows the medicine." (26-year-old aunt of 11-year-old boy)*
>
> *"The benefit is that the child will remind himself to take medicine and he will also remind you so you find that his health and mine continues to be good because we keep taking medicine together." (26-year-old mother of 6-year-old girl)*

For some, this expectation of better adherence and self-care was founded in prior experience with other children.

> *"The benefit is there; for example like my [other] daughter, before I told her I would give her medicine to take and instead she would hide it and throw it away and she would fall sick again. After disclosing to her I saw a big change, she now takes her medicine regularly and no longer falls sick. Now when it is time for taking medicine she takes it without me reminding her." (35-year-old mother of 9-year-old girl)*

Some caregivers discussed how disclosure will allow a child to take deliberate actions to protect his/her playmates and potential sexual partners, from accidental exposure to HIV.

> *"...the child should be told because if not told she may spread the HIV to other children, but if your child knows, if she uses a razor she throws it away so that others do not get in contact with it." (26-year-old mother of 6-year-old girl)*

The caregiver's responsibility to disclose. Most caregivers described disclosure as a responsibility the caregiver holds to the child. They were often preoccupied by feelings of this responsibility and the need to account to their children who, in most cases, were vertically infected. The desire to tell the child before the caregiver dies, as well as before other people tell the child, was frequently cited.

> *"I want to tell him because I do not know how long I am going to live. I may die before him..., so that is why I want to tell him so that even when I am already gone he knows that I am like this; Mum told me. ...So that I do not leave him in the dark. His friends might tell him and he would be like, 'my mother who gave birth to me, why could she not tell me this?'" (30-year-old mother of 12-year-old boy)*

Avoiding disclosure

Even though caregivers had strong desires to disclose, they had not yet embarked on the disclosure process. Analysis identified three main categories of reasons for avoiding disclosure, namely fear of negative outcomes, and a lack of self-efficacy.

Negative outcomes. Three sub-themes capture the most common harmful outcomes that caregivers feared might result from disclosure: the child's negative emotional reactions, anticipated stigma and discrimination, and harm to the parent-child relationship.

Most caregivers were very concerned that disclosure would lead to the child experiencing sadness, shame, hating himself, despair, hopelessness, social withdrawal, shock, collapse, and even self-harm and suicide.

> *"Some children I have heard who were disclosed to, some took poison after knowing. Some children lose hope and stop taking medicine; that after all they are going to die." (34-year-old mother of 8-year-old girl)*

Children receive negative messages in the community about HIV/AIDS, such as frightening media campaigns, and in some cases, children had negative, personal experiences, including loss of a parent. Caregivers therefore expressed concern that a child would have a very poor response to disclosure. For example:

> *"...especially if the child has somehow grown up. He goes to school and has learnt about HIV/AIDS and its effects. He has learnt that AIDS has no cure, it kills, and once the child already knows this information and you tell him that you have HIV, he can collapse. Some children have even hung themselves after being told... So it is very dangerous." (30-year-old aunt of 10-year-old boy)*

Such feelings were not considered irrational or unreasonable; caregivers extrapolated them from adult experiences with first learning the diagnosis.

> *"...it could be harmful to tell the child in that once he knows he can even run mad... Even an old person, when they go for testing and they are told that they have HIV/AIDS; some can even get a stroke..." (27-year-old mother of 6-year-old boy)*

Caregivers feared that the child and the family could be discriminated by the community, especially if the child disclosed intentionally or inadvertently to his/her friends, playmates, and/or schoolmates. This fear was commonly cited as a reason for avoiding disclosure.

> *"They are supposed to be told but to me I think they should be told when you see that the child understands what you are going to tell him, whether it is bad and he will not take it as a usual thing, and he goes spreading it around everywhere that he has HIV" (28-year-old mother of 12-year-old child)*

Many caregivers, especially biological parents, expressed feelings of guilt for infecting their children and feared that the disclosure could harm the parent-child relationship, in some cases with disastrous consequences.

> *"Telling the child that he got the disease from the parents, that is hard. That is something that usually annoys children. For example, back in our village there is a girl whose mother died of HIV. I think she might have been told, perhaps by the mother [that she has HIV]. Now the girl is in high school but she said she will hate her mother until she dies. You see, when you tell the child that he has HIV, inevitably, you have to tell him that you got it from me. It may not go well…" (Mother of 6-year-old child)*
>
> *"It is hard for me to tell the child that he got the disease from me because he might get annoyed with me and blame me for his status. It is difficult because how do you tell the child that I was promiscuous, that your father was promiscuous, that is how we got the disease? That is very hard to tell the child, there is no way I can explain it to you. This child does not know things of mature people…" (Mother of 7-year-old child)*

Feeling unable to disclose. When asked which aspects of disclosure they would find easy or difficult, caregivers' responses indicated they did not feel they had the skills necessary for handling the disclosure process and dealing with anticipated adverse outcomes. They felt that disclosure was a difficult undertaking; the anticipated adverse outcomes easily overrode any desired benefits from disclosure. These concerns were expressed across all aspects of disclosure, but particularly around naming the disease and discussing consequences of having HIV.

> *"Right now I am not at rest because she keeps asking me why she takes medicines… It would be good to tell her but where do you begin? You cannot tell her direct that you [the child] have HIV. I would tell her that you need to take medicine and it is important for your health, but it is very hard for me to tell her that you have HIV.*
> *I will try to tell her myself but if my heart fails then I will bring her to the doctors and they disclose to her. For them, they are experts" (34-year-old mother of 10-year-old girl)*

Coping before disclosure through deception

Caregivers were frequently presented with opportunities to begin disclosure; children often questioned why they needed to take regular medication, or occasionally, directly asked if they had HIV. Because of the above-noted fears, however, caregivers often created stories to tell HIV-infected children to avoid disclosure. Significantly, the majority spoke about these lies in the first person, meaning that they themselves had misled their children when confronted by questions about the child's HIV status or why the child was always taking medication. In some cases, such lies were told on a sustained basis and were expected to continue until disclosure finally happened. Caregivers suggested that this approach was justified if the child was too young or otherwise not ready for disclosure.

> *"When they are still young people deceive them that they have cough, or he might have a wound and I tell him that you are taking medicine because of this wound; and you keep deceiving him like that until he is of age and has grown to be told the real truth." (29-year-old mother of 6-year-old boy)*

The kinds of stories give some insight into the caregivers' fears regarding disclosure. Their purpose could be either concealment (e.g., sustaining the child's ignorance of his status) or denial (e.g., caregivers' own rejection of the reality of the HIV status). Importantly, some of stories would predictably make it more difficult for the caregivers to eventually disclose when the time comes. Thus:

> *"You tell the child that the medicine you are taking is not for HIV. The child might ask you that do I have the virus and you tell the children that no, you do not have it. HIV/AIDS is only contracted through sexual intercourse, and for you where would you get it from? (27-year-old mother of 6-year-old girl)*

Intentions for disclosure

All caregivers stated that they had intentions to disclose to their children in the future. The appropriate timing of disclosure was discussed mainly in terms of the child's age; the majority of caregivers intended to disclose when the children were between 12–15 years. When asked who they thought would be the best person to disclose to the child, most responded themselves, thus confirming their sense of personal responsibility to their children.

> *"I would do it myself because it is the right thing to do." (28-year old mother of 6-year-old boy)*
>
> *"I think I will do it myself because the child will not know whether the other person is telling the truth or lying. But once you tell her yourself she will know that what my mother is telling me is the truth." (34-year-old mother of 10-year-old girl)*

On the other hand, responses also revealed significant anxiety among some caregivers about their ability to handle the disclosure process. They wished for substantial support through the process, mostly from counsellors and health workers. These caregivers hoped that professional support would help them deal with any questions the children might ask, as well as difficult emotional reactions. Some caregivers also mentioned that getting support from peers and other children living with HIV/AIDS might be beneficial.

> *"You know, I have a friend in the neighbourhood. When she was going to disclose to her daughter she called me and I supported her. She recently asked me if I had disclosed to my child. I said, "No". She said to me "whenever you plan to disclose to her, call me and we shall counsel her together. Don't you recall how it went for me?" (28-year-old mother of 6-year-old boy)*

Discussion

In this study of caregivers in a rural Ugandan setting, we found that most perceived disclosure as a single momentous event of truth-telling that is usually preceded by a period of sustained avoidance and deliberate deception. Caregivers generally viewed disclosure as potentially beneficial to children and expressed a desire to derive a wide range of anticipated benefits, particularly improved medication adherence and better self-care, for their children through a properly timed and managed disclosure. They also viewed it as an opportunity and framework for accounting to the children for their own responsibility in the children's infection. However, most were preoccupied with fear of negative outcomes and did not feel able to disclose well. It was therefore easier for them to avoid disclosure even when presented with clear opportunities to tell.

Because children typically receive ART for a long time prior to disclosure and must develop sufficiently to understand their diagnosis, unique challenges arise that are best handled through a gradual disclosure process. World Health Organization and national guidelines recommend that disclosure consist of a gradual process in which information is delivered in a graded manner appropriate to the child's development. The child is given some, but not all, the information about their illness. The child may be told that he/she has a disease that is described in a way that is consistent with HIV/AIDS, but the disease not necessarily mentioned by name [10,30].

Caregivers in this study, however, perceived disclosure in a way similar to the post-test disclosure one would get with a first test for HIV. This finding reveals a lack of understanding of the concept of partial disclosure and suggests that children might be brought very quickly from a position of no disclosure to full disclosure. This phenomenon has been reported before; a qualitative study of 12 children in the Democratic Republic of the Congo who had received disclosure found that almost all children interviewed reported receiving their disclosure information through a single conversation with neither preparatory nor follow-on discussion after the event [19]. This approach is unlikely to be satisfactory, as it requires the child to absorb too much information, including reconciling the new knowledge with prior misinformation. Without the benefit of follow-on discussions to address questions and concerns, children could develop feelings of confusion, isolation and depression. Nonetheless, most caregivers independently described their understanding of full disclosure appropriately, even before hearing the interviewer's definition of essential components. This finding suggests that they may not need more counseling on the components of disclosure, but more on how to do it as a process.

We found that caregivers had important positive goals for disclosure including improved adherence to medication, better parent-child relationship, and community protection. Disclosure was, however, avoided because of a range of fears. Fears of negative emotional reactions by the child were similar to what has been reported in other studies [15,22,31,32]. These fears are perhaps not entirely unexpected. The vast majority of caregivers interviewed were themselves HIV-infected and had real-life experience going through the process of testing and learning for the first time that they were HIV-infected. This experience might have informed their expectation that receiving news of their HIV status would be distressing for the child.

Fears of negative emotional reactions are reinforced by a fatalistic view of HIV/AIDS in the community, media, and health education programs in school. As reported in other studies [33,34], caregivers feared that children would live in constant fear of dying once they were told they had HIV. However, such fears of adverse outcomes may be unduly exaggerated. Data from studies of the psychological impact of disclosure in children generally suggest that although some may experience some negative reactions initially, these are usually followed by more positive feelings of relief and empowerment [17,19,35]. Overall rates of depression, emotional and behavioural problems, for instance, are not higher among children who have been informed of their HIV status [26,34,36]. Helping parents understand this fact early may help mitigate these fears and get them to feel more positively about the prospect of disclosure.

Previous studies have reported that disclosure may be especially difficult for HIV-infected biological parents of HIV infected children [37,38], primarily due to feelings of guilt and fear of blame [25]. This study confirms this finding, but also suggests that concern about distressing the child, particularly for parents who may have experienced significant emotional distress following post-test disclosure, may play a significant role.

One fear frequently cited as a reason for delayed disclosure in previous studies is that HIV-infected caregivers fear revealing their own HIV status, and the attendant concern that the child might not be able to keep the diagnosis a secret [20,22,35]. Our data concurs, partly, with this finding. However, even caregivers who are open about their own HIV status can have difficulties disclosing their child's HIV status. In this study, a significant number of HIV-infected parents reported having disclosed their own status within their family and community and in some cases to the HIV-infected child in question. For these parents, at least, the delay to disclose may be more likely due to a genuine desire to protect the child from distress rather than a need to preserve secrecy of their own HIV status.

Caregivers are often presented with opportunities to begin the disclosure process, mostly when children begin questioning the need for taking regular medication. However, as a strategy to cope with fear they may deflect questions about HIV. This practice may be more pervasive than has previously been reported [10]. In our study, almost all caregivers indicated that they had told their children a lie when confronted by questions about the child's HIV status. Their justification of it and the expectation that they would continue until they felt ready for disclosure highlights the fact that, for many caregivers, pretense is a major strategy for coping through the pre-disclosure period. Unfortunately, some of the lies might make future disclosure more difficult. Interventions to support caregivers through disclosure should aim to provide viable alternative strategies for managing the pre-disclosure period and support caregivers through a managed process of partial disclosure.

Ultimately, whether and when disclosure happens will depend not only on caregivers' goals and desired outcomes, but also on their ability to act on them. Dematteo and others have argued that, for disclosure of the child's HIV diagnosis to occur, adult caregivers have first to trust in their own readiness and competency to disclose [39]. Our data revealed a lack of self-efficacy among caregivers; most felt that they lacked the skill to adequately communicate with their children about their HIV status and to deal with the anticipated negative reactions. Similar to other studies, caregivers frequently anticipated a need, and expressed a desire, for professional support when the time for disclosure comes [19,33,40,41].

Despite concerns about lack of ability to act independently, most caregivers still prefer that the parent or primary caregiver should be the one to disclose to children under their care. They perceived disclosure as a responsibility the caregiver holds to the child, and they see an opportunity to be accountable to their children and to foster a closer relationship of trust. Interventions to promote disclosure in this population should recognize caregivers' desire to personally conduct the disclosure process and offer support to help them overcome the barriers that hinder them from acting on this desire.

Considering caregivers' stated desire for guidance and support by health workers through the disclosure process, it is important that health workers are trained and supported with appropriate guidelines. Typically, this type of care is not routinely available in settings like this one. Even though most HIV-infected caregivers had disclosed their own status within their family or community following encouragement by health workers, they had received no specific support through the process. The suggestion of a possible role for peer counselling for the caregiver in preparation for disclosure, and the caregiver/child dyad during and after disclosure, offers potentially interesting implications for programs to support disclosure in this setting. Peer counsellors have been used to support HIV programs in African settings, particularly HIV prevention and treatment programs, with some success [42,43].

A major strength of this study is the depth of the interviews, which explored not only the caregivers' conceptualization of disclosure, but also their motivation, intentions, and barriers with disclosure. The study focused on caregivers who had not disclosed and thus allowed an exploration of caregivers' desires and needs prior to disclosure. This study also had some limitations. Because participants did not include caregivers who had disclosed, the study does not present comparative data that could have helped identify possible facilitators of disclosure among caregivers in similar circumstances. However, the exclusion of caregivers who had disclosed was deliberate; we sought to focus on antecedent attitudes and goals of disclosure among those caregivers who might be having difficulties with disclosing. We also included caregivers whose children were relatively young and who may therefore not be developmentally ready for disclosure; however, WHO and national guidelines suggest beginning the disclosure process even at this young age. The majority of participants in this study were biological mothers; opinions of other types of caregivers may vary. Furthermore, the study was restricted to caregivers of children who were plugged into care. Further work is needed to explore perspectives of families not receiving formal care and treatment. Studies exploring the perspective of the HIV-infected child would also provide additional insight into this important issue.

Conclusions

Caregivers of HIV-infected children mainly perceive disclosure as a single event rather than a process of gradual delivery of information about the child's illness. They anticipate a range of potential benefits to the children, as well as an opportunity for caregivers to clarify that they transmitted the virus to the child. However, most are over-whelmed with fear of negative outcomes, and reveal a lack of confidence to independently manage the disclosure process. Consequently, most did cope by deception to avoid (or delay) disclosure until they perceive readiness to disclose.

The results of this study have implications for future development of interventions to support families through disclosure-related communication. Such interventions should recognize caregivers' desire to disclose to children under their care, and the barriers that hinder them from acting on this desire. Caregivers should be empowered with practical skills to recognize opportunities to initiate the disclosure process early, and supported to manage it in a developmentally appropriate manner. Health care providers need to be equipped with skills and appropriate guidelines to be able to guide and support families towards satisfactory disclosure. The potential role for peer counselors in supporting caregivers and families through the disclosure process deserves further study.

Acknowledgments

The authors wish to thank the participants and staff of the HIV clinic, as well as Christine Tumuramye who assisted with the interviews. They are also grateful for the advice given by Sheana Bull, PhD from the University of Colorado, in the preparation of the manuscript. All data in this manuscript will be made available to interested individuals upon request to the corresponding author.

Author Contributions

Conceived and designed the experiments: JK EM JEH. Performed the experiments: JK EM. Analyzed the data: JK EM. Contributed reagents/materials/analysis tools: JK EM JEH. Wrote the paper: JK EM JEH.

References

1. World Health Organization, UNICEF, UNAIDS (2013) Global update on HIV treatment 2013: results, impact and opportunities. World Health Organization.
2. Ministry of Health Uganda (2012) Uganda AIDS Indicator Survey.
3. World Health Organization (2010) Antiretroviral therapy for HIV infection in infants and children: towards universal access. World Health Organization.
4. Judd A, Doerholt K, Tookey PA, Sharland M, Riordan A, et al. (2007) Morbidity, mortality, and response to treatment by children in the United Kingdom and Ireland with perinatally acquired HIV infection during 1996–2006: planning for teenage and adult care. Clin Infect Dis 45: 918–24.
5. Marston M, Zaba B, Salomon JA, Brahmbhatt H, Bagenda D (2005) Estimating the net effect of HIV on child mortality in African populations affected by generalized HIV epidemics. J Acquir Immune Defic Syndr 38: 219–27.
6. American Academy of Pediatrics Committee on Pediatrics AIDS (1999) Disclosure of illness status to children and adolescents with HIV infection. Pediatrics 103: 164–6.
7. Vreeman RC, Gramelspacher AM, Gisore PO, Scanlon ML, Nyandiko WM (2013) Disclosure of HIV status to children in resource-limited settings: a systematic review. Journal of the International AIDS Society 16: 18466.
8. Pinzon-Iregui MC, Beck-Sague CM, Malow RM (2013) Disclosure of their HIV status to infected children: a review of the literature. J Trop Pediatr 59: 84–9.
9. Chaudoir SF, Simoni JD (2011) Understanding HIV disclosure: A review and application of the Disclosure Processes Model. Social Science & Medicine 72: 1618–1629.
10. Funck-Brentano I, Costagliola D, Seibel N, et al. (1997) Patterns of disclosure and perceptions of the immunodeficiency virus in elementary school aged children. Arch Pediatr Adolesc Med 151: 978–985.
11. Kyaddondo D, Wanyenze RK, Kinsman J, Hardon A (2013) Disclosure of HIV status between parents and children in Uganda in the context of greater access to treatment. Sahara J 10 Suppl 1: S37–45.
12. Ministry of Health Uganda (2005) Uganda National Policy Guidelines for HIV Counseling and Testing. Ministry of Health.
13. World Health Organization (2011) Guideline on HIV disclosure counseling for children up to 12 years of age.
14. Butler AM, Williams PL, Howland LC, Storm D, Hutton N, et al. (2009) Impact of disclosure of HIV infection on health-related quality of life among children and adolescents with HIV infection. Pediatrics 123: 935–943.
15. Oberdorfer P, Puthanakit T, Louthrenoo O, Charnsil C, Sirisanthana V, et al. (2006) Disclosure of HIV/AIDS diagnosis to HIV-infected children in Thailand. J Paediatr Child Health 42: 283–288.
16. Wiener L, Mellins CA, Marhefka S, Battles HB (2007) Disclosure of an HIV diagnosis to children: history, current research, and future directions. J Dev Behav Pediatr 28: 155–166.
17. Petersen I, Bhana A, Myeza N, Alicea S, John S, et al. (2010) Psychosocial challenges and protective influences for socio-emotional coping of HIV+ adolescents in South Africa: a qualitative investigation. AIDS Care 22: 970–978.
18. Menon A GC, Campain N, Ngoma M (2007) Mental health and disclosure of HIV status in Zambian adolescents with HIV infection: implications for peer-support programs. J Acquir Immune Defic Syndr 1;46: 349–354.
19. Vaz LM, Eng E, Maman S, Tshikandu T, Behets F (2010) Telling children they have HIV: lessons learned from findings of a qualitative study in sub-Saharan Africa. AIDS Patient Care STDS 24: 247–256.
20. Biadgilign S, Deribew A, Amberbir A, Escudero HR, Deribe K (2011) Factors associated with HIV/AIDS diagnostic disclosure to HIV infected children receiving HAART: a multi-center study in Addis Ababa, Ethiopia. PLoS One 6(3): e17572. doi:10.1371/journal.pone.0017572.
21. Bikaako-Kajura W, Luyirika E, Purcell DW, Downing J, Kaharuza F, et al. (2006) Disclosure of HIV status and adherence to daily drug regimens among HIV-infected children in Uganda. AIDS Behav 10: S85–93.
22. Kallem S, Renner L, Ghebremichael M, Paintsil E (2011) Prevalence and Pattern of Disclosure of HIV Status in HIV-Infected Children in Ghana. AIDS Behav 15: 1121–1127.
23. Atwiine B (2012) Patterns and correlates of HIV diagnostic disclosure status among children attending MRRH Paediatric HIV Clinic. Mbarara University of Science and Technology. Unpublished thesis.
24. Flanagan-Klygis E, Ross LF, Lantos J, Frader J, Yogev R (2001) Disclosing the diagnosis of HIV in pediatrics. J Clin Ethics 12: 150–157.
25. Waugh S (2003) Parental views on disclosure of diagnosis to their HIV-positive children. AIDS Care 15: 169–176.

26. Wiener LS, Battles HB, Heilman N, Sigelman CK, Pizzo PA (1996) Factors associated with disclosure of diagnosis to children with HIV/AIDS. Pediatr AIDS HIV Infect 7: 310–324.
27. Strauss AL, Corbin JM (1998) Basics of qualitative research: Techniques and procedures for developing grounded theory: Sage Publications.
28. Hsieh H-F, Shannon SE (2005) Three Approaches to Qualitative Content Analysis. Qual Health Res 15: 1277.
29. Ryan GW, Bernard HR (2003) Techniques to Identify Themes. Field Methods: Sage Publications. pp. 85–109.
30. Melvin D (1999) Psychological issues, challenges and achievements. J HIV Ther 4: 77–81.
31. Hejoaka F (2009) Care and secrecy: being a mother of children living with HIV in Burkina Faso. Soc Sci Med 69: 869–76.
32. Kouyoumdjian F, Meyers T, Mtshizana S (2005) Barriers to disclosure to children with HIV. J Trop Pediatr 51: 285–287.
33. Madiba S, Mokwena K (2012) Caregivers' Barriers to Disclosing the HIV Diagnosis to Infected Children on Antiretroviral Therapy in a Resource-Limited District in South Africa: A Grounded Theory Study. AIDS Res Treat: 402–403.
34. Lester P, Chesney M, Cooke M, et al. (2002) Diagnostic disclosure to HIV-infected children: how parents decide when and what to tell. Clinical Child Psychology and Psychiatry 7: 85–99.
35. Vaz L, Maman S, Eng E, Barbarin O, Tshikandu T, et al. (2011) Patterns of disclosure of HIV status to infected children in a Sub-Saharan African setting. J Dev Behav Pediatr 32: 307–315.
36. Riekert KA, Wiener L, Battles HB (1999) Prediction of psychological distress in school-age children with HIV. Child Health Care 28: 201–220.
37. Ledlie SW (1999) Diagnosis disclosure by family caregivers to children who have perinatally acquired HIV disease: when the time comes. Nurs Res 48: 141–149.
38. Lee CL, Johann-Liang R (1999) Disclosure of the diagnosis of HIV/AIDS to children born of HIV-infected mothers. AIDS Patient Care STDS 13: 41–45.
39. DeMatteo D, Harrison C, Arneson C, Salter Goldie R, Lefebvre A, et al. (2002) Disclosing HIV/AIDS to children: the paths families take to truthtelling. Psychology, Health and Medicine 7: 339–356.
40. Heeren GA, Jemmott JB, 3rd, Sidloyi L, Ngwane Z (2012) Disclosure of HIV Diagnosis to HIV-Infected Children in South Africa: Focus Groups for Intervention Development. Vulnerable Child Youth Stud 7: 47–54.
41. Gerson AC, Joyner M, Fosarelli P, Butz A, Wissow L, et al. (2001) Disclosure of HIV diagnosis to children: when, where, why, and how. J Pediatr Health Care 15: 161–167.
42. Medley A, Ackers M, Amolloh M, Owuor P, Muttai H, et al. (2013) Early uptake of HIV clinical care after testing HIV-positive during home-based testing and counseling in western Kenya. AIDS Behav 17: 224–234.
43. Nor B, Ahlberg BM, Doherty T, Zembe Y, Jackson D, et al. (2012) Mother's perceptions and experiences of infant feeding within a community-based peer counselling intervention in South Africa. Matern Child Nutr 8: 448–458.

24

Progress in the Prevention of Mother to Child Transmission of HIV in Three Regions of Tanzania: A Retrospective Analysis

Ann M. Buchanan[1,2,3]*, Dorothy E. Dow[1,2], Charles G. Massambu[4], Balthazar Nyombi[5], Aisa Shayo[1], Rahma Musoke[1], Sheng Feng[6], John A. Bartlett[1,3,7], Coleen K. Cunningham[1], Werner Schimana[8]

1 Kilimanjaro Christian Medical Centre, Moshi, Tanzania, **2** Division of Infectious Diseases, Department of Pediatrics, Duke University Medical Center, Durham, North Carolina, United States of America, **3** Duke Global Health Institute, Duke University, Durham, North Carolina, United States of America, **4** Ministry of Health and Social Welfare, Dar es Salaam, Tanzania, **5** Kilimanjaro Christian Medical Centre Clinical Laboratory, Moshi, Tanzania, **6** Department of Biostatistics and Bioinformatics, Duke University, Durham, North Carolina, United States of America, **7** Division of Infectious Diseases, Department of Medicine, Duke University Medical Center, Durham, North Carolina, United States of America, **8** Elizabeth Glaser Pediatric AIDS Foundation, Dar es Salaam, Tanzania

Abstract

Background: Mother to child transmission (MTCT) of HIV-1 remains an important problem in sub-Saharan Africa where most new pediatric HIV-1 infections occur. Early infant diagnosis of HIV-1 using dried blood spot (DBS) PCR among exposed infants provides an opportunity to assess current MTCT rates.

Methods: We conducted a retrospective data analysis on mother-infant pairs from all PMTCT programs in three regions of northern Tanzania to determine MTCT rates from 2008–2010. Records of 3,016 mother-infant pairs were assessed to determine early transmission among HIV-exposed infants in the first 75 days of life.

Results: Of 2,266 evaluable infants in our cohort, 143 had a positive DBS PCR result at ≤75 days of life, for an overall transmission rate of 6.3%. Transmission decreased substantially over the period of study as more effective regimens became available. Transmission rates were tightly correlated to maternal regimen: 14.9% (9.5, 20.3) of infants became infected when women received no therapy; 8.8% (6.9, 10.7) and 3.6% (2.4, 4.8) became infected when women received single-dose nevirapine (sdNVP) or combination prophylaxis, respectively; the lowest MTCT rates occurred when women were on HAART, with 2.1% transmission (0.3, 3.9). Treatment regimens changed dramatically over the study period, with an increase in combination prophylaxis and a decrease in the use of sdNVP. Uptake of DBS PCR more than tripled over the period of study for the three regions surveyed.

Conclusions: Our study demonstrates significant reductions in MTCT of HIV-1 in three regions of Tanzania coincident with increased use of more effective PMTCT interventions. The changes we demonstrate for the period of 2008–2010 occurred prior to major changes in WHO PMTCT guidelines.

Editor: Paul Richard Harrigan, University of British Columbia, Canada

Funding: This research was supported by the President's Emergency Plan for AIDS Relief (PEPFAR) through a supplement to the National Institute of Allergy and Infectious Diseases (NIAID): NOT-A1-10-023 (3UO1 A1069484 A4S2); the Duke Clinical Trials Unit and Clinical Research Sites (U01 AI069484 to CKC, JAB, and AMB); the Duke Center for AIDS Research (5P30 AI064518 to CKC and AMB); the Eunice Kennedy Shriver National Institute of Child Health and Human Development (NICHD) training grant to the Division of Infectious Diseases, Department of Pediatrics, Duke University Medical Center (T32 HD060558 to DED); and HRSA grant T84HS21123 and NIH grants P30AI064518, D43CA153722, and D43TW06732 to JAB. The funders had no role in study design, data collection and analysis, decision to publish, or preparation of the manuscript.

Competing Interests: The authors have declared that no competing interests exist.

* E-mail: ann.buchanan@duke.edu

Introduction

More than 90% of the world's HIV-infected children reside in sub-Saharan Africa, where mother to child transmission (MTCT) of human immunodeficiency virus type 1 (HIV-1) remains the most important cause of pediatric HIV infection [1]. Furthermore, 50% of HIV-infected children will die by the age of two years without proper care and treatment [2]. Recent advances in prevention measures have resulted in vertical transmission rates in industrialized countries of less than 2% [3–5], and MTCT rates have decreased considerably in many resource-limited areas as well [6–10]. The international community has responded to the continued threat of MTCT of HIV-1 with the development of the Global Plan for elimination of MTCT by 2015 put forth by UNAIDS [11].

Tanzania is one of the 22 countries with the highest estimated numbers of pregnant women living with HIV, and as such is a focus country for MTCT elimination [11]. HIV prevalence among pregnant women is 6.8%, compared to an overall population prevalence of 5.7% [12]. As in other sub-Saharan African countries, tremendous progress has been made in Tanzania with regard to accessibility and uptake of prevention of mother to child transmission (PMTCT) services. Tanzanian PMTCT program data assessments for 2010 estimate that of the 119,000 HIV-infected women who give birth annually, approximately 70% receive some form of antiretroviral treatment for PMTCT [13]. Programs, however, vary widely, both across and within regions, and medications available to women and their infants vary as well.

Prior to 2011, HIV-infected pregnant women were eligible for highly active antiretroviral therapy (HAART) only if they had World Health Organization (WHO) Stage IV disease, or WHO Stage III disease *and* a CD4 count below 350 cells/uL. Pregnant women with stage I/II disease were eligible for HAART only when their CD4 count fell below 200 cells/uL. Women who did not qualify for HAART were eligible to start zidovudine (AZT) prophylaxis beginning at 28 weeks, along with single-dose nevirapine (sdNVP) and lamivudine (3TC) at labor/delivery and postpartum but where this was neither available nor feasible, single-dose nevirapine (sdNVP) alone was recommended. Exposed newborns were eligible to receive sdNVP within 72 hours of life and twice daily AZT for one week, or 4 weeks if the mother had received less than 4 weeks of prophylaxis; the use of daily nevirapine for breastfeeding infants had not yet been implemented.

In recent years, access to HIV early infant diagnosis (EID) has also increased in Tanzania. Prior to 2008 the country relied on antibody testing for infant diagnosis, making the diagnosis challenging due to the presence of maternal antibody up to 12–18 months of life. The country's current commitment to the provision of EID services using PCR on dried blood spots (DBS) in the first eight weeks of life not only allows for early diagnosis and treatment of infected infants, but can also be used as a tool to measure the effectiveness of PMTCT programs.

In order to determine uptake of PMTCT treatment regimens, prevalence of MTCT, and the relationship between these, we reviewed DBS PCR results from HIV-exposed infants, combined with PMTCT treatment information collected from national registries at all health facilities providing PMTCT services in three regions of northern Tanzania.

Methods

Design, Setting, and Data Collection

This study is a retrospective data analysis on mother-infant pairs from PMTCT program records in three regions of Tanzania, using stored DBS samples stored as standard of care from HIV-exposed infants to determine early MTCT prevalence rates from HIV-exposed children ≤75 days of age. "Early" MTCT in this context, therefore, encompasses in-utero transmission, intrapartum transmission, and early breast milk infection. This study was conceived and designed in conjunction with members from the Tanzanian Ministry of Health and Social Welfare Laboratory Services Division. Following Tanzanian national guidelines, HIV-exposed infants undergo DBS PCR testing at their first visit to a Reproductive Child Health (RCH) clinic, usually between 4–8 weeks of age. Using a heel prick, five circles are filled with blood on a specific filter paper (Whatman) and sent to a Zonal PCR Laboratory. The Kilimanjaro Christian Medical Centre Clinical Laboratory is one of four such laboratories in Tanzania responsible for processing, testing, and storing DBS results for the three regions we studied. In the laboratory, one DBS circle is used to run a DNA-PCR test and if positive, a second circle is analyzed to confirm the first result. Only if both PCR tests are positive does the result become classified as positive and this result is then sent back to the RCH clinic.

Every DBS card is labelled with the infant's name and a unique identifier which is also recorded in the EID and PMTCT Mother-Child Follow-up Register that remains at the clinical site. Other information recorded in the registry includes: date of birth, date sample taken, PMTCT regimen used by the mother, infant regimen, infant feeding option, and initiation of co-trimoxazole prophylactic therapy.

Three research assistants, each assigned to one region of northern Tanzania (Arusha, Kilimanjaro, and Tanga) visited all health facilities providing PMTCT and EID services within the regions. Using these national registries, de-identified information was collected from all mother-infant pairs where the infant received a first DBS PCR between January 1, 2008 and September 30, 2010. During this time period, possible maternal PMTCT regimens included either: 1) no medication; 2) sdNVP only; 3) combination prophylaxis (AZT, recorded as>or <4 weeks prior to delivery, and sdNVP and lamivudine (3TC) given at labor and delivery along with AZT plus 3TC for one week); or 4) HAART. The infant regimens provided during this time period included sdNVP at birth, with or without AZT (either for 1 week or 4 weeks depending on duration of maternal prophylaxis). After reviewing the registries of all facilities for the three regions as described, all positive DBS PCR results recorded at site registries were cross-checked by retrieving the original samples from the zonal laboratory (Kilimanjaro Christian Medical Centre). This enabled us to exclude any potential false positive PMTCT transcription errors from site PMTCT registries.

Statistical Analysis

Data were entered using the Cardiff Teleform system (Cardiff Inc., Vista, CA, USA) into an Access database (Microsoft Corp., Redmond, WA, USA). All data were manually reentered into a second Microsoft Access database and compared using Stata version 12 (StataCorp LP, College Station, TX, USA). All subsequent analyses were performed with Stata version 12, using a 5% level of significance (two-sided). Descriptive statistics were used to summarize demographic data. Categorical data were compared using the Chi-square test or Fisher's exact test, where appropriate.

Ethical Statement

The study was approved by the Duke University Institutional Review Board, the KCMC Research Ethics Committee, and the National Institute of Medical Research in Tanzania. All data collection was retrospective in nature and was collected as part of the routine delivery of PMTCT services in Tanzania. All ethical bodies approved the request for a waiver of informed consent due to the fact that all information collected was on de-identified patient information and PCR samples.

Results

Data from 3,016 mother-infant pairs were collected from 98 health facilities representing a total of 22 districts in the Arusha, Kilimanjaro, and Tanga Regions. Of these, 595 pairs were excluded due to a missing date of birth and/or date of test information, and 155 pairs were excluded due to missing test results (Figure 1). In total, data from 2,266 mother-infant pairs were used in the final analysis. The mean age of first infant PCR was 40 days, standard deviation (SD) 13. The median (range) maternal age at time of delivery was 28 years (16, 46), and 86.5% of infants were reported as exclusively breastfeeding at the time of first DBS PCR.

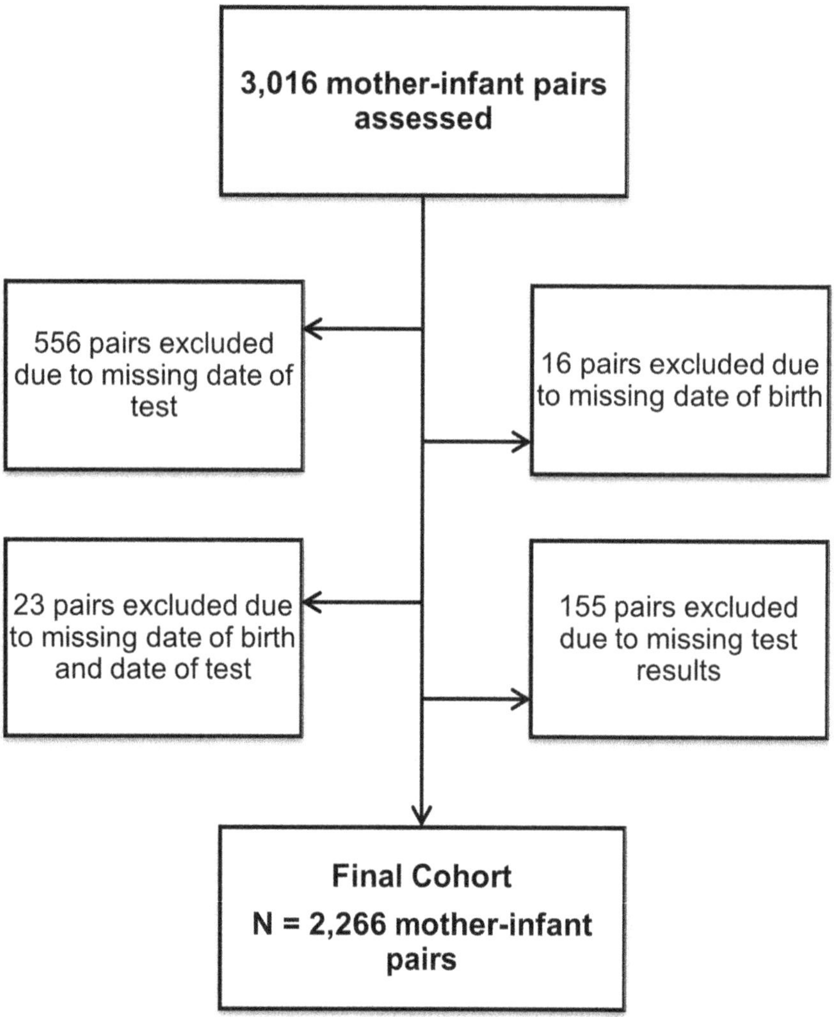

Figure 1. Population Flowchart.

During the study period, 7.4% of mothers received no medication, 36.1% received sdNVP only, 42.6% received combination prophylaxis, 10.7% received HAART, and 3.2% had no antiretroviral information recorded. Among infants, 9.0% received no medication, more than one-third (35.2%) received sdNVP only, and the majority (50.8%) received sdNVP with 1–4 weeks of AZT prophylaxis. An additional 5.0% had no information recorded.

Of the 2,266 infants in our cohort, a total of 143 tested positive on DBS PCR in the first 75 days of life, for an overall HIV-1 MTCT prevalence of 6.3% (95% CI: 5.3%, 7.3%). Transmission decreased substantially over the period of study, as more effective regimens were rolled out. Notably, uptake of DBS PCR testing more than tripled over the course of the study period, from 330 infants tested in 2008 to 1082 tested in the first 9 months of 2010 (Figure 2). Transmission rates were tightly correlated to maternal regimen; 14.9% (9.5%, 20.3%) of infants became infected when women received no therapy, compared to 8.8% (6.9%, 10.7%) and 3.6% (2.4%, 4.8%) when women received sdNVP or combination prophylaxis, respectively. The lowest MTCT rates occurred when women received HAART, with 2.1% transmission (0.3%, 3.9%) (Table 1). Women who received sdNVP only had a 41% decreased risk of MTCT (38%, 90%, $p = 0.01$) compared to women who received no antiretrovirals. Women who received combination prophylaxis had a 59% decreased risk of transmission compared to women receiving sdNVP alone (28%, 61%, $p < 0.01$).

Treatment regimens changed dramatically over the 33-month period of study. In 2008, 72.4% (67.6%, 77.2%) of women in the cohort received sdNVP only, decreasing to 14.6% (12.5%, 16.7%) in 2010. Conversely, just 7% (4.2%, 9.8%) of women received combination prophylaxis in 2008, increasing to 61.8% in 2010 (58.9%, 64.7%). Only 243 women received HAART although the proportion did increase over time with 5.5% of the cohort receiving HAART in 2008 and 14.4% in 2010 (Figure 3).

In addition to maternal prophylaxis, infant prophylaxis also plays a critical role in PMTCT. In this cohort, 11.3% (7%, 15.6%) of the 204 infants who received no therapy had a positive DBS PCR, compared to 9% (7%, 11%) of the 798 babies who received sdNVP. Over half of infants in the cohort received a combination of zidovudine and nevirapine, and this group represented the lowest MTCT transmission rate at 3.5% (2.4%, 4.6%) (Table 1).

Finally, analyzing mother and infant regimens together we see that when neither mother nor infant received any intervention, the transmission rate was 17.6% (8.9%, 26.3%). However, when the baby did receive prophylaxis in the form of sdNVP, transmission, as measured by the first DNA PCR, was reduced by more than 20% ($p = 0.61$). Table 1 shows results for each possible combina-

Table 1. Rates of Infant DBS PCR Results by 75 Days of Age According to Antiretroviral Regimen Received for Arusha, Kilimanjaro, Tanga Regions.

Maternal ARV Regimen (n)	Infant DBS PCR Positive (95% CI)*	Infant ARV Regimen				
		None	sdNVP	NVP+AZT	Not Recorded	Total
None (168)	14.9%	17.6%	14.0%	7.7%	25%	168
	(9.5, 20.3)	(8.9, 26.3)	(3.6, 24.4)	n = 39	n = 12	
		n = 74	n = 43			
sdNVP (818)	8.8%	11.1%	10.1%	4.9%	4.3%	818
	(6.9, 10.7)	(3.3, 18.9)	(7.6, 12.6)	(1.6, 8.2)	n = 47	
		n = 63	n = 546	n = 162		
Combination Prophylaxis (966)	3.6%	5.4%	5.5%	3.2%	3.6%	966
	(2.4, 4.8)	n = 37	(1.6, 9.5)	(2.0, 4.4)	n = 28	
			n = 128	n = 773		
HAART (243)	2.1%	0%	1.8%	2.6%	0%	243
	(0.3, 3.9)	n = 22	n = 55	n = 156	n = 10	
Other/Not Recorded (71)	8.7%	12.5%	11.5%	0%	12.5%	71
	(2.1, 15.3)	n = 8	n = 26	n = 21	n = 16	
Total (2,266)	6.3%	N = 204	N = 798	N = 1,151	N = 113	2,266
	(5.3, 7.3)					

*Where applicable.

tion of maternal and infant regimens. The majority of these combinations result in small numbers and p values are not significant. One exception, however, is comparing mothers and infants who received sdNVP only to mothers receiving sdNVP with infants receiving NVP+AZT. Here we see a 51% reduction in transmission from 10.1% to 4.9% ($p = 0.049$).

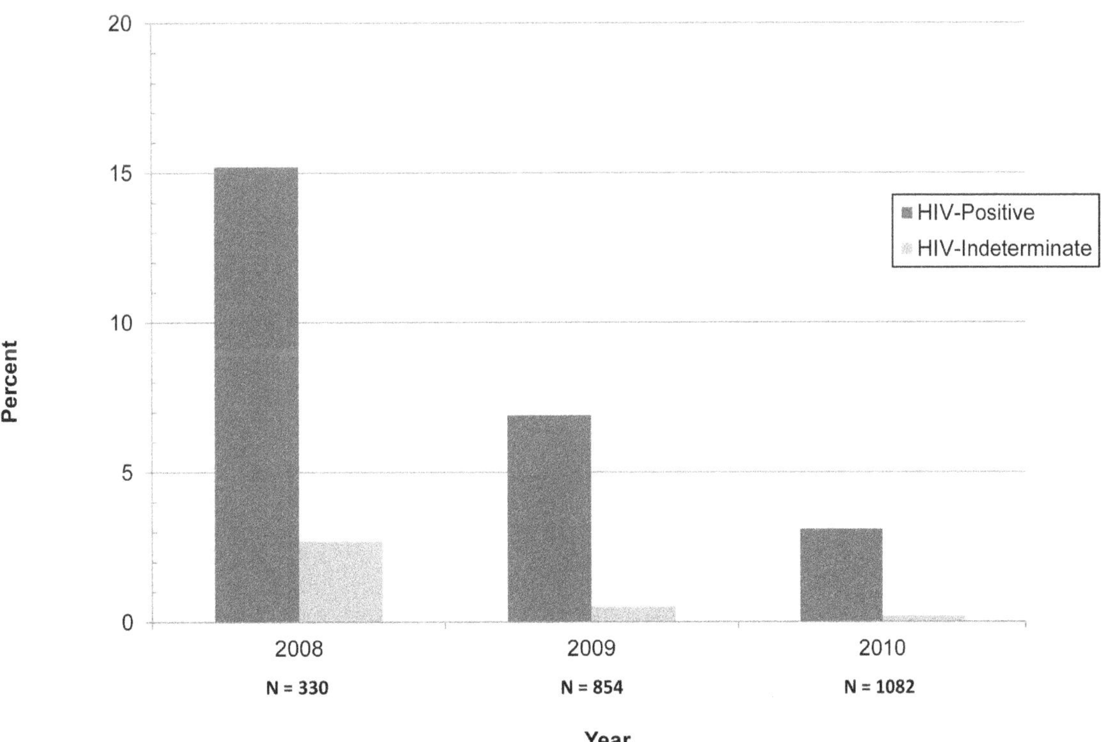

Figure 2. Positive Infant Dried Blood Spot PCR by Year for Arusha, Kilimanjaro, Tanga Regions.

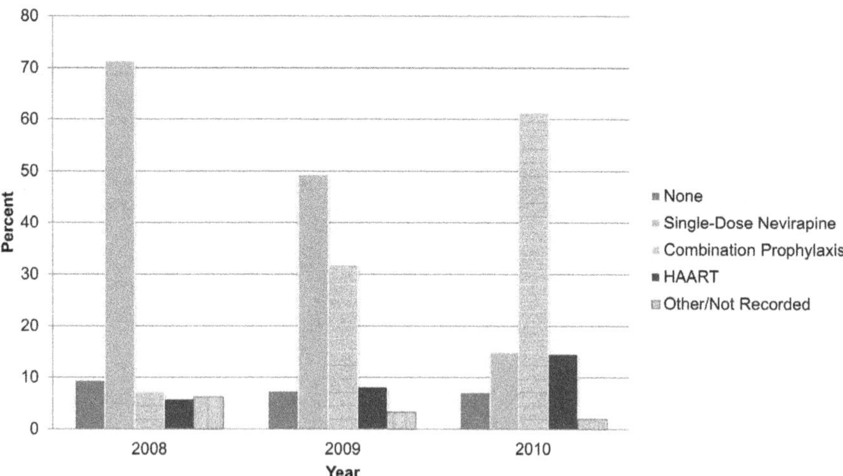

Figure 3. Maternal Antiretroviral Regimen by Year, Arusha, Kilimanjaro, Tanga Regions.

Discussion

These data, representing a comprehensive analysis from PMTCT programs providing EID services in three regions of northern Tanzania, show that MTCT has declined from 15.2% in 2008 to 3.1% in 2010, with an overall prevalence of 6.3% for this 33-month period. The change over time from primarily sdNVP use to a predominance of combination prophylaxis, combined with the dramatic increase in use of DBS PCR for EID, is a remarkable demonstration of PMTCT implementation and effective coordination of services. Tanzania has shown great success since its commencement of PMTCT services in 2000, with the development of newer guidelines and effective health policy implementation. By 2010, an estimated 94% of all Reproductive and Child Health facilities across the country were providing PMTCT services [13].

The revised Tanzanian HIV clinical guidelines introduced on a national level in 2011 include starting AZT prophylaxis twice daily beginning at 14 weeks gestation for HIV-infected pregnant women, with nevirapine and 3TC given peripartum for mothers who receive <4 weeks of AZT prior to delivery; or lifelong HAART for women with WHO Stage III or IV disease and/or an absolute CD4 count below 350 cells/μL [14]. Infants receive daily nevirapine for at least the first 6 weeks of life, and this continues until one week after complete breastfeeding cessation if the mother herself is not on HAART [14]. As new evidence on best PMTCT practices become available, guidelines continue to change. At present, Tanzania is rolling out the WHO B+ Option (which provides triple anti-retroviral therapy to all HIV-infected pregnant or breastfeeding women regardless of clinical stage or CD4 count – for life). Thus, the development and implementation of new guidelines demonstrate tremendous progress in the field of PMTCT in Tanzania; however, it is well known that the successful execution of services and the ability to reach all infected women and their infants takes time and will vary according to location and healthcare setting.

For our study, we found an MTCT rate of 14.9% when the mother received no ARV intervention. The MTCT rates we observed when no maternal or infant prophylaxis was reported (17.6%) are slightly lower than those of recently published clinical trials data, though direct comparisons are difficult. Among non-breastfeeding populations, the risk of MTCT of HIV-1 ranges from 15–30% when there is no maternal or infant ARV prophylaxis. Breastfeeding, however, increases the risk of transmission by anywhere from 5–20%, resulting in overall transmission rates of 20–45% [15]. Furthermore, non-exclusive breastfeeding is a well-established factor increasing transmission risk [16,17] compared with exclusive breastfeeding and this further complicates comparisons. More than 85% of the population we studied was reported to be exclusively breastfed at the time of the infant's first DBS PCR. The PETRA trial conducted in Tanzania, South Africa, and Uganda showed a transmission rate of 15.3% at 6 weeks of life among breastfed infants when no regimen was given to mother or infant – slightly lower than our cohort though ours also encompassed infants beyond the age of six weeks. [18] Recent studies conducted in Nigeria and Zambia showed higher transmission rates, of 19.5% and 21.8%, respectively, when there was no maternal or infant regimen given [19,20]; yet again, these were for infants up to the age of 6 weeks only.

Women who received combination prophylaxis had low HIV-1 transmission rates as would be expected, with an overall transmission rate of 3.6%. Clinical trials results have demonstrated transmission rates ranging from 2–9%, depending on length of regimen and whether or not the infant breastfed [18,21,22]. At the time our study cohort received PMTCT care, guidelines recommended AZT prophylaxis beginning at 28 weeks gestation for mothers who did not qualify for HAART. However, the women in our combination prophylaxis category included those who started as early as 28 weeks, as well as those who started just prior to delivery; thus, again, what we have observed in our field studies does seem to be lower than clinical trials results.

The number of women on HAART during the study period comprised only a small proportion of the entire cohort, making comparisons with this group difficult due to small sample size. Our MTCT rate observed of 2.1% among women on HAART is in line with other studies from developed countries, where maternal HAART among non-breastfed populations reduces MTCT to 2% or less [23–26]. In this analysis women receiving HAART actually comprise a group with higher transmission risk as it only includes women with WHO Stage IV disease, WHO Stage III disease *and* CD4<350 cells/ul, or a CD4 count<200 cells/uL regardless of WHO stage.

Finally, as a post-hoc analysis we evaluated the added benefit of infant AZT to reduce HIV transmission as compared to mother-infant pairs who received sdNVP only. The statistically significant reduction in transmission by 51% is interesting, but requires further study with a larger cohort.

With changing national guidelines we demonstrated a shift in maternal treatment regimens over time toward more women receiving combination prophylaxis and fewer receiving sdNVP (Figures 3 & 4). The decrease in transmission rates for this time period shows real progress for Tanzania (Figure 4). Furthermore, the number of women on HAART from 2008 to 2010 more than doubled. Perhaps most striking, the number of infants being tested for this time period, shortly after EID rollout began, more than tripled over the 33-months studied. Despite these successes, a number of challenges remain. The number of women in care who received no regimen did not decrease substantially over this time period and was still unacceptably high at 7% in 2010; this would represent more than 8000 untreated HIV-infected pregnant Tanzanian women if applied on a national level [13].

Our study had several limitations. First, a longitudinal prospective cohort study would have been a superior design for many reasons. Being a retrospective study on first DBS PCR results only, we were unable to determine transmission rates via breastfeeding, which contributes significantly to pediatric HIV infection in sub-Saharan Africa. Still, inferences about early MTCT in the first several weeks of life are useful. Second, as our cohort only represents those who received an HIV-1 DNA PCR within 75 days of life, it excludes the mother-infant pairs who accessed PMTCT services prior to delivery but were lost before testing. Third, we did not have access to data that may also influence MTCT, such as WHO clinical staging, maternal CD4 count and HIV-1 RNA levels, the latter not being part of routine care. We also did not have the ability to verify time of initiation nor adherence to documented PMTCT regimens for women or their infants. Fourth, data in national registries were occasionally missing or illegible and therefore, data from some individuals were incomplete. Finally, the women in our cohort are women who chose to receive PMTCT services and thus may be more likely to be adherent to medication, both for themselves and their babies, limiting generalizability to the population as a whole and suggesting that overall transmission might actually be higher than our data show.

The retrospective nature of our data collection represents a single point in time for each women and her infant while PMTCT policy, research, and guidelines have changed dramatically over these years. Tanzania is no exception. The changes demonstrated for the time period of 2008–2010 must be taken into context; namely, prior to major changes in the WHO PMTCT guidelines and in particular with the rollout of Option B/B+. Thus, the historical nature of our data does not reflect current practice in these settings. Still, however, the findings have both direct and indirect relevance to current practice. As we demonstrated, there were still women in 2010 who failed to receive any PMTCT services, and women who still received sdNVP only. With changing guidelines, improved access to care, and lower MTCT rates over time, we would expect that MTCT rates in Tanzania have now decreased even further. Today, Tanzania is rolling out option B+ and soon all HIV-infected pregnant women in the country should have access to lifelong HAART, offering the opportunity to decrease perinatal HIV transmissions even further.

Conclusions

In conclusion, our study demonstrates reductions in MTCT of HIV-1 in three regions of Tanzania coincident with increased use of more effective PMTCT interventions. The country's change in guidelines in recent years is seen at the field level by the change in treatment regimens over time, an increase in the uptake of maternal prophylaxis, and a subsequent decrease in the use of sdNVP. The use of infant DBS PCR is a valuable tool as an adjunct measurement of the effectiveness of PMTCT regimens and programs. The overall decrease in the proportion of positive

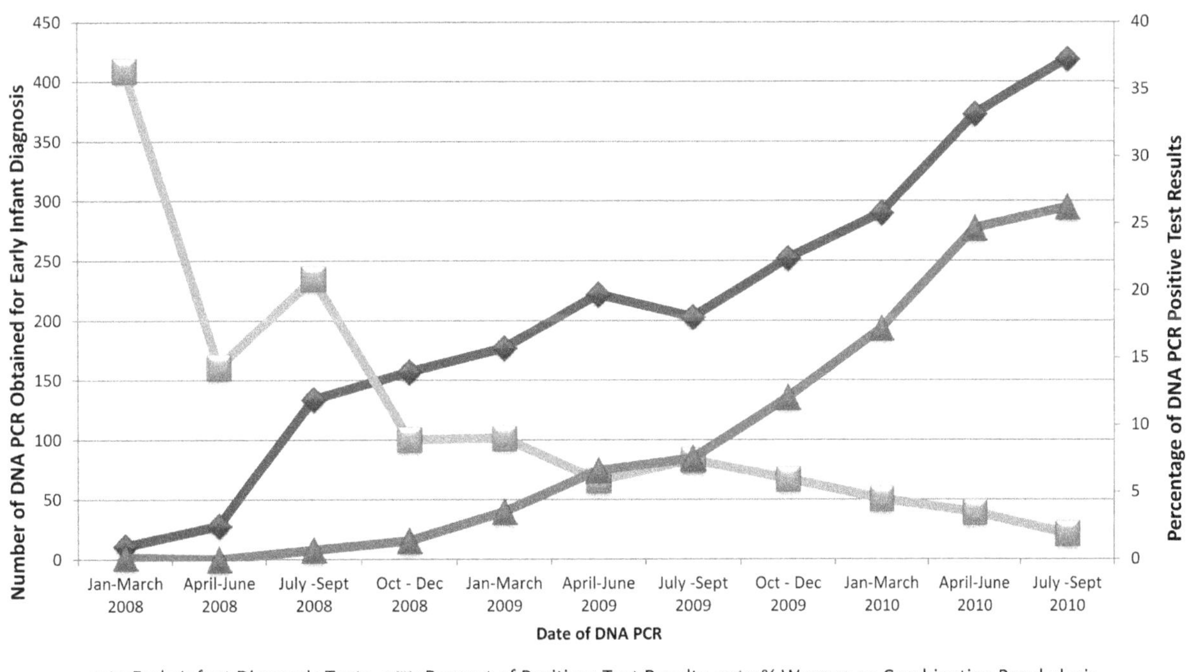

Figure 4. Changes in Early Infant Diagnosis Scale-Up and Percent HIV DNA PCR Positive over Study Period, January 2008–September 2010.

PCR over time, as well as the uptake of EID testing, are encouraging for Tanzania.

Acknowledgments

We would like to thank the Tanzanian Ministry of Health and PEPFAR with implementing partners for their support of this project. We thank our research assistants Jovita Jackson and Prisca Dominic who participated in data collection, organization, and cleaning. We are especially grateful to the staff and patients of the many health facilities visited throughout Arusha, Kilimanjaro, and Tanga Regions, Tanzania. This paper was presented in part as a poster at the XIX International AIDS Society Conference, Washington, DC, July 2012, Abstract # WEPE198.

Author Contributions

Conceived and designed the experiments: AMB JAB CKC CGM WS AS. Performed the experiments: BN RM. Analyzed the data: DED SF. Contributed reagents/materials/analysis tools: BN. Wrote the paper: AMB DED CGM BN AS RM SF JAB CKC WS.

References

1. UNAIDS (2012) UNAIDS Report on the Global AIDS Epidemic. Geneva: UNAIDS.
2. Obimbo EM, Mbori-Ngacha DA, Ochieng JO, Richardson BA, Otieno PA, et al. (2004) Predictors of early mortality in a cohort of human immunodeficiency virus type 1-infected african children. Pediatr Infect Dis J 23: 536–543.
3. Jamieson DJ, Clark J, Kourtis AP, Taylor AW, Lampe MA, et al. (2007) Recommendations for human immunodeficiency virus screening, prophylaxis, and treatment for pregnant women in the United States. Am J Obstet Gynecol 197: S26–32.
4. Jaspan HB, Garry RF (2003) Preventing neonatal HIV: a review. Curr HIV Res 1: 321–327.
5. Dao H, Mofenson LM, Ekpini R, Gilks CF, Barnhart M, et al. (2007) International recommendations on antiretroviral drugs for treatment of HIV-infected women and prevention of mother-to-child HIV transmission in resource-limited settings: 2006 update. Am J Obstet Gynecol 197: S42–55.
6. Dryden-Peterson S, Jayeoba O, Hughes MD, Jibril H, Keapoletswe K, et al. (2011) Highly active antiretroviral therapy versus zidovudine for prevention of mother-to-child transmission in a programmatic setting, Botswana. J Acquir Immune Defic Syndr 58: 353–357.
7. Shapiro RL, Hughes MD, Ogwu A, Kitch D, Lockman S, et al. (2010) Antiretroviral regimens in pregnancy and breast-feeding in Botswana. N Engl J Med 362: 2282–2294.
8. Kouanda S, Tougri H, Cisse M, Simpore J, Pietra V, et al. (2010) Impact of maternal HAART on the prevention of mother-to-child transmission of HIV: results of an 18-month follow-up study in Ouagadougou, Burkina Faso. AIDS Care 22: 843–850.
9. Ekouevi DK, Coffie PA, Becquet R, Tonwe-Gold B, Horo A, et al. (2008) Antiretroviral therapy in pregnant women with advanced HIV disease and pregnancy outcomes in Abidjan, Cote d'Ivoire. AIDS 22: 1815–1820.
10. Marazzi MC, Liotta G, Nielsen-Saines K, Haswell J, Magid NA, et al. (2010) Extended antenatal antiretroviral use correlates with improved infant outcomes throughout the first year of life. AIDS 24: 2819–2826.
11. UNAIDS (2011) Global Plan Towards the Elimination of New HIV Infections among Children by 2015 and Keeping Their Mothers Alive: 2011–2015. Geneva: UNAIDS.
12. National AIDS Control Programme, Ministry of Health and Social Welfare, The United Republic of Tanzania (2012) National Guidelines for the Management of HIV and AIDS. Available: http://www.nacp.go.tz/documents/nationalguideline42012.pdf. Accessed 3 May 2013.
13. Ministry of Health and Social Welfare, The United Republic of Tanzania (2012) Tanzania Elimination of Mother to Child Transmission of HIV Plan, 2012–2015. Available: http://www.emtct-iatt.org/wp-content/uploads/2012/11/Costed-eMTCT-Plan-Final-Nov-20121.pdf. Accessed 28 March 2013.
14. Ministry of Health and Social Welfare, The United Republic of Tanzania (2011) Prevention of Mother-to-Child Transmission of HIV: National Guidelines. Available: www.wavuti.com/4/post/2011/5/tanzania-pmtct-guideline-2011.html. Accessed 12 July 2011.
15. De Cock KM, Fowler MG, Mercier E, de Vincenzi I, Saba J, et al. (2000) Prevention of mother-to-child HIV transmission in resource-poor countries: translating research into policy and practice. JAMA 283: 1175–1182.
16. Olayinka B, Oni AO, Mbajiorgu FE (2000) Impact of infant feeding practices on the risk of mother to child transmission of HIV-1 in Zimbabwe. J Paediatr Child Health 36: 313–317.
17. Coutsoudis A (2000) Influence of infant feeding patterns on early mother-to-child transmission of HIV-1 in Durban, South Africa. Ann N Y Acad Sci 918: 136–144.
18. Petra Study Team (2002) Efficacy of three short-course regimens of zidovudine and lamivudine in preventing early and late transmission of HIV-1 from mother to child in Tanzania, South Africa, and Uganda (Petra study): a randomised, double-blind, placebo-controlled trial. Lancet 359: 1178–1186.
19. Torpey K, Mandala J, Kasonde P, Bryan-Mofya G, Bweupe M, et al. (2012) Analysis of HIV early infant diagnosis data to estimate rates of perinatal HIV transmission in Zambia. PLoS One 7: e42859.
20. Anoje C, Aiyenigba B, Suzuki C, Badru T, Akpoigbe K, et al. (2012) Reducing mother-to-child transmission of HIV: findings from an early infant diagnosis program in south-south region of Nigeria. BMC Public Health 12: 184.
21. Lallemant M, Jourdain G, Le Coeur S, Mary JY, Ngo-Giang-Huong N, et al. (2004) Single-dose perinatal nevirapine plus standard zidovudine to prevent mother-to-child transmission of HIV-1 in Thailand. N Engl J Med 351: 217–228.
22. Dabis F, Bequet L, Ekouevi DK, Viho I, Rouet F, et al. (2005) Field efficacy of zidovudine, lamivudine and single-dose nevirapine to prevent peripartum HIV transmission. AIDS 19: 309–318.
23. Cooper ER, Charurat M, Mofenson L, Hanson IC, Pitt J, et al. (2002) Combination antiretroviral strategies for the treatment of pregnant HIV-1-infected women and prevention of perinatal HIV-1 transmission. J Acquir Immune Defic Syndr 29: 484–494.
24. Dorenbaum A, Cunningham CK, Gelber RD, Culnane M, Mofenson L, et al. (2002) Two-dose intrapartum/newborn nevirapine and standard antiretroviral therapy to reduce perinatal HIV transmission: a randomized trial. JAMA 288: 189–198.
25. Mandelbrot L, Landreau-Mascaro A, Rekacewicz C, Berrebi A, Benifla JL, et al. (2001) Lamivudine-zidovudine combination for prevention of maternal-infant transmission of HIV-1. JAMA 285: 2083–2093.
26. Simpson BJ, Shapiro ED, Andiman WA (2000) Prospective cohort study of children born to human immunodeficiency virus-infected mothers, 1985 through 1997: trends in the risk of vertical transmission, mortality and acquired immunodeficiency syndrome indicator diseases in the era before highly active antiretroviral therapy. Pediatr Infect Dis J 19: 618–624.

Effect of a One-Off Educational Session about Enterobiasis on Knowledge, Preventative Practices, and Infection Rates among Schoolchildren in South Korea

Dong-Hee Kim[1], Hak Sun Yu[2,3]*

1 Department of Nursing, College of Nursing, Pusan National University, Yangsan, Gyeongsangnamdo, South Korea, **2** Department of Parasitology, School of Medicine, Pusan National University, Yangsan, Gyeongsangnamdo, South Korea, **3** Immunoregulatory therapeutics group in Brain Busan 21 project, Busan, South Korea

Abstract

Although health education has proven to be cost-effective in slowing the spread of enterobiasis, assessments of the effectiveness of health education to reduce infectious diseases specifically in children are rare. To evaluate the effect of health education on knowledge, preventative practices, and the prevalence of enterobiasis, 319 children from 16 classes were divided into experimental and control groups. Data were collected from May 2012 to March 2013. A 40-minute in-class talk was given once in the experimental group. There were significant differences over the time in the mean scores for children's knowledge of *Enterobius vermicularis* infection in the intervention group compared to the control group ($p < 0.001$). After the educational session, the score for knowledge about *E. vermicularis* infection increased from 60.2±2.32 to 92.7±1.19 in the experimental group; this gain was partially lost 3 months later, decreasing to 83.6±1.77 ($p < 0.001$). Children's enterobiasis infection prevention practice scores also increased, from 3.23±0.27 to 3.73±0.25, 1 week after the educational session, a gain that was partially lost at 3 months, decreasing to 3.46±0.36 ($p < 0.001$). The overall *E. vermicularis* egg detection rate was 4.4%; the rates for each school ranged from 0% to 12.9% at screening. The infection rate at 3 months after the treatment sharply decreased from 12.3% to 0.8% in the experimental group, compared to a decrease from 8.5% to 3.7% in the control group during the same period. We recommend that health education on enterobiasis be provided to children to increase their knowledge about enterobiasis and improve prevention practices.

Editor: David Joseph Diemert, The George Washington University Medical Center, United States of America

Funding: This research was supported by Basic Science Research Program through the National Research Foundation of Korea funded by the Ministry of Education, Science and Technology (NRF-2013R1A1A1A05012615). The funders had no role in study design, data collection and analysis, decision to publish, or preparation of the manuscript.

Competing Interests: The authors have declared that no competing interests exist.

* Email: hsyu@pusan.ac.kr

Introduction

Although most parasitic infectious diseases have disappeared in developed countries, enterobiasis (pinworm infection) has still often been reported in many developed countries [1–3]. In South Korea, the prevalence of total intestinal helminthic parasitic infection rates has sharply decreased from 84.3% in 1971 to 2.4% in 1997 [4,5]. However, a relatively high egg positive rate of *Enterobius vermicularis* ranging from 4% to 10% has been reported in Korean children during the last decade [6–9].

Enterobiasis is transmitted through direct contact with infected (or egg-contaminated) persons or objects. Transmission of *E. vermicularis* commonly occurs by ingesting infectious pinworm eggs. Eggs are transmitted from the anus to the finger, fingernails, or hands when an individual scratches the perianal area where the gravid female worms emerge and deposit eggs. Eggs are spread to underwear and night-clothing and further transmitted to other objects including food and books, desks, and chairs [10]. When dislodged from such objects, the eggs can enter another individual's mouth and nose, thereby being ingested [10,11]. As a result of this transmission process, children's personal and hygiene habits, such as thumb sucking, overcrowded conditions, and inadequate sanitation, contribute to the spread of enterobiasis in primary schools, where close contact between children occurs [2,7,9].

Medication against *E. vermicularis*, such as albendazole, is very effective in treating enterobiasis [12]. However, reinfection is also common in spite of treatment, as the medication only kills the adult worm but not the worm larvae [10]. An important aspect in the failure of single-dose chemotherapy is the continuing presence of infectious eggs in the environment, which facilitate rapid reinfection. Therefore, individuals with enterobiasis require repeated doses of medication to cover the time taken for the eggs to become adult worms. Importantly, most parents in South Korea believe that antihelminthic medications can easily cure every helminthic infection, including those by *E. vermicularis*, by just a one-time treatment [9]. In addition, most kindergarten directors and teachers have limited knowledge of *E. vermicularis* infection [2].

Knowledge of disease has successfully improved many different health outcomes [13]. However, there has been little emphasis on the impact of health education on the prevalence of enterobiasis, despite the incidence of enterobiasis being reduced by encouraging habits of cleanliness in children. Health education promoting knowledge of enterobiasis has proven to be cost-effective in decreasing reinfection rates in schoolchildren [14]. Previously, we evaluated the impact of a health education among pre-school children [2]. We provided brochures on prevention, transmission, and treatment of enterobiasis to parents, as they are in charge of their child's personal hygiene since children younger than 6 years of age are not old enough to be responsible for self-care [2].

In the present study, we conducted an experimental health education session on enterobiasis at primary schools in South Korea and assessed its effect on knowledge about *E. vermicularis* infection, enterobiasis infection prevention practices, and the incidence rate of enterobiasis among primary school children in Korea.

Subjects and Methods

Subject recruitment and screening evaluation

Participants were Grade 1 and Grade 2 primary school students (aged 7−9 years) from separate school districts in three distinct regions: an industrial city, an urban site, and a suburban area of South Korea. Recruitment was conducted through the Office of Education websites at each of these sites with a letter informing about the nature, significance, and objectives of the study. Schools were approached with the help of an assistant. Once the assistant had obtained verbal consent from the principal of a school, investigators met with the principal and class teachers of each school to describe the details of the study. The class teachers sent a consent form, a letter of information, and a questionnaire to the parents of each child. A total of 3,840 children from 183 classes in 27 schools underwent a screening for enterobiasis via the sellotape anal swab technique. The parents were each given two pieces of sellotape and written instructions showing how to swab the perianal area of their child with the sellotape and other aspects of the screening procedure. The investigators emphasized that the examinations should be done before the child washed or went to the toilet in the morning to prevent any pinworms eggs from being washed from the area. We cautioned that the chances of making an incorrect diagnosis of enterobiasis increased when the parents did not swab their child's anus first thing in the morning before the child washed. We asked the parents to do this twice, on separate days.

Sample size was determined on the basis of the primary outcome, the score in the knowledge test after education. To have an 80% chance of detecting as significant (at the two sided 5% level) a 10 point difference between the two groups in the knowledge test scores after education, with an assumed standard deviation of 15, the overall sample size required is 74 individuals (37 in each arm of the study). Since this study is cluster-randomized, the sample size had to be larger than if simple randomization had been performed, in order to take into account the design effect. Assuming that the inter-cluster correlation coefficient is 0.1, and a mean cluster size is 21 individuals, the design effect is 3. Therefore, the number of individuals required in each group is 111 ('Cochrane Consumers and Communication Review Group: cluster randomized controlled trials'. http://cccrg.cochrane.org, March 2014). Assuming the expected drop-out rate of 10%, the final sample size required is 246 (123 in each arm) with a minimum of 6 clusters per arm.

Study design

The study was designed as a pretest-posttest experiment, with an equivalent control group. We excluded schools that had classes with an incidence rate of 0% at the screening evaluation, and then selected classes in which all students were tested at the screening evaluation. Based on a combination of similar egg positive rates and geographical locations, 10 schools in different regions were involved this study; two schools were in an industrial city, four schools were in an urban site, and four schools were in a suburban area. One or two classes participated at each school. Each school was identified as either an intervention or control group in order to control for the contamination of the control group. The schools were assigned to either the intervention (8 classes from 5 schools) or control (8 classes from 5 schools) arms through a coin toss. A total of 346 children from 16 classes were included at baseline. At post-treatment examination, 319 children (130 for the experimental and 189 for the control group) participated (Fig. 1). Blinding of investigators was not possible as the intervention was educational; however, the investigators were blinded to the exposure status of participants during data collection. In the intervention group, an educational session was given once, for 40 minutes, in a group setting for each class. In the control group, children received an *E. vermicularis* infection brochure. Knowledge of *E. vermicularis* infection and enterobiasis infection prevention practice and the *E. vermicularis* infection rate among children were evaluated at baseline and at 3 months after the intervention. Children's knowledge of *E. vermicularis* infection was assessed on the day of the educational session in order to ensure that their knowledge of *E. vermicularis* infection increased.

Intervention

The educational program was developed based on the Dick & Carey's Systematic Design of Instruction model [15]. A comprehensive review of the literature, a pilot study, and a focus group interview were used to develop the educational session. The session was comprised of topics such as the lifecycle of *E. vermicularis*, diagnosis of enterobiasis, symptoms and signs, infection and transmission, and treatment and prevention of enterobiasis. A trained teacher provided a 30-minute lecture using visual aids to stimulate interest and support explanations of the educational contents. The lecture included an example situation, describing how one student became infected with a pinworm, and showing how enterobiasis spread to other students in the same classroom. Key messages were reinforced with an interactive quiz, and there was a 10-minute session to answer students' questions.

Measurement

The main outcome variable is the improvement of 15 or more points in children's knowledge of *E. vermicularis* infection. As there are no currently published scales for children's knowledge on *E. vermicularis* infection and children's preventative practice against enterobiasis infection, the investigators composed a scale, which was validated by experts (including parasitologists, pediatric doctors, internal medicine doctors, school nurses, and schoolteachers). Four pilot studies were conducted to assess comprehension of the questionnaire items. The instrument to measure children's knowledge of *E. vermicularis* infection included 10 dichotomous items (answered as either "correct" [1 point] or "incorrect" [0 points]).

The secondary outcome variables recorded are children's prevention practices and the infection rate 3 months later. The instrument to assess children's prevention practices consisted of 8 Likert-scale items; each Likert item ranged from 1 (never) to 4 (every time).

Study procedure

Children in both the education and control groups who tested positive for *E. vermicularis* eggs received medical treatment with 400 mg albendazole twice, at a 15-day interval. The pre-treatment structured questionnaire on knowledge of *E. vermicularis* infection was provided to the children by a class teacher. This questionnaire

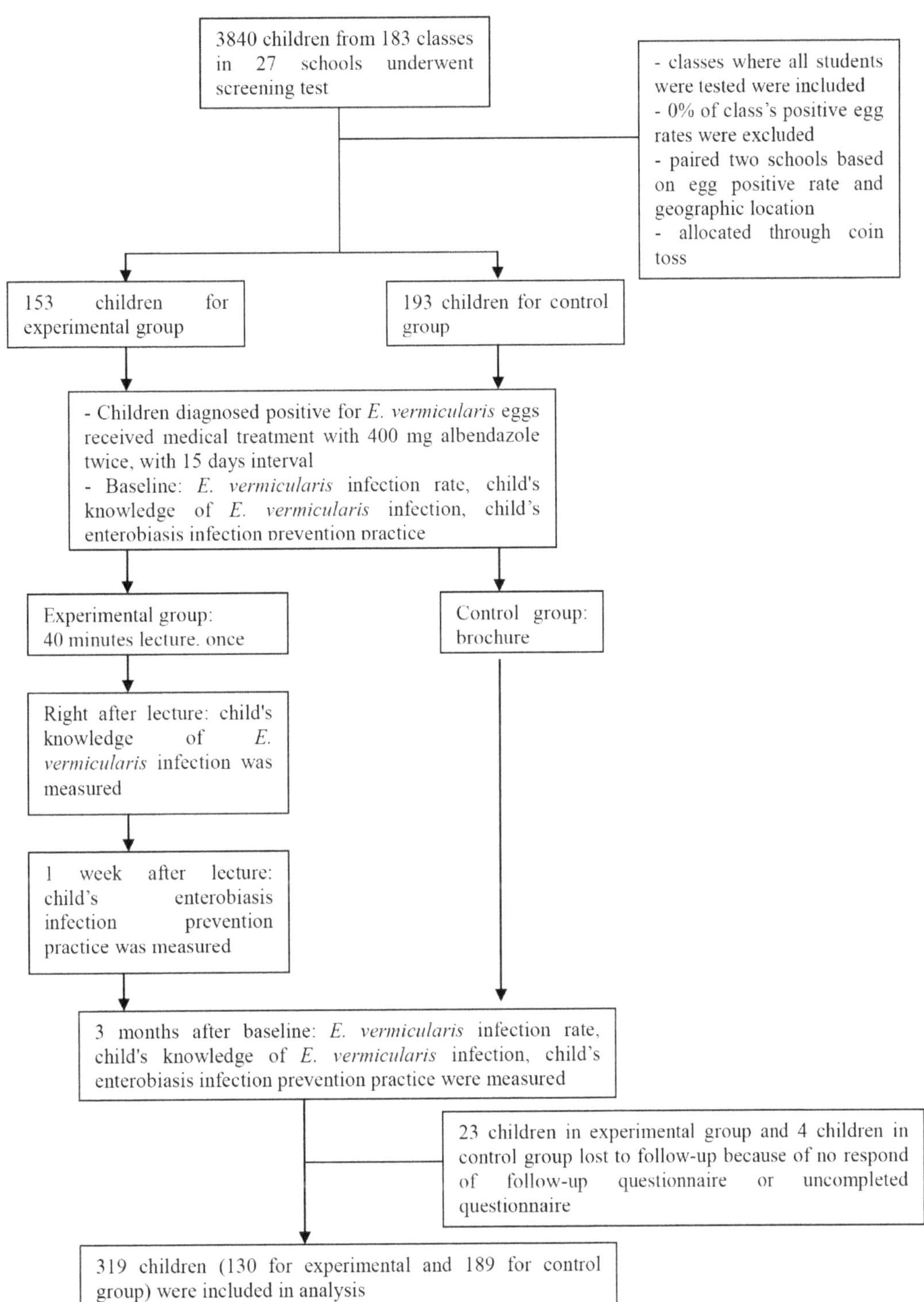

Figure 1. Study design including screening, group allocation, and follow-up. A total of 319 children from 16 classes were invited from among 3,840 children screened from 183 classes. The schools were assigned to either the intervention or the control arms by simple randomization using a coin toss.

was also provided to the parents of each child, enquiring about demographics and socioeconomic status, the child's enterobiasis infection prevention practices at home, and the parents' knowledge of enterobiasis. Children's knowledge of *E. vermicularis* infection was assessed the day they learned about enterobiasis and 3 months later. One week and three months after the intervention, parents were asked to complete another questionnaire on the children's enterobiasis infection prevention practices at home. *E. vermicularis* egg detection and the reinfection rates were evaluated using a sellotape anal swab 3 months after the intervention.

Ethics statement

The study was performed after receiving approval from the Ethical Review Committee of Yangsan Pusan National University Hospital, and after informed written consent was obtained from each participant before enrollment. Participation was entirely voluntary. Participants, including principals and teachers of schools, parents, and their children, were free to refuse to participate or withdraw from the study at any time, and were informed that only the aggregate data would be reported. Informed consent for the children in this study was provided by their parents or guardians and by the children. Once we obtained written consent from the parents or guardians to contact their children, the class teacher informed the children that permission to conduct the study had been granted. We briefed the individual children about the study and what they were being asked to do. Children who diagnosed positive for *E. vermicularis* eggs at screening received medical treatment with 400 mg albendazole twice, at a 15-day interval.

Statistical analysis

We report descriptive statistics for the characteristics of study sites and individual participants. To test the effectiveness of the education program in changing children's knowledge and prevention practices (continuous variables), we used multivariable mixed-effects analysis allowing random effects for clusters and controlling for gender and age. Each estimator was presented with its 95% confidence interval (95% CI). The prevalence of *E. vermicularis* eggs at baseline and after treatment in each group was compared using proportions and the McNemar test.

To examine the effectiveness of the education program in reducing infection (yes: 1; no: 0, binary response), we used multivariable logistic regression allowing random effects for clusters. All statistical analyses were performed using SAS 9.2 (SAS Institute, Inc., Cary, NC) statistical package and p values less than 0.05 were considered as statistically significant.

Results

Participant characteristics were compared between the experimental and control groups, most of which were similar. The small differences observed between groups were not statistically significant. Several characteristics of the participants are shown in Table S1. The overall *E. vermicularis* egg detection rate was 4.4%; the rate for each school ranged from 0% to 12.9% at screening (Table 1). Characteristics of study sites and individual participants are summarized in Table 2. Experimental and control groups enrolled 130 and 189 children, respectively. There were no statistically significant differences in children's baseline characteristics ($p>0.05$).

Between-group comparisons of knowledge of and prevention practices for *E. vermicularis* infection, as well as the prevalence of *E. vermicularis* egg positive rates, are show in Table 3. There were significant time effects in the mean scores for children's knowledge of *E. vermicularis* infection in the intervention group compared to the control group ($p<0.001$). Regarding *E. vermicularis* infection prevention practices, the experimental group increased from 3.22 to 3.45 (a difference of 0.23), whereas the control group increased from 3.19 to 3.23 (a difference of 0.04) between baseline and 3 months after treatment ($p<0.001$). The experimental group had a higher increase in knowledge test scores than the control group (adjusted difference = 1.95 [95% CI, 1.57–2.34]; $p<0.001$). The experimental group also had a higher increase in prevention practices than the control group (adjusted difference = 0.19 [95% CI, 0.13–0.25]; $p<0.001$). Clustering was considered in all logistic and multivariate regression models.

The incidence rate was lower in the experimental group, although this finding was not significant after adjustment for the clusters as random effects (adjusted odds ratio = 0.20, 95% CI = 0.02–2.41, $p=0.175$). The infection rate at 3 months after treatment sharply decreased from 12.3% to 0.8% in the experimental group ($p<0.001$), while that in the control group decreased from 8.5% to 3.7% ($p=0.049$) during the same period. Some children were diagnosed with new infections at 3 months after treatment; however, the number of new infections in the experimental group was lower than that in the control group. Moreover, although children who tested positive for *E. vermicularis* eggs were treated with antihelminthic drugs at baseline, *E. vermicularis* reinfection was observed in the control group.

We also jointly compared baseline, post-education, and 3-month changes in the experimental group. Correct answer rates on the *E. vermicularis* infection knowledge test in the experimental group are shown in Table 4. After the educational session, the score for knowledge about *E. vermicularis* infection increased from 60.2±2.32 to 92.7±1.19 in the experimental group; this gain was partially lost 3 months after the educational session, decreasing to 83.6±1.77 ($p<0.001$). The correct answer rate was 34.6% to 78.5% at baseline, 80.0% to 99.2% at post-education, and 75.4% to 93.1% 3 months after the intervention. At baseline, the item "Proper teeth brushing can prevent *E. vermicularis* infection" (34.6%) had the lowest rate of correct answers, followed by "Weekly change of underwear is important for preventing *E. vermicularis* infection" (36.9%), "*E. vermicularis* is not transmitted to other humans via hand contact" (47.7%), and "*E. vermicularis* infection can be treated by taking antihelminthic medication once" (50.0%); the rates for these items increased to over 80% correct responses at post-education, and over 75% correct 3 months later.

Results for children's practices for the prevention of *E. vermicularis* infection are shown in Table 5. Children's enterobiasis infection prevention practice scores also increased, from 3.23±0.27 to 3.73±0.25, 1 week after the educational session, and then partially decreased to 3.46±0.36 after 3 months ($p<0.001$). Items related to hand washing had lower scores than other items, such as keeping nails short and cleaning underwear. After 3 months, the item "My child does not bite his/her nails" had the lowest score of all items at both 1 week and 3 months after the health education session.

Discussion

Mass drug administration is the most effective means to control enterobiasis, but this method also has some limitations in that it does not prevent reinfections. In a previous study, we found new infection cases in the mass drug administration treatment group at both 3 and 6 months after treatment [2]. Moreover, reinfection increases the financial burden placed on preventative medicine programs. Consensus among government health employees and social workers might be necessary, because part of the cost of group treatment must be covered by the government. Furthermore, there is concern that mass drug administration might lead to the development of drug-resistant parasites [16]. The development of drug resistance in nematodes that infect humans is considered inevitable, given the number of species infecting livestock that are now resistant to antihelminthic agents due to continuous and extensive drug use [17,18]. Strategies to reduce the overall incidence of enterobiasis infection are likely to require an integrated approach, including pharmacological treatment to

Table 1. Egg positive rates of *E. vermicularis* infection among children in South Korea (n = 3840).

School	No. class	No. examined/total No. student (compliance %)	No. positive (%)
1	2	31/37 (83.8)	4(12.9)
2	11	260/287 (90.6)	21(8.1)
3	6	97/133 (72.9)	7(7.2)
4	2	15/19 (78.9)	1(6.7)
5	6	139/152 (91.4)	9(6.5)
6	6	122/136 (89.7)	7(5.7)
7	4	57/57 (100.0)	3(5.3)
8	13	317/361 (87.8)	16(5.0)
9	6	142/155 (91.6)	7(4.9)
10	10	238/256 (93.0)	11(4.6)
11	9	160/203 (78.8)	7(4.4)
12	6	115/149 (77.2)	5(4.3)
13	8	189/242 (78.1)	8(4.2)
14	10	288/309 (93.2)	12(4.2)
15	9	135/220 (61.4)	5(3.7)
16	10	202/259 (78.0)	7(3.5)
17	8	145/182 (79.7)	5(3.4)
18	8	134/189 (70.9)	4(3.0)
19	12	277/316 (87.7)	8(2.9)
20	9	272/272 (100.0)	8(2.9)
21	4	82/100 (82.0)	2(2.4)
22	6	127/158 (80.4)	3(2.4)
23	4	84/89 (94.4)	2(2.4)
24	7	134/169 (79.3)	1(0.7)
25	2	33/33 (100.0)	0(0.0)
26	2	17/17 (100.0)	0(0.0)
27	3	28/59 (47.5)	0(0.0)
Total	183	3840/4559 (84.2)	163
Mean positive rate			4.4%

reduce the infection rate and health education for prevention and sustainable control.

Our results showed that health-education increased students' knowledge about enterobiasis transmission and changed their behavior. Notably, students washed their hands more frequently and sucked their fingers or toys less after the health education session (Tables 4 and 5). Most instances of infection transmission could be effectively prevented by repeated hand washes; therefore, behavioral changes might contribute to a reduction in enterobiasis rates. Interestingly, most students remembered general facts about enterobiasis (life cycle, transmission route, prevention, etc.) 3 months after receiving an educational lecture (Table 4).

In Korea, over 80% of people were infected with intestinal helminthic parasites in the 1960s [19]. Most people at the time lived in poor environments in which parasitic infections were easily transmitted [20]. Additionally, farmers at the time used "Night-soil" (human feces and urine) as fertilizer on food crops. Furthermore, underground water was easily contaminated by parasite eggs found in human and animal feces; therefore, parasites were not easily eradicated in humans by mass drug administration. However, after the South Korean government launched a life environmental improvement project ("Saemaeul" [new village] Movement) and established the Korean Parasite Eradiation Association (KPEA), parasitic infection rates rapidly decreased. The Saemaeul Movement improved the drinking water supply system and sewage treatment system. The KPEA (now, Korea Association of Health Promotion) strived to eradicate parasite infections by conducting periodic examinations of the parasite infection rate, treating infected people, and providing preventative education for inhabitants in endemic areas. After the 1990s, most intestinal parasitic infection rates decreased to less than 3.0% in South Korea, with soil-transmitted helminthic infection rates decreasing to less than 1.0% [2,9].

However, in spite of the struggles of the government, enterobiasis has yet to be eliminated. One of the reasons for this is that there are misconceptions about enterobiasis in South Korea [2,9]. The first is the belief that parasitic infections, including enterobiasis, have already disappeared in South Korea; due to this belief, approximately half of children have not taken medication against helminthic parasites, including pinworms. The second misconception is that enterobiasis can easily be cured by a one-time anti-helminthic medication, as is the case for other intestinal nematodes. It was recently shown that the numbers of young children being cared for in group facilities, including private

Table 2. Characteristics of study sites and individual participants (n = 319).

Characteristic		Experimental (n = 130)	Control (n = 189)	P value
Site's characteristic				
Cluster size				
	mean ± SD	19.13±3.94	24.25±2.25	
No. of Conforming Requests/Total				
		11/14(78.6%)	25/26 (96.2%)	
		21/23 (91.3%)	21/21 (100.0%)	
		18/21 (85.7%)	27/27 (100.0%)	
		18/21 (85.7%)	21/21 (100.0%)	
		16/20 (80.0%)	23/24 (95.8%)	
		19/24 (79.2%)	23/24 (95.8%)	
		14/16 (87.5%)	26/26 (100.0%)	
		13/14 (92.9%)	23/25 (92.0%)	
Total		130/153 (85.0%)	189/194 (97.4%)	
Children's characteristics				
Sex				
	Male	69 (53.9%)	104 (57.1%)	0.581
	Female	59 (46.1%)	78 (42.9%)	
Age				
	Mean ± SD	8.22±0.70	8.24±0.67	0.827
House type				
	Apartment	109 (85.2%)	158 (86.8%)	0.823
	Non-apartment	19 (14.8%)	24 (13.2%)	
Job of parents				
	Single	71 (55.5%)	99 (54.4%)	0.261
	Both	57 (44.5%)	83 (45.6%)	
Family size				
	≤3 persons	96 (76.8%)	142 (78.5%)	0.583
	>4 persons	29 (23.2%)	39 (21.5%)	

educational institutes, have increased, and the employees and teachers of these facilities have such misconceptions [2]. Therefore, opportunities for infection and transmission from child to child have increased as a result. These misconceptions should be rectified through health education providing the correct information, which would be expected to result in a rapid decrease in infection rates [2,9].

Visual educational materials targeting schoolchildren have been shown to have a positive effect on knowledge and attitudes [18,21,22]. In this study, the educational information on enterobiasis included cartoon materials and real-life visual representations, such as microscopic images of pinworms, sellotape used for the diagnosis of enterobiasis, and the medications used to treat it. Most students who participated in this study were interested and immersed in the example situation as if he/she was the infected student. We believe that storytelling using cartoon materials was effective in helping children to focus on the educational contents. Moreover, descriptions of other aspects, such as the sellotape anal swab technique for diagnosis, elicited a response from the students, as they had themselves experienced this during the baseline data collection period. Finally, the interactive quiz emphasized the major educational content. This interactive health education session might lead to behavioral changes that result in decreasing the risk of *E. vermicularis* infection.

The health education session increased knowledge about enterobiasis. We were worried that at the 3-month follow-up assessment children would not remember the information acquired earlier. However, interestingly, the majority of children remembered most of the information they had learned on the subject. In addition, their prevention practices against *E. vermicularis* infection were maintained in their daily lives. Some children were administered the antihelminthic drug (albendazole) at the same time as their family members (personal communication), indicating that educating children may also have an indirect influence on their family members. These results could provide substantial gains in the elimination of enterobiasis in Korea, since Grade 1 and 2 primary school students are the most commonly infected population [6,23].

The prevalence of the *E. vermicularis* egg positive rate was not significant after adjusting for clusters as a random effect in this study, although the infection rates in the experimental group showed larger changes than in the control group. In a previous study, Gai et al. reported the negative relationship between the rate of parasitic infection and knowledge of prevention [24]. Enterobiasis was successfully treated with an anthelminthic agent.

Table 3. Comparison of the prevalence of *E. vermicularis* egg positive rates, knowledge, and prevention practices for *E. vermicularis* infection between groups (n = 319).

	Time	Experimental (n = 130)	Control (n = 189)	P value of Difference	Treatment Difference
		n (%)/mean ± SD	n (%)/mean ± SD		(95% CI)
Knowledge					
Baseline		6.02±2.32	6.12±2.09		
3 months after		8.36±1.77	6.45±2.04		
Difference		2.35±2.43	0.33±0.97	<0.001	1.96‡ (1.57–2.34)
Preventing Practice					
Baseline		3.22±0.28	3.19±0.43		
3 months after		3.45±0.36	3.23±0.40		
Difference		0.23±0.37	0.04±0.18	<0.001	0.19‡ (0.13–0.25)
Infection rate					
Baseline	Positive	16(12.3%)	16 (8.5%)	0.263	
3 months after	Positive	1(0.8%)*	7 (3.7%)*	0.175	0.20†(0.02–2.41)
Baseline - 3 months after	Positive - positive (re-infection case)	0(0.0%)	3(1.6%)		
	Negative - positive (New infected case)	1(0.8%)	4(2.1%)		

*Statistically significant between baseline and 3 months in experimental group ($p<0.001$) and control group ($p = 0.049$), based on the McNemar test.
†OR was adjusted for clusters as a random effect.
‡Mean difference was adjusted for clusters as a random effect, as well as gender and age.

Children in both the education and control groups who tested positive for *E. vermicularis* eggs received medical treatment with albendazole at baseline according to ethical considerations. Moreover, we evaluated the effect of the intervention for 3 months since participants changed classes as they advanced into the next grade. Future long-term evaluation studies need to assess whether health education increasing students' knowledge about enterobiasis transmission impacts infection rates.

Our study has a few limitations. First, there was potential confounding effect due to interaction between teachers in the experimental and control groups, despite our attempts to maintain a distance between groups by selecting them from different districts. Second, we asked the parents to assess their children's enterobiasis infection prevention practices, that is an indirect measure and might not be accurate. In addition, we asked the parents to do the Sellotape swab of their child's anus first thing in the morning, before the child had washed. There is a possibility that the children's parents decided to wash their child first, before preparing the swab, to show that their child had not become reinfected. This would influence the infection rates 3 months after the educational session. Third, as the study could not be double-blinded, other factors may have affected the results. Furthermore,

Table 4. Assessment of children's correct answer rates on *E. vermicularis* infection knowledge test (Experimental group: n = 130).

Items	Correct answer rate (%)		
	Baseline	After education	3 month after
E. vermicularis is parasitic worm that can live inside the human	74.6	99.2	88.5
E. vermicularis is not transmitted to other human via hands	47.7	86.9	88.5
Enterobius vermicularis infection can be diagnosed by using sellotape anal technique	68.5	98.5	83.1
Child with *E. vermicularis* may have anal itching	71.5	98.5	93.1
The habits of sucking fingers or biting nails is associated with *E. vermicularis* infection	65.4	93.1	89.2
Good hand hygiene can help prevent the spread of *E. vermicularis* infection	78.5	95.4	91.5
Proper brushing teeth can be preventive *E. vermicularis* infection	34.6	91.5	79.2
Anal cleansing can help prevent *E. vermicularis* infection	73.8	95.4	86.2
Weekly change of underwear is good for preventing *E. vermicularis* infection	36.9	80.0	75.4
E. vermicularis infection can be treated by taking antihelminthic medication once	50.0	88.5	80.0
Over all M± SD	60.2±2.32	92.7±1.19	83.6±1.77
Generalized linear mixed model test statistic (*p*)	157.230 (<0.001)		

Table 5. Children's prevention practices for *E. vermicularis* infection (Experimental group: n = 130).

Items	Baseline	1 week after	3 month after
My child practices hand washing after defecation	3.00±0.29	3.71±0.47	3.32±0.60
My child practices hand washing before eating	2.72±0.51	3.57±0.53	3.32±0.61
My child practices hand washing after coming in from outside	2.89±0.44	3.77±0.48	3.51±0.59
My child does not sucking fingers or toys	3.30±0.86	3.68±0.62	3.50±0.79
My child does not biting nails	3.12±0.97	3.45±0.82	3.28±0.96
My child keeps the nails short	3.58±0.75	3.78±0.54	3.40±0.55
My child practices proper anal cleansing	3.49±0.61	3.96±0.20	3.59±0.55
My child wears clean underwear	3.63±0.60	3.96±0.20	3.65±0.48
Over all M± SD	3.23±0.27	3.73±0.25	3.46±0.36
Generalized linear mixed model test statistic (*p*)		149.486 (<0.001)	

it was not clear whether the educational session would have an impact on infection rates due to lack of previous studies. That is why we tested children's knowledge as a primary outcome. To detect the infection rate difference of 2.9 derived in this study, the total number of clusters required is 117. Due to the lack of statistical power, the result regarding infection rates need to be interpreted with caution and future studies with large sample sizes are required.

In spite of these limitations, we believe that health education can be a cost-effective and safe strategy to decrease enterobiasis and other childhood diseases through to adulthood, as behaviors obtained early in life can result in long-term favorable sanitary habits later in life.

Acknowledgments

We would like to thank J. M. Choi at ACE statistical consulting for his valuable recommendations on statistical aspects of this paper.

Author Contributions

Conceived and designed the experiments: DHK HSY. Performed the experiments: DHK HSY. Analyzed the data: DHK HSY. Contributed reagents/materials/analysis tools: DHK HSY. Wrote the paper: DHK HSY.

References

1. Degerli S, Malatyali E, Ozcelik S, Celiksoz A (2009) Enterobiosis in Sivas, Turkey from past to present, effects on primary school children and potential risk factors. Turkiye Parazitol Derg 33: 95–100.
2. Kang IS, Kim DH, An HG, Son HM, Cho MK, et al. (2012) Impact of health education on the prevalence of enterobiasis in Korean preschool students. Acta Trop 122: 59–63.
3. Bager P, Vinkel Hansen A, Wohlfahrt J, Melbye M (2012) Helminth infection does not reduce risk for chronic inflammatory disease in a population-based cohort study. Gastroenterology 142: 55–62.
4. Report of Ministry of Health and Welfare of Republic of Korea and the Korea Association of Health (1971) Prevalence of intestinal parasitic infections in Korea—1st report. Ministry of Health and Welfare of Republic of Korea and the Korea Association of Health.
5. Report of Ministry of Health and Welfare of Republic of Korea and the Korea Association of Health (1997) Prevalence of intestinal parasitic infections in Korea -6th report. Ministry of Health and Welfare of Republic of Korea and the Korea Association of Health.
6. Kim BJ, Lee BY, Chung HK, Lee YS, Lee KH, et al. (2003) Egg positive rate of Enterobius vermicularis of primary school children in Geoje island. The Korean J Parasitol 41: 75–77.
7. Song HJ, Cho CH, Kim JS, Choi MH, Hong ST (2003) Prevalence and risk factors for enterobiasis among preschool children in a metropolitan city in Korea. Parasitol Res 91: 46–50.
8. Kang S, Jeon HK, Eom KS, Park JK (2006) Egg positive rate of Enterobius vermicularis among preschool children in Cheongju, Chungcheongbuk-do, Korea. Korean J Parasitol 44: 247–249.
9. Kim DH, Son HM, Kim JY, Cho MK, Park MK, et al. (2010) Parents' knowledge about enterobiasis might be one of the most important risk factors for enterobiasis in children. Korean J Parasitol 48: 121–126.
10. Roberts LS, Schmidt GD, Janovy J (2009) Foundations of parasitology. Boston: McGraw-Hill Higher Education. xvii, 701 p.
11. Cook GC (1994) Enterobius vermicularis infection. Gut 35: 1159–1162.
12. St Georgiev V (2001) Chemotherapy of enterobiasis (oxyuriasis). Expert Opin pharmacother 2: 267–275.
13. Owais A, Hanif B, Siddiqui AR, Agha A, Zaidi AK (2011) Does improving maternal knowledge of vaccines impact infant immunization rates? A community-based randomized-controlled trial in Karachi, Pakistan. BMC Public Health 11: 239.
14. Nithikathkul C, Akarachantachote N, Wannapinyosheep S, Pumdonming W, Brodsky M, et al. (2005) Impact of health educational programmes on the prevalence of enterobiasis in schoolchildren in Thailand. J Helminthol 79: 61–65.
15. Dick W, Carey L, Carey JO (2005) The systematic design of instruction. Boston; London: Pearson/Allyn & Bacon. xx, 376 p.
16. Keiser J, Utzinger J (2010) The drugs we have and the drugs we need against major helminth infections. Adv Parasitol 73: 197–230.
17. Albonico M (2003) Methods to sustain drug efficacy in helminth control programmes. Acta Trop 86: 233–242.
18. Bieri FA, Gray DJ, Williams GM, Raso G, Li YS, et al. (2013) Health-education package to prevent worm infections in Chinese schoolchildren. N Engl J Med 368: 1603–1612.
19. Seo BS, Rim HJ, Loh IK, Lee SH, Cho SY, et al. (1969) [Study On The Status Of Helminthic Infections In Koreans]. Kisaengchunghak chapchi 7: 53–70.
20. Kim CH, Park CH, Kim HJ, Chun HB, Min HK, et al. (1971) [Prevalence Of Intestinal Parasites In Korea]. Kisaengchunghak chapchi 9: 25–38.
21. Myint UA, Bull S, Greenwood GL, Patterson J, Rietmeijer CA, et al. (2010) Safe in the city: developing an effective video-based intervention for STD clinic waiting rooms. Health Promot Pract 11: 408–417.
22. Naldi L, Chatenoud L, Bertuccio P, Zinetti C, Di Landro A, et al. (2007) Improving sun-protection behavior among children: results of a cluster-randomized trial in Italian elementary schools. The "SoleSi SoleNo-GISED" Project. J Invest Dermatol 127: 1871–1877.
23. Lee KJ, Ahn YK, Ryang YS (2001) *Enterobius vermicularis* egg positive rates in primary school children in Gangwon-do (province), Korea. Korean J Parasitol 39: 327–328.
24. Gai L, Ma X, Fu Y, Huang D (1995) [Relationship between the rate of parasitic infection and the knowledge of prevention]. Zhongguo ji sheng chong xue yu ji sheng chong bing za zhi 13: 269–272.

Cost-Effectiveness of Early Infant HIV Diagnosis of HIV-Exposed Infants and Immediate Antiretroviral Therapy in HIV-Infected Children under 24 Months in Thailand

Intira Jeannie Collins[1,2,3*], John Cairns[4], Nicole Ngo-Giang-Huong[2,3,5], Wasna Sirirungsi[5], Pranee Leechanachai[5], Sophie Le Coeur[2,3,5,6], Tanawan Samleerat[5], Nareerat Kamonpakorn[7], Jutarat Mekmullica[8], Gonzague Jourdain[2,3,5], Marc Lallemant[2,3,5], for the Programme for HIV Prevention and Treatment (PHPT) Study Team

1 Faculty of Epidemiology and Population Health, London School of Hygiene & Tropical Medicine, London, United Kingdom, **2** Institut de Recherche pour le Développement (IRD)-Programs for HIV Prevention and Treatment (PHPT), Chiang Mai, Thailand, **3** Department of Immunology and Infectious Diseases, Harvard School of Public Health, Boston, Massachusetts, United States of America, **4** Faculty of Public Health and Policy, London School of Hygiene & Tropical Medicine, London, United Kingdom, **5** Department of Medical Technology, Faculty of Associated Medical Sciences, Chiang Mai University, Chiang Mai, Thailand, **6** Unité Mixte de Recherche 196 Centre Français de la Population et du Développement (INED-IRD-Paris V University), Paris, France, **7** Paediatrics Department, Somdej Prapinklao Hospital, Bangkok, Thailand, **8** Paediatrics Department, Bhumibol Adulyadej Hospital, Bangkok, Thailand

Abstract

Background: HIV-infected infants have high risk of death in the first two years of life if untreated. WHO guidelines recommend early infant HIV diagnosis (EID) of all HIV-exposed infants and immediate antiretroviral therapy (ART) in HIV-infected children under 24-months. We assessed the cost-effectiveness of this strategy in HIV-exposed non-breastfed children in Thailand.

Methods: A decision analytic model of HIV diagnosis and disease progression compared: EID using DNA PCR with immediate ART (Early-Early); or EID with deferred ART based on immune/clinical criteria (Early-Late); vs. clinical/serology based diagnosis and deferred ART (Reference). The model was populated with survival and cost data from a Thai observational cohort and the literature. Incremental cost-effectiveness ratio per life-year gained (LYG) was compared against the Reference strategy. Costs and outcomes were discounted at 3%.

Results: Mean discounted life expectancy of HIV-infected children increased from 13.3 years in the Reference strategy to 14.3 in the Early-Late and 17.8 years in Early-Early strategies. The mean discounted lifetime cost was $17,335, $22,583 and $29,108, respectively. The cost-effectiveness ratio of Early-Late and Early-Early strategies was $5,149 and $2,615 per LYG, respectively as compared to the Reference strategy. The Early-Early strategy was most cost-effective at approximately half the domestic product per capita per LYG ($4,420 in Thailand 2011). The results were robust in deterministic and probabilistic sensitivity analyses including varying perinatal transmission rates.

Conclusion: In Thailand, EID and immediate ART would lead to major survival benefits and is cost- effective. These findings strongly support the adoption of WHO recommendations as routine care.

Editor: Nicolas Sluis-Cremer, University of Pittsburgh, United States of America

Funding: Grant support: The Global Fund to fight AIDS, Tuberculosis and Malaria (Thailand Grant Round 1 sub recipient PR-A-N-008); Institut de Recherche pour le Développement (IRD), France; International Maternal Pediatric Adolescents Aids Clinical Trials Group (IMPAACT); The National Institutes of Health, US (R01 HD 33326; R01 HD 39615); Ministry of Public Health, Thailand; Oxfam Great Britain, Thailand; United Kingdom Medical Research Council Doctoral Training Account Studentship for Intira Collins. The funders had no role in study design, data collection and analysis, decision to publish, or preparation of the manuscript.

Competing Interests: The authors have declared that no competing interests exist.

* E-mail: jeannie.collins@ucl.ac.uk

Introduction

In 2011, there were an estimated 330,000 infants newly infected with HIV through mother-to-child transmission (MTCT), over 90% of whom were in sub-Saharan Africa and Asia [1]. Without antiretroviral therapy (ART), up to 50% will die by two years of age, in resource limited settings [2,3]. The scale up of ART has dramatically reduced HIV-related mortality in children [4–6]. However, the risk of early mortality on ART remains high among infants initiating therapy *after* presenting with symptoms or immunosuppression, with 14% to 27% deaths during the first year of therapy [7–9]. The landmark CHER trial in South Africa, which randomized asymptomatic HIV-infected infants with CD4>25% (at median of 7 weeks old) to immediate or deferred ART based on WHO 2006 clinical and immune criteria, reported a 76% reduction in mortality and 75% reduction in disease progression in the immediate ART strategy [10]. The WHO

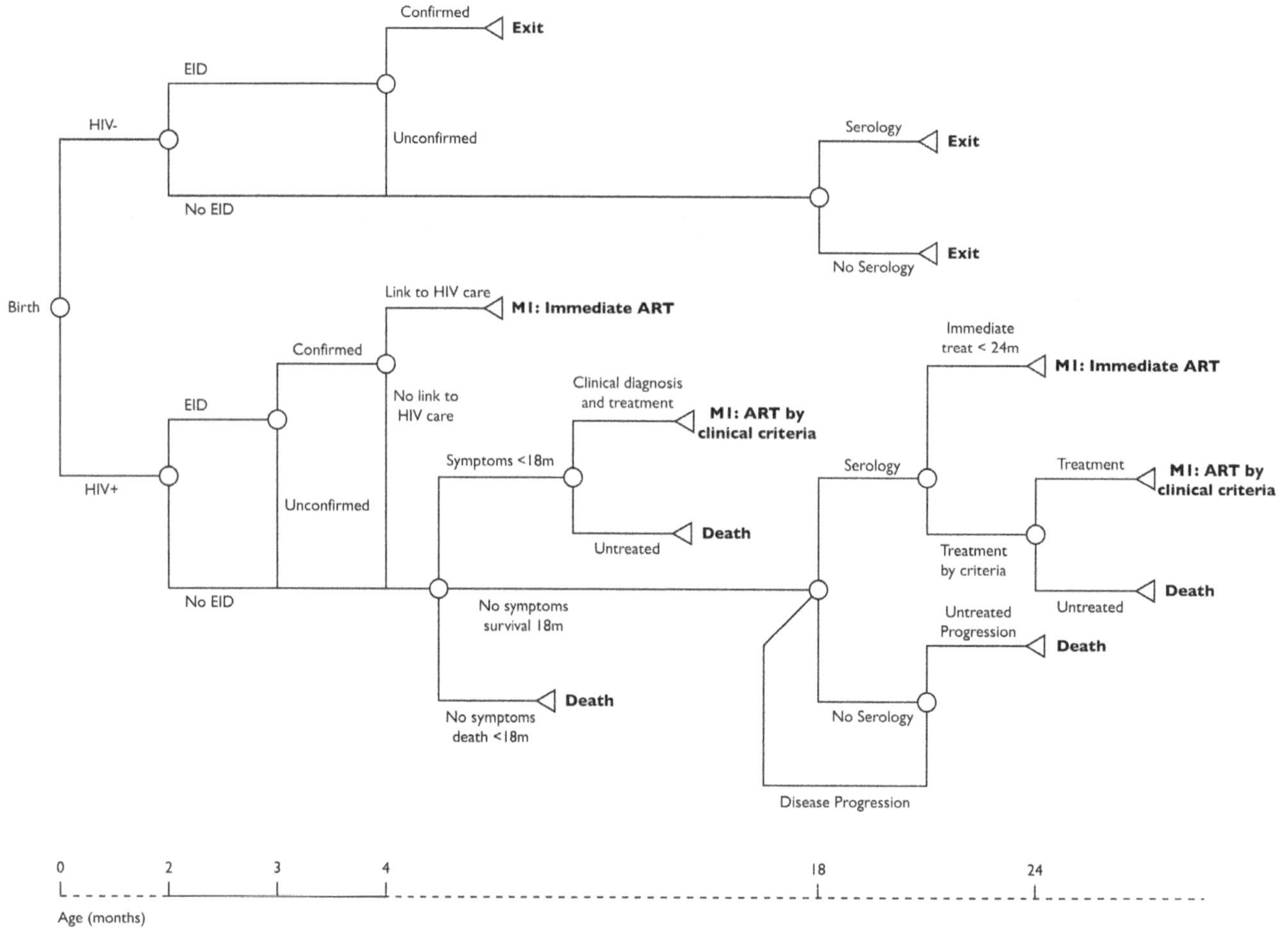

Figure 1. Decision tree for HIV diagnosis and treatment strategies.

guidelines were subsequently revised in 2008 to recommend immediate ART in all HIV-infected infants under 12-months, irrespective of clinical or immune status [11]. In 2010, this was extended to all HIV-infected children under 2-years [12] and in 2013, to all under 5-years [13].

Early initiation of ART during infancy, when risk of mortality is highest, requires access to early infant HIV diagnosis (EID) based on virologic assays (e.g. DNA PCR or RNA assays) rather than standard serology tests due to persistence of maternal anti-HIV antibodies for up to 18-months [11]. This requires access to a specialised laboratory and trained technicians. In 2011, it was estimated that only 28% of HIV-exposed infants in resource limited countries received EID within the first two months of life, as per recommendations [14], and coverage of ART among children eligible for treatment remains disproportionately low at 28% as compared to 57% among adults [1].

As part of the UN Global plan for the virtual elimination of paediatric AIDS through the scale up of prevention of MTCT (PMTCT) services, there is an urgent need to improve access to EID and ensure timely provision of ART in HIV-infected children. To date there are no data on the cost-effectiveness of early HIV diagnosis and treatment strategies in children in resource-limited settings to inform donors and policy makers facing competing public health demands.

This study examines the cost-effectiveness of EID of HIV-exposed infants and immediate ART of HIV-infected children under 24-months in the Thai setting. Thailand was one of the first middle-income countries to pilot a national EID programme from 2007 [15].

Methods

We examined the cost-effectiveness, from the health care provider's perspective, of: (i) EID of HIV-exposed infants using DNA PCR and immediate ART in HIV infected children <24-months (Early-Early); (ii) EID and deferred ART based on clinical and immune criteria (Early-Late); as compared to (iii) clinical based diagnosis and serology at 18-months with deferred initiation of ART based on clinical and immune criteria (Reference). The reference strategy represented standard of care in Thailand up to 2007 and reflects the current status in many resource-limited settings without access to EID. The Early-Late strategy represented the intermediate stage where EID is provided but with deferred ART as per 2008 WHO guidelines, before the results of the CHER trial [16]. This reflects current practice in some settings expanding EID, where immediate ART is not implemented due to poor referral systems or lack of readiness of parents/caregivers [17]. The Early-Early strategy reflects the 2010 WHO recommendations for best practice [12]. This is similar to current Thai guidelines which recommend EID and immediate ART in HIV infected children <12-months irrespective of immune/clinical status, although this has not yet been extended to all children <24 months [18].

Model Overview

We developed a cohort simulation model that incorporates data on perinatal transmission, natural history of HIV disease, treatment efficacy and cost of care from Thailand. The model was composed of a decision tree and a Markov model. The decision tree (Figure 1) presents the diagnostic component of the intervention and includes all HIV-exposed infants. The Markov model (Figure 2) presents the ART component of the intervention and includes only HIV-infected children initiated on therapy. Based on the current estimates in Thailand, we assumed a hypothetical cohort of 6,000 children born from HIV-infected mothers per year [14].

Decision Tree

HIV-exposed children entered the decision tree at birth with a probability of HIV infection through in-utero or intra-partum transmission. Post-partum transmission through breastfeeding was not considered as Thailand has very high coverage of formula feeding for this population.

Early HIV diagnosis was provided using DNA PCR on dried blood spots (DBS) with an assumed 100% sensitivity and specificity [19]. In the Early-Early and Early-Late strategies HIV-exposed children had probabilities of routine EID at 6–8 weeks of age, with confirmation EID as soon as possible in children who test positive (within one month). Among children who tested negative, the second confirmation test was conducted at 4 months [18]. HIV-infected children with confirmed diagnosis had monthly probabilities of: linkage to HIV care and initiation of ART (as per criteria in each strategy) or pre-ART death.

In the reference strategy, HIV-infected children had monthly probabilities of developing HIV symptoms; clinical diagnosis if < 18-months and serology thereafter; routine serology test at 18-months; initiation of ART based on clinical criteria or pre-ART death. Due to incomplete coverage of EID and linkage to HIV care, a proportion of HIV-infected children in the early diagnosis strategies would revert to the reference strategy with probabilities of disease progression and clinical based diagnosis but with access to EID for confirmation of HIV-infection if <18-months. The analytical time horizon for costs and life years among HIV-infected children in the absence of ART ran from birth until all children died or started therapy.

In all strategies, HIV-uninfected children were assumed to have the same probability of routine HIV diagnosis and exit the model at time of diagnosis or at 18-months if undiagnosed. They contributed only to the cost of EID and incurred no mortality as we assumed their survival to be unaffected by the different strategies.

Markov Model

HIV-infected children diagnosed and initiating ART entered the Markov model in one of the following three live states which represents their disease status at start of therapy:

- Asymptomatic/Mild: CD4>25% if <35 months or CD4> 15% if ≥36 months or Centre of Disease Control (CDC) clinical stage N or A
- Advanced: CD4 15–25% if <35 months, 7–15% if ≥36 months or CDC clinical stage B
- Severe: CD4<15% if <35 months, <7% if ≥36 months or CDC clinical stage C

The model was based on monthly cycles with a probability of remaining in the same health state, advancing to more severe health state or death. We assumed non reversibility of health states

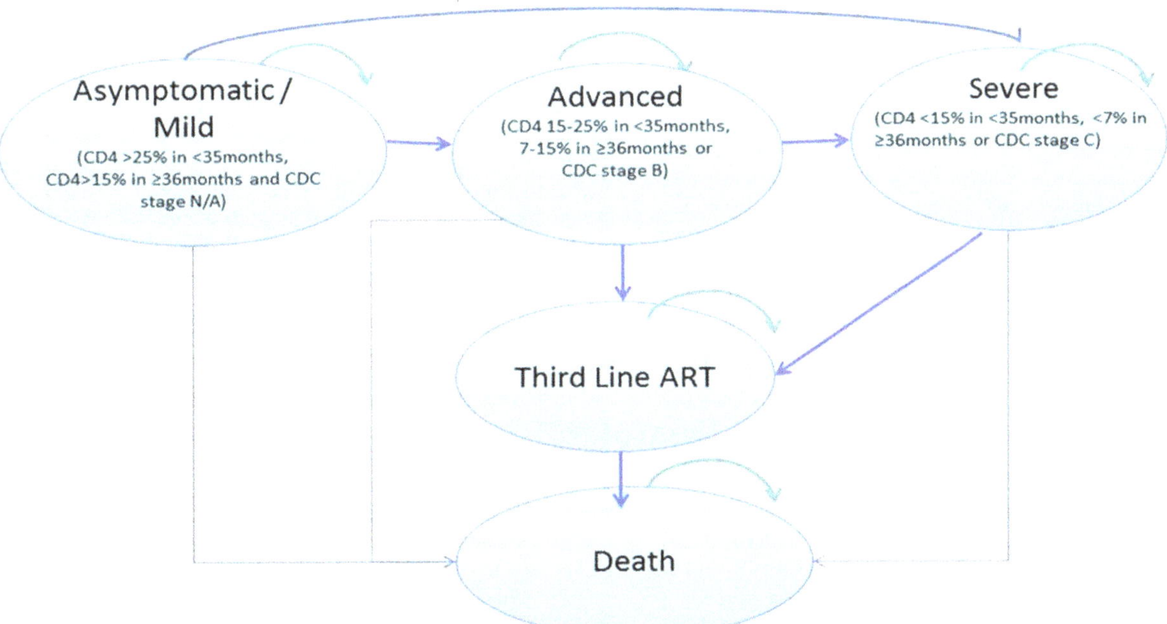

Figure 2. Markov model for HIV diagnosis and treatment strategies.

as children starting ART at more advanced disease stage are at higher risk of mortality during the first year of therapy [4,6,9], have lower probability of long-term immune reconstitution and experience longer duration in immunocompromised state despite ART [20,21].

The probability of death on ART by health state was based on the PHPT cohort (NCT00433030) with a median 5-years of follow up on therapy (described below) [9], and extrapolated using a Weibull distribution. The model projected unrealistically high long-term survival on therapy, most likely due to lack of treatment failures and long-term mortality captured during the follow up time. To allow for this, we assumed that after five years of ART, children in the advanced and severe disease stage had a probability of failing their first and second line therapy and progressing to the 'Third line ART' state, with a higher risk of mortality to reflect the increased risk of sub-optimal adherence and viremia over time on therapy. Children in the asymptomatic/mild stage were assumed to experience disease progression before progressing to Third line ART. The Markov model ran for up to 40 years on ART.

Population

As much as possible the modelling was based on data from Thailand, primarily from the PHPT paediatric observational cohort study, which has been described elsewhere [9,22]. In brief, HIV-infected children were enrolled through two modes of entry. First was the Birth cohort, children born to HIV-infected mothers enrolled in clinical trials on PMTCT [23,24] received EID at birth and at 6 weeks, HIV-infected children initiated ART based on WHO 2006 immune/clinical criteria [16]. Second was the Referred cohort: children without access to EID, who were diagnosed after presentation with HIV symptoms or through routine serology testing ≥18 months, they also initiated ART based on immune/clinical criteria. Due to limited data on long-term survival based on the Early-Early diagnosis and immediate ART strategy as part of routine care, this was modelled based on data from the CHER trial [10].

Input Parameters

Key input parameters are shown in Table 1. Coverage of EID using DNA PCR on DBS were based on data from the Thai national EID programme [15,25].

Survival Estimates and Disease Progression

Survival among untreated HIV-infected children was based on natural history data from the Birth cohort with children censored at date of death, last seen alive or start of ART, whichever was earliest (Table S1 in File S1). Due to few children alive and untreated after 2-years of age, the survival estimates after 2-years were based on adult natural history survival [26].

Survival estimates in HIV-infected children receiving ART were based on the Birth cohort for the Early-Late strategy and the Referred cohort for the Reference strategy. In both strategies, risk of death was highest during the first year of therapy and declined to low levels thereafter. Risk of mortality was substantially higher in children initiated on ART based on clinical/immune criteria < 12-months old (rapid progressors) as compared to older children who survived infancy without ART (slow progressors). To reflect this we weighted the experience of two subgroups (under and over 12-months at start of ART) to create a base case (Table S2 in File S1). In the Early-Early strategy, where infants receive immediate ART upon diagnosis, it is unknown what proportion of children would have been rapid or slow progressors, and this is likely to vary across settings according to different distributions of in-utero and intra-partum transmission [26–29]. We assumed a 50:50 distribution and in sensitivity analysis we tested different distribution assumptions. In the CHER trial, the 76% risk reduction in mortality observed in the immediate treatment strategy was driven by the reduction in pre-ART death (among untreated children) which is captured in the decision tree. There was no evidence of a difference in mortality after the start of therapy [10], therefore no reduced risk of mortality on ART was applied to the early-early strategy of the Markov model. However, a risk reduction on disease progression was applied for the first 12 months of therapy to reflect the results of the CHER study's 40 weeks follow up after the start of immediate ART.

The distribution of disease stage at start of therapy in the Reference and Early-Late strategies was based on that observed in the PHPT cohort (Table 1). The distribution in the Early-Early strategy was based on the Birth cohort with the risk reduction in disease progression of 0.24 observed in the CHER study applied to children in the Advanced and Severe stages starting ART <12-months-old. Although CDC stage B and C and CD4<25% were exclusion criteria in the CHER study, we wanted to allow for the natural disease progression in the pre-ART period to occur to avoid over-estimating the benefits of the intervention. Indeed, in the CHER trial, 22.5% of children were excluded from randomization (<12 weeks old) due to advanced disease at screening (2.9% CDC stage C, 19.6% had CD4<25%), who may still benefit from early treatment in routine care and therefore were included in the model.

Cost Parameters

The cost estimates used in this model are listed in Table 2. All costs were adjusted for inflation for Thailand up to 2011 and converted to US dollars using purchasing power parity (17.5 baht per international US dollar) [30]. As much as possible costs were based on data from the PHPT cohort (EID, hospitalization and ARV drug costs). The unit cost of EID was based on DNA PCR in-house assays [19], estimated at $57.14 (1000 baht) per test including cost of initial investment in equipment, reagents, DBS, transportation costs (DBS transported by regular postal mail), human resources and maintenance of equipment [25]. Standard serology test was estimated at $1 per test [31]. Mean cost of antiretroviral drugs (first, second and third line regimens) was based on annual average cost observed [19]. Cost of hospitalization of children on ART varied according to disease stage during the first year of therapy, and a mean cost thereafter [22]. The cost of pre-ART death was assumed to be equal to the cost of hospitalization during the first year of therapy of a child in the severe disease stage, as observed in adult studies [32]. We did not apply a cost of death on ART as we assumed this to be already incorporated in the hospitalization cost estimates.

Model Validation, Cost-effectiveness and Sensitivity Analyses

Model validation was based on model projections of survival at 1 and 5 years of ART as compared to the PHPT cohort data for the Early-Late and Reference strategies.

The modelled costs and outcome, in terms of life years gained were discounted at 3% per year [33]. We report the projected discounted and undiscounted life expectancy per HIV infected child, discounted total programme costs and lifetime costs per HIV infected child were compared across the three strategies. The incremental cost-effectiveness ratio (ICER) was defined as difference in discounted total programme cost divided by difference in discounted total life years gained (LYG). An ICER of less than one times the Gross Domestic Product (GDP) per

Table 1. Input parameters.

	Estimate	Distribution	Source
Perinatal HIV transmission and coverage of HIV diagnosis			
Rate of mother to child transmission of HIV in Thailand	3.9% (95% CI, 2.2–6.6)	Beta	[36].
Coverage of early infant HIV diagnosis	68% (range 47–79).	Normal	[15], Range [14]
Confirmation of EID	78% (range 47–85)	Normal	[15], Range [17]
Linkage to HIV care within 3 months of early diagnosis	73.1% (95% CI,64–82)	Beta	[25]
Initiated ART within 3 months of linkage to HIV care	85.4% (range 79–92)	Beta	[25]
Coverage of clinical diagnosis <18 months among symptomatic	80% (range 70–90)		Assumption
Coverage of serology testing >18 months among symptomatic	95% (range 90–97)		Assumption
Coverage of routine serology testing at 18 months	75.8% (range 70–80)		[36], Range assumption
Probability of developing symptoms when untreated (monthly)			
Probability of developing symptoms <12-months when untreated	6.4% (95% CI, 5.5–7.2)	Beta	[29]
Probability of developing symptoms between 12–23 months when untreated	3.2% (range, 2.8–3.6)		Assumption based on half rate of <12 months.
Distribution of disease stage at start of ART by strategy			
Reference strategy: Under 12 months; Over 12 months	A: 8%; 8%; B: 31%; 24%; C: 62%; 67%	Dirichlet	PHPT Referred cohort
Early-late strategy: Under 12 months; Over 12 months	A: 28%; 26%; B: 43%; 40%; C: 28%; 34%	Dirichlet	PHPT Birth cohort
Early-early strategy: Under 12 months; Over 12 months	A: 66%, 26%; B: 27%, 40%; C: 7%, 34%	Dirichlet	Assumption: based on PHPT Birth cohort* CHER study risk ratio 0.25 in <12 months [10]
Monthly probability of disease progression on ART			
Stage A to B	0.43%		[61]
Stage A to C	0.08%		
Stage B to C	0.14%		
Stage B or C to third line after 5 years of ART	0.83%		PHPT cohort
Third line to death			[62]
Risk reduction in disease progression	0.25 (95% CI, 0.15–0.41)		[10]

Note: EID; early infant HIV diagnosis, ART; antiretroviral therapy, CDC; centre of disease control.

capita for Thailand (US $4,420 in 2011, [30]) was considered as cost effective [34].

We conducted deterministic univariate sensitivity analysis using the high and low estimates of key input parameters to assess the impact on the cost-effectiveness estimates. Best and worse-case scenarios were assessed using high and low estimates of perinatal transmission combined with current and high estimated costs of EID and ART.

Probabilistic sensitivity analysis taking into account uncertainty of all input parameters was conducted using a Monte Carlo simulation with 1,000 random draws from the specified parameter distribution. Cholesky decomposition of the variance-covariance matrices was used to capture correlation between coefficients in the regression model for mortality on ART [35]. The results are presented in cost-effectiveness acceptability curves which represent the probability of the interventions being cost effective at various willingness to pay thresholds. In addition, sub-group analyses were conducted to assess the cost-effectiveness of the interventions by varying levels of access to PMTCT services and risk of perinatal transmission.

Results

Model Validation

Projected survival at 1 and 5 years of ART in the Reference and Early-Late strategy were compared to the survival estimates in the PHPT cohort according to age at start of therapy. Among children initiated on ART under 12-months old, the model projected poorer survival as compared to that observed in PHPT cohort, but projections were within the 95% confidence interval of the survival estimate, most likely due to the small sample size in this age group(Table S3 in File S1). Among children initiated on ART after 12-months of age, projected survival was within 2% of that observed in the PHPT cohort.

Projected Life Expectancy and Cost-effectiveness

In the reference strategy, the discounted life expectancy of an HIV-infected child was 13.3 years (undiscounted, 21.0 years), with a discounted lifetime cost of $17,335 per child. In the Early-Late strategy, the life expectancy increased to 14.3 years (undiscounted 22.8 years), with a lifetime cost of $22,583 per child. In the Early-

Table 2. Cost parameters.

Costs (2011 US$)	Unit cost	Source
Pre and post HIV test counselling		
HIV positive result	$9.53 (range 5.02–19.12)	[38]
HIV negative result	$3.61 (range 2.06–10.24)	
Cost of HIV diagnosis per test		
Early infant HIV diagnosis using DNA PCR and dried blood spots	$57.14	[25]
HIV rapid test by serology	$1	[31]
Mean cost of antiretroviral drugs per child per month		
Mean cost during the first five years of therapy (includes first and second line therapy)	$61.10 (SE 61.10)	[63]
Mean cost after five years of therapy (includes first and second line therapy)	$86.30 (SE 86.30)	[63]
Third line ART	$148.30 (SE 148.30)	[63]
Laboratory monitoring on ART	$26.09 (SE 26.09)	[52] and PHPT unpublished data.
Hospitalization during first year of ART in disease stage A or B	$24.9 (SE 24.90)	[22]
Hospitalization during first year of ART in CDC stage C	$43.0 (SE 43.0)	[22]
Hospitalization after first year of ART (all disease states)	$5.20 (SE 5.20)	[22]

Note. All cost estimates were adjusted for inflation up to 2011.

Early strategy, the life expectancy increased further to 17.8 years (undiscounted 29.1 years), with a lifetime cost of $29,108.

The Early-Late strategy had an incremental cost-effectiveness ratio of $5,149 per LYG as compared to the Reference strategy (Table 3). The Early-Early strategy had an ICER of $2,615 per LYG compared to the Reference strategy and $1,873 per LYG compared to the Early-Late strategy. The Early-Late strategy was extendedly dominated as compared to Early-Early strategy and therefore was not considered further (Figure S1 in File S1).

Based on the assumption of 6,000 HIV infected pregnant women delivering in Thailand per year and an overall risk of mother to child transmission of HIV of 3.9%, the total discounted programme cost was estimated at $4.0 million in the Reference strategy and increases to $6.8 million in the Early-Early strategy (Table 3). However, over 90% of the total cost of the Early-Early strategy was attributed to lifetime cost of ART for HIV infected children and less than 10% on the early infant HIV diagnosis component for all HIV-exposed infants.

Sensitivity Analyses

In univariate sensitivity analysis, the ICER of the Early-Early strategy was most sensitive to the discount rate, the cost of antiretroviral drugs, laboratory monitoring, cost of EID and rate of perinatal HIV transmission (Figure S2 in File S1). However, under all scenarios the ICER remained under $4,500 per LYG. These results were supported by the probabilistic sensitivity analysis allowing for uncertainty of all model parameters, the cost-effectiveness acceptability curve show a 99% probability of the Early-Early strategy being cost effective at $4,500 per LYG (Figure S3 in File S1).

In sub-group analyses, the cost-effectiveness of the Early-Early strategy was assessed according to varying levels of coverage of prophylaxis for PMTCT and risk of perinatal transmission as observed in Thailand [36]. The Early-Early strategy was most cost effective among children at highest risk of HIV infection, i.e. those who received no PMTCT, with 37.5% risk of perinatal transmission. The ICER of the Early-Early intervention in this population was $2,248 per LYG as compared to the Reference strategy. With improved prophylaxis for PMTCT and reduced risk of perinatal transmission, the ICER increased slightly, but the

Table 3. Cost and cost-effectiveness of the intervention strategies.

Programme model	Reference	Early-Late	Early-Early
Cost of HIV Diagnosis & pre-ART death	$23,754	$454,010	$458,433
Cost of ART including hospitalization	$4,009,804	$4,800,673	$6,314,682
Total Cost (All children)	$4,033,558	$5,254,683	$6,773,115
Total LY (HIV+child)	3,086	3,323	4,134
Incremental cost-effectiveness ratio per LY over Reference	-	$5,149	$2,615
Incremental cost-effectiveness ratio per LY over Early-Late	-	-	$1,873

Note: Model assumes 6,000 children born to HIV infected mothers with a risk of HIV transmission of 3.9% and provision of lifelong ART among HIV infected children diagnosed and initiated on therapy. All costs converted to USD using purchasing power parity (17.5 baht per international US dollar).

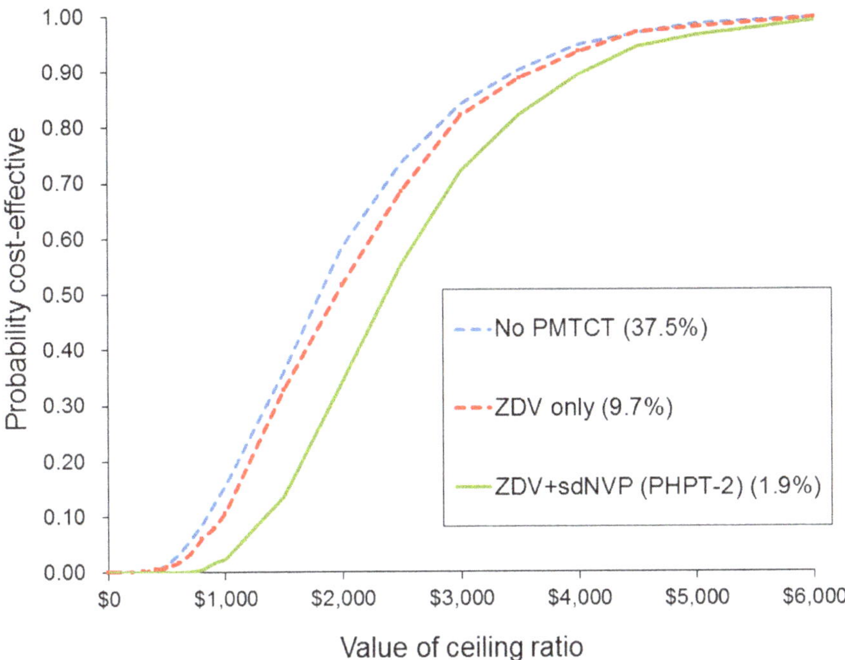

Figure 3. Cost-effectiveness acceptability curve of Early-Early versus Reference strategy by PMTCT prophylaxes and risk of perinatal transmission.

Early-Early strategy remained cost effective as compared to the Reference strategy at under $4,500 per LYG across all sub-groups (Figure 3).

In multi-way sensitivity analysis, we assumed the overall perinatal HIV transmission rate reduced to a target rate of 1.5% with the introduction of universal HAART for PMTCT [37], high estimates of EID coverage, confirmation and linkage to ART and current cost of EID and ART. In this scenario, the ICER increased to $3,470 per LYG, while the total programme cost reduced to $3.0 million due to fewer HIV-infected children requiring lifetime ART.

Discussion

In this study we modelled the survival and costs of providing EID using DNA PCR and immediate or deferred initiation of ART in HIV infected children aged <24-months as compared to late HIV diagnosis based on clinical status or serology at 18-months and deferred initiation of ART based on clinical and immune criteria in the Thai setting. The EID and immediate ART strategy increased the discounted life expectancy of HIV infected children from 13.3 to 17.8 years, at an incremental cost-effectiveness ratio of $2,615 per LYG in the base case. This is approximately half of Thailand's GDP per capita and would be considered as cost effective under WHO recommendations [34].

Importantly, these estimates were made by converting all costs to US dollars using purchasing power parity (17.5 baht per international USD). If we had used market exchange rates (34.3 baht per USD) as in other studies [38], with the rationale that the majority of costs are attributed to imported antiretrovirals and laboratory assays that are subject to market exchange rates, then the Early-Early strategy would have even lower incremental cost-effectiveness ratio and lower programme costs (Table S4 in File S1).

The benefits of the Early-Early strategy were observed in two main areas. Firstly, EID and immediate ART minimized the period in which HIV-infected children were untreated during infancy, resulting in a halving of pre-ART deaths from 42% in the Reference strategy down to 21% in the Early-Early strategy. This figure is not lower due to existing gaps in EID coverage and referral of HIV infected infants for ART initiation (data not shown). Second was the reduction in early mortality on ART due to fewer children initiating therapy at advanced disease stage. The cost-effectiveness estimate of this strategy is likely to be under-estimated as we assumed the benefit of immediate ART in reducing disease progression would only persist for the first year of therapy, based on the follow up duration of the CHER trial. It is likely that the benefits are longer lasting due to the preservation of the immune system; children are better able to maintain good long-term immunologic response to ART as reported in observational cohorts of infants who initiated therapy during the first 3 months of life while asymptomatic in Europe and the US [39,40]. Furthermore, we have not taken into account the benefits of averting damage to cognitive function and neurological development among children who progress to advanced disease when left untreated[41–44], nor have we included the benefits in terms of quality of life, of accessing early infant HIV diagnosis among HIV-uninfected infants.

The Early-Late strategy where EID was provided but ART deferred till after meeting clinical and immune criteria, as conducted in the PHPT birth cohort prior to WHO 2008 guidelines, was less cost effective when compared to the Reference Strategy. It resulted in a limited increase in the discounted life expectancy of HIV infected children (from 13.3 years in the reference strategy to 14.3 years). This is most likely due to the limited impact on reducing pre-ART deaths among infants who have high risk of rapid disease progression and death even at high CD4% [45], with no prior signs and symptoms [10,29]. In addition, infants who initiate therapy after disease progression remain at higher risk of mortality despite ART [7–9]. This highlights the importance of effective referral of HIV-infected infants as soon as they are diagnosed for immediate ART to maximize the potential benefits of early treatment.

To our knowledge, this is the first cost-effectiveness evaluation of early infant HIV diagnosis and different treatment strategies in children. Previous studies have examined the cost and acceptability of early HIV diagnosis using DNA PCR in low- and middle-income countries [17,46,47]. One study examined the cost-effectiveness of early infant HIV diagnosis using rapid antibody tests and clinical examination, primarily to screen out HIV-uninfected children at minimal cost, however that strategy had poor specificity among infants under 6 months and only assessed the cost-effectiveness per correct diagnosis and did not consider provision of ART for infected children [48]. An economic sub-study in the CHER trial reported that cost of earlier provision of ART to asymptomatic infants was more than offset by the reduced cost of inpatient care as compared to the deferred ART strategy, but did not include the cost of early HIV diagnosis of all exposed infants [49].

While there is a growing body of literature on the cost-effectiveness of different treatment strategies in HIV-infected adults [50], there are only two comparable studies on HIV care in children. One was on the cost-effectiveness of cotrimoxazole prophylaxis for prevention of opportunistic infections in untreated HIV infected children in Zambia ($74 per LYG) [51]. The second was on cost-effectiveness of virological monitoring and provision of second line therapy in HIV infected children in Thailand ($3,393 per year of virological failure averted) [52]. The latter is not directly comparable to our study as we assumed that HIV infected children on ART received routine CD4 and virological monitoring every 6 months and had access to second and third line regimen upon treatment failure as per national guidelines [18]. Based on these assumptions, the addition of EID and immediate treatment in all HIV-infected children <24-months was cost-effective, and is likely to be affordable in the Thai setting. Importantly, if the rate of mother-to-child transmission continues to decline further with introduction of HAART for PMTCT and more extensive provision of HAART to HIV-infected adults (including women during time of conception and pregnancy) [53], then the total programme cost of this strategy is likely to decrease over time as fewer children are infected and require lifelong treatment which accounts for over 90% of the programme costs.

In addition, on-going developments in low cost HIV laboratory services including EID at point of care in resource-limited settings are likely to further simplify collection and transportation of samples and make EID more affordable and feasible for routine use [54]. Maturing EID programmes have reported innovative strategies to improve uptake of EID and retention of HIV-exposed infants, although there remain scarce data on the follow-up and treatment status of newly diagnosed HIV-infected infants [15,55,56]. Such indicators are critical for the evaluation of PMTCT and paediatric HIV programmes and should be highlighted as an important goal as part of the campaign for a zero HIV generation.

There are a number of important limitations of this study. First, the survival estimates of children on ART were extrapolated from an observational study with five years of follow-up due to scarce long-term data from a low and middle income setting. Data from paediatric cohorts in the US or Europe were not used as they represented a different population with access to earlier treatment using more potent and costly drugs and lower estimates of mortality and hospitalization [5,57]. Second, the Markov model of children on ART assumed non reversibility of health states, as there remains limited data on long-term immunologic response and risk of mortality among infants/older children starting therapy at different disease stages to inform a more complex reversible model. However, the main benefits of EID and immediate ART were the reduction in pre-ART deaths and early mortality on ART, therefore a more detailed model of the long-term survival is unlikely to affect the overall findings.

Third, this study is based on data largely from the Thai setting and therefore the findings cannot be extended to other settings with different coverage of services, mortality rates, costs and thresholds for cost-effectiveness. Furthermore, this study was based on a non-breastfeeding population, most of the countries with the highest burden of HIV in sub-Saharan Africa, recommend exclusive breastfeeding and thus repeated early infant HIV diagnosis during the breastfeeding period and after weaning would be required. Fourth, in this study we assumed 100% sensitivity and specificity of DNA PCR testing from 2 months of life – based on data from the PHPT study where children were exposed to nevirapine and zidovudine prophylaxis for PMTCT. A study by Shapiro and colleagues suggests that early diagnosis of infants exposed to maternal or infant HAART for PMTCT may be less sensitive during the first months of life [58], which may have important implications for the recommended schedule for early diagnosis and may require more confirmation tests. However, when we assumed a doubling in the cost of EID – this intervention was still cost effective. Lastly, recent reports of a functional cure of an HIV-infected infant diagnosed and initiated ART at 30 hours of life in the United States [59] has generated much interest in the potential benefits of birth testing and very early ART in preventing seeding of the HIV reservoir [60]. However, the sensitivity of virological tests at birth with DBS and exposure to maternal HAART are not well described. Also, the birth test would only identify the in-utero transmissions, and the feasibility of such rapid return of test results and ART referral in resource-limited settings has yet to be determined; implementation studies and cost-effectiveness analyses of a birth test algorithm are needed to inform future policies and programmes.

Conclusion

Early infant HIV diagnosis combined with immediate ART of children under 24 months was cost effective in the Thai setting as compared to late diagnosis and deferred treatment. Expanding programmes for EID must place greater emphasis on retention of HIV infected infants identified and timely initiation of ART prior to disease progression to maximize the benefit in reducing HIV related morbidity and mortality in this highly vulnerable population.

Author Contributions

Conceived and designed the experiments: IJC JC ML. Analyzed the data: IJC. Contributed reagents/materials/analysis tools: JC. Wrote the paper: IJC JC NN SLC ML. Acquisition and analysis of data used in this analysis: NNGH WS PL TS NK JM SLC GJ. Provided a critical review of the manuscript and approved the final version: IJC JC NNGH WS PL SLC TS NK JM GJ ML.

References

1. UNAIDS (2012) Together we will end AIDS. Available on http://www.unaids.org/en/media/unaids/contentassets/documents/epidemiology/2012/20120725_Together_we_will_end_AIDS_en.pdf Accessed 2 February 2013.
2. Newell M-L, Coovadia H, Cortina-Borja M, Rollins N, Gaillard P, et al. (2004) Mortality of infected and uninfected infants born to HIV-infected mothers in Africa: a pooled analysis. The Lancet 364: 1236–1243.
3. Becquet R, Marston M, Dabis F, Moulton LH, Gray G, et al. (2012) Children who acquire HIV infection perinatally are at higher risk of early death than those acquiring infection through breastmilk: a meta-analysis. PLoS One 7: e28510.
4. Sutcliffe CG, van Dijk JH, Bolton C, Persaud D, Moss WJ (2008) Effectiveness of antiretroviral therapy among HIV-infected children in sub-Saharan Africa. The Lancet Infectious Diseases 8: 477–489.
5. Judd A, Doerholt K, Tookey PA, Sharland M, Riordan A, et al. (2007) Morbidity, mortality, and response to treatment by children in the United Kingdom and Ireland with perinatally acquired HIV infection during 1996–2006: planning for teenage and adult care. Clin Infect Dis 45: 918–924.
6. The KIDS-ART-LINC Collaboration (2008) Low Risk of Death, but Substantial Program Attrition, in Pediatric HIV Treatment Cohorts in Sub-Saharan Africa. JAIDS Journal of Acquired Immune Deficiency Syndromes 49: 523–531.
7. Sauvageot D, Schaefer M, Olson D, Pujades-Rodriguez M, O'Brien DP (2010) Antiretroviral therapy outcomes in resource-limited settings for HIV-infected children <5 years of age. Pediatrics 125: e1039–1047.
8. Bolton-Moore C, Mubiana-Mbewe M, Cantrell RA, Chintu N, Stringer EM, et al. (2007) Clinical outcomes and CD4 cell response in children receiving antiretroviral therapy at primary health care facilities in Zambia. JAMA 298: 1888–1899.
9. Collins IJ, Jourdain G, Hansudewechakul R, Kanjanavanit S, Hongsiriwon S, et al. (2010) Long-term survival of HIV-infected children receiving antiretroviral therapy in Thailand: a 5-year observational cohort study. Clin Infect Dis 51: 1449–1457.
10. Violari A, Cotton MF, Gibb DM, Babiker AG, Steyn J, et al. (2008) Early antiretroviral therapy and mortality among HIV-infected infants. New England Journal of Medicine 359: 2233–2244.
11. World Health Organization (2008) Paediatric HIV Antiretroviral Therapy and Care guideline review: Report of the WHO Technical Reference Group Paediatric HIV/ART Care Guideline Group Meeting. Available at http://www.who.int/hiv/pub/paediatric/WHO_Paediatric_ART_guideline_rev_mreport_2008.pdf. Accessed 10 April 2010.
12. World Health Organization (2010) Antiretroviral therapy of HIV infection in infants and children: Towards universal access. Recommendations for a public healthapproach. Available at http://whqlibdoc.who.int/publications/2010/9789241599801_eng.pdf. Accessed 19 February 2013.
13. World Health Organization (2013) Consolidated guidelines on the use of antiretroviral drugs for treating and preventing HIV infection: Recommendations for a public health approach. Available at http://www.who.int/hiv/pub/guidelines/arv2013/en/index.html. Accessed 14 August 2013.
14. World Health Organization (2011) Global HIV/AIDS Response: Epidemic update and health sector progress towards Universal Access Progress Report. Available at: http://www.who.int/hiv/pub/progress_report2011/summary_en.pdf. Accessed 10th February 2012.
15. Naiwatanakul T, Voramongkol N, Lolekha R, Kullerk N, Thaisri H, et al. (2012) Uptake of Thailand's National Program for early infant HIV diagnosis and infant HIV-infection outcomes, 2007–2010. Abstract no. WEPE159 19th International AIDS Conference. Washington D.C., USA.
16. World Health Organization (2006) Antiretroviral therapy of HIV infection in infants and children in resource-limited settings: towards universal access. Recommendations for a public health approach. Available at: http://www.who.int/hiv/pub/guidelines/WHOpaediatric.pdf. Accessed 10 April 2010.
17. Ciaranello AL, Park JE, Ramirez-Avila L, Freedberg KA, Walensky RP, et al. (2011) Early infant HIV-1 diagnosis programs in resource-limited settings: opportunities for improved outcomes and more cost-effective interventions. BMC Med 9: 59.
18. Puthanakit T, Tangsathapornpong A, Ananworanich J, Wongsawat J., Suntrattiwong P, et al. (2010) Thai national guidelines for the use of antiretroviral therapy in pediatric HIV infection in 2010. Asian Biomedicine 4: 505–513.
19. Ngo-Giang-Huong N, Khamduang W, Leurent B, Collins I, Nantasen I, et al. (2008) Early HIV-1 Diagnosis Using In-House Real-Time PCR Amplification on Dried Blood Spots for Infants in Remote and Resource-Limited Settings. JAIDS Journal of Acquired Immune Deficiency Syndromes 49: 465–471.
20. Lewis J, Walker AS, Castro H, De Rossi A, Gibb DM, et al. (2012) Age and CD4 Count at Initiation of Antiretroviral Therapy in HIV-Infected Children: Effects on Long-term T-Cell Reconstitution. Journal of Infectious Diseases 205: 548–556.
21. Patel K, Hernan MA, Williams PL, Seeger JD, McIntosh K, et al. (2008) Long-term effects of highly active antiretroviral therapy on CD4+ cell evolution among children and adolescents infected with HIV: 5 years and counting. Clin Infect Dis 46: 1751–1760.
22. Collins IJ, Cairns J, Jourdain G, Fregonese F, Nantarukchaikul M, et al. (2012) Hospitalization trends, costs, and risk factors in HIV-infected children on antiretroviral therapy. AIDS 26: 1943–1952.
23. Lallemant M, Jourdain G, Le Coeur S, Kim S, Koetsawang S, et al. (2000) A trial of shortened zidovudine regimens to prevent mother-to-child transmission of human immunodeficiency virus type 1. Perinatal HIV Prevention Trial (Thailand) Investigators. N Engl J Med 343: 982–991.
24. Lallemant M, Jourdain G, Le Coeur S, Mary JY, Ngo-Giang-Huong N, et al. (2004) Single-dose perinatal nevirapine plus standard zidovudine to prevent mother-to-child transmission of HIV-1 in Thailand. N Engl J Med 351: 217–228.
25. Sirirungsi W, Samleerat T, Ngo-Giang-Huong N, Collins IJ, Khamduang W, et al. (2013) Thailand National Program for Early Infant HIV Diagnosis: Six-year Experience using Real-time DNA PCR on Dried Blood Spots (Abstract no. O_16). 5th International Workshop on HIV Pediatrics. Kuala Lumpur, Malaysia.
26. Marston M, Zaba B, Salomon JA, Brahmbhatt H, Bagenda D (2005) Estimating the net effect of HIV on child mortality in African populations affected by generalized HIV epidemics. J Acquir Immune Defic Syndr 38: 219–227.
27. Tovo PA, de Martino M, Gabiano C, Cappello N, D'Elia R, et al. (1992) Prognostic factors and survival in children with perinatal HIV-1 infection. The Italian Register for HIV Infections in Children. Lancet 339: 1249–1253.
28. European Collaborative S (2001) Fluctuations in Symptoms in Human Immunodeficiency Virus-Infected Children: The First 10 Years of Life. Pediatrics 108: 116–122.
29. Chearskul S, Chotpitayasunondh T, Simonds RJ, Wanprapar N, Waranawat N, et al. (2002) Survival, Disease Manifestations, and Early Predictors of Disease Progression Among Children With Perinatal Human Immunodeficiency Virus Infection in Thailand. Pediatrics 110: e25–.
30. The World Bank (2011) World Development Indicators. Avalaible on http://databank.worldbank.org/data/home.aspx. Accessed 10 November 2012.
31. Clinton Foundation (2009) HIV/AIDS Diagnostic Pricing Outlook. Available http://www.who.int/hiv/topics/treatment/costing_clinton_diagnostic.pdf. Accessed 2 October 2012.
32. Harling G, Wood R (2007) The evolving cost of HIV in South Africa: changes in health care cost with duration on antiretroviral therapy for public sector patients. J Acquir Immune Defic Syndr 45: 348–354.
33. Teerawattananon Y, Chaikledkaew U., (2008) Thai health technology assessment guideline development. J Med Assoc Thai 91: S2: S11–15.
34. WHO-CHOICE (2003) Making Choices in Health: WHO Guide to Cost Effectiveness Analysis. In: Tan-Torres Edeger T, Baltussen R, Adam T, Hutubessy R, Acharya A et al., editors: WHO. Available: http://www.who.int/choice/publications/p_2003_generalised_cea.pdf. Accessed 20 January 2009.
35. Briggs A CK, Sculpher M (2006) Decision modelling for health economic evaluation: Oxford University Press.
36. Plipat T, Naiwatanakul T, Rattanasuporn N, Sangwanloy O, Amornwichet P, et al. (2007) Reduction in mother-to-child transmission of HIV in Thailand, 2001–2003: results from population-based surveillance in six provinces. AIDS 21: 145–151.
37. Phanuphak N, Lolekha R., Chokephaibulkit K., Voramongkol N., Boonsuk S., Limtrakul A., Limpanyalert P., Chasombat S., Thanprasertsuki S., Leechawengwong M., for the Thai National HIV Guidelines Working Group, (2010) Thai national guidelines for the prevention of mother to child transmission of HIV: March 2010. Asian Biomedicine 4: 529–540.
38. Teerawattananon Y, Vos T, Tangcharoensathien V, Mugford M (2005) Cost-effectiveness of models for prevention of vertical HIV transmission - voluntary counseling and testing and choices of drug regimen. Cost Effectiveness and Resource Allocation 3: 7.
39. Goetghebuer T, Le Chenadec J, Haelterman E, Galli L, Dollfus C, et al. (2012) Short- and long-term immunological and virological outcome in HIV-infected infants according to the age at antiretroviral treatment initiation. Clin Infect Dis 54: 878–881.
40. Judd A, European Pregnancy and Paediatric HIV Cohort Collaboration (EPPICC) study group in EuroCoord (2011) Early antiretroviral therapy in HIV-1-infected infants, 1996–2008: treatment response and duration of first-line regimens. AIDS 25: 2279–2287.
41. Ruel TD, Boivin MJ, Boal HE, Bangirana P, Charlebois E, et al. (2012) Neurocognitive and Motor Deficits in HIV-Infected Ugandan Children With High CD4 Cell Counts. Clinical Infectious Diseases 54: 1001–1009.
42. Smith R, Chernoff M, Williams PL, Malee KM, Sirois PA, et al. (2012) Impact of HIV Severity on Cognitive and Adaptive Functioning During Childhood and Adolescence. The Pediatric Infectious Disease Journal 31: 592–598 510.1097/INF.1090b1013e318253844b.
43. Puthanakit T, Ananworanich J, Vonthanak S, Kosalaraksa P, Hansudewechakul R, et al. (2013) Cognitive Function and Neurodevelopmental Outcomes in HIV-Infected Children Older than 1 Year of Age Randomized to Early Versus Deferred Antiretroviral Therapy: The PREDICT Neurodevelopmental Study. Pediatr Infect Dis J.
44. Laughton B, Cornell M, Grove D, Kidd M, Springer PE, et al. (2012) Early antiretroviral therapy improves neurodevelopmental outcomes in infants. AIDS 26: 1685–1690.

45. Dunn D, Woodburn P, Duong T, Peto J, Phillips A, et al. (2008) Current CD4 cell count and the short-term risk of AIDS and death before the availability of effective antiretroviral therapy in HIV-infected children and adults. Journal of Infectious Diseases 197: 398–404.
46. Sherman GG, Stevens G, Jones SA, Horsfield P, Stevens WS (2005) Dried blood spots improve access to HIV diagnosis and care for infants in low-resource settings. J Acquir Immune Defic Syndr 38: 615–617.
47. Hsiao NY, Stinson K, Myer L (2013) Linkage of HIV-infected infants from diagnosis to antiretroviral therapy services across the Western Cape, South Africa. PLoS One 8: e55308.
48. Menzies NA, Berruti AA, Berzon R, Filler S, Ferris R, et al. (2011) The cost of providing comprehensive HIV treatment in PEPFAR-supported programs. AIDS 25: 1753–1760.
49. Meyer-Rath G VA, Cotton M, et al. (2010) The cost of eary vs deferred paediatric antiretroviral treatment in South Africa - a comparative economic analysis of the first year of the CHER trial. 18th International AIDS Conference. Vienna.
50. Loubiere S, Meiners C, Sloan C, Freedberg KA, Yazdanpanah Y (2010) Economic evaluation of ART in resource-limited countries. Curr Opin HIV AIDS 5: 225–231.
51. Ryan M GS, Chitah B, Walker AS, Mulenga V, Kalolo D, Hawkins N, Merry C, Barry MG, Chintu C, Sculpher MJ, Gibb DM (2008) The cost-effectiveness of cotrimoxazole prophylaxis in HIV-infected children in Zambia. AIDS 22: 749–757.
52. Schneider K, Puthanakit T, Kerr S, Law MG, Cooper DA, et al. (2011) Economic evaluation of monitoring virologic responses to antiretroviral therapy in HIV-infected children in resource-limited settings. AIDS 25: 1143–1151.
53. UNAIDS (2012) A progress report on the Global Plan towards the elimination of new HIV infections among children by 2015 and keeping their mothers alive. http://www.unaids.org/en/media/unaids/contentassets/documents/unaidspublication/2012/JC2385_ProgressReportGlobalPlan_en.pdf Accessed 23 February 2013.
54. UNITAID (2012) HIV/AIDS Diagnostic Technology Landscape: 2nd Edition. Available at http://www.unitaid.eu/images/marketdynamics/publications/UNITAID-HIV_Diagnostics_Landscape-2nd_edition.pdf. Accessed 21 February 2013.
55. Kim M, Nanthuru D, Kanjelo K, Bhalakia A, Buck W, Kazembe PN, Paul ME, Wanless S, Kline M, Ahmed S, (2011) Using community health workers as case managers: creating a complete continuum of care between prevention of mother to child transmission (PMTCT), early infant diagnosis (EID), and pediatric HIV care and treatment services. 6th IAS Conference on HIV Pathogenesis and Treatment. Washington D.C., USA : Abstract no. TUPE291.
56. Binagwaho A, Mugwaneza P, Irakoze AA, Nsanzimana S, Agbonyitor M, et al. (2013) Scaling up early infant diagnosis of HIV in Rwanda, 2008–2010. J Public Health Policy 34: 2–16.
57. Brady MT, Oleske JM, Williams PL, Elgie C, Mofenson LM, et al. (2010) Declines in mortality rates and changes in causes of death in HIV-1-infected children during the HAART era. J Acquir Immune Defic Syndr 53: 86–94.
58. Shapiro D, Balasubramanian R, Fowler MG, et al for the International Collaborative Study of Pediatric HIV Diagnostic Tests, (2011) Time to HIV DNA-PCR positivity according to maternal/infant antiretroviral prophylactic regimen in non-breastfed HIV-infected infants in populations with predominantly non-B HIV subtype: a collaborative analysis. Abstract no. TUAB0203. 18th International AIDS Conference. Rome, Italy.
59. Persaud D, Gay H, Ziemniak C (2013) Functional HIV cure after very early ART of an HIV infected infant. 20th Conference on Retroviruses and Opportunistic Infections (CROI 2013). Atlanta, GA, USA.
60. Deeks SG, Lewin SR, Havlir DV (2013) The end of AIDS: HIV infection as a chronic disease. The Lancet.
61. Sturt AS, Halpern MS, Sullivan B, Maldonado YA (2012) Timing of antiretroviral therapy initiation and its impact on disease progression in perinatal human immunodeficiency virus-1 infection. Pediatr Infect Dis J 31: 53–60.
62. Ananworanich J, Prasitsuebsai W, Kosalaraksa P, et al. (2012) Outcomes of third-line antiretroviral therapy containing darunavir, etravirine or raltegravir in Thai children with HIV infection. Abstract no. MOPE038 19th International AIDS Conference. Washington D.C., USA.
63. Collins IJ, Cairns J, Le Coeur S, Pagdi K, Ngampiyaskul C, et al. (2013) Five-year trends in antiretroviral usage and drug costs in HIV-infected children in Thailand J Acquir Immune Defic Syndr 64: 95–102.

Permissions

All chapters in this book were first published in PLOS ONE, by The Public Library of Science; hereby published with permission under the Creative Commons Attribution License or equivalent. Every chapter published in this book has been scrutinized by our experts. Their significance has been extensively debated. The topics covered herein carry significant findings which will fuel the growth of the discipline. They may even be implemented as practical applications or may be referred to as a beginning point for another development.

The contributors of this book come from diverse backgrounds, making this book a truly international effort. This book will bring forth new frontiers with its revolutionizing research information and detailed analysis of the nascent developments around the world.

We would like to thank all the contributing authors for lending their expertise to make the book truly unique. They have played a crucial role in the development of this book. Without their invaluable contributions this book wouldn't have been possible. They have made vital efforts to compile up to date information on the varied aspects of this subject to make this book a valuable addition to the collection of many professionals and students.

This book was conceptualized with the vision of imparting up-to-date information and advanced data in this field. To ensure the same, a matchless editorial board was set up. Every individual on the board went through rigorous rounds of assessment to prove their worth. After which they invested a large part of their time researching and compiling the most relevant data for our readers.

The editorial board has been involved in producing this book since its inception. They have spent rigorous hours researching and exploring the diverse topics which have resulted in the successful publishing of this book. They have passed on their knowledge of decades through this book. To expedite this challenging task, the publisher supported the team at every step. A small team of assistant editors was also appointed to further simplify the editing procedure and attain best results for the readers.

Apart from the editorial board, the designing team has also invested a significant amount of their time in understanding the subject and creating the most relevant covers. They scrutinized every image to scout for the most suitable representation of the subject and create an appropriate cover for the book.

The publishing team has been an ardent support to the editorial, designing and production team. Their endless efforts to recruit the best for this project, has resulted in the accomplishment of this book. They are a veteran in the field of academics and their pool of knowledge is as vast as their experience in printing. Their expertise and guidance has proved useful at every step. Their uncompromising quality standards have made this book an exceptional effort. Their encouragement from time to time has been an inspiration for everyone.

The publisher and the editorial board hope that this book will prove to be a valuable piece of knowledge for researchers, students, practitioners and scholars across the globe.

List of Contributors

Ludmila Khailova, Benjamin Petrie, Christine H. Baird, Jessica A. Dominguez Rieg and Paul E. Wischmeyer
Department of Anesthesiology, University of Colorado School of Medicine, Aurora, Colorado, United States of America

Nguyen Tien Huy
Department of Immunogenetics, Institute of Tropical Medicine (NEKKEN), Nagasaki University, Nagasaki City, Japan

Kenji Hirayama
Department of Immunogenetics, Institute of Tropical Medicine (NEKKEN), Nagasaki University, Nagasaki City, Japan
Global COE Program, Nagasaki University, Nagasaki City, Japan

Nguyen Thanh Hong Thao
Department of Pediatrics, University of Medicine and Pharmacy at Ho Chi Minh City, Ho Chi Minh City, Vietnam

Nguyen Anh Tuan and Doan Thi Ngoc Diep
Department of Pediatrics, University of Medicine and Pharmacy at Ho Chi Minh City, Ho Chi Minh City, Vietnam
Children's Hospital No.1, Ho Chi Minh City, Vietnam

Nguyen Tuan Khiem
Department of Pediatrics, Pham Ngoc Thach University of Medicine, Ho Chi Minh City, Vietnam

Christopher C. Moore
Division of Infectious Diseases and International Health, Department of Medicine, University of Virginia, Charlottesville, Virginia, United States of America

Sameena Nawaz, David J. Allen, Farah Aladin, Christopher Gallimore and Miren Iturriza-Gómara
Virus Reference Department, Health Protection Agency, London, United Kingdom

Xiaobing Wang, Linxiu Zhang and Renfu Luo
Center for Chinese Agricultural Policy, Institute for Geographical Sciences and Natural Resources Research, Chinese Academy of Sciences, Beijing, China

Guofei Wang and Yingdan Chen
National Institute of Parasitic Diseases, Chinese Center for Disease Control and Prevention, Shanghai, China

Alexis Medina, Karen Eggleston and Scott Rozelle
Freeman Spogli Institute, Stanford University, Stanford, California, United States of America

D. Scott Smith
Stanford University School of Medicine, Stanford, California, United States of America
Department of Internal Medicine, Kaiser Permanente Medical Group, Redwood City, California, United States of America

Gyaviira Nkurunungi, Jimreeves E. Lutangira, Swaib A. Lule, Hellen Akurut, Robert Kizindo, Dennison Kizito, Ismail Sebina and Lawrence Muhangi
Co-infection Studies Programme, Medical Research Council/Uganda Virus Research Institute Uganda Research Unit on AIDS, Entebbe, Uganda

Stephen Cose and Alison M. Elliott
Co-infection Studies Programme, Medical Research Council/Uganda Virus Research Institute Uganda Research Unit on AIDS, Entebbe, Uganda
Department of Clinical Research, London School of Hygiene and Tropical Medicine, London, United Kingdom

Joseph R. Fitchett
Department of Clinical Research, London School of Hygiene and Tropical Medicine, London, United Kingdom

Emily L. Webb
Department of Infectious Disease Epidemiology, London School of Hygiene and Tropical Medicine, London, United Kingdom

Filemón Bucardo and Yaoska Reyes
Department of Microbiology, University of León (UNAN-León), León, Nicaragua

Lennart Svensson and Johan Nordgren
Division of Molecular Virology, Department of Clinical and Experimental Medicine, Linköping University, Linköping, Sweden

Simone Cesaro, Gloria Tridello, Irene Sara Panizzolo and Rita Balter
Pediatric Hematology Oncology, Azienda Ospedaliera Universitaria Integrata, Verona, Italy

Francesca Nesi
Pediatric Hematology Oncology, Ospedale Infantile Regina Margherita, Torino, Italy

Massimo Abate
Chemotherapy Unit, Istituto Ortopedico Rizzoli, Bologna, Italy

Elisabetta Calore
Department of Pediatrics, Pediatric Hematology Oncology, Padova, Italy

Marta Alonso and María Ercibengoa
Microbiology Department, Hospital Universitario Donostia-Instituto Biodonostia, San Sebastián, Spain

José M. Marimon
Microbiology Department, Hospital Universitario Donostia-Instituto Biodonostia, San Sebastián, Spain
Biomedical Research Center Network for Respiratory Diseases, San Sebastián, Spain

Emilio Pérez-Trallero
Microbiology Department, Hospital Universitario Donostia-Instituto Biodonostia, San Sebastián, Spain
Biomedical Research Center Network for Respiratory Diseases, San Sebastián, Spain
Faculty of Medicine, University of the Basque Country, San Sebastián, Spain

Eduardo G. Pérez-Yarza
Pediatric Department, Hospital Universitario Donostia-Instituto Biodonostia, San Sebastián, Spain
Faculty of Medicine, University of the Basque Country, San Sebastián, Spain

Nobuoki Eshima and Kiyo Uruma
Department of Biostatistics, Faculty of Medicine, Oita University, Yufu, Oita, Japan

Osamu Tokumaru
Department of Neurophysiology, Faculty of Medicine, Oita University, Yufu, Oita, Japan

Shohei Hara
Editorial Bureau, The Yomiuri Shimbun Osaka (newspaper), Osaka, Japan

Kira Bacal
Medical Programme Directorate, Faculty of Medical and Health Sciences, University of Auckland, Auckland, New Zealand

Seigo Korematsu
Department of Pediatrics and Child Neurology, Faculty of Medicine, Oita University, Yufu, Oita, Japan

Shigeru Karukaya and Toyojiro Matsuishi
Department of Pediatrics and Child Health, Kurume University School of Medicine, Kurume, Fukuoka, Japan

Nobuhiko Okabe
Infectious Disease Surveillance Center, National Institute of Infectious Diseases, Shinjuku, Tokyo, Japan

Patricia Quincó
Pós-Graduaçóo em Medicina Tropical, Universidade do Estado do Amazonas/Fundação de Medicina Tropical Dr. Heitor Vieira Dourado, Manaus, Amazonas, Brazil

Marlucia da Silva Garrido
Pós-Graduaçóo em Medicina Tropical, Universidade do Estado do Amazonas/Fundação de Medicina Tropical Dr. Heitor Vieira Dourado, Manaus, Amazonas, Brazil
Programa de Controle da Tuberculose, Departamento de Vigilância Epidemiológica, Fundação de Vigilância em Saúde do Estado do Amazonas, Manaus, Amazonas, Brazil

Samira Bührer-Sékula
Pós-Graduaçóo em Medicina Tropical, Universidade do Estado do Amazonas/Fundação de Medicina Tropical Dr. Heitor Vieira Dourado, Manaus, Amazonas, Brazil
Instituto de Patologia Tropical e Saúde Pública, Universidade Federal de Goiás, Goiânia, Goiás, Brazil

Flor Ernestina Martinez-Espinosa
Pós-Graduaçóo em Medicina Tropical, Universidade do Estado do Amazonas/Fundação de Medicina Tropical Dr. Heitor Vieira Dourado, Manaus, Amazonas, Brazil
Instituto Leônidas e Maria Deane - Fiocruz Amazônia, Fundação Oswaldo Cruz, Manaus, Amazonas, Brazil

Tomàs M. Pérez-Porcuna
Pós-Graduaçóo em Medicina Tropical, Universidade do Estado do Amazonas/Fundação de Medicina Tropical Dr. Heitor Vieira Dourado, Manaus, Amazonas, Brazil
Departament de Salut Pblica, Facultat de Medicina, Universitat de Barcelona, Barcelona, Catalunya, Spain
Servei de Pediatria, CAP Valldoreix, Unitat de Investigació Fundació Mútua Terrassa, Hospital Universitari Mútua Terrassa, Terrassa, Catalunya, Spain

Rosa Abellana
Departament de Salut Pblica, Facultat de Medicina, Universitat de Barcelona, Barcelona, Catalunya, Spain

Carlos Ascaso
Departament de Salut Pblica, Facultat de Medicina, Universitat de Barcelona, Barcelona, Catalunya, Spain
Institut d'Investigacions Biomèdiques August Pi i Sunyer, Barcelona, Catalunya, Spain

Adriana Malheiro
Laboratório de Imunologia Básica e Aplicada, Fundação de Hematologia e Hemoterapia do Amazonas, Manaus, Amazonas, Brazil

Universidade Federal do Amazonas. Manaus, Amazonas, Brazil

Marilaine Martins and José Felipe Jardim Sardinha
Fundação de Medicina Tropical Dr. Heitor Vieira Dourado, Manaus, Amazonas, Brazil

Irineide Assumpção Antunes
Centro de Referência da Tuberculose, Policlı´nica Cardoso Fontes, Manaus, Amazonas, Brazil

Sarah Korup, Janita Rietscher, Franziska Trusch, Sebastian Voigt and Bernhard Ehlers
Division of Viral Infections, Robert Koch Institute, Berlin, Germany

Sébastien Calvignac-Spencer
Research Group Emerging Zoonoses, Robert Koch Institute, Berlin, Germany

Jörg Hofmann
Institute of Virology, Charité - Universitätsmedizin Berlin, Berlin, Germany

Ugo Moens
Department of Medical Biology, University of Tromsø, Tromsø, Norway

Igor Sauer and Rosa Schmuck
General, Visceral, and Transplantation Surgery, Experimental Surgery and Regenerative Medicine, Charité-Campus Virchow, Charité Universitätsmedizin Berlin, Germany

Masashi Mizuguchi
Department of Developmental Medical Sciences, School of International Health, Graduate School of Medicine, The University of Tokyo, Tokyo, Japan

Shoko Okitsu and Hiroshi Ushijima
Department of Developmental Medical Sciences, School of International Health, Graduate School of Medicine, The University of Tokyo, Tokyo, Japan
Division of Microbiology, Department of Pathology and Microbiology, Nihon University, School of Medicine, Tokyo, Japan

Dinh Nguyen Tran
Department of Developmental Medical Sciences, School of International Health, Graduate School of Medicine, The University of Tokyo, Tokyo, Japan
Department of Pediatrics, University of Medicine and Pharmacy at Ho Chi Minh City, Ho Chi Minh City, Vietnam
Children's Hospital 2, Ho Chi Minh City, Vietnam

Thi Minh Hong Pham
Department of Pediatrics, University of Medicine and Pharmacy at Ho Chi Minh City, Ho Chi Minh City, Vietnam

Manh Tuan Ha, Thi Thu Loan Tran and Thi Kim Huyen Dang
Children's Hospital 2, Ho Chi Minh City, Vietnam

Lay-Myint Yoshida
Institute of Tropical Medicine, Nagasaki University, Nagasaki, Japan

Satoshi Hayakawa
Division of Microbiology, Department of Pathology and Microbiology, Nihon University, School of Medicine, Tokyo, Japan

Nico Marr, Aaron F. Hirschfeld, Angie Lam, Shirley Wang, Pascal M. Lavoie and Stuart E. Turvey
Department of Pediatrics, University of British Columbia, Child and Family Research Institute, Vancouver, British Columbia, Canada

Sonia Prot-Labarthe
Pharmacie, AP-HP Hôpital Robert-Debré, Paris, France

Thomas Weil
Pharmacie, AP-HP Hôpital Robert-Debré, Paris, France
Pharmacie Clinique, Université Paris Descartes, Paris, France

Olivier Bourdon
Pharmacie, AP-HP Hôpital Robert-Debré, Paris, France
Pharmacie Clinique, Université Paris Descartes, Paris, France
Laboratoire Educations et Pratiques de Santé, Université Paris XIII, Bobigny, France

François Angoulvant
Service d'Accueil des Urgences, AP-HP Hôpital Robert-Debré, Paris, France

Rym Boulkedid
Unité d'Epidémiologie Clinique, AP-HP Hôpital Robert Debré, Paris, France
Inserm U 1123 et CIC 1426, Paris, France

Corinne Alberti
Unité d'Epidémiologie Clinique, AP-HP Hôpital Robert Debré, Paris, France
Inserm U 1123 et CIC 1426, Paris, France
Sorbonne Paris Cité UMRS 1123, Université Paris Diderot, Paris, France

Chi-Hui Cheng
Division of Pediatric Nephrology, Department of Pediatrics, Chang Gung Children's Hospital, Chang Gung Memorial Hospital, Taoyuan, Taiwan
College of Medicine, Chang Gung University, Taoyuan, Taiwan

Tzou-Yien Lin
College of Medicine, Chang Gung University, Taoyuan, Taiwan
Division of Pediatric Infectious Diseases, Department of Pediatrics, Chang Gung Children's Hospital, Chang Gung Memorial Hospital, Taoyuan, Taiwan

Yun-Shien Lee
Genomic Medicine Research Core Laboratory (GMRCL), Chang Gung Memorial Hospital, Taoyuan, Taiwan
Department of Biotechnology, Ming-Chuan University, Taoyuan, Taiwan

Chee-Jen Chang
Statistical Center for Clinical Research, Chang Gung Memorial Hospital, Taoyuan, Taiwan

Paul Schnitzler
Department of Infectious Diseases, Virology, University of Heidelberg, Heidelberg, Germany

Julia Tabatabai
Department of Infectious Diseases, Virology, University of Heidelberg, Heidelberg, Germany
London School of Hygiene and Tropical Medicine, London, United Kingdom

Christiane Prifert
Institute of Virology and Immunobiology, University of Würzburg, Würzburg, Germany

Jürgen Grulich-Henn
Department of Pediatrics, University of Heidelberg, Heidelberg, Germany

Johannes Pfeil
Department of Pediatrics, University of Heidelberg, Heidelberg, Germany
German Centre for Infectious Diseases (DZIF), Heidelberg, Germany

Wenjing Ying, Jinqiao Sun, Danru Liu, Xiaoying Hui, Yeheng Yu, Jingyi Wang and Xiaochuan Wang
Department of Clinical Immunology, Children's Hospital of Fudan University, Shanghai, China

Maren Johanne Heilskov Rytter and Henrik Friis
Department of Nutrition, Exercise and Sports, Faculty of Science, University of Copenhagen, Frederiksberg, Denmark

André Briend
Department of Nutrition, Exercise and Sports, Faculty of Science, University of Copenhagen, Frederiksberg, Denmark
Department for International Health, University of Tampere, School of Medicine, Tampere, Finland

Lilian Kolte
Department of Infectious Diseases, Copenhagen University Hospital, Hvidovre, Denmark

Vibeke Brix Christensen
Department of Paediatrics, Copenhagen University Hospital Rigshospitalet, Copenhagen, Denmark

King Pan Chan, Chit Ming Wong and Xi Ling Wang
School of Publish Health, The University of Hong Kong, Hong Kong Special Administrative Region, China

J. S. Malik Peiris
School of Publish Health, The University of Hong Kong, Hong Kong Special Administrative Region, China
HKU - Pasteur Research Centre, Hong Kong Special Administrative Region, China

Lin Yang
School of Publish Health, The University of Hong Kong, Hong Kong Special Administrative Region, China
Squina International Centre for Infection Control, School of Nursing, The Hong Kong Polytechnic University, Hong Kong Special Administrative Region, China

Susan S. S. Chiu and Eunice L. Y. Chan
Department of Paediatrics and Adolescent Medicine, The University of Hong Kong, Hong Kong Special Administrative Region, China,

Kwok Hung Chan
Department of Microbiology, The University of Hong Kong, Hong Kong Special Administrative Region, China

Meridith Blevins and Bryan E. Shepherd
Vanderbilt Institute for Global Health, Vanderbilt University School of Medicine, Nashville, Tennessee, United States of America
Department of Biostatistics, Vanderbilt University School of Medicine, Nashville, Tennessee, United States of America

Philip J. Ciampa
Vanderbilt Institute for Global Health, Vanderbilt University School of Medicine, Nashville, Tennessee, United States of America

Department of Medicine, Vanderbilt University School of Medicine, Nashville, Tennessee, United States of America

José A. Tique
Vanderbilt Institute for Global Health, Vanderbilt University School of Medicine, Nashville, Tennessee, United States of America
Friends in Global Health, Quelimane and Maputo, Mozambique

Sten H. Vermund and Troy D. Moon
Vanderbilt Institute for Global Health, Vanderbilt University School of Medicine, Nashville, Tennessee, United States of America
Department of Pediatrics, Vanderbilt University School of Medicine, Nashville, Tennessee, United States of America
Friends in Global Health, Quelimane and Maputo, Mozambique

Lara M. E. Vaz
Vanderbilt Institute for Global Health, Vanderbilt University School of Medicine, Nashville, Tennessee, United States of America
Department of Preventive Medicine, Vanderbilt University School of Medicine, Nashville, Tennessee, United States of America
Friends in Global Health, Quelimane and Maputo, Mozambique

Eurico José and Linda Moiane
Friends in Global Health, Quelimane and Maputo, Mozambique

Mohsin Sidat
School of Medicine, Universidade Eduardo Mondlane, Maputo, Mozambique

Emily White Johansson and Katarina Ekholm Selling
International Maternal and Child Health, Department of Women's and Children's Health, Uppsala University, Uppsala, Sweden

Stefan Swartling Peterson
International Maternal and Child Health, Department of Women's and Children's Health, Uppsala University, Uppsala, Sweden
Global Health, Department of Public Health Sciences, Karolinska Institutet, Stockholm, Sweden
School of Public Health, College of Health Sciences, Makerere University, Kampala, Uganda

Peter W. Gething and Bonnie Mappin
Spatial Ecology and Epidemiology Group, Department of Zoology, University of Oxford, Oxford, United Kingdom

Helena Hildenwall
Global Health, Department of Public Health Sciences, Karolinska Institutet, Stockholm, Sweden

Max Petzold
Center for Applied Biostatistics, University of Gothenburg, Gothenburg, Sweden

Chyong-Hsin Hsu, Chia-Ying Lin, Jui-Hsing Chang, Han-Yang Hung, Hsin-An Kao, Chun-Chih Peng and Wai-Tim Jim
Department of Pediatrics, Division of Neonatology, Mackay Memorial Hospital, Taipei, Taiwan

Hsin Chi
Department of Pediatrics, Division of Infectious Disease, Mackay Memorial Hospital, Taipei, Taiwan

Julius Kiwanuka
Department of Paediatrics and Child Health, Mbarara University of Science and Technology, Mbarara, Uganda

Edgar Mulogo
Department of Community Health, Mbarara University of Science and Technology, Mbarara, Uganda

Jessica E. Haberer
Massachusetts General Hospital, Center for Global Health, Boston, Massachusetts, United States of America
Harvard Medical School, Boston, Massachusetts, United States of America

Aisa Shayo, Rahma Musoke and Coleen K. Cunningham
Kilimanjaro Christian Medical Centre, Moshi, Tanzania

Dorothy E. Dow
Kilimanjaro Christian Medical Centre, Moshi, Tanzania
Division of Infectious Diseases, Department of Pediatrics, Duke University Medical Center, Durham, North Carolina, United States of America

Ann M. Buchanan
Kilimanjaro Christian Medical Centre, Moshi, Tanzania
Division of Infectious Diseases, Department of Pediatrics, Duke University Medical Center, Durham, North Carolina, United States of America
Duke Global Health Institute, Duke University, Durham, North Carolina, United States of America

John A. Bartlett
Kilimanjaro Christian Medical Centre, Moshi, Tanzania
Duke Global Health Institute, Duke University, Durham, North Carolina, United States of America
Division of Infectious Diseases, Department of Medicine, Duke University Medical Center, Durham, North Carolina, United States of America

Charles G. Massambu
Ministry of Health and Social Welfare, Dar es Salaam, Tanzania

Balthazar Nyombi
Kilimanjaro Christian Medical Centre Clinical Laboratory, Moshi, Tanzania

Sheng Feng
Department of Biostatistics and Bioinformatics, Duke University, Durham, North Carolina, United States of America

Werner Schimana
Elizabeth Glaser Pediatric AIDS Foundation, Dar es Salaam, Tanzania

Dong-Hee Kim
Department of Nursing, College of Nursing, Pusan National University, Yangsan, Gyeongsangnamdo, South Korea

Hak Sun Yu
Department of Parasitology, School of Medicine, Pusan National University, Yangsan, Gyeongsangnamdo, South Korea
Immunoregulatory therapeutics group in Brain Busan 21 project, Busan, South Korea

Intira Jeannie Collins
Faculty of Epidemiology and Population Health, London School of Hygiene and Tropical Medicine, London, United Kingdom
Institut de Recherche pour le Développement (IRD)-Programs for HIV Prevention and Treatment (PHPT), Chiang Mai, Thailand
Department of Immunology and Infectious Diseases, Harvard School of Public Health, Boston, Massachusetts, United States of America

Nicole Ngo-Giang-Huong, Gonzague Jourdain and Marc Lallemant
Institut de Recherche pour le Développement (IRD)-Programs for HIV Prevention and Treatment (PHPT), Chiang Mai, Thailand
Department of Immunology and Infectious Diseases, Harvard School of Public Health, Boston, Massachusetts, United States of America
Department of Medical Technology, Faculty of Associated Medical Sciences, Chiang Mai University, Chiang Mai, Thailand

Sophie Le Coeur
Institut de Recherche pour le Développement (IRD)-Programs for HIV Prevention and Treatment (PHPT), Chiang Mai, Thailand
Department of Immunology and Infectious Diseases, Harvard School of Public Health, Boston, Massachusetts, United States of America
Department of Medical Technology, Faculty of Associated Medical Sciences, Chiang Mai University, Chiang Mai, Thailand
Unité Mixte de Recherche 196 Centre Français de la Population et du Développement (INED-IRD-Paris V University), Paris, France

John Cairns
Faculty of Public Health and Policy, London School of Hygiene and Tropical Medicine, London, United Kingdom

Wasna Sirirungsi, Pranee Leechanachai and Tanawan Samleerat
Department of Medical Technology, Faculty of Associated Medical Sciences, Chiang Mai University, Chiang Mai, Thailand

Nareerat Kamonpakorn
Paediatrics Department, Somdej Prapinklao Hospital, Bangkok, Thailand

Jutarat Mekmullica
Paediatrics Department, Bhumibol Adulyadej Hospital, Bangkok, Thailand

Index

www.ingramcontent.com/pod-product-compliance
Lightning Source LLC
Chambersburg PA
CBHW080510200326
41458CB00012B/4156
9781632417343